CONTENTS

Countries

ABOUT THE AUTHOR

Sarah E. Boslaugh, Ph.D., M.P.H., has over 20 years of experience in statistical analysis, grant writing, and teaching; her employers and clients have included the New York City Public Schools, Montefiore Medical Center, Saint Louis University, and Washington University School of Medicine. She served as editor-in-chief for the *Encyclopedia of Epidemiology* (SAGE, 2007), and has published three additional books: *An Intermediate Guide to SPSS Programming: Using Syntax for Data Management* (SAGE, 2004), *Secondary Data Sources for Public Health: A Practical Guide* (Cambridge University Press, 2007), and *Statistics in a Nutshell* (O'Reilly, 2nd ed., 2012).

Boslaugh received her Ph.D. in measurement and evaluation from the City University of New York Graduate Center and her M.P.H. from Saint Louis University. She is currently a grant writer and journalist for the Center for Sustainable Journalism at Kennesaw State University (Georgia); as a journalist, she specializes in data-based articles and explaining statistical principles to the general public. Her research interests include comparative health care delivery systems, quality of life measurement, and gender and sexuality issues in health care delivery. In her spare time, she reviews films and books for PopMatters (http://www.popmatters.com) and Playback St. Louis (http://www.playbackstl.com).

INTRODUCTION

Everyone has an interest in health, as reflected in truisms such as "at least you've got your health" and "if you've got your health, you've got just about everything." If all people have an interest in health, at least their own health and that of their families, it then follows that every government has an interest in health care delivery because the many wonderful achievements of modern medicine are only useful when they are delivered to the people who need them.

There are many different ways to organize and deliver health care to a population, and to some extent, each country's method of organizing health care delivery is unique and based on its specific situation, including its history and culture, the amount of money it has to spend, and the value it places on different outcomes. It is not surprising that public discussions about health care often become heated because the demand for health services is theoretically unlimited, yet no government has unlimited resources. Designing and running a health care system therefore requires making difficult choices that are almost guaranteed not to please everyone, at least not all the time.

Discussions about health and health care often draw on two key statements from international organizations that formed after the conclusion of World War II. The first is the definition of health, as stated in the Preamble to the Constitution of the World Health Organization (WHO), adopted in 1946 and entering into force in 1948:

Health is a state of complete physical, mental, and social well-being and not merely the absence of disease or infirmity.

This broad definition of health has been adopted in principle by many nations that have integrated social services systems including not only medical care but also other services, such as old-age pensions and income support. Other nations prefer to maintain a number of separate services, each with its own sources of funding and eligibility requirements. Both systems can produce good results or bad results—the details of how a specific system is organized and executed are crucial when making comparisons.

The second statement comes from the Universal Declaration of Human Rights proclaimed in 1948 by the United Nations General Assembly:

Everyone has the right to a standard of living adequate for the health and well-being of himself and of his family, including food, clothing, housing, and medical care and necessary social services and the right to security in the event of unemployment, sickness, disability, widowhood, old age or other lack of livelihood in circumstances beyond his control.

Some governments include the right to health in their constitutions, while in others it is a tacit expectation that those who need medical care will receive it. Again, it would be incorrect to assume that the population whose constitution declares health to be a human right do in fact fare better than people living in countries where this is not explicitly stated: Instead, it is necessary to look at how each nation's health care delivery functions in practice and at the health outcomes for each nation.

Making comparisons across countries is always a tricky matter because any two nations may differ on a vast number of characteristics, including level of development, geography and climate, political history, and social values. Looking at how different countries organize their health care systems, and what kind of results they achieve, is no different—some countries simply have more resources than others, and some have enjoyed long periods of peace and prosperity, while others have been engaged in lengthy wars or periods of civil unrest or subject to periodic environmental threats (hurricanes, earthquakes, extended periods of drought), which play little or no role elsewhere, and so on. National values also play a role—in some nations, equal access to services is a first principle, while in others, values such as choice or personal responsibility are considered more important.

Many studies comparing health care systems have been published, but for the reasons cited above, these studies usually confine themselves to a small group of countries that are similar to each other. For instance, many useful studies have been published comparing health care delivery systems and outcomes in western European countries or comparing systems and outcomes in developing countries in sub-Saharan Africa. This book takes a different approach to the subject: It provides basic information about health care organization and outcomes, organized into 10 categories, for 193 countries around the world:

- Emergency health services
- Insurance
- Costs of hospitalization
- Access to health care
- Cost of drugs
- Health care facilities
- Major health issues
- Health care personnel
- Government role in health care
- Public health programs

The purpose is not to provide the final answer on any question regarding health care delivery but to facilitate comparisons among countries and raise questions that may lead to further, more detailed, investigations.

Characterizing the health care delivery system for any country is a tricky task because, not only is every country different, but many countries use a mix of systems adapted to the needs and values of their populations as well as the availability of resources. However, several basic models have been identified, and keeping these in mind may help in understanding the choices made within a particular country, as well as when making comparisons across countries.

One way to deliver health care services is through a national health service such as that of the United Kingdom (which, strictly speaking, is four national health services, for England, Scotland, Wales, and Northern Ireland, respectively). A national health service is typically funded out of general tax revenues and organized at the national level. A second way to organize health care is through a social insurance system, funded through payroll taxes; this type of health care system began in Germany in the 1880s and is used in many European countries today. Canada provides a good example of a national health insurance or single-payer system: Health care is delivered by independent providers and institutions but is paid for through tax revenues; some single-payer systems also allow individuals to hold private insurance to supplement that provided by the state.

In a private insurance system, individuals and households purchase insurance from private providers, and care is paid for through some combination of insurance payments and copayments. This system may show the greatest variation across countries—for instance, in the United States, most people with private insurance receive it as a benefit of employment, coverage is optional, insurance companies can refuse to cover individuals, and there are great variations in terms of the costs of insurance and what services are covered, while in the Netherlands, purchase of a health insurance policy is mandatory, insurance companies are tightly regulated by the national government, and companies are required to provide insurance for anyone who lives in a coverage area.

Even within a specific model, many other questions remain. For instance, how should those who provide health care services be paid? In some countries, doctors, nurses, and other professionals are employed by the state and receive salaries; in other countries, some or all of these professionals may be paid according to the number of patients they see and the services they provide. Similarly, there are many ways hospitals are funded, from global budgets to payments based on services provided (often based on a schedule of payments for different diagnoses) to simple payments based on the number of beds occupied over the period of a year.

There are also many ways to provide medicines to people, and to pay for them—in some systems, prescription drugs are provided without charge (this is often limited to drugs listed on a national formulary) as part of the national health system; in some systems, some or all medicines are heavily subsidized, but patients are still required to pay something for them; and in some systems, the marketplace is allowed to set the price for each drug. Some countries tightly regulate which drugs may be sold within their borders, while others accept any drug that has achieved basic standards for health and efficacy. As with the different models for providing care, there is not a single best way to answer any of these questions, but consideration of the different options may help clarify the advantages and disadvantages of each.

Health care delivery seems fated to remain a topic of interest in the future, and more rather than less attention will be focused on the different ways to organize care and the strong and weak points of each type of system. Rising costs are an issue around the world as the advances of medical science provide more and more ways to improve health but at a cost that may be unsustainable. Improvements in a nation's health can also create more issues that must be dealt with—for instance, as many developing countries have adopted effective measures to prevent and treat infectious disease, thus reducing the toll taken by diseases such as tuberculosis and influenza, they find themselves facing a much higher incidence of chronic diseases, such as cancer and diabetes, and their health systems must adapt to this new reality. Even industrialized countries with high standards of care face questions of resource allocation, requiring them to decide what services take priority over others. Ultimately, however, the necessity to make such decisions is based on what can only be called a positive trend—thanks in large part to modern systems of health care, life expectancy is increasing globally, and that is something to be thankful for.

SARAH E. BOSLAUGH

COUNTRY RANKINGS

The country rankings provide a list of the top 10 and bottom 10 countries in rank order on different measures related to health and health care systems. The purpose is to give the reader opportunities to compare how different countries, which are similar in some factors, provide health care to their citizens, with the proviso that many factors may influence both a country's health care system and the health of its population. Unless otherwise noted, all information is from the *CIA World Factbook* (2012 edition).

OUTCOMES

Life Expectancy at Birth (Highest)
Monaco
Japan
Singapore
San Marino
Andorra
Australia
Italy
Liechtenstein
Canada
France

Life Expectancy at Birth (Lowest)
Chad
Guinea-Bissau
South Africa
Swaziland
Afghanistan
Central African Republic
Somalia
Zimbabwe

Lesotho
Mozambique

Infant Mortality (Highest)
Afghanistan
Niger
Mali
Somalia
Central African Republic
Guinea-Bissau
Chad
Angola
Burkina Faso
Malawi

Infant Mortality (Lowest)
Monaco
Japan
Singapore
Sweden
Iceland
Italy
Spain

France
Finland
Norway

Maternal Mortality (Highest)
Afghanistan
Somalia
Chad
Guinea-Bissau
Liberia
Burundi
Sierra Leone
Central African Republic
Nigeria
Mali

Maternal Mortality (Lowest)
Greece
Ireland
Austria
Sweden
Belgium
Denmark
Iceland
Italy
Spain
Slovakia

Children Under Age 5 Underweight (Highest)
India
Yemen
Bangladesh
Timor-Leste (East Timor)
Niger
Burundi
Nepal
Burkina Faso
Madagascar
Ethiopia

Children Under Age 5 Underweight (Lowest)
Chile
Germany
United States
Belarus
Bulgaria
Bosnia and Herzegovina
Macedonia
Serbia

Czech Republic
Jamaica

Adult HIV Prevalence Rate (Highest)
Swaziland
Botswana
Lesotho
South Africa
Zimbabwe
Zambia
Namibia
Mozambique
Malawi
Uganda

Adult HIV Prevalence Rate (Lowest)
(Countries with the lowest HIV prevalence rates are not listed because there are so many tied at the low end)

Adult Prevalence of Obesity (Highest)
Tonga
Kiribati
Saudi Arabia
United States
United Arab Emirates
Egypt
Kuwait
New Zealand
Seychelles
Fiji

Adult Prevalence of Obesity (Lowest)
Vietnam
Laos
Madagascar
Indonesia
China
Japan
South Korea
Eritrea
Philippines
Singapore

HEALTH SERVICES

Physician Density per 1,000 (Highest)
San Marino
Cuba
Greece

Monaco
Belarus
Austria
Georgia
Russia
Italy
Norway

Physician Density per 1,000 (Lowest)

Tanzania
Liberia
Sierra Leone
Malawi
Niger
Ethiopia
Bhutan
Rwanda
Mozambique
Burundi

Hospital Bed Density per 1,000 (Highest)

Japan
North Korea
South Korea
Belarus
Russia
Ukraine
Germany
Azerbaijan
Austria
Barbados

Hospital Bed Density per 1,000 (Lowest)

Cambodia
Ethiopia
Madagascar
Guinea
Niger
Senegal
Uganda
Sierra Leone
Côte d'Ivoire
Mauritania

Percent of Births Attended by Skilled Health Personnel (Lowest)

(Data from the Population Reference Bureau)
Ethiopia
Afghanistan
Chad

Bangladesh
Timor-Leste (East Timor)
Nepal
Laos
Haiti
Eritrea
Niger

Percent of Births Attended by Skilled Health Personnel (Highest)

(Countries with the highest percent of births attended by skilled personnel are not listed because many countries are tied at 100 percent)

Total Health Expenditure as a Percentage of GDP (Highest)

Malta
United States
Mexico
Niue
Lesotho
Sierra Leone
Burundi
Timor-Leste (East Timor)
Kenya
Nauru

Total Health Expenditure as a Percentage of GDP (Lowest)

North Korea
Burma
Equatorial Guinea
Turkmenistan
India
Qatar
Marshall Islands
Pakistan
United Arab Emirates
Syria
Congo, Republic of the

DEMOGRAPHICS

Birth Rate (Highest)

Niger
Uganda
Mali
Zambia
Burkina Faso

Ethiopia
Somalia
Burundi
Malawi
Congo, Republic of the

Birth Rate (Lowest)
Monaco
Hong Kong
Singapore
Germany
Japan
South Korea
Czech Republic
Austria
Slovenia
Taiwan

Death Rate (Highest)
South Africa
Russia
Ukraine
Lesotho
Chad
Guinea-Bissau
Central African Republic
Afghanistan
Somalia
Bulgaria

Death Rate (Lowest)
Qatar
United Arab Emirates
Kuwait
Bahrain
Jordan
Saudi Arabia
Brunei
Singapore
Libya
Oman

Population Growth Rate (Highest)
Qatar
Zimbabwe
Niger
Uganda
Ethiopia
Burundi
Burkina Faso

United Arab Emirates
Zambia
Madagascar

Population Growth Rate (Lowest)
Moldova
Jordan
Syria
Bulgaria
Estonia
Montenegro
Ukraine
Latvia
Russia
Serbia

Human Development Index (Highest)
(Data from the United Nations Development Programme)
Norway
Australia
Netherlands
United States
New Zealand
Canada
Ireland
Liechtenstein
Germany
Sweden

Human Development Index (Lowest)
(Data from the United Nations Development Programme)
Congo, Democratic Republic of the
Niger
Burundi
Mozambique
Chad
Liberia
Burkina Faso
Sierra Leone
Central African Republic
Guinea

The Global Gender Gap (Most Equal)
(Data from the World Economic Forum)
Iceland
Norway
Finland
Sweden

Ireland
New Zealand
Denmark
Philippines
Lesotho
Switzerland

The Global Gender Gap (Least Equal)
(Data from the World Economic Forum)
Yemen
Chad
Pakistan
Mali
Saudi Arabia
Côte d'Ivoire
Morocco
Benin
Oman
Nepal

GDP per Capita (Purchasing Power Parity Basis, Highest)
Liechtenstein
Qatar
Luxembourg
Bermuda
Singapore
Norway
Brunei
United Arab Emirates
United States
Switzerland

GDP per Capita (Purchasing Power Parity Basis, Lowest)
Congo, Democratic Republic of the
Liberia
Burundi
Zimbabwe
Somalia
Eritrea
Sierra Leone
Niger
Central African Republic
Madagascar
Malawi

Distribution of Family Income (Most Equal)
Sweden
Montenegro

Hungary
Denmark
Norway
Austria
Malta
Luxembourg
Slovakia
Kazakhstan

Distribution of Family Income (Most Unequal)
Namibia
South Africa
Lesotho
Botswana
Sierra Leone
Central African Republic
Haiti
Bolivia
Honduras
Colombia

Population (Largest)
China
India
United States
Indonesia
Brazil
Pakistan
Nigeria
Bangladesh
Russia
Japan

Population (Smallest)
Nauru
Tuvalu
Palau
Monaco
San Marino
Liechtenstein
Saint Kitts and Nevis
Dominica
Andorra
Antigua and Barbuda

Urbanization (High)
(Data from the Population Reference Bureau)
Singapore
Malta
Nauru

Qatar
Bahrain
Monaco
Belgium
Kuwait
Venezuela
Argentina

Urbanization (Low)
(Data from the Population Reference Bureau)
Burundi
Papua New Guinea
Trinidad and Tobago
Malawi
Uganda
Liechtenstein
Sri Lanka
Niger
Ethiopia
Nepal

Rate of Urbanization (Highest)
(Data from the Population Reference Bureau)
Burundi
Liberia
Laos
Eritrea
Afghanistan
Maldives
Malawi
Congo, Democratic Republic of the
Timor-Leste (East Timor)
Burkina Faso

Rate of Urbanization (Lowest)
(Data from the Population Reference Bureau)
Moldova
Montenegro
Ukraine
Georgia
Slovenia
Russia
Latvia
Lithuania
Poland
Armenia

Geographic Area (Largest)
Russia
Canada

United States
China
Brazil
Australia
India
Argentina
Kazakhstan
Algeria

Geographic Area (Smallest)
Monaco
Nauru
Tuvalu
San Marino
Liechtenstein
Saint Kitts and Nevis
Maldives
Malta
Grenada
Saint Vincent and the Grenadines

COMPARATIVE HEALTH SYSTEM INFORMATION

(From the World Health Report 2000*)*
The World Health Organization's (WHO's) World Health Report 2000 included rankings of the health systems of its member countries on a number of factors. Although these rankings should be interpreted with caution due to their age, they represent an unprecedented effort to evaluate the world's health systems and provide a useful snapshot of their functioning at that time.

WHO Overall Health System Performance (Best)
France
Italy
San Marino
Andorra
Malta
Singapore
Spain
Oman
Austria
Japan

WHO Overall Health System Performance (Worst)
Myanmar
Central African Republic
Congo, Democratic Republic of the
Nigeria

Liberia
Malawi
Mozambique
Lesotho
Zambia
Angola

WHO Disability-Adjusted Life Expectancy (Highest)

Japan
Australia
France
Sweden
Spain
Italy
Greece
Switzerland
Monaco
Andorra

WHO Disability-Adjusted Life Expectancy (Lowest)

Sierra Leone
Niger
Malawi
Zambia
Botswana
Uganda
Rwanda
Zimbabwe
Mali
Ethiopia

WHO Responsiveness of Health System (Highest)

United States
Switzerland
Luxembourg
Denmark
Germany
Japan
Canada

Norway
Netherlands
Sweden

WHO Responsiveness of Health System (Lowest)

Somalia
Niger
Mozambique
Uganda
Mali
Eritrea
Nepal
Guinea-Bissau
Central African Republic
Chad

WHO Fairness of Financial Contribution to Health Systems (Highest)

Colombia
Luxembourg
Belgium
Djibouti
Denmark
Ireland
Germany
Norway
Japan
Finland

WHO Fairness of Financial Contribution to Health Systems (Lowest)

Sierra Leone
Myanmar
Brazil
China
Viet Nam
Nepal
Russian Federation
Peru
Cambodia
Cameroon

CHRONOLOGY

2635–2155 B.C.E.: During the Old Kingdom in Egypt, texts contain the names of at least 50 physicians.

ca. 1700 B.C.E.: The Code of Hammurabi includes sections on the liability of physicians for failed surgical procedures and also on physicians' compensation; in both cases, the amount of the penalty or payment is based on the status of the patient, not the difficulty of the medical procedure.

ca. 1600 B.C.E.: Tablets believed to be a collection of Mesopotamian medical knowledge over several centuries include guides for diagnosing diseases and conditions including fevers, worms, venereal disease, neurological conditions, and skin lesions.

ca. 1500 B.C.E.: An ancient Egyptian text, the *Ebers Papyrus*, describes illnesses resembling schizophrenia, dementia, and depression.

ca. 1400 B.C.E.: An ancient Indian text, the *Atharva Veda*, describes mental illness as being caused by an imbalance of humors.

ca. 1000 B.C.E.: In China, the *Yellow Emperor's Classic of Internal Medicine* describes epilepsy and dementia.

5th century B.C.E.: The Greek philosopher Empedocles, writing in his treatise *On Nature*, says that the human body is created out of the elements of earth, ether, fire, and water and that health was created by the appropriate mixture of wet and dry and hot and cold.

460–377 B.C.E.: The Greek physician Hippocrates, sometimes termed the father of medicine, attributes human illness to natural factors, including environmental conditions, rather than divine intervention; the Hippocratic Oath is still used today.

ca. 312 B.C.E.: The Romans construct an aqueduct to supply potable water from distant streams and springs to the city of Rome.

ca. 1st century C.E.: Several Roman writers mention *valetudinaria*, rooms in imperial households reserved for the care of ill or exhausted slaves; archeological excavations later confirm these reports and also the existence of *valetudinaria* within military facilities.

ca. 1st century: The Greek physician Dioscorides writes an encyclopedia of medicinal substances, *De Material Medica*.

ca. 200: The Roman physician Galen writes works that form the foundation of Western medicine for the next millennium.

314: The Church of the Synod of Ankyra creates a religious ritual to sanctify the separation of lepers from the rest of society.

499: Eusebius, bishop of Edessa (a city in Anatolia), orders that the city's poor be provided with food, shelter, and nursing care.

6th century: A leper house is established in Franconia in southern Gaul to house and care for lepers.

ca. 530: The Rule of St. Benedict includes the specification that monks should care for the ill and disabled among them; this principle is later extended to providing medical care for laypersons.

603: Pope Gregory I founds a hospice in Jerusalem to care for ill pilgrims.

ca. 707: An Islamic hospital is founded in Damascus, Syria.

830: Plans for a monastery for the monks of St. Gall include an infirmary with separate rooms for monks requiring different levels of care and a guesthouse for lay visitors.

874: A *bimaristan* (hospital) is founded in Cairo, Egypt.

918: A *bimaristan* (hospital) is founded in western Baghdad; a second *bimaristan* is founded in eastern Baghdad in 981.

ca. 980–1027: During his lifetime, the Iranian physician Abu Ali Sina (Avicenna) writes numerous books, including the *Canon of Medicine* and *The Book of Healing.*

ca. 1080: Founding of a hospice, staffed by Benedictine monks, in Jerusalem; it is dedicated to St. John the Baptist.

ca. 1100: The Knights of St. Lazarus establish a hospice to care for lepers in Jerusalem; similar houses subsequently established throughout Europe are referred to as "lazarrettos" or Houses of St. Lazarus.

ca. 1136: Founding of the Pantocrator monastery in Constantinople, including five separate wards or dormitories for persons with different levels of disease.

1179: The Third Lateran Council reinforces the segregation of lepers, banning them from attending parish churches and from burial in parish cemeteries.

1247: The Order of the Star of Bethlehem builds a priory in London; it begins to admit mentally ill patients in the 1350s, making it the oldest psychiatric hospital in Europe; it is colloquially known as "Bedlam."

1257: Founding of the "Bürgerspital," the oldest hospital in Vienna, Austria.

1300s: In some European countries, craft guilds create mutual assistance associations, an early form of social insurance.

1311: At the Council of Ravenna, one topic of discussion is the increasing corruption of monastic hospitals; Pope Clement V later prohibits clerics from profiting personally from the operation of these hospitals.

1348: In response to the plague pandemic sweeping Europe, Jehan Jacme publishes a tractate exhorting European city leaders to assume responsibility for safeguarding the population against disease outbreaks.

1348–1350: The Black Death (bubonic plague) sweeps Europe, killing an estimated quarter of the population.

1496: Pox houses are established in several German cities to care for people suffering from *morbus gallicus*, probably a form of syphilis.

1505: The city of Paris, France, assumes control of the Hotel Dieu, a hospital with more than 1,000 beds.

1518: In Great Britain, King Henry VIII orders the founding of the Royal College of Physicians.

1530: Emperor Charles V cedes Malta to the order of the Knights Hospitallers, an order founded to provide care for pilgrims to Jerusalem.

1592: In response to a plague outbreak, public officials in London begin publishing the *Bills of Mortality*, listing the cause of death for deaths within the city.

1637: Construction begins on the first hospital in Canada, the Hotel-Dieu de Quebec; it begins operation in 1639, staffed by members of the Augustines de la Misericorde de Jesus from France and, in 1644, is moved to its current site on the Rue du Palais.

1644: The Hotel-Dieu de Montreal in Canada is founded by Jeanne Mance; the building is completed in 1645 and is run by Mance until it is taken over in 1659 by the Hospitallers of St. Joseph.

1647: The Massachusetts Bay Colony establishes a quarantine for ships arriving in Boston harbor.

1656: In an effort to control the plague, Roman officials quarantine Trastavere, a community on the Tiber floodplain in Rome, Italy.

1659: The first known typhus outbreak in Canada.

1720: Westminster Infirmary, the first voluntary hospital in England, opens.

1736: Creation of the New York City Almshouse including a six-bed hospital ward; this facility will later become Bellevue Hospital.

1747: James Lind demonstrates that consumption of citrus fruits is the best remedy for scurvy in small-sample clinical trials with British seamen comparing oranges and lemons with other substances, including seawater, garlic, and horseradish.

1776: In order to encourage enlistment in the army, the U.S. Continental Congress provides pensions for disabled soldiers.

1780s: Institutional mortality of more than 21 percent is reported for the Hospice de Charité and almost 25 percent for the Hotel Dieu, both in Paris, France.

1784: Opening of the Allgemeines Krankenhaus (General Hospital) in Vienna, Austria.

1792: In France, Philippe Pinel leads a reform effort for more humane treatment of people in mental hospitals.

1796: Edward Jenner successfully vaccinates a child against smallpox using the cowpox virus.

1811: The United States creates the first federal medical facility for disabled veterans.

1821: Massachusetts General Hospital opens in Boston; from the start, founders emphasize the hospital's multiple roles of educating physicians, conducting research, and caring for the sick.

1831: Canada creates a sanitation committee and strengthens quarantine laws in response to the threat of cholera being spread by immigrants from Europe.

1832: La Grosse Ile, an island in the St. Lawrence River near Quebec City in Canada, becomes a quarantine station during a cholera epidemic; immigrants are examined at the island before being permitted to enter the mainland, but despite these efforts, the disease spreads to Montreal and Quebec City.

1839: A group of physicians in Toronto, Canada, many of whom had been educated in Great Britain, are incorporated as the College of Physicians and Surgeons of Upper Canada.

1840s: Working at the General Hospital of Vienna, Austria, Ignaz Semmelweis successfully reduces deaths from puerperal fever by requiring physicians to disinfect their hands between performing autopsies and delivering babies.

1842: In England, Edwin Chadwick publishes the *Report . . . on Inquiry Into the Sanitary Condition of the Laboring Population of Great Britain*, calling for city engineers to create more healthful conditions in order to control disease.

1846: Physicians successfully use ether to render patients unconscious during surgery.

1847: A typhus epidemic in Ireland spreads to Canada as many Irish emigrate due to the so-called potato famine; despite efforts to examine immigrants at La Grosse Ile quarantine station, the disease spreads to Montreal and Quebec City.

1851: The first International Sanitary Conference meets in Paris, France, to harmonize quarantine requirements among European countries.

1854: During a cholera epidemic in London, England, John Snow traces the source of infection to a specific water pump in the city.

1860: Florence Nightingale founds a training school for nurses at St. Thomas' Hospital in London, England.

1861–1865: During the Civil War, American hospitals develop several innovative methods for treating patients, including the ward system (grouping beds for patients with similar ailments together in order to treat them more easily) and the development of specialty orthopedic care and the use of prosthetic limbs.

1863: Founding of the International Committee of the Red Cross in Geneva, Switzerland, prompted by Henry Dunant's desire to aid those wounded in war without reference to which side they fought on.

1863: During the American Civil War, the U.S. federal government creates the Invalid Corps to employ disabled veterans in war-related tasks; the name is change in 1864 to the Veteran Reserve Corps.

1865: London, England, completes its sewage system.

1866: In the United States, New York City creates the Metropolitan Board of Health, which later becomes the New York City Health Department.

1867: Founding of the Canadian Medical Association.

1867: Joseph Lister publishes a series of articles arguing for the use of carbolic acid to prevent infection during surgery.

1867: In Great Britain, passage of the Metropolitan Poor Act requires workhouses (institutions housing the poor) to maintain hospitals separately from the main workhouse site.

1867: In Canada, jurisdiction over public health is divided by the Constitution Act into federal and provincial responsibilities, the former being responsible for border quarantine and the latter for creating and running hospitals.

1869: Massachusetts creates the first state public health department in the United States.

1872: Dr. Stephen Smith, commissioner of the Metropolitan Health Board of New York City, founds the American Public Health Association.

1873: In the United States, the federal government creates the Marine Health Service, the forerunner of the U.S. Public Health Service.

1874: The first nursing school in Canada is established at the General and Marine Hospital in St. Catharines, Ontario.

1881: A nursing school based on the principles established by Florence Nightingale is founded at the Toronto General Hospital in Canada.

1881: Founding of the U.S. American Red Cross by Clara Barton; the same year, the first local chapter is founded in Dansville, New York, and the American Red Cross delivers its first disaster relief services to victims of forest fires in Michigan.

1882: Ontario, Canada, establishes a provincial board of health.

1883: Germany enacts a mandatory national health insurance program.

1883: Sir Francis Galton coins the term *eugenics*.

1885: A major smallpox epidemic in Montreal leads to riots, as some believe the disease was spread by vaccination, a practice not yet universal in Canada.

1887: The U.S. Marine Hospital creates one of the world's first bacteriological laboratories.

1890: A nursing school based on the principles established by Florence Nightingale is founded at the Montreal General Hospital in Canada.

1893: Lillian Wald creates the profession of public health nursing by founding the Henry Street Settlement in New York City in the United States.

1896: In Germany, Emil Kraepelin begins the modern process of classifying mental illness by distinguishing between mania and paranoia.

1906: The U.S. Congress passes the Pure Food and Drug Act, authorizing the government to monitor purity and safety of food and drugs.

1908: The United States creates a workmen's compensation system for federal employees.

1909: The U.S. insurance company Metropolitan Life hires Lee Frankel, an industrial social worker, to write pamphlets promoting health education; the first, centering on tuberculosis prevention, is distributed to more than 10,000 individuals.

1910: About half of all U.S. physicians are members of the American Medical Association (AMA); the approximately 70,000 members of the AMA at this time comprise a substantial increase from the approximately 8,000 members in 1901.

1910: Abraham Flexner issues a report highly critical of the state of American medical education, which leads to the creation of higher standards and the closing of numerous medical schools.

1912: In the United States, the Progressive Party and its candidate Teddy Roosevelt endorse social and health insurance as part of its platform.

1913: Founding of the American College of Surgeons.

1916: In the United States, the Council on Medical Education recommends that medical schools require students to have completed one year of college; in 1918, this is increased to two years of college.

1917: As the United States enters World War I, the federal government establishes a new system of benefits for veterans, including insurance, vocational rehabilitation, and disability compensation.

1918: In the United States, the federal government makes its first state grants for public health services.

1918: A report by the American College of Surgeons states that only 13 percent of U.S. hospitals meet its standards; by 1932, more than 90 percent meet them.

1919: Canada creates a federal department of health to set standards for food and medicines, enforce quarantines, and cooperate with voluntary organizations and the provinces; the department was created in part in response to the influenza pandemic of 1918.

1919: The International Federation of Red Cross and Red Crescent Societies is founded in Paris, France (as the League of Red Cross Societies).

1919: In the United States, a commission from the state of Illinois reports that, for most people, the primary cost of illness is not medical treatment but lost wages.

1919: The University of British Columbia creates Canada's first university degree program for nurses.

1926: Joseph Goldberger demonstrates that pellagra, a disease endemic in the American South, is caused by a deficiency of niacin, after previously establishing that consumption of a diet based primarily on corn (typical of the poor in the South) was associated with pellagra.

1928: In London, Sir Andrew Fleming discovers penicillin and observes that it destroys colonies of bacteria; however, regular use of the drug does not begin until the 1940s.

1929: Baylor University develops a health insurance plan for hospital care for a group of Dallas, Texas, teachers; this plan is a precursor of the Blue Cross system.

1929: Atlantic City, New Jersey, hosts the first International Hospital Congress; observers note that American hospitals provide more clinical education and are used by a broader range of social classes than those in Europe.

1930: In the United States, Congress creates the Veterans Administration to consolidate services provided to military veterans.

1930: In the United States, 70 percent of graduates from medical schools also hold bachelor's degrees; by 1945, this is increased to 80 percent.

1932: The U.S. Public Health Service begins the Tuskegee Study, observing the course of syphilis in African Americans while not informing them of their disease nor providing medical treatment; the study ends in 1972, long after penicillin had become available, and prompts creation of the National Research Act in 1974.

1933: The American Hospital Association approves private hospital insurance.

1933: In the United States, the hospital bed occupancy rate falls to 55 percent as fewer people can pay for care due to the Great Depression.

1935: In the United States, passage of the Social Security Act creates a system of old-age and survivors' pensions funded by contributions from employees and employers, but it does not include health insurance.

1938: The U.S. Technical Committee on Medical Care publishes its report, *A National Health Program.*

1938: In Italy, the physician Ugo Cerletti begins using electroshock therapy to treat depression.

1941: The American Red Cross begins collecting blood for the military under the National Blood Donor Services, directed by Dr. Charles Drew.

1941: The Netherlands adopts a mandatory national social health insurance system.

1941–1945: Wage and price controls on American employers during World War II prompt many to offer health benefits as additional compensation.

1943: In the United States, clinical trials begin for penicillin; once proven effective, production is scaled up in the next few years to supply the military, and the price drops substantially ($0.55 in 1946 for one dose versus $20.00 for one dose in 1943).

1944: U.S. President Franklin Roosevelt mentions the right to medical care in his State of the Union address.

1945: U.S. President Harry Truman proposes creation of a national universal health insurance program; it is opposed by the American Medical Association and denounced by a subcommittee of the House of Representatives as a communist plot.

1945: The United Nations (UN) creates the United Nations Children's Fund (UNICEF) to provide food, clothing, and health care to impoverished children.

1945: During meetings to establish the UN, representatives from Brazil and China propose creation of an international health organization, first called the Interim Commission; in 1948, it becomes the World Health Organization (WHO).

1946: In the United States, creation of the Communicable Disease Center (CDC), later the Centers for Disease Control and Prevention.

1947: Writing in the *British Medical Journal*, Austin Bradford Hill argues that medical practices should be evaluated using statistical methods.

1948: The first modern clinical trial is conducted in the United Kingdom; it demonstrates that streptomycin is an effective therapy for tuberculosis.

1948: The American Red Cross opens a blood collection center in Rochester, New York. It is the first such center created in the United States under the civilian National Blood Program.

1948: Great Britain founds the National Health Service (NHS).

1949: In the United States, the National Labor Relations Board rules that unions are permitted to negotiate benefit packages for their members, including health insurance and pension plans.

1950: Dr. Jonas Salk introduces the Salk vaccine for polio.

1952: In the United Kingdom, the NHS begins charging one shilling for prescriptions.

1954: In Boston, Massachusetts, physicians Joseph Murray and John Merrill carry out the first successful living donor transplant with a kidney obtained from the patient's identical twin.

1957: Canada passes the Hospital Insurance and Diagnostic Act of 1957, giving the Canadian government authority to create a universal coverage plan for hospital, laboratory, and radiology services; this is the first part of the current Canadian national health insurance plan.

1958: In the United States, almost three-quarters of citizens have private health insurance.

1958: In the United Kingdom, the NHS launches a program to immunize everyone aged 14 and younger against polio and diphtheria.

1960s: Development of antipsychotic drugs allows many psychiatric patients to be released from asylums and treated in community mental health facilities instead.

1961: In Canada, the Royal Commission on Health Services is created to study the Canadian health care system; its 1964 report becomes the cornerstone of the contemporary health system in Canada.

1962: In the United States, the Migrant Health Act funds medical clinics for migrant workers.

1964: The U.S. Surgeon General's report on smoking and health lends weight to efforts to control the advertising and sale of tobacco products.

1965: In the United States, the Medicare and Medicaid programs are created as part of the Social Security Act of 1965; Medicare provides federal funding for health insurance for persons age 65 and older, the disabled, and those with end-stage renal disease, while Medicaid is a joint federal–state program providing funding for insurance for the poor.

1965: In the United Kingdom, the NHS drops charges for prescriptions; the charges are reinstated in 1968.

1965: In the United States, only 37 percent of U.S. physicians are general practitioners versus 84 percent in 1940.

1966: Henry Beecher publishes a research article in the *New England Journal of Medicine* identifying 22 biomedical studies he believed were unethical due to issues such as lack of consent and harm caused to the subject of the research.

1966: In the United States, the first collection of the Household Component of the Medical Expenditure Panel Study (MEPS) occurs; data collected includes health status, conditions, and utilization; health care expenditures; and health insurance coverage.

1966: Canada passes the Medical Care Act of 1966, extending health insurance to cover physician services; this is the second part of the current Canadian national health insurance plan.

1971: Founding of Doctors Without Borders (Médicins sans Frontières) in France to respond to flooding in Bangladesh and war and famine in Biafra (Nigeria).

1971: In the United States, tobacco advertising is banned on television.

1973: In the United States, the federal Health Maintenance Organization Act spurs the development of health maintenance organizations (HMOs) across the country.

1974: In response to the Tuskegee Study, which became public knowledge in 1974, the U.S. Congress passes the National Research Act, requiring creation of Institutional Review Boards (IRBs) to ensure ethical conduct of research.

1974: In the United States, the federal government establishes the Women, Infants, and Children (WIC) program to provide nutritious food to low-income women, infants, and children.

1975: Doctors Without Borders establishes its first large-scale program to aid Cambodians fleeing the Pol Pot regime.

1979: The National Commission for the Protection of Research Subjects of Biomedical and Behavioral Research (United States) publishes the *Belmont Report,* identifying three basic principles necessary for the ethical conduct of research: respect for persons, beneficence, and justice.

1979: Announcement of the successful eradication of smallpox, a fact confirmed by WHO in 1980.

1980: In the United Kingdom, the *Black Report* finds that social class remains related to health outcomes, such as life expectancy and infant mortality, despite the efforts of the National Health Services (NHS).

1981: The *Morbidity and Mortality Weekly Report,* published by the U.S. Centers for Disease Control and Prevention, reports five cases of a rare type of pneumonia; these patients are among the first identified cases of acquired immune deficiency syndrome (AIDS).

1983: San Francisco General Hospital establishes a ward for AIDS patients dedicated to research on the disease as well as patient care.

1984: In the United States, the Centers for Disease Control and Prevention begins collecting data in 15 states with the Behavioral Risk Factor Surveillance System, a survey designed to collect information on health behaviors such as smoking, exercise, and eating habits;

by 1995, all 50 states plus Puerto Rico, Guam, and the U.S. Virgin Islands take part in the annual survey.

1984: In Canada, physicians are prohibited from charging fees greater than those specified in provincial benefit schedules.

1986: In the United States, the Emergency Medical Treatment and Active Labor Act (EMTALA) requires hospitals to treat patients with medical emergencies without regard to their insurance status or ability to pay.

1986: Ian Chalmers and colleagues at Oxford University in the United Kingdom publish the first medical systematic review of perinatal interventions.

1987: Fluoxetine (Prozac) offers better, safer treatment for depression and other mental illnesses, including panic disorder and anxiety disorders; it is the first of many selective serotonin reuptake inhibitor (SSRI) drugs introduced to the pharmaceutical marketplace.

1988: Doctors Without Borders establishes its first mental health program to serve survivors of an earthquake in Armenia.

1988: The NHS in the United Kingdom introduces a national program of screening for breast cancer.

1990: In the United States, tobacco smoking is banned on all domestic airplane flights.

1993: Founding of the *Cochrane Review*, a leading source of information about clinical effectiveness and controlled trials of medical interventions.

1993: In the United States, the Family and Medical Leave Act mandates large employers to allow 12 weeks of unpaid leave for employees for reasons such as the birth of a child, a serious health condition, or the need to care for an ill family member; the law covers approximately 40 to 50 percent of the population.

1996: In the United States, the first collection of the Insurance Component of the Medical Expenditure Panel Survey (MEPS) occurs. It gathers information from households and employers about employer-based health insurance.

1999: Doctors Without Borders launches a campaign to increase access to essential medicines by the world's poor.

2000: Doctors Without Borders begins providing antiretroviral therapy to persons with human immunodeficiency virus and acquired immune deficiency syndrome (HIV/AIDS) in Thailand; the following year, the program is extended to Cambodia, Guatemala, Cameroon, Kenya, Malawi, and South Africa.

2001: WHO launches the Measles Initiative in partnership with UNICEF, the Centers for Disease Control and Prevention, the United Nations Foundation, and the American Red Cross.

2001: In the United Kingdom, tobacco advertising on billboards is banned, and tobacco companies are banned from sponsoring most sporting activities by 2003.

2004: WHO adopts a Global Strategy on Diet, Physical Activity, and Health.

2005: The European Commission creates the Executive Agency for Public Health Programs to improve community health programs in the European Union through means such as supporting scientific research and collaboration, implementing public health programs, and awarding grants and contracts.

2006: Doctors Without Borders creates a surgical program in Jordan to care for victims of the Iraq War as physicians are unable to operate safely in Iraq.

2008: In the United Kingdom, patients are allowed to seek treatment in any clinic or hospital that meets NHS standards.

2010: In the United States, the Affordable Care Act becomes law; 2010 changes include tax credits for small businesses and nonprofit organizations, creation of a program to provide insurance to individuals with preexisting conditions, allowing young adults to remain covered by a parent's health plan until they turn 26, prohibition of the practice of rescission (retroactively cancelling insurance coverage) in the absence of fraud, and broadening of Medicaid eligibility; various other phases become active from 2011 to 2014.

2011: In the United States, a Center for Medicare & Medicaid Innovation is created to develop methods to provide quality care at lower cost.

2012: The U.S. Supreme Court hears arguments on the constitutionality of the Affordable Care Act.

2012: In the United Kingdom, the British Social Attitudes Survey estimates that public satisfaction with the NHS fell from 70 percent in 2010 to 58 percent in 2011, the largest fall since the survey began in 1983.

2012: In the United States, the medical loss ratio (MLR) requires insurance companies to spend at least 80 percent (85 percent for large plans) of collected premiums on providing care or making quality improvements.

2013: In the United States, states are required to pay physicians for services delivered to Medicaid patients at rates at least as high as the rate for Medicare patients.

2014: In the United States, the final provisions of the Affordable Care Act are scheduled to take effect, including the creation of insurance exchanges to offer health insurance policies to people who do not receive coverage from their employers and requiring most people to purchase a basic health insurance policy or pay a penalty.

AFGHANISTAN

Afghanistan is a landlocked Asian country with an area of 251,827 square miles (652,230 square kilometers, similar to Texas) and a July 2012 estimated population of 30.4 million. In 2010, 23 percent of the population lived in urban areas, and the 2010 to 2015 annual rate of urbanization is estimated at 4.7 percent. Kabul is the capital and largest city (with a 2009 population of 3.6 million). The population is growing at 2.2 percent, the 39th-highest rate in the world, due to a fertility rate of 5.6 births per woman (the ninth-highest in the world) and birth rate of 39.3 births per 1,000 population; the July 2012 population growth rate was the 13th-highest in the world despite a negative net migration rate (negative 2.51 migrants per 1,000 population) and low life expectancy. The United Nations High Commissioner for Refugees (UNHCR) estimates that, in 2010, there were 6,434 refugees and persons in refugee-like situations in Afghanistan in addition to 351,907 internally displaced persons and persons in internally displaced-person-like situations.

Afghanistan became independent from the United Kingdom in 1919 and has suffered a series of civil wars, invasions, and other types of unrest since the

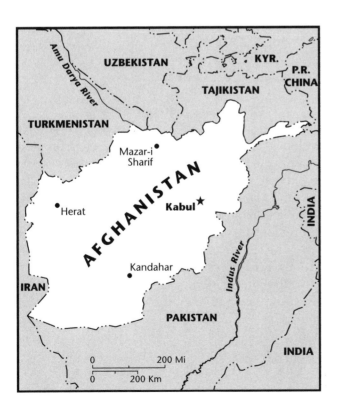

1970s. Afghanistan ranked near the bottom in 2011 (180th out of 183 countries) on Transparency International's *Corruption Perceptions Index*, with a score of 1.5 (on a scale where 0 indicates highly corrupt and 10 very clean).

In 2011, Afghanistan was classified as a country with low human development (the lowest of four categories) on the United Nations Development Programme's (UNDP's) Human Development Index (HDI), with a score of 0.398 (on a scale where 1 denotes high development and 0 low development). The World Food Programme estimated in 2012 that 2.6 million people in Afghanistan's northern provinces were severely food insecure. Life expectancy at birth in 2012 was estimated at 49.72 years, among the five lowest in the world. Estimated gross domestic product (GDP) per capita in 2011 was $1,000, among the 20 lowest in the world, and unemployment in 2008 was estimated at 35.0 percent, among the highest rates in the world. In 2008, the Gini Index (a measure of dispersion, in which perfect equality is denoted by 0 and maximum inequality is denoted by 100) for family income was 29.4.

Emergency Health Services

According to the World Health Organization (WHO), as of 2007, Afghanistan did not have a formal and publicly available system for providing prehospital care (emergency care). Doctors Without Borders (Médecins Sans Frontières, or MSF) began working in Afghanistan in 1984, ceased services in the country in 2004 due to continued violence (MSF projects were transferred to national or local authorities), and returned to Afghanistan in 2009; at the close of 2010, MSF had 200 staff working in the country. In October 2009, a small inpatient department and apartment theater were established in Ahmed Shah Baba Hospital in Kabul, and 5,500 patients were treated that month. Services continued to expand, and in 2010, more than 118,200 patients were treated in the Ahmed Shah Baba Hospital. In 2010, MSF restored Boost Hospital in Lashkargah to functioning status and treated more than 26,000 patients between May and December.

Insurance

Despite continuing conflict and widespread poverty within Afghanistan, the country has made progress in providing health coverage; for instance, a 2010 WHO report noted that a Basic Package of Health Services (BPHS) was available in 85 percent of the country.

Selected Health Indicators: Afghanistan Compared With the Global Average (2010)

	Afghanistan	Global Average
Male life expectancy at birth* (years)	47	66
Female life expectancy at birth* (years)	50	71
Under-5 mortality rate, both sexes (per 1,000 live births)	149	57
Adult mortality rate, both sexes* (probability of dying between 15 and 60 years per 1,000 population)	399	176
Maternal mortality ratio (per 100,000 live births)	460	210
Tuberculosis prevalence (per 100,000 population)	352	178

Source: World Health Organization Global Health Observatory Data Repository.
*Data refers to 2009.

Extension of the BPHS to all residents is a national priority, with an intermediate goal of 95 percent coverage by 2015; another priority is strengthening the hospital referral network in order to facilitate the provision of the Essential Package of Hospital Services (EPHS) to patients in need of hospital care. As of 2010, much (60 to 80 percent) of the health care operating budget in Afghanistan was provided by external donors, and provision of the BPHS was largely contracted out to nongovernmental organizations (NGOs) working in the country. Provision of services in some areas remains problematic due to continuing violence, sparse populations, and poor infrastructure; other problems include tensions between the NGOs and provincial health authorities, governmental corruption, and questions about the cost and quality of services provided.

It is difficult to locate or verify current information about social health insurance (for example, cash benefits for sickness and maternity) in Afghanistan due to the disrupted functioning of governmental entities within the country. The most recent information available in the International Social Security Database about social health insurance in Afghanistan dates from 1989. (While the database was updated in 2008, much of the information is older.) Under public health law passed in 1985 and an ordinance passed in 1987, all Afghani citizens are covered by a social insurance system providing sickness leave benefits (20 days with salary) and maternity leave benefits (90 days, or

105 days for twins, both with salary). The Ministry of Finance administers the program. Employed personnel are also provided a work injury benefit in the form of a lump sum payment, depending on the degree of disability and whether it is permanent or temporary; survivors are also eligible for a lump sum benefit.

Costs of Hospitalization

As of 2010, most hospitals in Afghanistan were supported by NGOs or donors, including the United States Agency for International Development (USAID) and the European Commission.

Access to Health Care

Despite continuing conflict and widespread poverty within Afghanistan, the country has made progress in providing health coverage; a 2010 WHO report noted that a BPHS was available in 85 percent of the country. Some services required payment, with different mechanisms around the country offering some exemptions for the poor. In addition, some services were provided free to all citizens, including immunizations, prenatal care and delivery, family planning, nutrition interventions, and treatment of tuberculosis. Using as a goal that primary health care services should be available to everyone at no more than two hours' walking distance, considerable improvement has been made since 2000, when this standard was met for only 9 percent of the population; by 2006, it was met for 65 percent of the population, and by

2010, for 90 percent. In 2010, an estimated 3 percent of persons with advanced human immunodeficiency virus (HIV) infection were receiving antiretroviral therapy in accordance with 2010 WHO guidelines.

A 2003 survey conducted by the Ministry of Health determined that access to hospital services was in need of improvement. A large percentage of the population had no access to referral hospitals. The hospitals were poorly maintained and lacked access to regular electricity and water supplies, they were underutilized (average occupancy below 50 percent), and some were overstaffed (particularly in urban areas). However, they often lacked sufficient female staff, and insufficient emergency obstetric care was available. In response, an EPHS was developed to aid in standardizing the referral process and provision of services.

According to WHO, in 2003 (the most recent data available), 14 percent of births in Afghanistan were attended by skilled personnel (for example, physicians, nurses, or midwives). In 2008, 36 percent of pregnant women received at least one prenatal care visit. The 2010 immunization rates for 1-year-olds were 66 percent for diphtheria and pertussis (DPT3), 62 percent for measles (MCV), and 66 percent for Hib (Hib3).

Cost of Drugs

According to Omid Ameli and William Newbrander, in April 2006 and 2007, mean annual drug costs per capita for 21 NGO contracts to deliver the BPHS in 355 health facilities in 13 provinces of Afghanistan were $0.65; the average drug cost per visit was $0.30 (8.5 percent of the total cost of the visit). Most of this cost was fixed, with little relationship to utilization or security. A 1999 survey in Jalalabad found wide variation in the prices of paracetamol, chloroquine, metronidazole, ampicillin, and levamizole sold in 10 pharmacies located in the vicinity of the teaching hospital. For instance, the mean price for levamizole tables was AFN 110, with a range of AFN 30 to 500, and the mean price for chloroquine ampules was AFN 412, with a range of AFN 250 to 1020.

Health Care Facilities

Afghanistan's focus is providing a BPHS to all residents, with a goal of 95 percent coverage by 2015. Services are provided by contract with NGOs within the country and are supported by three major donors: the World Bank, USAID, and the European Commission. The BHPS system includes four levels: a health post with two community health workers (one male and one female) covering a catchment area of about 1,000 to 1,500 people; a basic health center, including a nurse, midwife, and staff trained to administer vaccinations, serving a catchment area of 15,000 to 30,000 people; a comprehensive health center, including male and female physicians and nurses, midwives, and lab and pharmacy technicians, serving a catchment area of 30,000 to 60,000 people; and a district hospital staffed with specialized physicians, including a female obstetrics and gynecology (OB/GYN) specialist, midwives, technicians, and a dentist, serving a catchment area of 100,000 to 300,000 people.

In 2009, Afghanistan had 0.40 hospital beds per 1,000 population, one of the 10 lowest rates in the world. As of 2010, according to WHO, Afghanistan had 2.87 health posts per 100,000 population, 1.19 health centers per 100,000, 0.18 district or rural hospitals per 100,000, 0.10 provincial hospitals per 100,000, and 0.08 specialized hospitals per 100,000. According to WHO, in 2010, Afghanistan had 0.11 magnetic resonance imaging (MRI) machines per 1 million population and 0.22 computer tomography (CT) machines per 1 million.

Major Health Issues

Compared to other countries at a similar level of development, Afghanistan ranked last among the 43 least-developed countries on the 2011 Mothers' Index, produced by the international NGO Save the Children, based on a number of health and social factors relating to women, children, and maternal and child care. Afghanistan's maternal mortality rate (death from any cause related to or aggravated by pregnancy) is the highest in the world, estimated at 1,400 per 100,000 live births (2008 data). The infant mortality rate, defined as the number of deaths of infants younger than 1 year, is also the highest in the world at 121.63 per 1,000 live births (2012 data). Child malnutrition is a serious problem: In 2004, 32.9 percent of children under age 5 were underweight (defined as 2 kilograms [kg] below standard weight-for-age at age 1, 3 kg below for ages 2 to 3, and 4 kg below for ages 4 to 5), one of the 20 highest rates in the world.

Afghanistan's health indicators are among the lowest in the world, and they are below those of any neighboring country. As of 2010, an estimated 4.5 million people faced food insecurity, and chronic malnutrition and micronutrient deficiency were prevalent in many areas. Poor nutrition is one among several factors implicated in high infant and maternal mortality rates and low life expectancy; other factors include widespread poverty; shortages of medical equipment, supplies, and trained personnel; and continuing violent conflict within the country. Rates of communicable disease are high: In 2007, eight of the 10 most common diseases were communicable, including pneumonia, acute diarrhea, malaria, and urinary tract infections, while the remaining two were psychiatric disorders and trauma. Violence against women is a continuing problem, as is kidnapping and forced marriage. Despite being prohibited by Afghan law, an estimated 70 to 80 percent of women are forced into marriage, and 57 percent of Afghan girls are married at age 15 or younger.

In 2008, WHO estimated that 74 percent of years of life lost were due to communicable diseases, 18 percent to noncommunicable diseases, and 9 percent to injuries. In 2008, the age-standardized estimate of cancer deaths was 108 per 100,000 for men and 97 per 100,000 for women; for cardiovascular diabetes, 765 per 100,000 for men and 578 per 100,000 for women; and for chronic respiratory disease, 89 per 100,000 for men and 55 per 100,000 for women.

Afghanistan is one of three countries in the world in which polio is endemic; most cases occur in the provinces of Helmand, Kandahar, and Uruzgan, where ongoing conflict and insecurity make it difficult to deliver medical services to children. In 2010, 69,397 cases of malaria were reported. The burden of tuberculosis is high at 161 per 100,000 population, and tuberculosis-related mortality is 32 per 100,000. WHO estimated that the case detection rate in 2010 was 47 percent. The rate of tuberculosis is unusually high among women, who constitute two-thirds of the cases. Access to potable water is less common in rural (26 percent) than in urban areas (64 percent), and in some provinces, less than 10 percent of the population have access to potable water. Modern sanitary methods to dispose of excreta are rare, and almost one-fourth (24.9 percent) have no access to any kind of sanitary facilities; this creates an environment favoring outbreaks of waterborne diseases, such as cholera, particularly during the summer. Malaria is endemic, with more than 4.6 million cases reported in 2008. Leishmaniasis is endemic, particularly in Kabul, where incidences in 2010 were estimated at 70,000 (up from 15,000 in 1995).

The prevalence of HIV/acquired immune deficiency syndrome (AIDS) in Afghanistan is somewhat unknown due to social stigma; only 417 cases have been reported, but some estimate there could be 1,000 to 2,000 Afghans currently infected, primarily injecting drug users (IDUs) and their partners. Polio still exists in Afghanistan; 31 cases were reported in 2010 (as of November). Maternal and neonatal tetanus remain a high risk in some districts of the country. However, routine coverage for some vaccines is high; coverage with the DPT3/HepB3 vaccine was reported at 83 percent in 2008 (up from 41 percent in 2001), and MCV vaccine coverage was reported at 75 percent in 2008; reported measles cases have fallen from 88,762 in 2001 to 1,149 in 2008, although small measles outbreaks still occur.

Mental health is a major concern in Afghanistan, as it is estimated that most residents suffer from some type of stress disorder due to continuing violent conflicts within the country, and more than 2 million are estimated to suffer from conditions such as schizophrenia, depression, or bipolar disorder. The mental health of women has been found to vary according to whether they live in an area controlled by the Taliban or not; a 2000 study found 78 percent of women living in Taliban-controlled areas suffered from depression versus 28 percent of women living in non-Taliban-controlled areas, and suicidal ideation and suicide attempts were higher among women living in Taliban-controlled areas (65 percent and 16 percent, respectively) than in women living in non-Taliban-controlled areas (18 percent and 9 percent, respectively).

Health Care Personnel

In 2006, WHO identified Afghanistan as one of 57 countries with a critical deficit in the supply of skilled health workers. As of 2010, Afghanistan had six medical schools enrolling about 8,000 medical students, with most physicians and dentists coming from Kabul Medical University. The basic course of medical training, including practical training, lasts seven years and results in a degree of doctor of medicine (M.D.). Work in government service after graduation is obligatory. Foreign physicians require no official permission to practice, but graduates of foreign medical schools must have their degrees validated by an internationally recognized agency. Afghanistan has nine Institutes of Health Sciences, enrolling approximately 3,500 students as of 2010, which train nurses, midwives, and professionals in allied health fields. A community midwifery program, begun in 2002, has produced 140 community midwives since 2002 and currently has 640 students enrolled.

Afghanistan has a five-year plan to develop its health workforce over the years 2012 to 2016. Objectives include increasing the number of health workers to 39 per 10,000 population and the number of doctors, nurses, and midwives to 13 per 10,000. An additional goal is to improve the gender balance among health workers (that is, increase the number of female health workers).

In 2009, Afghanistan had 0.21 physicians per 1,000 population, 0.50 nurses and midwives per 1,000, and 0.03 dentists per 1,000. Many professionals, including those trained in medicine and health care, left the country during periods of civil unrest, and training more medical workers is a priority of the 2008 to 2013 country cooperation strategy developed jointly by WHO and the Afghan Ministry of Health; an estimated 7,000 additional physicians, 20,000 nurses, and other health professionals are needed to provide basic medical and hospital care.

Resources are poorly distributed, with rural and remote areas underserved (36 public health workers per 10,000 in urban areas, 16.7 per 10,000 in rural areas, with more than three-quarters of the population living in rural areas). Only 28 percent of the health workforce are female (and that figure includes unqualified support staff), and female health workers are particularly scarce in rural areas, yet are necessary due to national customs if women are to receive adequate care. In 2006, about 38 percent of health care workers in the country were from NGOs.

Government Role in Health Care

Data about health care financing in Afghanistan are difficult to locate and often contradictory. However, it is clear that the government plays only a small role in financing health care, while international donors play large roles, providing services and managing infrastructure; in addition, much care must be paid for out of pocket. The 2010 WHO report on the country cooperation strategy for health care estimated that 60 percent or more of health care in Afghanistan were financed by donors, that health spending by the government was 0.6 percent of the total spending, and that per capita government spending on health was less than $4, while out-of-pocket spending on health was approximately $29 per household. In 2009, according to WHO, official development assistance (ODA) for health in Afghanistan came to $11.69 per capita.

Public Health Programs

The Afghan Public Health Institute (APHI) is located in Kabul and directed by Bashir Noormal. APHI trained more than 3,000 health professionals in 2009 in areas including epidemiology, biostatistics, research methodology, public health management, health care financing, conflict management, and human resource management. The APHI also coordinates with researchers from around the world to conduct research in Afghanistan. According to the World Higher Education Database (WHED), one university in Afghanistan offers programs in epidemiology or public health: Balkh University, located in Mazar-e-Sharif.

Afghanistan faces many challenges in developing public health programs, including a lack of infrastructure, widespread poverty, destruction caused by ongoing violence, a lack of trained personnel, and government corruption. As of 2010, only 37 percent of the population had access to improved sanitation facilities (30 percent in rural areas), and 42 percent of the population had access to improved drinking water sources (42 percent in rural areas). However, the Afghan Ministry of Public Health (MoPH) has several plans focused on improving the nation's health, including a national health and nutrition strategy for 2008 through 2013 that emphasizes developing effective institutions and reducing morbidity and mortality and a plan based on the Millennium Development Goals (MDGs) focused on wider social indicators including poverty reduction. The Afghanistan National Development Strategy, developed in conjunction with WHO, provides a road map for the country to develop its human resources and transition toward self-sustaining growth and greater stability.

One priority area for Afghanistan has been the provision of a BPHS to all residents; as of 2010, the BPHS was available to about 85 percent of the population. However, Afghanistan's health structure is largely (60 to 80 percent) funded by outside donors, and BPHS is largely provided by contract with NGOs working within the country. In the medium term (2008–2013), the country cooperation strategy for WHO and Afghanistan is focused on human resource development, information systems, financing, improving the social and environmental determinants of health, control of communicable diseases, mental health care, reproductive and child health, and emergency preparedness and response.

ALBANIA

Albania is a southeastern European country with an area of 11,071 square miles (28,674 square kilometers, similar to Maryland) and a July 2012 estimated population of 3 million. In 2010, 52 percent of the population lived in urban areas, and the 2010 to 2015 annual rate of urbanization is estimated at 2.3 percent. Tirana is the capital and largest city (2009 population estimated at 433,000). Total fertility is below replacement levels (1.5 children per woman), and the July 2012 population growth rate is low (0.3 percent), due in part to a negative migration rate (negative 3.3 migrants per 1,000 population). The United Nations High Commissioner for Refugees (UNHCR) estimates that, in 2010, there were 76 refugees and persons in refugee-like situations in Albania.

Albania became independent from the Ottoman Empire in 1912, was occupied by Italy in 1939, and was allied with the Soviet Union until 1960 and China until 1978. Albania ranked in the midrange in 2011 (95th out of 183 countries) on Transparency International's *Corruption Perceptions Index*, with a score of 3.1 (on a scale where 0 indicates highly corrupt and 10 very clean). In 2011, Albania was classified as a country with high human development (the second-highest category) on the United Nations Development Programme's (UNDP's) Human Development Index (HDI), with a score of 0.739 (on a scale where 1 denotes high development and 0 low development). However, it is one of the poorest countries in Europe, with a per capita gross domestic product (GDP) of $7,800 in 2011. In 2008, the Gini Index (a measure of dispersion, in which perfect equality is denoted by 0 and maximum inequality is denoted by 100) for family income was 34.5. According to the World Economic Forum's *Global Gender Gap Index 2011*, Albania ranked 78th out of 135 countries on gender equality with a score of 0.675 (on a scale with a theoretical range of 1 for equality to 0 for inequality and an actual range in 2011 from 0.8530 to 0.4873).

Emergency Health Services

According to the World Health Organization (WHO), in 2007, Albania had a formal and publicly available emergency care (prehospital care) system accessible by regional telephone numbers but not a universal national access number. In 2010 to 2011, Albania

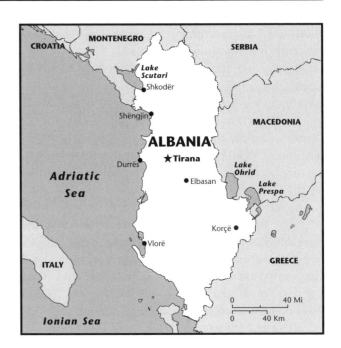

worked with the WHO Regional Office for Europe to create a national version of the Public Health and Emergency Management course and to assess the crisis preparedness and response capabilities of the national health system.

Insurance

Albania's social insurance program dates to 1947, with the current laws regulating sickness and maternity benefits dating to 1993 and 1994. Everyone residing in Albania is entitled to medical benefits; employed persons are eligible for cash sickness benefits, and employers, employed persons, and the self-employed are entitled to cash maternity benefits. The maternity benefit is based on the insured's income and pays for up to 365 days (390 days for multiple births). A flat birth grant is also paid if either parent is insured and has been working for at least one year. Sickness benefits are based on the insured's wages and last for up to six months, with a three-month extension possible. Compensation is paid if a person must change employment due to health reasons or pregnancy.

The social insurance system is funded through taxes on employees and employers. Private insurance is also available. General medical services are free, with a copayment required for some medicines (0 to 65 percent copay) and some types of examinations (10 percent copay). Some population groups are provided with entirely free services, including children younger than 1 year, disabled people, veterans and invalids of World War II, and people with certain illnesses. The social insurance system is supervised by the Ministry of Finance and the Ministry of Health Protection.

Costs of Hospitalization

According to its national accounts report, in 2010, Albania spent 31.3 percent of its total health expenditures on secondary care.

Access to Health Care

In 2007, Albania had 2.92 hospital beds per 1,000 population, ranking 78th in the world. According to WHO, in 2010, Albania had 2.55 magnetic resonance imaging (MRI) machines per 1 million population, 5.41 computer tomography (CT) machines per 1 million, 0.32 telecolbalt units per 1 million, and 0.32 radiotherapy machines per 1 million. According to WHO, in 2003, 99.3 percent of births in Albania were attended by skilled personnel (for example, physicians, nurses, or midwives). In 2009, 67 percent of pregnant women received at least four prenatal care visits. The 2010 immunization rates for 1-year-olds were 99 percent for diphtheria and pertussis (DPT3), 99 percent for measles (MCV), and 99 percent for Hib (Hib3).

Cost of Drugs

According to Douglas Ball, since 2005, drug prices, markups, and reimbursement levels in Albania are set annually by the Pharmaceutical Directorate and the Drugs Pricing Commission. A positive list of medicines specifies which are eligible for reimbursement by the Health Insurance Institute; the price of most medicines on this list are set by internal reference pricing, with the price for more expensive drugs negotiated with manufacturers. Patients pay a lower copayment for lower-priced generics. Hospital medicines are purchased centrally and provided at no charge. As of 2007, reimbursed medicines had a 12 percent wholesale and a 29 percent retail markup, while non-reimbursed medicines had an 18 percent wholesale markup and a 33 percent retail markup. According to its national accounts report, in 2010, Albania spent 40.6 percent of its total health expenditures on medical goods, a relatively high proportion.

Health Care Facilities

In 2007, Albania had 2.92 hospital beds per 1,000 population. As of 2010, according to WHO, Albania had 12.95 health posts per 100,000 population, 0.72 district and rural hospitals per 100,000, 0.34 provincial hospitals per 100,000, and 0.28 specialized hospitals per 100,000.

Major Health Issues

In 2008, WHO estimated that 9 percent of years of life lost in Albania were due to communicable diseases, 76 percent to noncommunicable diseases, and 14 percent to injuries. In 2008, the age-standardized estimate of cancer deaths was 172 per 100,000 for men and 126 per 100,000 for women; for cardiovascular disease and diabetes, 469 per 100,000 for men and 417 per 100,000 for women; and for chronic respiratory disease, 29 per 100,000 for men and 18 per 100,000 for women.

In 2010, tuberculosis incidence was 14.0 per 100,000 population, tuberculosis prevalence 16.0 per 100,000, and deaths due to tuberculosis among human immunodeficiency virus (HIV)-negative people 0.38 per 100,000. Compared to other countries at a similar level of development, Albania ranked last (43rd) on the 2011 Mothers' Index produced by the international nongovernmental organization (NGO) Save the Children, based on a number of health and social factors relating to women, children, and maternal and child care. Albania's maternal mortality rate (death from any cause related to or aggravated by pregnancy) in 2008 was 31 maternal deaths per 100,000 live births. The infant mortality rate, defined as the number of deaths of infants younger than 1 year, was 14.12 per 1,000 live births as of 2012.

Health Care Personnel

Albania has one medical school, the Fakulteti I Mjerkësisë at the Universitetii Tiranës in Tirana, founded in 1952. The basic medical degree course, including practical training, lasts six years, with a further year of supervised clinical practice required for the degree. The license to practice medicine is granted by the Ministry of Health (after submission of the applicant's diploma and grades), and physicians must register with the Order of Albanian Physicians. There is no required government service work after graduation. In 2007, Albania had 1.15 physicians per 1,000 population, 0.39 pharmaceutical personnel per 1,000, 0.33 dentistry personnel per 1,000, and 4.03 nurses and midwives per 1,000.

Government Role in Health Care

According to WHO, in 2010, Albania spent $777 million on health care, or $241 per capita. About two-thirds of this total (61 percent) was spent by households, with the remaining 39 percent spent by the government. Almost all (98 percent) of the funding for Albania's health care system is provided domestically, with the remaining 2 percent coming from abroad. About 8 percent of Albania's government resources are allocated to health. Albania ranks relatively low among upper- and middle-income European countries in terms of total government expenditure on health, share of government spending allocated to health, and government expenditure on health as a percent of GDP. In 2009, according to WHO, official development assistance (ODA) for health in Albania came to $7.15 per capita.

Public Health Programs

According to its national accounts report, in 2010, Albania spent 3.7 percent of its total health expenditures on public health. According to the World Higher Education Database (WHED), one university in Albania offers training in epidemiology or public health: the University of Vlora 'Ismail Qemali,' located in Vlore. The Institute of Public Health, founded in 1935 and located in Tirana, works with other organizations to develop health promotion and education programs, conduct surveillance activities, identify and monitor health risks, train personnel to work in public health, conduct research, and help develop public health policy. The 2012 director was Enver Roshi. Centers within the Institute of Public Health include the National Center for Training in Public Health, the National Center for Research and Study in Public Health, the National Reference Center for Public Health, the National Operations Center for Public Health, the National Technical Center for Expertise in Public Health, and the National Center of Quality Control and Safety and Public Health Laboratory. As of 2010, access to improved sanitation facilities (94 percent) and improved drinking water sources (95 percent) was nearly universal.

ALGERIA

Algeria is a north African country with a northern coastline on the Mediterranean Sea, an area of 919,595 square miles (2,381,741 square kilometers), making it the 10th-largest country in the world and the largest in Africa (about 3.5 times the size of Texas), with a population of 35.4 million (based on a July 2012 estimate, the 35th-largest in the world). In 2010, 66 percent of the population lived in urban areas, and the 2010 to 2015 annual rate of urbanization is estimated at 2.3 percent. Algiers is the capital and largest city (with the 2009 population estimated at 2.74 million). Population growth in 2012 was estimated at 1.165 percent, below replacement levels, due in part to a low total fertility rate (estimated at 1.74 children per woman in 2012) and a negative migration rate (estimated at negative 0.27 migrants per 1,000 population in 2012), meaning that more people were leaving Algeria than moving to it. The United Nations High Commissioner for Refugees (UNHCR) estimates that, in 2010, there were 94,144 refugees and persons in refugee-like situations in Algeria.

Algeria achieved independence from France in 1962 and has had a multiparty system of elections since 1988. Algeria ranks low on measures of gender equality: According to the World Economic Forum's *Global Gender Gap Index 2011*, Algeria ranked 121st out of 135 countries on gender equality, with a score of 0.599 (on a scale with a theoretical range of 1 for equality to 0 for inequality and an actual range in 2011 from 0.8530 to 0.4873). According to the Ibrahim Index, in 2011, Algeria ranked 18th among 53 African countries in terms of governance performance, with a score of 55 (out of 100). Algeria ranked in the middle range in 2011 (112th out of

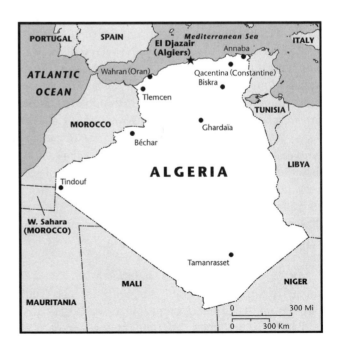

183 countries) on Transparency International's *Corruption Perceptions Index*, with a score of 2.9 (on a scale where 0 indicates highly corrupt and 10 very clean). In 2011, Algeria was classified as a country with medium human development (the second from the lowest of four categories) on the United Nations Development Programme's (UNDP's) Human Development Index (HDI), with a score of 0.698 (on a scale where 1 denotes high development and 0 low development). Life expectancy at birth in 2012 was estimated at 74.73 years.

Estimated gross domestic product (GDP) per capita in 2011 was $7,200. In 1995 the Gini Index (a measure of dispersion, in which perfect equality is denoted by 0 and maximum inequality is denoted by 100) for family income was 35.3. Unemployment in 2011 was estimated at 9.7 percent, and in 2006, 23 percent of families lived below the poverty line.

Emergency Health Services

According to the U.S. State Department, Algeria has several sets of phone numbers for emergency assistance, depending on whether one is calling from a landline or mobile phone and depending on the type of emergency and assistance required (ambulance, police, or fire).

Insurance

The law establishing Algeria's current social insurance program was passed in 1983 and implemented in 1984. Cash and medical benefits are available to people who are employed, while medical benefits are not universal but are provided to many classes of people, including the employed, self-employed, and those receiving unemployment benefits; pensioners; some disabled persons (with at least 50 percent disability); unemployed students and their dependents; national liberation war pensioners; those receiving social assistance; and the dependents of some prisoners. The system is paid for by a combination of employee, self-employed, and employer contributions.

Medical benefits for those included in the system include hospitalization, surgery, drugs, lab services, rehabilitation, medical treatment, some specialized treatments, transportation, prostheses, eye care, and some dental care. Persons with some categories of illness are provided with free care in government hospitals, while for others, there is a copayment required. Maternity care is completely reimbursed, including up to eight days hospitalization. Dependents receive the same benefits as the insured. The system is supervised by the Ministry of Labor and Social Security.

Costs of Hospitalization

No data available.

Access to Health Care

According to the World Health Organization (WHO), in 2006, 95.0 percent of births in Algeria were attended by skilled personnel (for example, physicians, nurses, or midwives). In 2006, 89 percent of pregnant women received at least one prenatal care visit. The 2010 immunization rates for 1-year-olds were 95 percent for diphtheria and pertussis (DPT3), 95 percent for measles (MCV), and 95 percent for Hib (Hib3). In 2010, an estimated 32 percent of persons with advanced human immunodeficiency virus (HIV) infection were receiving antiretroviral therapy in accordance with 2010 WHO guidelines.

Cost of Drugs

No data available.

Health Care Facilities

In 2004, Algeria had 1.70 hospital beds per 1,000 population.

Major Health Issues

In 2008, WHO estimated that 43 percent of years of life lost in Algeria were due to communicable diseases, 45 percent to noncommunicable diseases, and 12 percent to injuries. In 2008, the age-standardized estimate of cancer deaths was 98 per 100,000 for men and 79 per 100,000 for women; for cardiovascular disease and diabetes, 279 per 100,000 for men and 275 per 100,000 for women; and for chronic respiratory disease, 75 per 100,000 for men and 39 per 100,000 for women.

In 2010, tuberculosis incidence was 90.0 per 100,000 population, tuberculosis prevalence 11,360 per 100,000, and deaths due to tuberculosis among HIV-negative people 12.0 per 100,000. As of 2009, an estimated 0.1 percent of adults age 15 to 49 were living with HIV or acquired immune deficiency syndrome (AIDS). Algeria's maternal mortality rate (death from any cause related to or aggravated by pregnancy) was estimated in 2008 as 120 maternal deaths per 100,000 live births. The infant mortality rate, defined as the number of deaths of infants younger than 1 year, was estimated at 24.90 per 1,000 live births as of 2012.

Health Care Personnel

Algeria has 11 medical schools: the Institut National d'Enseignement Supérieur en Sciences Médicales of the University of Algiers, the Institut National d'Enseignement Supérieur en Sciences Médicales in Annaba, the Institut de Sciences Médicales of the University of Batna, the Institut de Sciences Médicales of the University of Blida, the Institut National d'Enseignement Supérieur en Sciences Médicales in Constantine, the Institut National d'Enseignement Supérieur en Sciences Médicales in Mostaganem, the Institut National d'Enseignement Supérieur en Sciences Médicales in Oran, the Institut de Sciences Médicales of the University of Sétif, the Institut de Sciences Médicales of the University of Sidi Bel Abbes, the Institut de Sciences Médicales of the University of Tizi-Ouzou, and the Institut de Sciences Médicales of the University of Tlemcen.

The course of training for the basic medical degree lasts six or seven years, and the degree awarded is the Docteur en Médecine (doctor of medicine), with the license to practice medicine granted by the Ministère de la Santé de la Population.

In 2007, Algeria had 1.21 physicians per 1,000 population, 0.24 pharmaceutical personnel per 1,000, 0.33 dentistry personnel per 1,000, 0.03 community and traditional health workers per 1,000, and 1.95 nurses and midwives per 1,000. The global "brain drain" (international migration of skilled personnel) plays a role in this relative undersupply of medical personnel in Algeria: Michael Clemens and Bunilla Petterson estimate that 44 percent of Algerian-born physicians and 9 percent of Algerian-born nurses are working in one of nine developed countries, primarily in France.

Government Role in Health Care

According to WHO, in 2010, Algeria spent $6.3 billion on health care, or $178 per capita. The Algerian health care system is funded entirely domestically, with the government funding over three-quarters (78 percent) of health care expenditures; households purchase 21 percent of the total, with the remaining 1 percent being purchased by other entities. Government and total spending on health have increased in recent years, while out-of-pocket household spending has remained fairly constant. In 2010, about 8 percent of government resources were allocated to health care. Compared to other upper-middle-income African countries, Algeria ranks low in terms of total government expenditure on health as a percent of gross domestic product (GDP) and share of government spending allocated to health. In 2009, according to WHO, official development assistance (ODA) for health in Algeria came to $0.33 per capita.

Public Health Programs

According to WHO, in 2007, Algeria had 0.07 environmental and public health workers per 1,000 population. As of 2010, access to improved sanitation facilities (95 percent) and improved drinking water sources (83 percent) was common, although not universal; access to both was lower in rural than in urban areas, with only 88 percent of people in rural areas having access to improved sanitation facilities and 79 percent to improved drinking water sources. According to C. B. Ijsselmuiden and colleagues, in 2007, Algeria had four institutions offering postgraduate public health programs.

ANDORRA

Andorra is a mountainous, landlocked southwestern European country sharing borders with France and Spain. It is one of the smallest countries in Europe, with a total area of 181 square miles (468 square kilometers, about 2.5 times the size of Washington, D.C.) and population (2012 estimate) of 85,082. In 2010, 88 percent of the population lived in urban areas, and the 2010 to 2015 annual rate of urbanization is estimated at 1.1 percent. The capital and largest city is Andorra La Vella (with a 2009 population estimated at 25,000). The population growth rate in 2012 was 0.3 percent, the birth rate 9.3 births per 1,000 population, the net migration rate 0.0 migrants per 1,000, and the total fertility rate 1.4 children per woman, among the 20 lowest rates in the world.

Until 1993, Andorra was ruled as a coprincipality of Spain and France; in 1993, it became a parliamentary democracy. In 2011, Andorra was classified as a country with very high human development (the highest of four categories) on the United Nations Development Programme's (UNDP's) Human Development Index (HDI), with a score of 0.838 (on a scale where 1 denotes high development and 0 low development). Life expectancy at birth in 2012 was estimated at 82.50 years, among the highest in the

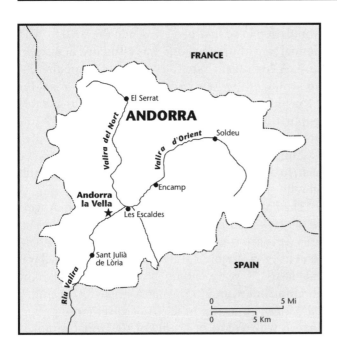

FRANCE

El Serrat

ANDORRA

Valira del Nort

Valira d'Orient

Soldeu

Andorra
la Vella

Encamp

Les Escaldes

Sant Julià
de Lòria

SPAIN

Riu Valira

0   5 Mi

0   5 Km

world, and per capita gross domestic product (GDP) in 2011 was estimated at $37,200.

Emergency Health Services

Andorra has a dedicated phone number, 116, for emergency health care.

Insurance

The law establishing Andorra's first social insurance program dates to 1966 (implemented 1968); it was amended in 2006. The current law governing medical benefits was passed in 2008 and implemented in 2009. The system covers the employed, self-employed, and their dependents. The system is paid for by contributions from employees, the self-employed, and employers: Employed people pay 3 percent of gross earnings for disability, maternity, survivors, sickness, and work injury coverage, and a choice of 2.5 percent, 5 percent, or 7.5 percent for old-age coverage. A self-employed person pays 10 percent of gross earnings for sickness, maternity, disability, survivors, and work injury coverage, and a choice of 10 percent, 12.5 percent, or 15 percent of average monthly earnings to the National Social Security Fund. Employers pay 7 percent of gross earnings for disability, survivors, sickness, and work injury coverage, and 7.5 percent of gross earnings for old-age coverage.

Medical benefits covered include hospitalization, primary and secondary medical care, maternity care,

and some transportation. Maternity care is covered 100 percent, while hospitalization requires a 10 percent copay and other medical expenses a 25 percent copay. Dependents receive the same care and pay the same copayments as the insured. The cash maternity benefit for mothers is 100 percent of the insured's average daily wage for up to 16 weeks, with additional weeks for multiple births; for fathers, the benefit is paid for 14 days. The cash sickness benefit is based on the average salary of the insured over the past year; for the first 30 days, the benefit is 53 percent of that average, while after 30 days, it is 70 percent of that average. Both maternity and sickness cash benefits require specified periods of coverage before a benefit can be paid. The National Social Security Fund manages Andorra's social insurance program.

Costs of Hospitalization

No data available.

Access to Health Care

According to the World Health Organization (WHO), the 2010 immunization rates for 1-year-olds in Andorra were 99 percent for diphtheria and pertussis (DPT3), 99 percent for measles (MCV), and 98 percent for Hib (Hib3).

Cost of Drugs

No data available.

Health Care Facilities

In 2007, Andorra had 2.62 hospital beds per 1,000 population. Andorra has one general hospital, the Hospital Nostra Senyora de Meritxell, and a geriatric hospital, the Clinica Geriatrica St. Vicenc d'Enclar.

Major Health Issues

In 2008, WHO estimated that 4 percent of years of life lost in Andorra were due to communicable diseases, 84 percent to noncommunicable diseases, and 12 percent to injuries. In 2008, the age-standardized estimate of cancer deaths was 144 per 100,000 for men and 70 per 100,000 for women; for cardiovascular disease and diabetes, 146 per 100,000 for men and 87 per 100,000 for women; and for chronic respiratory disease, 46 per 100,000 for men and 15 per 100,000 for women.

The infant mortality rate, defined as the number of deaths of infants younger than 1 year, was 3.76 per 1,000 live births as of 2012. No information is available from WHO on the maternal mortality rate in Andorra. In 2010, tuberculosis incidence was 7.4 per 100,000 population, tuberculosis prevalence 9.8 per 100,000, and deaths due to tuberculosis among human immunodeficiency virus (HIV)-negative people 0.66 per 100,000.

Health Care Personnel

Andorra does not have a medical school but has offered nurse's training since 1988. The School of Nursing is now part of the University of Andorra (created in 1997) and offers midwife training as well as a bachelor's degree in nursing. In 2007, Andorra had 3.72 physicians per 1,000 population, 1.09 pharmaceutical personnel per 1,000, 0.70 dentistry personnel per 1,000, and 4.18 nurses and midwives per 1,000.

Government Role in Health Care

According to WHO, in 2010, Andorra spent $263 million on health care or $3,099 per capita. Health care in Andorra was entirely funded by domestic spending, with 70 percent being purchased by the government, 22 percent by private households, and 8 percent by other entities. About 21 percent of government resources were spent on health. Compared with other high-income European countries, Andorra's total government expenditure as a percent of gross domestic product (GDP) is low, as is the share of government spending allocated to health care.

Public Health Programs

As of 2010, access to improved sanitation facilities and improved drinking water sources was universal. According to the World Higher Education Database (WHED), one university in Andorra offers training in epidemiology or public health: the University of Andorra. The primary language of instruction is Catalan.

ANGOLA

Angola is a country in southwestern Africa that shares borders with Namibia, Zambia, and the Democratic Republic of the Congo (DRC) and that has an Atlantic coastline. Total area is 481,354 square miles (1,246,700 square kilometers, just under twice the size of Texas), and the population in 2012 was estimated at 18.0 million. In 2010, 59 percent of the population lived in urban areas, and the 2010 to 2015 annual rate of urbanization was estimated at 4.0 percent. A high birth rate (39.4 per 1,000 population) and total fertility rate (5.54 children per woman, the 11th-highest in the world) contributed to a rapid population growth rate of 2.8 percent in 2012, the 16th-highest in the world. The United Nations High Commissioner for Refugees (UNHCR) estimated that, in 2010, there were 15,155 refugees and persons in refugee-like situations in Angola.

The Portuguese established trading posts in Angola in the 16th century, and the country was an important area for slave trading; the country became independent in 1975. Angola is still recovering from a civil war that lasted 27 years, ending in 2002. According to the Ibrahim Index, in 2011, Angola ranked 41st among 53 African countries in terms of governance performance, with a score of 41 (out of 100). Angola ranked tied for 168th among 183 countries on the *Corruption Perceptions Index 2011,* with a score of 2.0 (on a scale where 0 indicates highly corrupt and 10 very clean).

In 2011, Angola was classified as a country with low human development (the lowest of four categories) on the United Nations Development Programme's (UNDP's) Human Development Index (HDI), with a score of 0.486 (on a scale where 1 denotes high development and 0 low development). In 2011, the International Food Policy Research Institute (IFPRI) classified Angola as a country with an "alarming" hunger

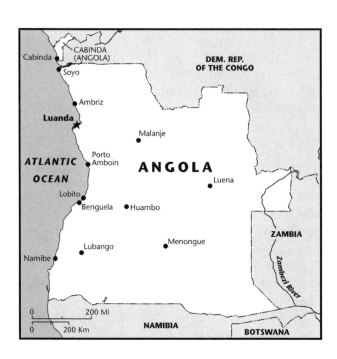

Selected Health Indicators: Angola Compared With the Global Average (2010)

	Angola	Global Average
Male life expectancy at birth* (years)	51	66
Female life expectancy at birth* (years)	53	71
Under-5 mortality rate, both sexes (per 1,000 live births)	161	57
Adult mortality rate, both sexes* (probability of dying between 15 and 60 years per 1,000 population)	364	176
Maternal mortality ratio (per 100,000 live births)	450	210
HIV prevalence* (per 1,000 adults aged 15 to 49)	20	8
Tuberculosis prevalence (per 100,000 population)	411	178

Source: World Health Organization Global Health Observatory Data Repository.
*Data refers to 2009.

problem and the country received a Global Hunger Index (GHI) score of 24.2 (where 0 reflects no hunger and higher scores more hunger). Life expectancy at birth in 2012 was estimated at 54.59 years, among the 30 lowest in the world, and estimated gross domestic product (GDP) per capita in 2011 was $5,900. According to the World Economic Forum's *Global Gender Gap Index 2011*, Angola ranked 87th out of 135 countries on gender equality with a score of 0.662 (on a scale with a theoretical range of 1 for equality to 0 for inequality and an actual range in 2011 from 0.8530 to 0.4873).

Emergency Health Services

According to the World Health Organization (WHO), as of 2007, Angola did not have a formal and publicly available system for providing prehospital care (emergency care).

Insurance

Angola's National Health Services (NHS) was established in the same year the country became independent, 1975. Universal, free primary care was provided until 1992, when user fees were introduced and private health services became legal.

Costs of Hospitalization

No data available.

Access to Health Care

A 2011 report on the quality and availability of health services in Luanda and Uige (Froystad) found major differences in the available services. In Luanda, all health facilities provided immunization and nutritional services for children, and 90 percent provided prenatal care for women; in Uige, only 80 percent of facilities provided immunization services and 60 percent nutritional services, and only 50 percent provided prenatal care. However, almost all facilities provided testing for malaria, although drugs to treat malaria were often not available. Facilities in Uige were less likely than those in Luanda to be staffed by a general practitioner or specialized nurse and also less likely to have a pharmacist and trained lab technician available. Even basic equipment, such as a stethoscope or thermometer, was not available in all health facilities in Uige.

The availability of medications also varied by location: Mona Froystad found that 75 percent of the facilities in Luanda had antibiotics in stock, while only 50 percent of the facilities in Uige did. Antimalarials were available in 80 percent of facilities in Luanda, but only 65 percent of facilities in Uige had them. Over half of the facilities in Uige were lacking one or more basic childhood vaccines (for measles, polio, diphtheria, and so on), while only 25 percent of facilities in Luanda were not fully stocked with these vaccines.

The quality of care was also lower in Uige than in Luanda, as measured both by tests of staff ability to make correct diagnoses and the frequency with which physician examinations were performed to aid diagnosis. Use of and knowledge about health care were strongly associated with household income: For instance, almost three-quarters (72 percent of women in the lowest-wealth quintile) gave birth at home, as compared to 11 percent in the highest quintile, and 97 percent of those in the highest-wealth quintile were aware of human immunodeficiency virus (HIV), while only 44 percent of those in the lowest quintile were. Persons living in urban areas in both provinces had better access to care in terms of the distance and time necessary to travel to the nearest clinical post (providing primary care), health center, or hospital. Seeking medical care for illness or an accident was almost equal between the two provinces for children (73 percent for Luanda, 68 percent for Uige) but substantially different for adults (73 percent for Luanda, 52 percent for Uige).

According to WHO, in 2009, 49.4 percent of births in Angola were attended by skilled personnel (for example, physicians, nurses, or midwives). In 2009, 47 percent of pregnant women received at least four prenatal care visits. The 2010 immunization rates for 1-year-olds were 91 percent for diphtheria and pertussis (DPT3), 93 percent for measles (MCV), and 91 percent for Hib (Hib3). In 2010, an estimated 33 percent of persons with advanced HIV infection were receiving antiretroviral therapy in accordance with the 2010 WHO guidelines. According to WHO, in 2010, Angola had 0.06 magnetic resonance imaging (MRI) machines per 1 million population and 0.50 computer tomography (CT) machines per 1 million population.

Cost of Drugs

The supply and distribution of drugs and medical products is regulated by the National Directorate of Medical Supplies; the priority in the Angolan system is to supply the entire population with safe access to medicines at an affordable price. However, many parts of the country regularly experience shortages of essential drugs. Some products, such as antiretrovirals, reproductive health kits, vaccines, and mosquito nets, are provided by donor agencies such as the United Nations Children's Fund (UNICEF).

Health Care Facilities

In 2005, Angola had 0.8 hospital beds per 1,000 population, one of the 30 lowest rates in the world, less than 0.01 provincial hospitals per 100,000 population, and less than 0.01 specialized hospitals per 100,000. Almost all hospitals are located in the cities, and the lengthy civil war destroyed much of the country's infrastructure, making it difficult for individuals in rural areas to travel to receive health care.

Major Health Issues

In 2008, WHO estimated that 79 percent of years of life lost in Angola were due to communicable diseases, 14 percent to noncommunicable diseases, and 7 percent to injuries. In 2008, the age-standardized estimate of cancer deaths was 88 per 100,000 for men and 83 per 100,000 for women; for cardiovascular disease and diabetes, 477 per 100,000 for men and 489 per 100,000 for women; and for chronic respiratory disease, 133 per 100,000 for men and 175 per 100,000 for women.

In 2010, tuberculosis incidence was 304.0 per 100,000 population, tuberculosis prevalence 411.0 per 100,000, and deaths due to tuberculosis among human immunodeficiency virus (HIV)-negative people 34.0 per 100,000. Angola has recently suffered from epidemics of Marburg virus (2005) and cholera (2006). As of 2009, an estimated 2.0 percent of adults age 15 to 49 were living with HIV or acquired immune deficiency syndrome (AIDS). In 2010, 32 percent of pregnant women tested positive for HIV. The mother-to-child transmission rate for HIV in 2010 was estimated at 33 percent, and in 2009, 19 percent of deaths to children under age 5 were attributed to HIV. In 2008, the age-standardized death rate from malaria was 51.5 per 100,000 population.

Angola's maternal mortality rate (death from any cause related to or aggravated by pregnancy) was quite high by global standards as of 2008, estimated at 610 maternal deaths per 100,000 live births. The infant mortality rate, defined as the number of deaths of infants younger than 1 year, was the eighth-highest in the world as of 2012, at 83.53 per 1,000 live births. In 2001, 27.5 percent of children under age 5 were underweight (defined as 2 kilograms [kg] below standard weight-for-age at age 1, 3 kg below for ages 2 to 3, and 4 kg below for ages 4 to 5).

Health Care Personnel

In 2006, WHO identified Angola as one of 57 countries with a critical deficit in the supply of skilled health workers. Angola has one medical school, the Faculdade de Medecina in Luanda. Instruction is in

Portuguese, and a 6-year course of study leads to a degree of Doctor em Medicine (doctor of medicine). Angola has 2.24 public-sector health workers per 1,000 inhabitants, slightly below the WHO limit of a severe health worker shortage; in addition, health workers are unevenly distributed throughout the country, with 2.78 per 1,000 population in Luanda but only 1.61 in Uige.

In 2004, Angola had 0.08 physicians per 1,000 population, 0.07 pharmaceutical personnel per 1,000, 0.14 laboratory health workers per 1,000, 0.02 dentistry personnel per 1,000, 0.02 health management and support workers per 1,000, and 1.35 nurses and midwives per 1,000. The global "brain drain" (international migration of skilled personnel) plays a role in this relative undersupply of medical personnel in Angola: Michael Clemens and Bunilla Petterson estimate that 70 percent of Angola-born physicians and 12 percent of Angola-born nurses are working in one of nine developed countries, primarily in Portugal. Although the number of physicians in Angola tripled between 2005 and 2009, there is still a shortage of doctors; the government has dealt with this in part by hiring physicians from Cuba on short-term contracts.

Government Role in Health Care

The 2010 Angola constitution states that the government is responsible for providing universal, free primary care. In 2003, the law established a system of health services provided at three levels: primary, secondary, and tertiary, corresponding to the district, provincial, and national levels of government. The primary level of health care includes health clinics, health posts, referral health centers, and district hospitals; the second includes general hospitals; and the third level includes central hospitals. In 2008, the districts were given the primary responsibility for managing health services delivery. Angola has a National Medicines Policy (NMP) and an Essential Medicines List (EML).

Public spending on health in Angola increased dramatically in the early 21st century, with the greatest percentage increase seen in spending on primary care, from $5.80 per capita in 2001 (20 percent of public spending on health) to $31.20 in 2005 (40.7 percent of public spending on health). Public spending on secondary and tertiary care almost tripled during this time, from $21.60 in 2001 to $57.70 in 2005.

According to WHO, in 2010, Angola spent $2.4 billion on health care, which comes to $123 per capita.

Almost all (97 percent) of this health care was funded domestically, with only 3 percent of the funding coming from abroad. Most health care (82 percent) was purchased by the government, with 18 percent purchased by individual households. Household out-of-pocket expenditures have risen only gradually in recent years, while government expenditures on health rose sharply from 2005 to 2009 before falling sharply in 2010. About 7 percent of government resources are allocated to health care, which is low compared to other lower-middle-income African countries. Total government expenditure on health as a percent of gross domestic product (GDP) is also low compared to other lower-middle-income African countries. In 2009, according to WHO, official development assistance (ODA) for health in Angola came to $5.36 per capita.

Public Health Programs

The National Institute of Public Health for Angola recently became a member institute of Angola's National Institute of Health. However, according to the World Higher Education Database (WHED), as of 2011, no universities in Angola offered programs in epidemiology or public health. As of 2010, access to improved sanitation facilities and drinking water sources in Angola was much lower in rural than in urban areas; 85 percent of the urban population had access to improved sanitation facilities, as compared to only 19 percent of the rural population, and 60 percent of the urban population had access to improved drinking water sources, as opposed to 38 percent of the rural population.

ANTIGUA AND BARBUDA

Antigua and Barbuda is a small Caribbean country consisting of two major islands (Antigua and Barbuda) and a number of smaller islands. The total area is 171 square miles (442.6 square kilometers, 2.5 times the size of Washington, D.C.), and the population in 2012 was estimated at 89,018. In 2010, 30 percent of the population lived in urban areas, and the 2010 to 2015 annual rate of urbanization was estimated at 1.4 percent. The capital and largest city is St. Johns (with a 2009 population estimated at 27,000). The population growth rate in 2012 was 1.3 percent, the birth rate 16.2 births per 1,000 population, the total fertility rate 2.0 children per woman, and the net migration 2.3 migrants per 1,000 population (the 35th-highest in the world).

A former British colony, Antigua and Barbuda became independent in 1981. In 2011, Antigua and Barbuda was classified as a country with high human development (the second-highest category) on the United Nations Development Programme's (UNDP's) Human Development Index (HDI), with a score of 0.764 (on a scale where 1 denotes high development and 0 low development). Life expectancy at birth in 2012 was estimated at 75.69 years, and per capita gross domestic product (GDP) in 2011 was estimated at $22,100. According to the 2005 to 2006 Survey of Living Conditions and Household Budget Survey, Antigua and Barbuda was characterized by large gaps in spending power.

Emergency Health Services

According to the U.S. State Department, Antigua and Barbuda has a specific phone number, 911, to call in case of emergency. Holberton Hospital in St. Johns, Antigua, provides emergency medical services. In 2005, Antigua and Barbuda had 13 emergency medical technicians and three first responders.

Insurance

Antigua and Barbuda's social insurance system was created in 1972 and 1973, and the laws regulating it were amended in 2000. All registered residents are covered for specified illnesses under the Medical Benefits Scheme (MBS), which provides care in public health facilities. Maternity benefits and cash sickness benefits are available to private-sector employees and the self-employed. Medical benefits are paid for by employers, the self-employed, and employee contributions, with lower and upper caps on income subject to this tax.

Cash sickness and maternity benefits require periods of enrollment before benefits can be claimed. Maternity benefits pay 60 percent of the average weekly wages of the insured for up to 13 weeks, while cash sickness benefits pay the same rate for up to 26 weeks, with a possible extension of 13 weeks.

General supervision for the social insurance system is provided by the Ministry of Finance, with the MBS supervised by the Ministry of Health and the cash sickness and maternity schemes by the Antigua and Barbuda Social Security Board.

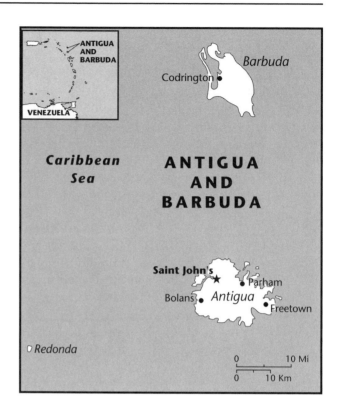

Costs of Hospitalization

Antigua and Barbuda's MBS provides free services to beneficiaries who are hospitalized and treated in a general hospital ward for any disease; services covered include medical and surgical care, lab tests, X-rays, prescription drugs, electrocardiograms (EKGs), and similar services.

Access to Health Care

According to the World Health Organization (WHO), in 2008, 100 percent of births in Antigua and Barbuda were attended by skilled personnel (for example, physicians, nurses, or midwives). Also in 2008, 100 percent of pregnant women received at least one prenatal care visit. The 2010 immunization rates for 1-year-olds were 98 percent for diphtheria and pertussis (DPT3), 98 percent for measles (MCV), and 98 percent for Hib (Hib3). According to WHO, in 2010, Antigua and Barbuda had 11.54 magnetic resonance imaging (MRI) machines per 1 million population, and 23.09 computer tomography (CT) machines per 1 million population. Treatment for human immunodeficiency virus and acquired immune deficiency syndrome (HIV/AIDS) is provided universally and without charge. Some outpatient services, including lab tests, X-rays, and EKGs, are provided free for beneficiaries of the MBS if the services are obtained at Holberton Hospital; if received at other facilities, the individual may claim reimbursement.

Cost of Drugs

Antigua and Barbuda's Ministry of Health regulates and controls the supply of pharmaceutical products, and the country has a National Drug Formulary Committee to regulate their purchase and use. Antigua and Barbuda receives assistance from the Eastern Caribbean Drug Service. Beneficiaries of Antigua and Barbuda's MBS are provided with free drugs while being treated in the general ward of a hospital and free drugs to treat nine chronic diseases (asthma, cancer, cardiovascular disease, certified lunacy [sic], diabetes, glaucoma, hypertension, leprosy, and sickle cell anemia) when in outpatient care. Prescription drugs formed the largest single expense for Antigua and Barbuda's MBS in 2010 (ECD 15.2 million), with by far the greatest expense for cancer drugs (26.8 percent of the total, although only 1.2 percent of the total prescriptions filled were for cancer patients). The second-highest expenditure among prescription drug expenses was for hypertension drugs (23.5 percent of the total).

Health Care Facilities

Holberton Hospital in St. Johns, Antigua, provides general, specialized, and rehabilitation services; the Adelin Medical Centre on Antigua provides both outpatient and inpatient care; and the Hannah Thomas Hospital on Barbuda provides mostly outpatient care. Antigua and Barbuda has 26 health clinics providing care and making referrals for hospital care. As of 2010, according to WHO, Antigua and Barbuda had 222.07 specialized hospitals per 100,000 population in the public sector (the only hospital statistic reported).

Major Health Issues

In 2008, WHO estimated that 17 percent of years of life lost in Antigua and Barbuda were due to communicable diseases, 69 percent to noncommunicable diseases, and 14 percent to injuries. In 2008, the age-standardized estimate of cancer deaths was 123 per 100,000 for men and 134 per 100,000 for women; for cardiovascular disease and diabetes, 301 per 100,000 for men and 283 per 100,000 for women; and for chronic respiratory disease, 19 per 100,000 for men and 14 per 100,000 for women. The infant mortality rate, defined as the number of deaths of infants younger than 1 year, was 14.17 per 1,000 live births as of 2012. No information is available from WHO on the maternal mortality ratio in Antigua and Barbuda. In 2010, tuberculosis incidence was 4.9 per 100,000 population, tuberculosis prevalence 3.1 per 100,000, and deaths due to tuberculosis among HIV-negative people 0.43 per 100,000.

Health Care Personnel

Antigua and Barbuda has one medical school, the University of Health Sciences Antigua in St. Johns, founded in 1983. The language of instruction is English; the basic medical degree course last four years and leads to a degree of doctor of medicine (M.D.). Foreign students are allowed to attend. Graduates must register with the Ministry of Health, and the license to practice medicine is granted by the Medical Board of Antigua and Barbuda. The degrees of graduates of foreign medical schools must be validated by Antiguan authorities. In 1999, Antigua and Barbuda had 0.17 physicians per 1,000 population and 3.28 nurses and midwives per 1,000. Alok Bhargava and colleagues placed Antigua and Barbuda sixth among countries most affected by medical "brain drain" (international migration of skilled personnel) in 2004.

Government Role in Health Care

According to WHO, in 2010, Antigua and Barbuda spent $61 million on health care, which comes to $690 per capita. All health care funding is domestic, with no funding coming from abroad. Most health care purchasing (71 percent) is done by the government, with private households purchasing 26 percent and other entities the remaining 3 percent. About 17 percent of government resources are allocated to health care, and health care expenditures represent about 4 percent of Antigua and Barbuda's GDP. Compared to other middle-income countries in the Americas, Antigua and Barbuda ranks low on both share of government spending allocated to health care and government expenditure on health as a percent of GDP.

Public Health Programs

According to the World Higher Education Database (WHED), in 2011, no university in Antigua and Barbuda offered programs in epidemiology or public health. As of 2010, access to improved sanitation facilities (98 percent) and improved drinking water sources (95 percent) was nearly universal.

ARGENTINA

Argentina is a country in southeastern South America that shares borders with Bolivia, Brazil, Chile, Paraguay, and Uruguay and that has an Atlantic coastline. Total area is 1,073,518 square miles (2,780,400 square kilometers, the eighth-largest in the world and second-largest in South America or about 30 percent of the size of the United States), and the population in 2012 was estimated at 42.2 million. In 2010, 92 percent of the population lived in urban areas, and the 2010 to 2015 annual rate of urbanization was estimated at 1.1 percent. Buenos Aires is the capital and largest city (with a 2009 estimated population of 13.0 million). The population growth rate in 2012 was 1.0 percent, the birth rate 17.3 births per 1,000 population, and the total fertility rate 2.3 children per woman. The United Nations High Commissioner for Refugees (UNHCR) estimated that, in 2010, there were 3,276 refugees and persons in refugee-like situations in Argentina.

Argentina ranked tied for 100th among 183 countries on the *Corruption Perceptions Index 2011*, with a score of 3.0 (on a scale where 0 indicates highly corrupt and 10 very clean). In 2011, Argentina was classified as a country with very high human development (the highest of four categories) on the United Nations Development Programme's (UNDP's) Human Development Index (HDI), with a score of 0.797 (on a scale where 1 denotes high development and 0 low development). Life expectancy at birth in 2012 was estimated at 77.14 years, and per capita gross domestic product (GDP) in 2011 was estimated at $17,400; in 2009, the Gini Index (a measure of dispersion, in which perfect equality is denoted by 0 and maximum inequality is denoted by 100) for family income was 45.8. Argentina ranks relatively high on gender equality: According to the World Economic Forum's *Global Gender Gap Index 2011*, Argentina ranked 28th out of 135 countries on gender equality, with a score of 0.724 (on a scale with a theoretical range of 1 for equality to 0 for inequality and an actual range in 2011 from 0.8530 to 0.4873).

Emergency Health Services

According to the World Health organization (WHO), as of 2007, Argentina had a formal and publicly available emergency care (prehospital care) system, accessible through regional access telephone numbers, but not a universal national access number.

Insurance

Argentina's first laws regulating maternity and sickness benefits were written in 1934 and 1944, respectively; current laws date from 1971 and later. The country has a combination of a social insurance program and employer-related benefits. Medical benefits are provided to employed persons, the self-employed, the unemployed, retired people, and household workers, with special insurance programs covering groups such as the military, police, public-sector employees, and university professors and dependents (spouses, cohabiting partners, unmarried children under 21, and children enrolled in school to age 25). The medical benefits system is paid for through a payroll and self-employment tax and employer contributions. Cash benefits for insured workers provide 100 percent of salary for three to six months, depending on years of service; the amount is doubled for those with dependents. The maternity benefit provides for payment equal to average gross income for 45 days before and after the birth. The Superintendent of Health Services administers the social insurance system; the medical benefits system is supervised by the Ministry of Health, and the maternity benefits system is supervised by the National Social Security Administration.

As of 2001, about 48 percent of the population were covered by the public health services delivery system, which is organized primarily at the provincial level; 47.2 percent were covered by the social security system (publicly funded but with most care provided by private providers), and 7.5 percent had private health insurance (some of these were also covered by the social security system). According to Ke Xu and colleagues, in 2003, 5.8 percent of households in Argentina experienced catastrophic health expenditures annually; "catastrophic" was defined as exceeding 40 percent of household income remaining after basic needs were met.

Costs of Hospitalization

No data available.

Access to Health Care

Responsibility for health care is, by Argentina's constitution, the responsibility of the provinces, and some of this responsibility has been delegated further to the municipal level, so the level of access and care is not uniform across the country.

According to Latinobarometer, an annual public opinion survey conducted in Latin America, 55 percent of citizens in Argentina are satisfied with the level of health care available to them (the regional average is 51.9 percent). High-quality care is available to those who can pay (medical tourism is a growing industry in Argentina).

Compared to other countries at a similar level of development, Argentina ranked fourth among 80 less-developed countries on the 2011 Mothers' Index produced by the international nongovernmental organization (NGO) Save the Children, based on a number of health and social factors relating to women, children, and maternal and child care. According to WHO, in 2007, 99.4 percent of births in Argentina were attended by skilled personnel (for example, physicians, nurses, or midwives). In 2005, 89 percent of pregnant women received at least one prenatal care visit. The 2010 immunization rates for 1-year-olds were 94 percent for diphtheria and pertussis (DPT3), 99 percent for measles (MCV), and 94 percent for Hib (Hib3). In 2010, an estimated 79 percent of persons with advanced human immunodeficiency virus (HIV) infection were receiving antiretroviral therapy in accordance with the 2010 WHO guidelines.

Cost of Drugs

Argentina provides some medicines, including prescription drugs, free of charge to its population through primary health care units and hospitals. Categories of persons authorized to receive free medicines include children under age 5, pregnant women, the elderly, and the poor. Some essential medicines are provided free through the REMEDIAR program, and in addition, drugs to treat certain conditions are provided free of charge, such as drugs for human immunodeficiency virus and acquired immune deficiency syndrome (HIV/AIDS) and opportunistic diseases, sexually transmitted diseases (STDs), tuberculosis, malaria, and some chronic disease (including arthritis, hypertension, diabetes, and asthma). Drugs used for care within public hospitals are also free. The pharmaceuticals market grew 25 percent in 2010.

Pharmaceutical products must be evaluated and registered before appearing on the market, following explicit, publicly available criteria; as of 2010, more than 55,000 pharmaceuticals were authorized in Argentina. Although there are no laws controlling drug prices, the government has negotiated some voluntary pricing arrangements and publishes the Average Drug Price Index (IPPM). The government also publishes Standard Treatment Guidelines (STGs) for common illnesses and an Essential Medicines List (EML); drugs are placed on the EML through a standard, written process.

Health Care Facilities

In 2005, Argentina had 4.00 hospital beds per 1,000 population, among the 50 highest rates in the world. Medical tourism is a growing industry, as people from industrialized countries seek treatment in Argentina, where costs are much lower than they are in, for example, the United States.

Major Health Issues

In 2008, WHO estimated that 18 percent of years of life lost in Argentina were due to communicable diseases, 67 percent to noncommunicable diseases, and 16 percent to injuries. In 2008, the age-standardized estimate of cancer deaths was 168 per 100,000 for men and 107 per 100,000 for women; for cardiovascular disease and diabetes, 263 per 100,000 for men and 153 per 100,000 for women; and for chronic respiratory disease, 73 per 100,000 for men and 41 per 100,000 for women. Argentina's maternal mortality rate (death from any cause related to or aggravated by pregnancy) was estimated in 2008 as 94 maternal deaths per 100,000 live births. The infant mortality rate, defined as the number of deaths of infants younger than 1 year, was 10.52

per 1,000 live births as of 2012. In 2010, tuberculosis incidence was 27.0 per 100,000 population, tuberculosis prevalence 40.0 per 100,000, and deaths due to tuberculosis among HIV-negative people 1.9 per 100,000. As of 2009, an estimated 0.5 percent of adults age 15 to 49 were living with HIV or AIDS.

Health Care Personnel

Argentina has 16 medical schools, the oldest of which is the Facultad de Ciencias Médicas of the Universidad Austral in Buenos Aires, which began offering instruction in 1852. The course of study is six or seven years, and a further year of practice is required. Foreign students are allowed to attend. The degree awarded is Médico (physician). Physicians must register with the Dirección Nacional de Fiscalización Sanitaria in Buenos Aires and with the secretariat of one of the provincial health authorities. Graduates of foreign medical schools must have their degrees validated. Argentina has cooperative agreements with Bolivia, Colombia, and Ecuador. All medical schools in Argentina offer instruction in Spanish, and the Escuela de Medicina of the Universidad Favaloro (formerly the Instituto Universitario de Ciencias Biomédicas or IUCB) in Buenos Aires also offers instruction in English. In 2004, Argentina had 3.16 physicians per 1,000 population, 0.50 pharmaceutical personnel per 1,000, 0.51 laboratory health workers per 1,000, and 0.48 nurses and midwives per 1,000.

Government Role in Health Care

Health care in Argentina is primarily organized and delivered at the provincial level. Three sectors provide care: public, private, and social security, with many private providers contracted to provide care under the social security system. The system in 2006 was characterized by the Pan American Health Organization (PAHO) as fragmented, with poor coordination and many inequalities across the country. In 2003, 47.2 percent of the population (17.5 million people) were covered through the social security system, 48 percent (17.8 million) through the public sector, and about 2.8 million had private insurance (with about 1 million having both social security and private coverage).

According to WHO, in 2010, Argentina spent $30 billion on health care or $742 per capita. All health care was funded domestically, with 30 percent of the expenditures made by households, 55 percent by government spending, and 16 percent spending by other entities. About 15 percent of government resources are allocated to health care, and government expenditure on health represents 4 percent of GDP. Argentina ranks low in both categories as compared to other upper-middle-income countries in the Americas region. In 2009, according to WHO, official development assistance (ODA) for health in Argentina came to $0.91 per capita.

Public Health Programs

Argentina's National Laboratories and Health Institutes Administration (ANLIS) is located in Buenos Aires and directed by Gustavo Rios. ANLIS oversees Argentina's National Reference Laboratory and works with other governmental entities within Argentina, as well as international organizations, to promote public health. Specific duties of ANLIS include ensuring diagnosis quality, coordinating investigations, supervising the development of biological products, and conducting research to develop new products. According to the World Higher Education Database (WHED), eight universities in Argentina offer programs in epidemiology or public health: ISALUD University, the National University of Cordoba, the National University of Cuyo, the National University of Lanús, the National University of Rosario, the National University of Salta, the National University of the Littoral, and the National University of Buenos Aires.

The Federal Health Plan of 2005 to 2007 prioritized primary care, health promotion, and preventive care activities. Argentina has national programs to combat tuberculosis, Chagas disease, parasites, and STDs, including HIV/AIDS, and to control tobacco use and provide reproductive health services. As of 2005, most (90 percent) of Argentina's population had access to improved sanitation facilities, although access was lower among the rural population (77 percent) than for people living in urban areas (91 percent). Access to improved sources of drinking water was nearly universal (98 percent) for people living in urban areas but only 80 percent for those living in rural areas; the national average was 96 percent.

ARMENIA

Armenia is a landlocked country in southwestern Asia, sharing borders with Azerbaijan, Georgia, Iran, and Turkey. Total area is 11,484 square miles (29,743 square

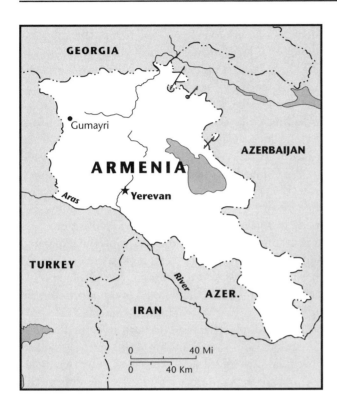

Life expectancy at birth in 2012 was estimated at 73.49 years, and estimated gross domestic product (GDP) per capita in 2011 was $5,400. In 2008, the Gini Index (a measure of dispersion, in which perfect equality is denoted by 0 and maximum inequality is denoted by 100) for family income was 30.9. According to the World Economic Forum's *Global Gender Gap Index 2011*, Armenia ranked 84th out of 135 countries on gender equality, with a score of 0.665 (on a scale with a theoretical range of 1 for equality to 0 for inequality and an actual range in 2011 from 0.8530 to 0.4873).

Emergency Health Services

According to the World Health Organization (WHO), as of 2007, Armenia had a formal and publicly available emergency care (prehospital care) system, accessible through a universal national access number. Doctors Without Borders (Médecins Sans Frontières, or MSF) began working in Armenia in 1984 and had 200 staff members in the country at the close of 2010. MSF's primary focus in Armenia is diagnosing and treating drug-resistant tuberculosis; some aspects of MSF's program in Yerevan (the national capital) were transferred to the Armenian Red Cross in 2010, while MSF expanded the program to the rural provinces of Lori and Shirak.

Insurance

Current laws regulating Armenia's social insurance and medical benefits system date to 2005. Everyone residing in Armenia is covered by the medical benefits system, while the employed and self-employed are also eligible for maternity and cash sickness benefits. The sickness and medical benefits system is funded by wage taxes and employer contributions. Medical services, including physician care, hospitalization, dental care, lab services, and maternity care, are provided by government health providers; copayments are required for some services. Maternity benefits do not depend on the period of covered employment, but sickness benefits do differ depending on the length of covered employment. The maternity benefit is 100 percent of average earnings for 70 days before and after birth, with longer periods for multiple births or birth complications. A child-care benefit is paid until the age of 2 years. A lump sum benefit is also paid for childbirth or adoption. The cash sickness benefit is 100 percent of average earnings if the insured has been in covered employment for at least eight years, with 80 percent of average earnings otherwise.

kilometers, similar to Maryland), and the population in 2012 was estimated at 3.0 million. In 2010, 64 percent of the population lived in urban areas, and the 2010 to 2015 annual rate of urbanization was estimated at 0.5 percent. Yerevan is the capital and largest city (with a 2009 population estimated at 1.11 million). In 2012, the total fertility rate in Armenia was 1.38 children per woman, one of the 20 lowest in the world; this and a negative migration rate (negative 3.35 migrants per 1,000 population in 2012), have resulted in slow population growth (0.1 percent in 2012). The United Nations High Commissioner for Refugees (UNHCR) estimated that, in 2010, there were 3,296 refugees and persons in refugee-like situations in Armenia.

Armenia became independent from the Soviet Union in 1991 and has been engaged in ongoing conflict with Azerbaijan over the Nagorno–Karabakh area. Armenia ranked 129th among 183 countries on the *Corruption Perceptions Index 2011,* with a score of 2.6 (on a scale where 0 indicates highly corrupt and 10 very clean). In 2011, Armenia was classified as a country with high human development (the second-highest category) on the United Nations Development Programme's (UNDP's) Human Development Index (HDI), with a score of 0.716 (on a scale where 1 denotes high development and 0 low development).

Costs of Hospitalization

Armenia's service delivery system is dominated by hospitals, as is typical of former Soviet republics. Determining how care is funded is difficult because of the common practice of requiring unofficial cash payments to receive services. Matthew Jowett and Elizabeth Danielyan estimate that, of the 40 percent of medical expenses paid out of pocket in Armenia, 10 percent are official patient charges, most of which are required to receive care in hospitals. They estimate that hospital treatment in Yerevan, in a department of general surgery, would have required unofficial payments of $260 to $530 in 2010.

Access to Health Care

Armenia's hospitals and ambulatory care services are organized at the provincial level. In addition, a private sector of health care services exists alongside the public-sector services. According to WHO, in 2005, 98.0 percent of births in Armenia were attended by skilled personnel (for example, physicians, nurses, or midwives). In 2005, 71 percent of pregnant women received at least four prenatal care visits. The 2010 immunization rates for 1-year-olds were 94 percent for diphtheria and pertussis (DPT3), 97 percent for measles (MCV), and 48 percent for Hib (Hib3). In 2010, an estimated 30 percent of persons with advanced human immunodeficiency virus (HIV) infection were receiving antiretroviral therapy in accordance with the 2010 WHO guidelines. According to WHO, in 2010, Armenia had 2.27 magnetic resonance imaging (MRI) machines per 1 million population, 2.92 computer tomography (CT) machines per 1 million population, 0.97 telecolbalt units per 1 million, and 0.97 radiotherapy machines per 1 million.

Cost of Drugs

In 2008, total pharmaceutical expenditure in Armenia was AMD 23.103 billion ($75.5 million); total pharmaceutical expenditure per capita was AMD 7,030 ($23). Pharmaceutical expenditures accounted for 16.9 percent of total health expenditures and 0.6 percent of GDP. Most pharmaceuticals were paid for privately, with public expenditures representing 17.8 percent of the total. Armenia has a National Medicines Policy (NMP), which is part of its National Health Policy, and covers selection of essential medicines: pricing, financing, procurement, distribution, and regulation; pharmacovigilance; human resource development; research; monitoring and evaluation; and traditional medicine. Access to essential medicines is recognized by national legislation as part of the right to health, but there is no implementation plan for the NMP. Armenia provides medicines at no charge to children under age 5 and to treat specified conditions, including malaria, tuberculosis, and human immunodeficiency virus and acquired immune deficiency syndrome (HIV/AIDS); vaccines for children listed on the WHO Expanded Programme on Immunization (EPI) list are also provided for free. Medicines on the national Essentials Medicines List (including 293 medicines as of 2007) are also provided for free.

Any pharmaceutical products must be evaluated and registered before they can be marketed in Armenia; there are explicit and publicly available specifications for this procedure, and 3,900 pharmaceutical products were registered in Armenia in 2007. Promotion and advertising of prescription medications is regulated by Armenian law. Armenia has no laws or regulations regarding the price of pharmaceuticals and does not maintain a monitoring system for the price of medications. A 2001 WHO survey found that prices for medicines in private pharmacies in Armenia were much higher than international reference prices: over 10 times as high for brand-name drugs and over three times as high for generics.

Health Care Facilities

Armenia's health care system is dominated by hospital care and is heavily centered in Yerevan, which has 52 percent of all hospital beds and 32 percent of all inpatient care facilities. However, utilization is relatively low (inpatient admissions in 2007 were about half the European average) due in part to the practice of collecting unofficial payments for hospital care. As of 2010, according to WHO, Armenia had 7.70 health posts per 100,000 population, 0.52 health centers per 100,000, 1.75 district or rural hospitals per 100,000, 1.52 provincial hospitals per 100,000, and 0.61 specialized hospitals per 100,000. In 2007, Armenia had 4.07 hospital beds per 1,000 population, among the 50 highest rates in the world.

Major Health Issues

In 2008, WHO estimated that 14 percent of years of life lost in Armenia were due to communicable diseases, 77 percent to noncommunicable diseases, and 9 percent to injuries. In 2008, the age-standardized estimate of cancer deaths was 232 per 100,000 for men and 131 per 100,000 for women; for cardiovascular disease and diabetes, 709 per 100,000 for men and 388 per 100,000 for women; and for chronic respiratory disease, 77 per 100,000 for men and 54 per 100,000 for women.

Armenia's maternal mortality rate (death from any cause related to or aggravated by pregnancy) in 2008 was 29 maternal deaths per 100,000 live births. The infant mortality rate, defined as the number of deaths of infants younger than 1 year, was estimated at 18.21 per 1,000 live births as of 2012. In 2010, tuberculosis incidence was 73.0 per 100,000 population, tuberculosis prevalence 114.0 per 100,000, and deaths due to tuberculosis among HIV-negative people 11.0 per 100,000. Armenia is classified by WHO as having a high burden of multidrug-resistant tuberculosis: An estimated 9.4 percent of new cases are multidrug resistant, as are 43 percent of retreatment cases. As of 2009, an estimated 0.1 percent of adults age 15 to 49 were living with HIV or AIDS.

Health Care Personnel

Armenia has one medical school, Yerevan State Medical University in Yerevan, founded in 1922. The duration of the basic medical degree course is six years, with a further year of supervised clinical practice required, and instruction is offered in Armenian and Russian. The degree awarded is doctor of medicine (M.D.) and the license to practice medicine is granted by the Ministry of Health. Government service work is obligatory after graduation. Armenia has agreements with universities in several other countries, including the Catholic University of Louvain, Belgium; the Mediterranean University in Marseilles, France; the Aristotle University in Thessalonica, Greece; McGill University in Montreal, Canada; and Aleppo University in Syria. In 2007, Armenia had 3.70 physicians per 1,000 population, 0.05 pharmaceutical personnel per 1,000, 0.39 dentistry personnel per 1,000, and 4.87 nurses and midwives per 1,000.

Government Role in Health Care

Armenia provides access to health care for its entire population through primary care centers, but many types of services and drugs include copayments that must be paid at the point of service. According to WHO, in 2010, Armenia spent $413 million on health care, coming to $133 per capita. Most (86 percent) of this health care was provided with domestic funding, while 14 percent were provided through funding from abroad. Just over half (55 percent) of expenditures for health care were spent by households, with 41 percent government expenditures, and the remaining 4 percent spent by other entities. The Armenian government spent 6 percent of its budget on health care, representing 2 percent of Armenia's GDP; both figures are low by the standards of other countries in the lower middle-income European region. In 2009, according to WHO, official development assistance (ODA) for health in Armenia came to $9.76 per capita.

Public Health Programs

As of 2010, most (90 percent) of Armenia's population had access to improved sanitation facilities, although access was lower among the rural population (80 percent) than for people living in urban areas (95 percent). Access to improved sources of drinking water was nearly universal (99 percent).

According to the World Higher Education Database (WHED), in 2011, no universities in Armenia offered programs in epidemiology or public health.

AUSTRALIA

Australia is a country located between the south Pacific and Indian Oceans, consisting of one large island (Australia), the island of Tasmania, and a number of smaller islands. With an area of 2,988,902 square miles (7,741,220 square kilometers, a bit smaller than the 48 contiguous U.S. states), it is the sixth-largest country in the world; the population of 22.0 million, as of 2012, was largely concentrated in urban areas clustered along the coastline. In 2010, 89 percent of the population lived in urban areas, and the 2010 to 2015 annual rate of urbanization was estimated at 1.2 percent. Canberra is the capital; the largest cities are Sydney (with a 2009 estimated population of 4.43 million) and Melbourne (3.85 million). Population growth in 2012 was 1.1 percent. The birth rate was 12.3 births per 1,000 population, the total fertility rate 1.8 children per woman, and net migration 5.9 migrants per 1,000 population (the 17th-highest in the world). The United Nations High Commissioner for Refugees (UNHCR) estimated that, in 2010, there were 21,805 refugees and persons in refugee-like situations in Australia.

A former British colony, in 1907, Australia became a dominion of the British Empire, and in 1986, the Australia Act ended any British role in Australia's government. Australia's government is noted for its transparency, ranking least corrupt among 183 countries on the *Corruption Perceptions Index 2011,* with a score of 8.8 (on a scale where 0 indicates highly corrupt and 10 very clean). Australia also ranks high on gender equality: According to the World Economic Forum's *Global Gender Gap Index 2011*, Australia ranked 23rd out of 135 countries on gender equality with a score of 0.729 (on a scale with a theoretical range of 1 for equality to 0 for inequality and an actual range in 2011 from 0.8530 to 0.4873).

Australia ranked second in 2011 on the United Nations Development Programme's (UNDP's) Human Development Index (HDI), with a score of 0.929 (on a scale where 1 denotes high development and 0 low development). Life expectancy at birth in 2012 was estimated at 81.90 years, among the highest in the world, and per capita gross domestic product (GDP) in 2011 was estimated at $40,800. In 2006, the Gini Index (a measure of dispersion, in which perfect equality is denoted by 0 and maximum inequality is denoted by 100) for family income was 30.5. Australia has a high net migration rate (5.93 migrants per 1,000 population, the 17th-highest in the world in 2012) and a low birth rate (12.28 births per 1,000 population), combining for a moderate July 2012 population growth rate (1.13 percent in 2012).

Emergency Health Services

The availability of after-hours care in clinics varies, although the Royal Australian College of General Practitioners stipulates that "reasonable" arrangements for care outside normal opening hours should be provided. The Australian government offers grants to physicians to provide after-hours care in order to reduce the number of nonemergency patients using hospital emergency departments for after-hours care. In 2009, according to a Commonwealth Fund survey, half (50 percent) of Australian primary care physicians had some kind of after-hours arrangement for their practices; often, after-hours care is provided by a private company that contracts with the physician's practice. According to the World Health Organization (WHO), as of 2007, Australia's emergency care (prehospital care) system included a universal national access number.

Insurance

Australia has universal public health insurance called Medicare, administered at the regional level, that covers most medical care, including physician services, hospital services, and prescriptions. Limited dental coverage is provided under Medicare, while services such as optometry, podiatry, and complementary medical services are not covered. Mental health care is covered when it is provided in a hospital, and community-based health care is subsidized in whole or in part. Preventive services such as cancer screening and vaccinations are provided through public programs.

Citizens, permanent residents, visitors, and people on temporary visas from some countries (those with reciprocal agreements with Australia) are covered. Asylum seekers receive temporary coverage, and overseas students are covered under a special arrangement. The government provides health care for migrants in detention centers, but many documented migrants are not eligible for Medicare, and their care may be covered by organizations such as the Australian Red Cross.

Medicare is financed by general tax revenue and earmarked income tax. Individuals are allowed to buy additional insurance that provides extra benefits, including access to private health facilities; about 50 percent do so. Out-of-pocket expenses are subsidized if they exceed a set level (AUSD 1,158, or $1,204, in

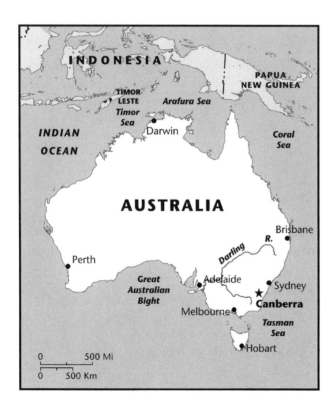

Selected Health Indicators: Australia Compared With the Organisation for Economic Co-operation and Development (OECD) Country Average

	Australia	OECD average (2010 or nearest year)
Male life expectancy at birth, 2010	79.5	77
Female life expectancy at birth, 2010	84	82.5
Total expenditure on health (percent of GDP), 2009	9.1	9.5
Total expenditure on health (per capita, USD purchasing power parity), 2009	3,670.2	3,265
Public expenditure on health (per capita, USD purchasing power parity), 2009	2,514.6	2,377.8
Public expenditure on health (percent total expenditure on health), 2009	68.5	72.2
Doctor consultations (number per capita), 2011	6.7	6.4
Practicing physicians (per 1,000 population), 2009	3.1	3.1
MRI units (per 1,000,000 population), 2011	5.7	12.5
CT scanners (per 1,000,000 population), 2011	44	22.6
Hospital beds (per 1,000 population), 2009	3.7	4.9

Source: OECD Health Data 2012 (Organisation for Economic Co-operation and Development, 2012).

2011), with the subsidy beginning at a lower set level for the elderly and low-income people. Prescription drugs are subsidized for war veterans and their dependents through the Repatriation Pharmaceutical Benefits Scheme. Primary care is paid for on a fee-for-service basis, while hospital payments are handled through a combination of global budgets and, in some states, case-based payments; hospital payments include physician costs. Patients are not required to register with a general practitioner.

Costs of Hospitalization

Public hospital care is free to the Australian population, as specified in the National Health Act of 1953. However, people may also choose to pay for private hospital care. According to Organisation for Economic Co-operation and Development (OECD) data, in 2009, hospital spending per capita in Australia was $1,356 (adjusted for differences in the cost of living), and hospital spending per discharge came to $8,350 in 2011. The average length of stay in acute care was

5.9 days (in 2008), and there were 162 hospital discharges per 1,000 population.

Access to Health Care

In 2009, according to OECD data, Australians had an average of 6.5 physician visits. In 2010, 65 percent of Australians reported that, when sick, they were able to get a medical appointment the same day or the next day. A slightly lower proportion (59 percent) reported it was very or somewhat difficult to get medical care after usual office hours. For those who needed particular types of care, 28 percent reported they waited two or more months to see a specialist (of those who needed to see a specialist in the prior two years), 18 percent reported waiting four or more months for elective surgery (of those who required elective surgery in the prior two years), and 22 percent reported they had experienced an access barrier due to cost in the previous two years; an access barrier was defined as failing to fill or refill a prescription, failing to visit a physician, or failing to get recommended care. In 2010, fewer than one in seven Australians (14 percent) reported experiencing a medical, medication, or lab test error in the previous two years, and 19 percent of those who needed to visit a specialist in the previous two years reported that the specialist did not have information about their medical history at the time of the appointment. Over half (61 percent) reported experiencing a gap in hospital discharge planning in the previous two years (did not receive a written plan for care, did not have arrangements made for follow-up visits, did not know whom to contact with questions, or did not receive instruction about when to seek further care).

A 2011 Commonwealth Fund Survey compared access to health care for sicker adults (those 18 and older in self-reported poor or fair health who had been treated for a serious illness or injury in the past year or been hospitalized in the past two years) in 11 OECD countries. This survey found that 30 percent of sicker Australians surveyed reported experiencing an access problem related to cost in the previous year; the most common result was skipping a treatment or follow-up. Other problems reported include having serious problems paying medical bills (8 percent), waiting six days or longer for needed care (10 percent), having difficulty getting after-hours care except in an emergency room (56 percent), and experiencing coordination gaps in care (36 percent).

Australia ranked second (tied with Iceland) among more-developed countries in the 2011 Mothers' Index produced by the international nongovernmental organization (NGO) Save the Children, based on a number of health and social factors relating to women, children, and maternal and child care. According to WHO, in 2008, 99.1 percent of births in Australia were attended by skilled personnel (for example, physicians, nurses, or midwives). In 2008, 92 percent of pregnant women received at least one prenatal care visit. The 2010 immunization rates for 1-year-olds were 92 percent for diphtheria and pertussis (DPT3), 94 percent for measles (MCV), and 92 percent for Hib (Hib3).

Cost of Drugs

The Pharmaceutical Benefits Scheme (PBS) maintains a list of drugs subsidized by Medicare; this list includes drugs considered to be cost-effective to treat health conditions (a determination reached, in part, by comparing a given mediation with alternatives to treat the same condition on the grounds of safety and effectiveness). The PBS is determined by the Pharmaceutical Benefits Advisory Committee (PBAC), an independent advisory body. Pharmaceutical manufacturers are required to submit detailed information regarding the effectiveness and cost-effectiveness of a drug they wish to be included on the PBS, and the PBAC then contracts with independent researchers to investigate the claims. The price of each drug on the PBS list is fixed and is determined through negotiation between the Australian government and the drug's supplier. Drugs not on the PBS list are paid for out of pocket. There was also a standard copayment of AUSD 33 ($34) in 2011, although some were eligible for subsidy or waiver of this copayment.

In 2009, according to OECD data, pharmaceutical spending per capita in Australia was $503 (adjusted for differences in the cost of living). According to Douglas Ball, Australia does not charge a value-added tax (VAT) for medicines (the standard VAT is 15 percent). There is no regulated dispensing fee, and the wholesale and pharmacy markup for medicines is not fixed. Real annual growth in pharmaceutical expenditures in Australia grew 7.6 percent from 1997 to 2005, faster than the 5.4 percent growth of total health expenditure (minus pharmaceutical expenditures) over those years. As of 2011, Australia did not charge VAT for prescribed medicines and charged 10 percent for over-the-counter medicines. The pharmacy dispensing fee is fixed at AUD 5.44, the wholesale markup is 7.52 percent for most items (with a maximum of $69.94), and the retail markup is between 4 and 10 percent (with a maximum of $40.00).

Health Care Facilities

Hospitals in Australia include both private and public facilities; the latter constitute about two-thirds of the total and are managed by state or territory governments, while the former may be either for-profit or nonprofit. Patients receive public hospital care for free but may choose to be treated as a private patient in either a public or private hospital; salaried physicians working in public hospitals may treat private patients as well. Most elective surgery is performed in private hospitals, while most emergency surgery is provided in public hospitals. According to Donald West and colleagues, Australia has about 750 public hospitals and 290 private hospitals; just under one-third (33.2 percent) of all hospital beds in Australia are in private hospitals. Australia has 20 public psychiatric hospitals with 2,560 beds (3.2 percent of total beds). In 2009, Australia had 3.82 hospital beds per 1,000 population, 5.9 magnetic resonance imaging (MRI) machines per 1 million population, and 23.3 MRI exams were performed per 100,000 population. Most (95 percent) of primary care physicians used electronic medical records in 2009.

Major Health Issues

In 2008, WHO estimated that 6 percent of years of life lost in Australia were due to communicable diseases, 79 percent to noncommunicable diseases, and 15 percent to injuries. In 2008, the age-standardized estimate of cancer deaths was 154 per 100,000 for men and 95 per 100,000 for women; for cardiovascular disease and diabetes, 166 per 100,000 for men and 89 per 100,000 for women; and for chronic respiratory disease, 26 per 100,000 for men and 16 per 100,000 for women.

The maternal mortality rate (death from any cause related to or aggravated by pregnancy) in Australia in 2008 was eight maternal deaths per 100,000 live births, among the lowest in the world. The infant mortality rate, defined as the number of deaths of infants younger than 1 year, was 4.55 per 1,000 live births as of 2012. In 2010, tuberculosis incidence was 6.3 per 100,000 population, tuberculosis prevalence 8.0 per 100,000, and deaths due to tuberculosis among human immunodeficiency virus (HIV)-negative people 0.20 per 100,000. As of 2009, an estimated 0.1 percent of adults age 15 to 49 were living with HIV or acquired immune deficiency syndrome (AIDS).

Health disparities are a problem in Australia: Poor people, those living in remote areas, and indigenous people are in general less healthy than others in the population. A number of programs are underway to address this problem, including increased outreach to indigenous communities, an improved health care safety net for the poor, and government subsidies to provide more outreach and services for people in rural or remote areas.

Health Care Personnel

Australia has 11 medical schools, the oldest of which is the Faculty of Medicine of the University of Melbourne, founded in 1862. Basic medical training lasts four to six years, and an additional year of clinical practice in a teaching hospital is required before the degree is awarded. The degree awarded is a bachelor of medicine (M.B.) and a bachelor of surgery (B.S.). The Australian Medical Council (AMC) grants the license to practice medicine following satisfactory completion of the clinical internship, while graduates of foreign medical schools must pass a two-part examination administered by the AMC, with the exception of graduates of AMC-accredited New Zealand medical schools. In 2009, Australia had 2.99 physicians per 1,000 population, 1.04 pharmaceutical personnel per 1,000, 0.69 dentistry personnel per 1,000, and 9.59 nurses and midwives per 1,000. In 2000, 21.4 percent of practicing physicians in Australia were trained in another country, primarily the United Kingdom. Overall, Australia imports about twice as many physicians as it exports in a given year.

Government Role in Health Care

According to WHO, in 2010, Australia spent $108 billion on health care, coming to $4,775 per capita. Australian health care was entirely funded by domestic sources. More than two-thirds (68 percent) of Australia's health care expenditures represent government expenditures, with 21 percent by household spending and the remaining 11 percent by other entities. The Australian government allocates 17 percent of its budget to health care, which comes to 6 percent of GDP; both figures are low in comparison to other high-income Western Pacific Region countries. According to Donald West and colleagues, the federal government funds about 40 percent of the costs of health care services, while the rest is supplied by the states.

The Australian Register of Therapeutic Goods lists therapeutic goods (including medical devices, drugs, and therapies) determined to be safe and efficacious; high-risk products are also evaluated for cost-effectiveness. Listing of goods on the register is determined by the Therapeutic Goods Administration, which has the authority to withdraw a manufacturer's license.

Public Health Programs

Australia has a modern infrastructure, and as of 2010, access to improved sanitation facilities and improved sources of drinking water was essentially universal in Australia. The country also has an advanced system of public health programs, and according to the World Higher Education Database (WHED), 20 universities in Australia offer programs in epidemiology or public health.

AUSTRIA

Austria is a landlocked country in central Europe, sharing borders with eight countries. The area is

32,383 square miles (83,871 square kilometers, similar to Maine), and the July 2012 population was estimated at 8.2 million. In 2010, 68 percent of the population lived in urban areas, and the 2010 to 2015 annual rate of urbanization was estimated at 0.6 percent. The capital and largest city is Vienna (with a 2009 population estimated at 1.69 million). Population growth is very low at 0.03 percent annually, as is the birth rate (8.69 births per 1,000 population). The United Nations High Commissioner for Refugees (UNHCR) estimates that, in 2010, there were 42,630 refugees and persons in refugee-like situations in Austria.

Austria was part of the Austro–Hungarian Empire and became a distinct country after World War I. It was annexed and occupied by Germany in 1938, and after the conclusion of World War II, the status of the two countries became unclear until 1955, when a treaty recognized Austria's independence. The Austrian government has a reputation for transparency and honesty, ranking tied for 16th among 183 countries on the *Corruption Perceptions Index 2011*, with a score of 7.8 (on a scale where 0 indicates highly corrupt and 10 very clean). In 2011, Austria was classified as a country with very high human development (the highest of four categories) on the United Nations Development Programme's (UNDP's) Human Development Index (HDI), with a score of 0.885 (on a scale where 1 denotes high development and 0 low development). Life expectancy at birth in 2012 was estimated at 79.91

years, and per capita gross domestic product (GDP) in 2011 was estimated at $41,700. Income distribution is among the most equal in the world: In 2007, the Gini Index (a measure of dispersion, in which perfect equality is denoted by 0 and maximum inequality is denoted by 100) for family income was 26.0. According to the World Economic Forum's *Global Gender Gap Index 2011*, Austria ranked 34th out of 135 countries on gender equality, with a score of 0.717 (on a scale with a theoretical range of 1 for equality to 0 for inequality and an actual range in 2011 from 0.8530 to 0.4873).

Emergency Health Services

Austria's laws governing emergency health systems date from the 2000s, as does Austrian recognition of emergency medicine as a medical specialty; by law, free access to hospitals for emergency care is provided for all persons, including the uninsured. Funding for the emergency system is provided from multiple sources, and different states within the country organize the provision of ambulance services differently. Austria has two national telephone numbers for medical emergencies, 112 (the European Union standard) and 144, and has 52 dispatch centers; a secure Internet connection provides information on the availability of intensive-care beds.

Insurance

Austria has a social insurance system funded by contributions from the employed, the self-employed, employers, pensioners, and the government; there are caps on the maximum level of contributions from wages and floors below which individuals do not pay into the system. In general, wage earners pay 3.95 percent of covered wages, 3.82 percent of covered salary, and 5.10 percent of pension; the self-employed pay 7.65 percent of covered earnings. To receive medical benefits, maternity benefits, or cash sickness benefits, the individual must be in covered employment or fall into some other covered category, such as a pensioner or the dependent or wife of an insured person. Public-sector employees, railway employees, and the self-employed working in agriculture and trade are covered by separate systems. Medical benefits include physician care, maternal coverage, dental care, hospitalization, drugs, home care, preventive services, and transportation; some copayments are required for some services, with exceptions for the poor.

A 2004 study by the World Health Organization (WHO) found that 0.2 percent of the Austrian

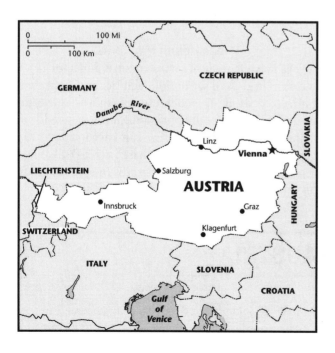

population had substitutive voluntary health insurance (covering services that would otherwise be available from the state), 18.8 percent had complementary voluntary health insurance (for services not covered, or not fully covered, by the state), and 12.9 percent had supplementary health insurance (providing increased choice or faster access to services); the subscription rate for voluntary health insurance varied substantially by district, from more than 50 percent in Carinthia to 17.5 percent in Burgenland.

The maternity benefit is 100 percent of average earnings for 8 weeks before and after the birth. The cash benefit is 100 percent of earnings for up to 12 weeks, then 50 percent for up to 4 weeks. Cash benefits for sickness are paid by employers for a period depending on length of employment; after the employer ceases to pay full benefits, sickness funds pay 60 percent of the assessment base (based on average earnings plus family supplements) for 26 to 52 weeks. The Federal Ministry of Health provides general supervision for the system, with sickness funds managed by elected representatives of employers and those covered by the plans.

Costs of Hospitalization

In 2008, according to the Organisation for Economic Co-operation and Development (OECD), hospital spending represented 38.8 percent of total spending on health, or $1,393 per capita; 47 percent of payments were based on Diagnosis Related Groups (DRGs), and 48 percent were based on retrospective reimbursement of costs.

Access to Health Care

According to WHO, in 2010, Austria had 16.91 magnetic resonance imaging (MRI) machines per 1 million population and 2.76 positron emission tomography (PET) machines per 1 million. According to WHO, in 1993 (the most recent year for which data was available), 100 percent of births in Austria were attended by skilled personnel (for example, physicians, nurses, or midwives). The 2010 immunization rates for 1-year-olds were 83 percent for diphtheria and pertussis (DPT3), 76 percent for measles (MCV), and 83 percent for Hib (Hib3).

Cost of Drugs

In 2007, total pharmaceutical expenditure in Austria was 2,648,000 euros ($4,997,000), with per capita pharmaceutical expenditure 439 euros ($601);

pharmaceutical expenditure came to 1.35 percent of GDP and 13.3 percent of total health expenditures. Almost two-thirds (65.4 percent) of the total expenditure on pharmaceuticals came from the public sector. Real annual growth in pharmaceutical expenditures in Austria grew 3.9 percent from 1997 to 2005, faster than the 2.3 percent growth of total health expenditure (minus pharmaceutical expenditures) over those years.

Austria has a National Health Policy, and a number of separate laws and regulations constitute the equivalent of a National Medicines Policy (NMP). Austria's NMP covers selection of essential medicines: pricing, financing, procurement, distribution, and regulation of medicines; pharmacovigilance; human resource development; research; and monitoring and evaluation. Access to essential medicines is recognized in national legislation as a part of the right to health, and the Austrian government publishes a positive list (*Erstattungskodex*) that is entirely publicly funded, although the patient must pay a small prescription fee. In addition, children under age 4, pregnant women, elderly people, and the poor are provided with free medicines. Medicines provided in hospitals are also free.

Any pharmaceutical products must be evaluated and registered before they can be marketed; there are explicit and publicly available specifications for this procedure, and 13,168 pharmaceutical products were registered in Austria in 2010. Promotion and advertising of prescription medications is regulated by Austrian law, and prescription drugs may not be marketed directly to the public. As of 2011, Austria charged a 20 percent value-added tax (VAT) for prescribed and over-the-counter medicines. The pharmacy-dispensing fee is fixed at 15 percent, the wholesale markup is based on reimbursement categories (with a maximum of 23.74 euros), and the retail markup is between 3.9 and 37 percent, with high markups for nonreimbursed medicines and lower markups for reimbursed. According to Elizabeth Docteur, in 2004, generic drugs represented 8 percent of the market share by value and 12 percent of the market share by volume of the total pharmaceutical market.

Health Care Facilities

In 2008, Austria had 7.71 hospital beds per 1,000 population, the ninth-highest ratio in the world.

Major Health Issues

In 2008, WHO estimated that 4 percent of years of life lost in Austria were due to communicable diseases, 84 percent to noncommunicable diseases, and 12 percent to injuries. In 2008, the age-standardized estimate of cancer deaths was 154 per 100,000 for men and 95 per 100,000 for women; for cardiovascular disease and diabetes, 188 per 100,000 for men and 124 per 100,000 for women; and for chronic respiratory disease, 22 per 100,000 for men and nine per 100,000 for women.

The maternal mortality rate (death from any cause related to or aggravated by pregnancy) in Austria in 2008 was five maternal deaths per 100,000 live births, among the lowest in the world. The infant mortality rate, defined as the number of deaths of infants younger than 1 year, was 4.26 per 1,000 live births as of 2012. In 2010, tuberculosis incidence was 5.0 per 100,000 population, tuberculosis prevalence 5.8 per 100,000, and deaths due to tuberculosis among human immunodeficiency virus (HIV)-negative people 0.26 per 100,000. As of 2009, an estimated 0.3 percent of adults age 15 to 49 were living with HIV or acquired immune deficiency syndrome (AIDS).

Health Care Personnel

Austria has three medical schools, located in Graz, Innsbruck, and Vienna; the oldest is the Medizinische Fakultät of the University of Vienna, founded in 1365. The basic medical course lasts six to eight years, including a compulsory internship lasting 16 weeks. The degree granted is Medicinae Universalis Doctor (doctor of medicine). Physicians must register with the Österreichische Ärztekammer (Austrian General Medical Council), and graduates of foreign medical schools must have their degrees validated.

Austria, as a member of the European Union, cooperates with other countries in recognizing physicians qualified to practice in other European Union countries, as specified by Directive 2005/36/EC of the European Parliament. This allows qualified professionals to practice in other European Union states on a temporary basis and requires that the host country automatically recognize qualifications for certain professions, including physicians, nurses, dentists, midwives, and pharmacists, if certain conditions have been met (for instance, facility in the language of the host country may be required). In 2009, Austria had 4.75 physicians per 1,000 population, 0.56 dentistry personnel per 1,000, and in 2008, had 0.61 pharmaceutical personnel and 7.84 nurses and midwives per 1,000. In 2001, 3.3 percent of practicing physicians in Austria were trained abroad, primarily in Germany.

Government Role in Health Care

According to WHO, in 2010, Austria spent $42 billion on health care, or $4,958 per capita. This health care was entirely provided through domestic funding, with about three-fourths (78 percent) representing government expenditures, 15 percent by households, and the remaining 8 percent by other entities. Government expenditures on health represented 16 percent of government spending and 9 percent of GDP; both are high as compared to other high-income European countries.

Public Health Programs

As of 2010, access to improved sanitation facilities and improved sources of drinking water was essentially universal in Austria. According to the World Higher Education Database (WHED), two universities in Austria offer programs in epidemiology or public health: the Private University for Health Sciences, Medical Informatics, and Techniques, located in Hall in Tirol; and the University of Veterinary Medicine, located in Vienna.

AZERBAIJAN

Azerbaijan is a country in central Asia that shares borders with Armenia, Georgia Iran, Russia, and Turkey and has a coastline on the Caspian Sea. It has an area of 31,892 square miles (82,600 square kilometers, similar to Maine), and the July 2012 population was estimated at 9.5 million. In 2010, 52 percent of the population lived in urban areas, and the 2010 to 2015 annual rate of urbanization was estimated at 1.4 percent. The capital and largest city is Baku (with a 2009 population estimated at 1.95 million). Population growth in 2012 was 1.0 percent, the birth rate 17.3 births per 1,000 population, the net migration rate 0.0 migrants per 1,000, and the total fertility rate 1.9 children per woman. The United Nations High Commissioner for Refugees (UNHCR) estimated that, in 2010, there were 1,891 refugees and persons in refugee-like situations in Azerbaijan, and 592,860 internally displaced persons and persons in internally displaced-person-like situations.

Azerbaijan became independent of the Soviet Union in 1991 and is currently involved in a dispute with Armenia over the Nagorno–Karabakh region. Azerbaijan ranked 143rd among 183 countries on the *Corruption Perceptions Index 2011,* with a score of 2.4 (on a scale where 0 indicates highly corrupt and 10 very clean). In 2011, Azerbaijan was classified as a country with high human development (the second-highest category) on the United Nations Development Programme's (UNDP's) Human Development Index (HDI), with a score of 0.700 (on a scale where 1 denotes high development and 0 low development). Life expectancy at birth in 2012 was estimated at 71.32 years, and per capita gross domestic product (GDP) in 2011 was estimated at $10,200. In 2008, the Gini Index (a measure of dispersion, in which perfect equality is denoted by 0 and maximum inequality is denoted by 100) for family income was 33.7. According to the World Economic Forum's *Global Gender Gap Index 2011*, Azerbaijan ranked 91st out of 135 countries on gender equality with a score of 0.658 (on a scale with a theoretical range of 1 for equality to 0 for inequality and an actual range in 2011 from 0.8530 to 0.4873).

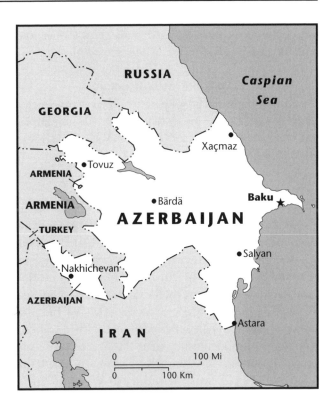

Emergency Health Services

According to the World Health Organization (WHO), as of 2007, Azerbaijan had a formal and publicly available emergency care (prehospital care) system, accessible through both a universal national access telephone number and subnational access numbers. Doctors Without Borders (Médecins Sans Frontières, or MSF) began working in Azerbaijan in 1990 and completed operations in the county in March 2010. While working in the country, MSF provided medical care for people displaced due to the war with Armenia, rehabilitated the public health structure, and carried out immunization programs; MSF programs have been transferred to other organizations whose missions include long-term development.

Insurance

Current laws governing social insurance in Azerbaijan date from 1997 and health insurance from 1999. All citizens of Azerbaijan are covered by the medical benefits system, while all workers residing in Azerbaijan (including citizens of other countries) are covered by the cash benefits system. The system is funded by earnings taxes (3 percent of gross earnings) and payroll taxes on employers (22 percent of total payroll). Medical benefits are provided by public and private facilities that contract with health insurance agencies. The medical benefits system is administered by the Ministry of Health, while the State Social Protection Fund manages the social insurance program.

To receive maternity benefits or cash sickness payments, the insured must have contributed to the system for at least six months. The sickness benefit is 100 percent of wages for the last month of earnings for someone with at least eight years of employment, with lower rates for shorter periods of employment (80 percent for those employed for five to eight years and 50 percent for less than five years). However, certain groups receive 100 percent benefits regardless of length of employment: These include the survivors of soldiers killed in combat, those who participated in containing the Chernobyl disaster, and those wounded in certain military conflicts. Sickness benefits are paid by the employer for the first 14 days, then by the State Social Protection Fund. Maternity benefits pay 100 percent of average monthly earnings for 70 days before birth and 56 days after, and maternity leave is also provided for this period (with longer periods for multiple births or complications of childbirth).

The entire population of Azerbaijan is covered by the public health service, but there is no national insurance system. Most expenditures on health are paid for through private, out-of-pocket spending. According to Ke Xu and colleagues, in 2003, 7.2 percent of households in Azerbaijan experienced catastrophic health expenditures annually; "catastrophic" was defined as exceeding 40 percent of household income remaining after basic needs were met.

Costs of Hospitalization

Treatment in public hospitals and clinics is free to citizens; however, some prefer to pay for treatment in private facilities, which may have better staff and more up-to-date equipment.

Access to Health Care

According to WHO, in 2006, 89.0 percent of births in Azerbaijan were attended by skilled personnel (for example, physicians, nurses, or midwives). In 2006, 45 percent of pregnant women received at least four prenatal care visits. The 2010 immunization rates for 1-year-olds were 72 percent for diphtheria and pertussis (DPT3) and 67 percent for measles (MCV). In 2010, an estimated 32 percent of persons with advanced human immunodeficiency virus (HIV) infection were receiving antiretroviral therapy in accordance with the 2010 WHO guidelines. According to WHO, in 2010, Azerbaijan had 0.57 magnetic resonance imaging (MRI) machines per 1 million population.

Cost of Drugs

Azerbaijan does not have a national medicines policy and does not regulate drug prices. However, some other aspects of pharmaceutical policies are regulated, covering a selection of essential medicines: financing, procurement, distribution, and regulation; pharmacovigilance; human resource development; research; monitoring and evaluation; and traditional medicine. Azerbaijan is not a member of the World Trade Organization (WTO), but legal provisions to grant patents to drug and medical equipment manufacturers do exist. The total public expenditure on pharmaceuticals in Azerbaijan in 2010 was AZN 102,500,000 ($129.60); per capita expenditure was $14.40. There are no publicly reported data on total pharmaceutical expenditures in Azerbaijan. There are no classes of people entitled to receive medicines free of charge, but medicines are free for some conditions, including tuberculosis, human immunodeficiency virus and acquired immune deficiency syndrome (HIV/AIDS), diabetes, and epilepsy; vaccines on the WHO Expanded Programme on Immunization (EPI) list are also provided free, as are drugs on the Essential Medicines List (EML). Medicine pricing is not regulated by the government, and the government does not monitor medication prices. Direct advertising of prescription medications to the public is prohibited by law, and advertisements for over-the-counter medications must be approved by the Ministry of Health.

Health Care Facilities

In 2007, Azerbaijan had 7.93 hospital beds per 1,000 population, the eighth-highest ratio in the world, reflecting the heritage of the hospital-centered system typical of former Soviet republics. As of 2010, according to WHO, Azerbaijan had 7.62 health centers per 100,000, 5.44 district or rural hospitals per 100,000, 2.18 provincial hospitals per 100,000, and 0.08 specialized hospitals per 100,000.

Major Health Issues

In 2008, WHO estimated that 26 percent of years of life lost in Azerbaijan were due to communicable diseases, 66 percent to noncommunicable diseases, and 8 percent to injuries. In 2008, the age-standardized estimate of cancer deaths was 155 per 100,000 for men and 121 per 100,000 for women; for cardiovascular disease and diabetes, 655 per 100,000 for men and 583 per 100,000 for women; and for chronic respiratory disease, 40 per 100,000 for men and 31 per 100,000 for women.

Azerbaijan's maternal mortality rate (death from any cause related to or aggravated by pregnancy) in 2008 was 38 maternal deaths per 100,000 live births. The infant mortality rate, defined as the number of deaths of infants younger than 1 year, was estimated at 28.76 per 1,000 live births as of 2012. In 2010, tuberculosis incidence was 110.0 per 100,000 population, tuberculosis prevalence 166.0 per 100,000, and deaths due to tuberculosis among HIV-negative people 10.0 per 100,000. Azerbaijan is classified by WHO as having a high burden of multidrug-resistant tuberculosis: An estimated 22.0 percent of new cases are multidrug resistant, as are 56 percent of retreatment cases. As of 2009, an estimated 0.1 percent of adults age 15 to 49 were living with HIV or AIDS.

Health Care Personnel

Azerbaijan has two medical schools, the Azerbaijan State Medical Institute N. Narimanov in Baku, which began offering instruction in 1919, and the School of Medical Sciences of Khazar University, also in Baku, which began offering instruction in 1997. In 2007, Azerbaijan had 3.79 physicians per 1,000 population, 0.19 pharmaceutical personnel per 1,000, 0.30 dentistry personnel per 1,000, and 8.42 nurses and midwives per 1,000. Salaries for medical personnel in public facilities are relatively low, causing some to seek employment in private facilities.

Government Role in Health Care

Azerbaijan has a National Health Policy, updated in 2008, but no implementation plan for it. It does not have a national medicines policy, although there are policies and regulations governing pharmaceuticals. According to WHO, in 2010, Azerbaijan spent $3.0 billion on health care, which came to $332 per capita. Almost all (99 percent) of this health care was provided with domestic funding, with only 1 percent funded from abroad. Most (70 percent) of health care purchasing was done by households, with 20 percent representing government expenditures, and 10 percent purchases by other entities. Azerbaijan ranks low compared to other upper-middle-income Asian countries in terms of the share of government spending allocated to health care (4 percent) and government expenditure on health as a percent of GDP (1 percent). In 2009, according to WHO, official development assistance (ODA) for health in Azerbaijan came to $1.53 per capita.

Public Health Programs

As of 2010, 82 percent of Azerbaijan's population had access to improved sanitation facilities, although access was lower among the rural population (78 percent) than for people living in urban areas (86 percent). Access to improved sources of drinking water was also higher (88 percent) for people living in urban areas than for those living in rural areas (71 percent); the national average was 80 percent. According to the World Higher Education Database (WHED), two universities in Azerbaijan offer programs in epidemiology or public health: Azerbaijan University and Khazar University, both located in Baku.

BAHAMAS

The Bahamas is an island nation in the Caribbean Sea, with an area of 5,359 square miles (13,880 square kilometers, similar to Connecticut) and a July 2012 population estimated at 316,182. In 2010, 84 percent of the population lived in urban areas, and the 2010 to 2015 annual rate of urbanization was estimated at 1.3 percent. Nassau is the capital and largest city (with a 2009 population estimated at 248,000). In 2012, the population growth rate was 0.9 percent, the birth rate 16.0 births per 1,000 population, the net migration rate 0.0 migrants per 1,000, and the total fertility rate 2.0 children per woman. The United Nations High Commissioner for Refugees (UNHCR) estimated that, in 2010, there were 28 refugees and persons in refugee-like situations in the Bahamas.

A former British colony, the Bahamas became independent in 1973. The Bahamas are noted for government honesty and transparency, ranking 21st among 183 countries on the *Corruption Perceptions Index 2011,* with a score of 7.3 (on a scale where 0 indicates highly corrupt and 10 very clean). In 2011, the Bahamas was classified as a country with high human development (the second-highest category) on the United Nations Development Programme's (UNDP's) Human Development Index (HDI), with a score of 0.771 (on a scale where 1 denotes high development and 0 low development). Life expectancy at birth in 2012 was estimated at 71.44 years. According to the World Economic Forum's *Global Gender Gap Index 2011,* the Bahamas ranked 22nd out of 135 countries on gender equality, with a score of 0.734 (on a scale with a theoretical range of 1 for equality to 0 for inequality and an actual range in 2011 from 0.8530 to 0.4873).

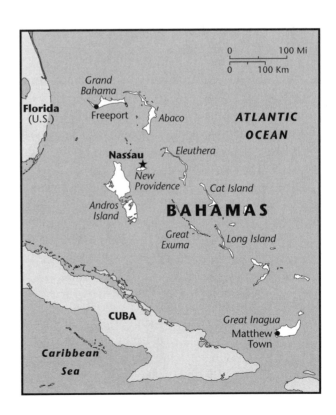

Emergency Health Services

The Bahamas began an ambulance service in 1949, and services were substantially upgraded in 1993 so that a single-response system is used throughout the country for prehospital emergencies. The system is most advanced on the islands of Grand Bahama and New Providence. A first responder program to train volunteers to provide emergency care is in place in Andros, Bimini, Exuma, Eleuthera, Long Island, and Grand Bahama.

Insurance

The Bahamas has a social insurance system regulated by the National Insurance Act No. 21 of 1972 and amended in 1999 and 2010; all workers in the public and private sectors are required to participate. Employed and self-employed people are covered by the system, with the government subsidizing care for children, the elderly, and the poor. Funding for the system is provided through a tax on wages and employer contributions; there is a cap on earnings taxed for this purpose.

To receive maternity, cash sickness, or funeral benefits, the individual must have been paying into the system for a specified number of weeks. A sickness benefit of 60 percent of covered earnings is paid for up to 26 weeks, with a possible extension for an additional 14 weeks; those who do not qualify for the sickness benefit and who meet means-tested criteria are eligible for a flat sickness allowance. Lump sum benefits are paid for the birth of a child or for a funeral, and maternity benefits amounting to 66.6 percent of average covered earnings are paid for 13 weeks, with a possible 2-week extension. The National Insurance Board administers the social insurance program with general supervision from the Ministry of Finance.

Since at least 2002, there have been proposals for the Bahamas to adopt a universal National Health Insurance scheme; however, as of 2012, no such plan has been implemented. In 2008, an estimated 51 percent of Bahamians had private health insurance.

Costs of Hospitalization

Health care in the Bahamas is financed through a combination of government support, private health insurance, users' fees, social health insurance, and external sources. In 2003 and 2004, about 65 percent of the Ministry of Health's expenditures went to the Public Hospitals Authority.

Access to Health Care

In 2003, the Bahamas had five public and private hospitals, 55 health centers or clinics, 59 satellite clinics, and 286 privately owned health care facilities offering primary care and diagnostic services. The Public Health Authority of the Bahamas manages the Princess Margaret Hospital, a tertiary care facility, and the Sandilands Rehabilitation Centre, providing psychiatric and geriatric care. The Grand Bahama Health System includes Rand Memorial Hospital, located in Freeport, as well as nine rural health clinics.

According to the World Health Organization (WHO), in 2007, 99.0 percent of births in the Bahamas were attended by skilled personnel (for example, physicians, nurses, or midwives). In 2007, 98 percent of pregnant women received at least one prenatal care visit. The 2010 immunization rates for 1-year-olds were 99 percent for diphtheria and pertussis (DPT3), 94 percent for measles (MCV), and 98 percent for Hib (Hib3). According to WHO, in 2010, the Bahamas had 2.96 magnetic resonance imaging (MRI) machines per 1 million population and 14.81 computer tomography (CT) machines per 1 million.

Cost of Drugs

The Bahamas National Drug Agency was established in 1994 and is responsible for regulating and managing pharmaceuticals in the public sector; it maintains the Bahamas National Drug Formulary and produces drugs for the public health care institutions. Wholesalers who wish their product to be considered for the formulary must take part in an annual tender process and must also provide information showing that they follow the Good Manufacturing Practice guidelines specified by WHO. The National Prescription Drug Plan subsidizes drugs for children and the elderly.

Health Care Facilities

Hospitals in the Bahamas are governed by the Public Hospitals Authority, created in 1999. The Public Hospitals Authority governs three institutions: the Princess Margaret Hospital, the Sandilands Rehabilitation Centre, and Rand Memorial Hospital. In 2008, the Bahamas had 3.10 hospital beds per 1,000 population. As of 2010, according to WHO, the Bahamas had 43.75 health posts per 100,000 population, 0.87 provincial hospitals per 100,000, and 0.29 specialized hospitals per 100,000.

Major Health Issues

In 2008, WHO estimated that 24 percent of years of life lost in the Bahamas were due to communicable diseases, 57 percent to noncommunicable diseases, and 18 percent to injuries. In 2008, the age-standardized estimate of cancer deaths was 130 per 100,000 for men and 95 per 100,000 for women; for cardiovascular disease and diabetes, 274 per 100,000 for men and 206 per 100,000 for women; and for chronic respiratory disease, 28 per 100,000 for men and 12 per 100,000 for women. The rate of maternal mortality in the Bahamas (death from any cause related to or aggravated by pregnancy) was estimated in 2008 as 49 maternal deaths per 100,000 live births. The infant mortality rate, defined as the number of deaths of infants younger than 1 year, was 13.09 per 1,000 live births as of 2012. In 2010, tuberculosis incidence was 110.0 per 100,000 population, tuberculosis prevalence 9.2 per 100,000, and deaths due to tuberculosis among human immunodeficiency virus (HIV)-negative people 0.86 per 100,000. As of 2009, an estimated 3.1 percent of adults age 15 to 49 were living with HIV or acquired immune deficiency syndrome (AIDS).

Health Care Personnel

There are no medical schools in the Bahamas, but the country has informal agreements with the University of the West Indies and the Caribbean Region Medical Boards to educate Bahamian students, and in 2009, Ross University announced plans to open a branch campus in Freeport, Grand Bahama (the main medical campus of Ross University is located in Portsmouth, Dominica). Physicians wishing to practice in the Bahamas must register with the Bahamas Medical Council in Nassau, with a license to practice medicine granted to those who have graduated from a recognized medical school and completed an approved internship. Foreigners also require a work permit from the Department of Immigration before they can practice medicine in the Bahamas. In 2002, the Ministry of Health created a nursing task force to address the nursing shortage in the Bahamas. In 2003, the Bahamas had 16.8 physicians per 10,000 population, 2.5 dentists per 10,000, 26.9 nurses and nurse practitioners per 10,000, and 4.2 pharmacists per 10,000.

Government Role in Health Care

According to WHO, in 2010, the Bahamas spent $595 million on health care, amounting to $1,735 per capita. This health care was entirely funded by domestic sources and was divided among spending by households (29 percent), government expenditures (46 percent), and other expenditures (25 percent). Although the Bahamas allocates a relatively high proportion of total government spending toward health care (14 percent), compared to other high-income countries in the Americas region, government expenditure on health care as a percent of gross domestic product (GDP) is low (4 percent) compared to other comparable countries in the region.

Public Health Programs

The Department of Public Health's program areas include maternal and child health, immunization, nutrition services, disease surveillance, and training and development. Public health laboratories at Princess Margaret Hospital and Rand Memorial Hospital provide testing services. As of 2005, access to improved sanitation facilities was essentially universal in the Bahamas, and 98 percent of the population had access to improved sources of drinking water. According to the World Higher Education Database (WHED), no universities in the Bahamas offer programs in epidemiology or public health. As of 2002, the Bahamas had 2.0 public or environmental health inspectors per 10,000 population.

BAHRAIN

Bahrain is an island nation located in the Persian Gulf, consisting of one large island and a number of smaller islands. The area is 293 square miles (760 square kilometers, about 3.5 times the size of Washington, D.C.), and the July 2012 population was estimated at 1.25 million. In 2010, 89 percent of the population lived in urban areas, and the 2010 to 2015 annual rate of urbanization was estimated at 1.8 percent. Manama is the capital and largest city (with a 2009 population estimated at 163,000). Net migration to Bahrain in 2012 was 14.74 migrants per 1,000 population, the eighth-highest in the world; the 2012 population growth rate of 2.65 percent was the 20th-highest in the world, the total fertility rate was 1.9 children per woman, and the birth rate was 14.4 births per 1,000 population. The United Nations High Commissioner for Refugees (UNHCR) estimated that, in 2010, there were 165 refugees and persons in refugee-like situations in Bahrain.

Bahrain became a British protectorate in the 19th century and became independent in 1971. Originally relying on its oil reserves, Bahrain is also involved in petroleum processing and refining, and is an international banking center. Bahrain ranked 46th among 183 countries on the *Corruption Perceptions Index 2011*, with a score of 5.1 (on a scale where 0 indicates highly corrupt and 10 very clean). In 2011, Bahrain was classified as a country with very high human development (the highest of four categories) on the United Nations Development Programme's (UNDP's) Human Development Index (HDI), with a score of 0.806 (on a scale where 1 denotes high development and 0 low development). Life expectancy at birth in 2012 was estimated at 78.29 years, and per capita gross domestic product (GDP) in 2011 was estimated at $27,300. Gender equality is relatively low: According to the World Economic Forum's *Global Gender Gap Index 2011*, Bahrain ranked 110th out of 135 countries on gender equality with a score of 0.623 (on a scale with a theoretical range of 1 for equality to 0 for inequality and an actual range in 2011 from 0.8530 to 0.4873).

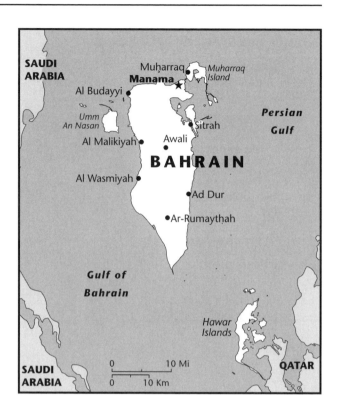

Emergency Health Services

According to the World Health Organization (WHO), as of 2007, Bahrain had a formal and publicly available emergency care (prehospital care) system, accessible through a universal national access number.

Insurance

Bahrain has had a national health system since 1960, funded through taxation and governed by the Ministry of Health. As of 2008, about 90 percent of primary health care services and about 80 percent of secondary care services were provided through the national system. Citizens also pay user fees and may also belong to private health insurance plans, while multiple public insurance schemes cover different segments of the population.

Costs of Hospitalization

Hospital care is provided without charge in public hospitals, but because patients must sometimes wait several months for care, some choose to be treated in private hospitals or overseas.

Access to Health Care

Bahrain has both public and private health care facilities, with the preponderance of care being provided through the public system. According to WHO, in 2008, 97.4 percent of births in Bahrain were attended by skilled personnel (for example, physicians, nurses, or midwives). In 2007, 100 percent of pregnant women received at least four prenatal care visits. The 2010 immunization rates for 1-year-olds were 99 percent for diphtheria and pertussis (DPT3), 99 percent for measles (MCV), and 99 percent for Hib (Hib3).

Cost of Drugs

The pharmaceutical sector in Bahrain is regulated by the Ministry of Health through the Drug Regulatory Authority. Most pharmaceutical products are obtained through group-purchasing tenders, and generally only generic drugs are purchased; exceptions can be made for lifesaving products when no substitute is available. In 2004, 20 percent of total health expenditures were spent on drugs. Drugs listed on the national formulary are provided free in public facilities; for drugs not on the formulary, patients must pay full price unless they have private insurance to cover the expense.

Health Care Facilities

In 2011, the public health care system in Bahrain included 20 primary care centers, three clinics, the Salmaniya Medical Complex (the main secondary

Selected Health Indicators: Bahrain Compared With the Global Average (2010)

	Bahrain	Global Average
Male life expectancy at birth* (years)	73	66
Female life expectancy at birth* (years)	76	71
Under-5 mortality rate, both sexes (per 1,000 live births)	10	57
Adult mortality rate, both sexes* (probability of dying between 15 and 60 years per 1,000 population)	112	176
Maternal mortality ratio (per 100,000 live births)	20	210
Tuberculosis prevalence (per 100,000 population)	25	178

Source: World Health Organization Global Health Observatory Data Repository.
*Data refers to 2009.

and tertiary care facility), a psychiatric hospital, five maternity hospitals, and a geriatric hospital. There were also 11 private hospitals and 42 private clinics and polyclinics. In 2008, Bahrain had 1.90 hospital beds per 1,000 population.

Major Health Issues

In 2008, WHO estimated that 13 percent of years of life lost in Bahrain were due to communicable diseases, 57 percent to noncommunicable diseases, and 20 percent to injuries. In 2008, the age-standardized estimate of cancer deaths was 98 per 100,000 for men and 85 per 100,000 for women; for cardiovascular disease and diabetes, 357 per 100,000 for men and 311 per 100,000 for women; and for chronic respiratory disease, 61 per 100,000 for men and 36 per 100,000 for women.

The maternal mortality rate (death from any cause related to or aggravated by pregnancy) in Bahrain in 2008 was 19 maternal deaths per 100,000 live births. The infant mortality rate, defined as the number of deaths of infants younger than 1 year, was 10.20 per 1,000 live births as of 2012. In 2010, tuberculosis incidence was 23.0 per 100,000 population, tuberculosis prevalence 25.0 per 100,000, and deaths due to tuberculosis among human immunodeficiency virus (HIV)-negative people 0.90 per 100,000. As of 2009, an estimated 0.2 percent of adults age 15 to 49 were living with HIV or acquired immune deficiency syndrome (AIDS).

Health Care Personnel

Bahrain has two medical schools: the college of Medicine and Medical Sciences of the Arabian Gulf University in Manama, which began offering instruction in 1985, and the Faculty of Medicine of the Medical University of Bahrain, also in Manama, which began offering instruction in 2004 and was granted provisional accreditation in January 2006. The basic course of medical study lasts for x years, and an additional year of supervised clinical practice is also required. The title awarded is doctor of medicine (M.D.). Graduates must pass a licensure examination and register with the Licensure Office of the Ministry of Health in Manama. Bahrain has agreements with all Gulf Arab states and the Arab Board of Medical Specialties. In 2008, Bahrain had 1.44 physicians per 1,000 population, 0.24 pharmaceutical personnel per 1,000, 0.50 laboratory health workers per 1,000, 0.36 dentistry personnel per 1,000, and 3.73 nurses and midwives per 1,000.

Government Role in Health Care

According to WHO, in 2010, Bahrain spent $1.1 billion on health care, which comes to $864 per capita. Health care in Bahrain was provided entirely by domestic funding, with about three-quarters (73 percent) of expenditures representing government expenditures, 14 percent household spending, and 12 percent other entities. About 11 percent of government spending was allocated to health care, and government expenditure on health represented 4 percent of GDP; both figures rank Bahrain high among other high-income countries in the eastern Mediterranean region.

Public Health Programs

According to WHO, in 2004, Bahrain had 0.40 environmental and public health workers per 1,000 population. In 2010, access to improved sanitation facilities and improved drinking water resources was essentially universal. According to the World Higher Education Database (WHED), no universities in Bahrain offer programs in epidemiology or public health.

BANGLADESH

Bangladesh is a country in southern Asia, sharing borders with India and Burma and having a coastline on the Bay of Bengal. The area of 55,598 square miles (143,998 square kilometers, similar to Iowa) is mostly alluvial plain, and the July 2012 population was estimated at 161.1 million, the eighth largest in the world. In 2010, 28 percent of the population lived in urban areas, and the 2010 to 2015 annual rate of urbanization was estimated at 3.1 percent. Dhaka is the capital and largest city (with a 2009 population estimated at 14.25 million). Net migration is negative (negative 1.04 migrants per 1,000 population), and the July 2012 population growth rate was moderate (1.6 percent). The United Nations High Commissioner for Refugees (UNHCR) estimated that, in 2010, there were 229,253 refugees and persons in refugee-like situations in Bangladesh. Europeans began creating trading posts in Bangladesh in the 16th century, and it became part of British India until 1947, when it became the independent country of Pakistan, consisting of East Pakistan and West Pakistan. In 1971, West Pakistan seceded from Pakistan and became Bangladesh. Bangladesh ranked 120th among 183 countries on the *Corruption Perceptions Index 2011*, with a score of 2.7 (on a scale where 0 indicates highly corrupt and 10 very clean).

In 2011, Bangladesh was classified as a country with low human development (the lowest of four categories) on the United Nations Development Programme's (UNDP's) Human Development Index (HDI), with a score of 0.500 (on a scale where 1 denotes high development and 0 low development). In 2011, the International Food Policy Research Institute (IFPRI) classified Bangladesh as a country with

an "alarming" hunger problem, and a Global Hunger Index (GHI) score of 24.5 (where 0 reflects no hunger and higher scores more hunger). Life expectancy at birth in 2012 was estimated at 70.06 years, and estimated gross domestic product (GDP) per capita in 2011 was $1,700. In 2005, the Gini Index (a measure of dispersion, in which perfect equality is denoted by 0 and maximum inequality is denoted by 100) for family income was 33.2. According to the World Economic Forum's *Global Gender Gap Index 2011*, Bangladesh ranked 69th out of 135 countries on gender equality with a score of 0.681 (on a scale with a theoretical range of 1 for equality to 0 for inequality and an actual range in 2011 from 0.8530 to 0.4873).

Emergency Health Services

According to the World Health Organization (WHO), as of 2007, Bangladesh did not have a formal and publicly available system for providing prehospital care (emergency care). Doctors Without Borders (Médecins Sans Frontières, or MSF) began working in Bangladesh in 1985 and had 291 staff members in the country at the close of 2010. MSF currently operates several programs there. MSF provides care to an estimated 30,000 refugees living on the borders of a United Nations High Commissioner for Refugees

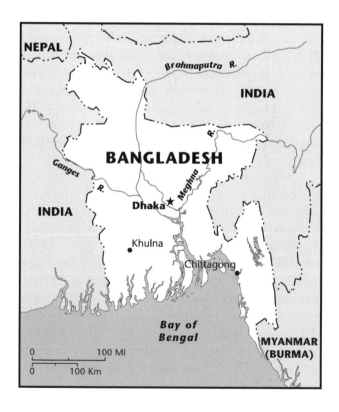

(UNHCR) camp in Cox's Bazaar, an area on the Bangladesh–Myanmar border. In the Chittagong Hill Tracts in southern Bangladesh, MSF operates eight health centers providing prenatal care and outpatient services, including treatment for malaria. MSF operates the only clinic in Bangladesh devoted to treating *kala azar* (leishmaniasis), the second deadliest parasitic disease in the world (after malaria). In Kamrangirchar, an area in the national capital of Bangladesh, MSF operates a health clinic and feeding center focusing on maternal and child care, which provided approximately 10,000 consultations in 2010.

Insurance

Bangladesh has a social insurance system governed by the 2006 Bangladesh Labour Act. Employed women are entitled to cash maternity benefits, and workers in manufacturing and companies with at least five employees are entitled to cash sickness benefits. Some employers also provide medical facilities on-site, and workers are allowed to use some public hospitals. If a company does not provide medical facilities, workers are entitled to a medical allowance of 100 taka per month. Employers cover the entire cost of the sickness benefits system, while the government funds public hospitals. The cash sickness benefit is 100 percent of earnings for up to 14 days per year; the maternity benefit, based on earnings, is paid for eight weeks before and after childbirth.

Many people are excluded from the social insurance system, including self-employed people, household workers, and those working in the informal sector. According to Ke Xu and colleagues, in 2003, 1.2 percent of households in Bangladesh experienced catastrophic health expenditures annually; "catastrophic" was defined as exceeding 40 percent of household income remaining after basic needs were met.

Costs of Hospitalization

No data available.

Access to Health Care

According to WHO, in 2008, 18.0 percent of births in Bangladesh were attended by skilled personnel (for example, physicians, nurses, or midwives). In 2007, 21 percent of pregnant women received at least one prenatal care visit. The 2010 immunization rates for 1-year-olds were 95 percent for diphtheria and pertussis (DPT3), 94 percent for measles (MCV), and 95 percent for Hib (Hib3). In 2010, an estimated 33 percent

of persons with advanced human immunodeficiency virus (HIV) infection were receiving antiretroviral therapy in accordance with the 2010 WHO guidelines.

Cost of Drugs

Drugs are generally provided without charge in the public sector in Bangladesh. However, a 2007 study found serious problems with the availability of 32 essential medicines in a sample of 20 public- and 20 private-sector facilities in Bangladesh: Median availability ranged from 0 to 5 percent in the public sector. The drugs were more available in the private sector (median availability from 20 to 30 percent), with median price ratios from 1.14 for the lowest price generics to 1.31 for innovator brands.

Health Care Facilities

In 2005, Bangladesh had 0.40 hospital beds per 1,000 population, one of the 10th-lowest rates in the world. As of 2010, according to WHO, Afghanistan had 6.54 health posts per 100,000 population, 0.02 health centers per 100,000, 0.04 district or rural hospitals per 100,000, 0.09 provincial hospitals per 100,000, and 0.05 specialized hospitals per 100,000.

Major Health Issues

In 2008, WHO estimated that 52 percent of years of life lost in Bangladesh were due to communicable diseases, 34 percent to noncommunicable diseases, and 14 percent to injuries. In 2008, the age-standardized estimate of cancer deaths was 105 per 100,000 for men and 107 per 100,000 for women; for cardiovascular disease and diabetes, 447 per 100,000 for men and 388 per 100,000 for women; and for chronic respiratory disease, 92 per 100,000 for men and 73 per 100,000 for women.

Bangladesh's maternal mortality rate (death from any cause related to or aggravated by pregnancy) is high by global standards, estimated at 340 maternal deaths per 100,000 live births in 2008. The infant mortality rate, defined as the number of deaths of infants younger than 1 year, was estimated at 48.99 per 1,000 live births as of 2012. Child malnutrition is a serious problem: In 2007, 41.3 percent of children under age 5 were underweight (defined as 2 kilograms [kg] below standard weight-for-age at age 1, 3 kg below for ages 2 to 3, and 4 kg below for ages 4 to 5), one of the highest rates in the world.

In 2010, tuberculosis incidence was 225.0 per 100,000 population, tuberculosis prevalence 411.0 per

100,000, and deaths due to tuberculosis among HIV-negative people 43.0 per 100,000. WHO estimated that the case detection rate in 2010 was 47 percent. Bangladesh is classified by WHO as having a high burden of multidrug-resistant tuberculosis: An estimated 2.1 percent of new cases are multidrug resistant, as are 28 percent of retreatment cases. As of 2009, an estimated 2.1 percent of adults age 15 to 49 were living with HIV or acquired immune deficiency syndrome (AIDS). In 2008, the age-standardized death rate from malaria was 1.6 per 100,000 population.

Health Care Personnel

In 2006, WHO identified Bangladesh as one of 57 countries with a critical deficit in the supply of skilled health workers. Bangladesh has 22 medical schools, including several that began offering instruction in the 1990s or 2000s. In 2007, Bangladesh had 0.30 physicians per 1,000 population, 0.06 pharmaceutical personnel per 1,000, 0.03 laboratory health workers per 1,000, 0.02 dentistry personnel per 1,000, 0.33 community and traditional health workers per 1,000, and 0.27 nurses and midwives per 1,000.

Government Role in Health Care

According to WHO, in 2010, Bangladesh spent $3.5 billion on health care, a total that represents expenditures of $23 per capita. Most (92 percent) of this care was funded domestically, with 8 percent of funding coming from abroad. About two-thirds (64 percent) of health care expenditures represent spending by households, with 34 percent being government expenditures and 2 percent other expenditures. Bangladesh allocated 7 percent of government spending to health, representing 1 percent of GDP; both figures are low for low-income countries in the southeast Asia region. In 2009, according to WHO, official development assistance (ODA) for health in Bangladesh came to $1.16 per capita.

Public Health Programs

The Bangladesh Institute of Epidemiology, Disease Control and Research (IEDCR) and National Influenza Center (NIC) are located in Dhaka, directed by Mahmudur Rahman. The IEDCR, founded in 1976, is the leading public health institution in Bangladesh and was made an NIC by WHO in 2007. IEDCR has 115 employees, organized into eight departments: biostatistics, epidemiology, medical entomology, medical social science, microbiology, parasitology, virology, and zoonoses. Major areas of research within IEDCR include parasitic diseases, viral diseases, bacterial diseases, skin diseases, and mass psychogenic illness (the spread of symptoms lacking in an organic origin within a cohesive group). In 2008, the IEDCR conducted 29 outbreak investigations; goals for the future include expanding the current surveillance system for flu-like illness, improving capacity to respond to emergencies such as floods, and improving IEDCR's capacity to detect and investigate disease outbreaks.

According to WHO, in 2005, Bangladesh had 0.04 environmental and public health workers per 1,000 population. In 2010, only 56 percent of people in Bangladesh had access to improved sanitation facilities, and 81 percent had access to improved drinking water sources. According to the World Higher Education Database (WHED), three universities in Bangladesh offer programs in epidemiology or public health: the Northern University of Bangladesh, located in Dhaka; the State University of Bangladesh, located in Dhaka; and Sylhet Agricultural University, located in Shamimabad.

BARBADOS

Barbados is an island nation in the Caribbean. The area is 166 square miles (430 square kilometers, about 2.5 times the size of Washington, D.C.), and the July 2012 population was estimated at 287,733. In 2010, 44 percent of the population lived in urban areas, and the 2010 to 2015 annual rate of urbanization was estimated at 1.7 percent.

The capital and largest city is Bridgetown (with a 2009 population estimated at 112,000). The population growth rate in 2012 was 0.4 percent, the net migration rate negative 0.3 migrants per 1,000 population, the birth rate 12.2 births per 1,000, and the total fertility rate 1.7 children per woman.

A former British colony, Barbados became independent in 1966. The government has a reputation for transparency and honesty, tied for 16th among 183 countries on the *Corruption Perceptions Index 2011,* with a score of 7.8 (on a scale where 0 indicates highly corrupt and 10 very clean). In 2011, Barbados was classified as a country with very high human development (the highest of four categories) on the United Nations Development Programme's (UNDP's)

Human Development Index (HDI), with a score of 0.796 (on a scale where 1 denotes high development and 0 low development). Life expectancy at birth in 2012 was estimated at 74.52 years, and per capita gross domestic product (GDP) in 2011 was estimated at $23,600. According to the World Economic Forum's *Global Gender Gap Index 2011*, Barbados ranked 33rd out of 135 countries on gender equality with a score of 0.717 (on a scale with a theoretical range of 1 for equality to 0 for inequality and an actual range in 2011 from 0.8530 to 0.4873).

Emergency Health Services

According to the World Health Organization (WHO), as of 2007, Barbados had a formal and publicly available emergency care (prehospital care) system, accessible through a national universal access number. Queen Elizabeth Hospital in Bridgetown has an Accident and Emergency Department.

Insurance

Barbados has a social insurance system governed by the National Insurance and Social Security Act No. 15 of 1966. Persons age 16 to 66 who are employed or self-employed are included in the system; the upper age of coverage was designated to rise to 67 by 2018. Those working in unpaid family labor are not included in the system. The system is funded through a tax on earnings (with a floor and ceiling on the amount of income taxed) and employer contributions (based on payroll). Free medical care is provided in public hospitals and public health centers, so the system does not pay medical benefits per se. Eligibility for cash sickness benefits and maternity benefits are dependent on a period of paying into the system; for example, 26 weeks for employed women and 39 weeks for self-employed women are required in order to receive maternity benefits. Women who do not meet these conditions, but whose husbands do, are entitled to maternity grants.

The sickness cash benefit is 66.6 percent of covered weekly earnings for up to 26 weeks, with a possible extension for another 26 weeks, depending on how long the insured has been paying into the system. Lump sum grants for childbirth and funerals are also provided. The social insurance program is administered by the National Insurance Office, and policy is set by the Ministry of Finance. As of 2007, an estimated 20 to 25 percent of the population had private health insurance.

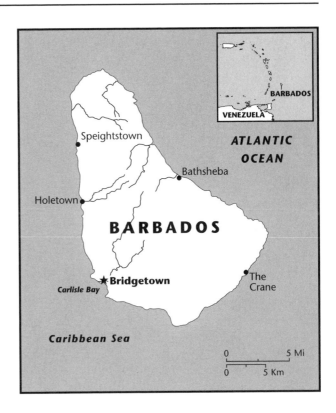

Costs of Hospitalization

From 2005 to 2006, Barbados spent an estimated $136.6 million for hospital services. Additional funds were spent on improving Queen Elizabeth Hospital, including $3.5 million to improve the cardiac unit and $2.75 million to develop the hospital's information services network.

Access to Health Care

Most health services in Barbados are provided by the Ministry of Health, including care at Queen Elizabeth Hospital (including specialty services, such as neurosurgery and cardiovascular surgery), mental health services at the psychiatric hospital, and four long-term care institutions. Primary care services are provided by eight polyclinics and two satellite clinics, and dental care is provided for children under age 18 at public clinics. In 1998, the private sector provided just over half of all medical and surgical ambulatory services, most dental services, as well as services such as in vitro fertilization, complementary and alternative medicine, cosmetic surgery, stem-cell therapy, renal dialysis, and some long-term and elderly care.

Compared to other countries at a similar level of development, Barbados ranked fifth (tied with South Korea) among 80 less-developed countries on the

2011 Mothers' Index, produced by the international nongovernmental organization (NGO) Save the Children, based on a number of health and social factors relating to women, children, and maternal and child care. According to WHO, in 2007, 100 percent of births in Barbados were attended by skilled personnel (for example, physicians, nurses, or midwives). In 2007, 100 percent of pregnant women received at least one prenatal care visit. The 2010 immunization rates for 1-year-olds were 86 percent for diphtheria and pertussis (DPT3), 85 percent for measles (MCV), and 86 percent for Hib (Hib3).

Cost of Drugs

The Barbados Drug Service obtains essential drugs from a local manufacturer and from sources in Europe, South America, the United States, and Canada. Barbados maintains a national Drug Formulary, and some medications are provided free to children under age 16, persons over age 65, and for treatment of asthma, cancer, diabetes, epilepsy, and hypertension. Vaccines are purchased through the Pan American Health Organization's (PAHO's) Revolving Fund for Vaccine Procurement. From 2004 to 2005, Barbados spent $11.7 million providing drug benefits to the population.

Health Care Facilities

Queen Elizabeth Hospital, located in Bridgetown, is the main hospital in Barbados and is also the teaching hospital for the Cave Hill Campus of the University of the West Indies. In 2008, Barbados had 7.60 hospital beds per 1,000 population, the 10th-highest ratio in the world. As of 2010, according to WHO, Barbados had 4.02 health posts per 100,000 population, 0.73 provincial hospitals per 100,000, and 0.37 specialized hospitals per 100,000. Primary, preventive, and ambulatory care is provided in both the public and private sectors.

Major Health Issues

In 2008, WHO estimated that 16 percent of years of life lost in Barbados were due to communicable diseases, 73 percent to noncommunicable diseases, and 11 percent to injuries. In 2008, the age-standardized estimate of cancer deaths was 194 per 100,000 for men and 100 per 100,000 for women; for cardiovascular disease and diabetes, 293 per 100,000 for men and 174 per 100,000 for women; and for chronic respiratory disease, 35 per 100,000 for men and 10 per 100,000 for women.

The maternal mortality rate (death from any cause related to or aggravated by pregnancy) in Barbados was estimated in 2008 as 64 maternal deaths per 100,000 live births. The infant mortality rate, defined as the number of deaths of infants younger than 1 year, was 11.63 per 1,000 live births as of 2012. In 2010, tuberculosis incidence was 1.7 per 100,000 population, tuberculosis prevalence 1.9 per 100,000, and deaths due to tuberculosis among human immunodeficiency virus (HIV)-negative people 0.24 per 100,000. As of 2009, an estimated 1.4 percent of adults age 15 to 49 were living with HIV or acquired immune deficiency syndrome (AIDS). In 2008, the age-standardized death rate from malaria was 0.1 per 100,000 population.

Health Care Personnel

Barbados has one medical school, the School of Clinical Medicine and Research of the University of the West Indies, located in Bridgetown, an institution supported by 17 English-speaking Caribbean territories and countries. The language of instruction is English and studies for the basic medical degree last five years. The degree awarded is bachelor of medicine and surgery (M.B., B.S.). Physicians must register with the Medical Council of the Ministry of Health, and the license to practice is granted to medical school graduates after completion of an 18-month internship. Graduates of foreign medical schools wishing to practice in Barbados are required to complete a 15-month internship. Physicians are required to work in government service after graduation.

In 2005, Barbados had 1.81 physicians per 1,000 population, 0.93 pharmaceutical personnel per 1,000, 0.05 laboratory health workers per 1,000, 0.02 health management and support workers per 1,000, 0.35 dentistry personnel per 1,000, and 4.86 nurses and midwives per 1,000. Alok Bhargava and colleagues place Barbados 11th among countries most affected by the medical "brain drain" (international migration of skilled personnel) in 2004.

Government Role in Health Care

According to WHO, in 2010, Barbados spent $274 million on health care, or $1,003 per capita. Health care was entirely funded by domestic sources, and about two-thirds (65 percent) was paid for by the government, with most of the remainder (28 percent) representing spending by households and 7 percent spending by other entities. Barbados allocated 9 percent of government expenditures to health spending, representing 5 percent of GDP; both figures are low in comparison to other high-income countries in the Americas region.

Public Health Programs

According to WHO, in 2005, Barbados had 0.72 environmental and public health workers per 1,000 population. The Environmental Protection Department monitors groundwater, springs, and near-shore bathing water, and in 2010, access to improved sanitation facilities and improved sources of drinking was essentially universal. Current public health efforts include human immunodeficiency virus and acquired immune deficiency syndrome (HIV/AIDS) prevention and care, tuberculosis protection and care, and cancer screening, and the National Epidemiologist leads a team responsible for communicable disease surveillance. According to the World Higher Education Database (WHED), one university in Barbados offers programs in epidemiology or public health: the University of the West Indies in Bridgetown.

BELARUS

Belarus is a landlocked country in eastern Europe, sharing borders with Latvia, Lithuania, Poland, Russia, and Ukraine. The area is 80,155 square miles (207,600 square kilometers, similar to Kansas), and the July 2012 population was estimated at 9.5 million. In 2010, 75 percent of the population lived in urban areas, and the 2010 to 2015 annual rate of urbanization was estimated at 0.1 percent. The capital and largest city is Minsk (with an estimated 2009 population of 1.84 million). The July 2012 population growth rate was negative (negative 0.4 percent), although net migration is positive (0.38 migrants per 1,000 population) due in part to a low birth rate (9.73 births per 1,000 population) and one of the lowest total fertility rates in the world (1.27 women per children). The United Nations High Commissioner for Refugees (UNCHR) estimated that, in 2010, there were 589 refugees and persons in refugee-like situations in Belarus.

Belarus became independent from the Soviet Union in 1991. Belarus ranked tied for 143rd among 183 countries on the *Corruption Perceptions Index 2011,* with a score of 2.4 (on a scale where 0 indicates

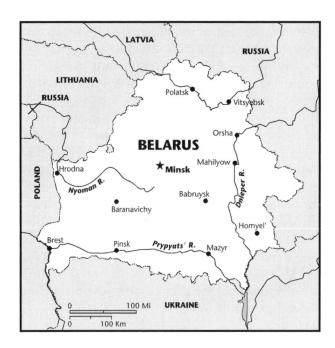

highly corrupt and 10 very clean). In 2011, Belarus was classified as a country with high human development (the second-highest category) on the United Nations Development Programme's (UNDP's) Human Development Index (HDI), with a score of 0.756 (on a scale where 1 denotes high development and 0 low development). Life expectancy at birth in 2012 was estimated at 71.48 years, and per capita gross domestic product (GDP) in 2011 was estimated at $14,900. Income distribution is among the most equal in the world: In 2008, the Gini Index (a measure of dispersion, in which perfect equality is denoted by 0 and maximum inequality is denoted by 100) for family income was 27.2.

Emergency Health Services

According to the World Health Organization (WHO), as of 2007, Belarus had a formal and publicly available emergency care (prehospital care) system, accessible through a national universal access number.

Insurance

Belarus has a social insurance system that pays cash benefits and a universal system for medical benefits; the latter covers everyone residing in Belarus. Funds are provided through payroll taxes paid by the employer (6 percent of payroll) and income tax on self-employed workers (6 percent of declared income). Medical care is provided by government employees in government facilities, including clinics, hospitals, and maternity homes; medical services provided in this way include general and specialist care, medication, hospitalization, and prostheses. Cash sickness benefits are 80 percent of average earnings for six days, then 100 percent of average earnings, with a monthly maximum benefit of 300 percent of the average national wage. Foreign nationals are also eligible for cash sickness benefits. Maternity benefits pay 100 percent of average monthly earnings, and a lump sum payment for prenatal care is provided during the first trimester. Sickness and maternity benefits are supervised by the Ministry of Labor and Social Protection, medical care is supervised and coordinated by the Ministry of Health and local health departments, and the Ministry of Labor and Social Protection provides general supervision for the system.

Costs of Hospitalization

No data available.

Access to Health Care

According to WHO, in 2005, 100 percent of births in Belarus were attended by skilled personnel (for example, physicians, nurses, or midwives). The 2010 immunization rates for 1-year-olds were 98 percent for diphtheria and pertussis (DPT3) and 99 percent for measles (MCV). In 2010, an estimated 51 percent of persons with advanced human immunodeficiency virus (HIV) infection were receiving antiretroviral therapy in accordance with the 2010 WHO guidelines. According to WHO, in 2010, Belarus had 2.48 magnetic resonance imaging (MRI) machines per 1 million population.

Cost of Drugs

Belarus created an essential drug list in 1991, and it is reviewed annually; the costs of medicines on this list are reimbursed for both inpatient and outpatient care. The Ministry of Health Care authorizes medicines to be marketed in Belarus, and prices are regulated according to Presidential Edict No. 366 of 2005.

Health Care Facilities

In 2007, Belarus had 11.23 hospital beds per 1,000 population, the fourth-highest ratio in the world, reflecting the hospital-centered health care system typical of former Soviet republics. As of 2010, according to WHO, Belarus had 14.98 health posts per 100,000 population, 2.79 health centers per 100,000,

4.01 district or rural hospitals per 100,000, 2.72 provincial hospitals per 100,000, and 0.53 specialized hospitals per 100,000.

Major Health Issues

In 2008, WHO estimated that 5 percent of years of life lost in Belarus were due to communicable diseases, 72 percent to noncommunicable diseases, and 23 percent to injuries. In 2008, the age-standardized estimate of cancer deaths was 206 per 100,000 for men and 88 per 100,000 for women; for cardiovascular disease and diabetes, 701 per 100,000 for men and 371 per 100,000 for women; and for chronic respiratory disease, 58 per 100,000 for men and 1 per 100,000 for women.

The maternal mortality rate (death from any cause related to or aggravated by pregnancy) in Belarus in 2008 was 15 maternal deaths per 100,000 live births. The infant mortality rate, defined as the number of deaths of infants younger than 1 year, was 6.16 per 1,000 live births as of 2012. In 2010, tuberculosis incidence was 70.0 per 100,000 population, tuberculosis prevalence 98.0 per 100,000, and deaths due to tuberculosis among HIV-negative people 11.0 per 100,000. An estimated 26.0 percent of new cases are multidrug resistant, as are 69 percent of retreatment cases. As of 2009, an estimated 0.3 percent of adults age 15 to 49 were living with HIV or acquired immune deficiency syndrome (AIDS).

Health Care Personnel

Belarus has four medical schools, one each in Gomel, Grodno, Minsk, and Vitebsk. The basic medical course lasts five or sxix years with an additional one or two years of supervised clinical practical also required. The degree awarded is Kvalifikacija (physician). One or two years of government service is required after graduation, and after completing this, physicians must pass an examination and register with the Executive Committee on Health in one of Belarus's oblasts. Foreign medical graduates must have their degrees certified by the Examination Board of the Republic of Belarus. Degrees granted in other members of the Commonwealth of Independent States (11 countries that were formerly part of the Soviet Union) are recognized in Belarus.

In 2007, Belarus had 4.87 physicians per 1,000 population, 0.31 pharmaceutical personnel per 1,000, 0.50 dentistry personnel per 1,000, and 12.86 nurses and midwives per 1,000.

Government Role in Health Care

According to WHO, in 2010, Belarus spent $3.1 billion on health care, or $320 per capita. Almost all (99 percent) of this health care was funded domestically, with only 1 percent being funded from abroad. More than three-quarters (78 percent) represents government expenditures, with most of the remainder (20 percent) being household spending and 2 percent spending by other entities. Belarus allocated about 10 percent of government spending to health in 2010, and government spending on health represented 4 percent of gross domestic product (GDP); both figures rank Belarus low in comparison to other upper middle-income European countries. In 2009, according to WHO, official development assistance (ODA) for health in Belarus came to $0.56 per capita.

Public Health Programs

In 2010, 93 percent of the Belarus population had access to improved sanitation facilities, and almost 100 percent had access to improved sources of drinking water. According to the World Higher Education Database (WHED), three universities in Belarus offer programs in epidemiology or public health: the Belarusian State Medical University, located in Minsk; the International Environmental University 'A.D. Sakharov,' located in Minsk; and Vitebsk State Medical University, located in Vitebsk.

estimated that, in 2010, there were 17,892 refugees and persons in refugee-like situations in Belgium.

Belgium became independent from the Netherlands in 1830. Brussels is the seat of both the North Atlantic Treaty Organization (NATO) and the European Union (EU), and the Belgian government has a reputation for honesty and transparency, ranking tied for 19th among 183 countries on the *Corruption Perceptions Index 2011,* with a score of 7.5 (on a scale where 0 indicates highly corrupt and 10 very clean). In 2011, Belgium was classified as a country with very high human development (the highest of four categories) on the United Nations Development Programme's (UNDP's) Human Development Index (HDI), with a score of 0.886 (on a scale where 1 denotes high development and 0 low development). Life expectancy at birth in 2012 was estimated at 79.65 years, and per capita gross domestic product (GDP) in 2011 was estimated at $37,600. Income distribution is among the most equal in the world: In 2005, the Gini Index (a measure of dispersion, in which perfect equality is denoted by 0 and maximum inequality is denoted by 100) for family income was 28.0. According to the World Economic Forum's *Global Gender Gap Index 2011,* Belgium ranked 13th out of 135 countries on gender equality, with a score of 0.753 (on a scale with a theoretical range of 1 for equality to 0 for inequality and an actual range in 2011 from 0.8530 to 0.4873).

BELGIUM

Belgium is a western European country sharing borders with France, Luxembourg, Germany, and the Netherlands and having a coastline on the North Sea. The area is 11,787 square miles (30,528 square kilometers, about the size of Maryland), and the July 2012 population was estimated at 10.4 million. In 2010, 97 percent of the population lived in urban areas, and the 2010 to 2015 annual rate of urbanization was estimated at 0.4 percent. The capital and largest city is Brussels (with a 2009 population estimated at 1.9 million). The population growth rate in 2012 was less than 0.1 percent, the birth rate 10.0 births per 1,000 population, the total fertility rate 1.6 children per woman, and the net migration rate 1.2 migrants per 1,000 population. The United Nations High Commissioner for Refugees (UNHCR)

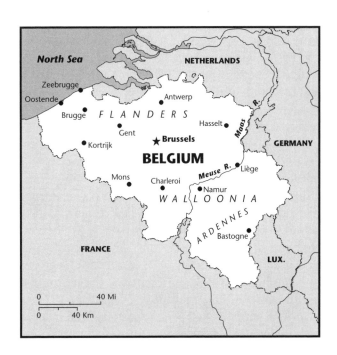

Emergency Health Services

Belgium's laws governing the emergency health system date from the 1960s, the oldest such laws in the European Community; emergency medicine became recognized as a medical specialty in the 1990s. In Belgium, by law, free access to hospitals for emergency care is provided for all persons, including the uninsured. Funding for the emergency system is provided from multiple sources. Belgium has two national telephone numbers for medical emergencies, 112 (the EU standard) and 100, and the country has 10 dispatch centers.

Insurance

Belgium has a social insurance system based on a law passed in 1994 (the Coordinating Law of 14 July), although the system of mutual benefit societies dates back to 1894. Employed people are members of a mutual benefit society or an auxiliary sickness and disability insurance fund; this also covers their dependents, and recipients of social security benefits, including retired people, are also covered by the system; special systems cover the self-employed and seamen. The social insurance system covers medical benefits, cash benefits, and disability pensions, and it is paid for through contributions from wage earners, pensioners, and employers. There is no qualifying period to receive medical benefits in most cases, but to receive cash maternity or sickness benefits, the insured must have met several requirements during the prior period of employment. Medical benefits include general and specialist care, nursing care, hospitalization, surgery, medicines, lab services, dental services, rehabilitation services, and appliances; copayments are required, based on income and status. Contributions are collected through the National Social Security Office; the National Sickness and Invalidity Insurance Institute coordinates the cash and medical benefits system, and general supervision is provided by the Social Security Public Federal Service.

A 2004 study by the World Health Organization (WHO) found that 7.1 percent of the Belgian population had substitutive voluntary health insurance (covering services that would otherwise be available from the state), and 30 to 50 percent had complementary voluntary health insurance (covering services not covered, or not fully covered, by the state). According to Ke Xu and colleagues, in 2003, less than 0.1 percent of households in Belgium experienced catastrophic health expenditures annually; "catastrophic" was defined as exceeding 40 percent of household income remaining after basic needs were met.

Costs of Hospitalization

In 1994, Belgium introduced an all-payer diagnosis-related group (DRG) system intended to improve efficiency and make resource allocations more equitable; one feature of the program is that hospitals receive lower payments for bed days two or more days over the average length of stay for a DRG. In 2008, according to the Organisation for Economic Co-operation and Development (OECD), hospital spending represented 31.2 percent of total spending on health, and $11,147 per capita; 45 percent of payments were based on DRGs, 41 percent on retrospective reimbursement of costs, and 14 percent for drugs.

Access to Health Care

According to WHO, in 1999 (the most recent year for which data was available), 99.0 percent of births in Belgium were attended by skilled personnel (for example, physicians, nurses, or midwives). The 2010 immunization rates for 1-year-olds were 99 percent for diphtheria and pertussis (DPT3), 94 percent for measles (MCV), and 97 percent for Hib (Hib3). According to WHO, in 2010, Belgium had 25.02 computer tomography (CT) machines per 1 million population and 1.98 positron emission tomography (PET) machines per 1 million.

Cost of Drugs

As of 2011, Belgium charged a lower rate of value-added tax (6 percent) than is charged for most other purchases (20 percent). The wholesale markup is 13.1 percent of the ex-factory price (the manufacturer's list price before discounts), with a ceiling of 2.18 euros, and the retail markup is 31 percent of the wholesale price, with a ceiling of 7.44 euros. According to Elizabeth Docteur, in 2004, Belgium ranked fifth-lowest among OECD countries in terms of the use of generics; generic drugs represented 6 percent of the market share by value and 9 percent of the market share by volume of the total pharmaceutical market.

Health Care Facilities

In 2008, Belgium had 6.60 hospital beds per 1,000 population, among the 20 highest ratios in the world.

Major Health Issues

In 2008, WHO estimated that 7 percent of years of life lost in Belgium were due to communicable diseases, 78 percent to noncommunicable diseases, and 15 percent to injuries. In 2008, the age-standardized

Selected Health Indicators: Belgium Compared With the Organisation for Economic Co-operation and Development (OECD) Country Average

	Belgium	OECD average (2010 or nearest year)
Male life expectancy at birth, 2010	77.6	77
Female life expectancy at birth, 2010	83	82.5
Total expenditure on health* (percent of GDP), 2010	10.5	9.5
Total expenditure on health* (per capita, USD purchasing power parity), 2010	3,968.8	3,265
Public expenditure on health* (per capita, USD purchasing power parity), 2010	2,999.8	2,377.8
Public expenditure on health* (percent total expenditure on health), 2010	75.6	72.2
Average length of hospital stay, all causes (days), 2008	8.1	7.1
Total expenditure on pharmaceuticals and other medical nondurables (percent total expenditure on health), 2010	15.8	16.6
Total expenditure on pharmaceuticals and other medical nondurables (per capita, USD purchasing power parity), 2010	626.2	495.4

Source: *OECD Health Data 2012* (Organisation for Economic Co-operation and Development, 2012).
*Excluding investments

estimate of cancer deaths was 163 per 100,000 for men and 93 per 100,000 for women; for cardiovascular disease and diabetes, 161 per 100,000 for men and 102 per 100,000 for women; and for chronic respiratory disease, 43 per 100,000 for men and 17 per 100,000 for women.

Belgium ranked eighth among more developed countries in the 2011 Mothers' Index, produced by the international nongovernmental organization (NGO) Save the Children, based on a number of health and social factors relating to women, children, and maternal and child care. The maternal mortality rate (death from any cause related to or aggravated by pregnancy) in Belgium in 2008 was 5 maternal deaths per 100,000 live births, among the lowest in the world. The infant mortality rate, defined as the number of deaths of infants younger than 1 year, was 4.28 per 1,000 live births as of 2012. In 2010, tuberculosis incidence was 8.7 per 100,000 population, tuberculosis prevalence 11.0 per 100,000, and deaths due to tuberculosis among human immunodeficiency virus (HIV)-negative people 0.48 per 100,000. As of 2009, an estimated

0.2 percent of adults age 15 to 49 were living with HIV or acquired immune deficiency syndrome (AIDS).

Health Care Personnel

Belgium has 11 medical schools that offer instruction in Dutch or French. The basic course of medical training lasts seven years, and the degrees awarded are Docteur en Médecine, Chirurgie et Accouchement (doctor of medicine, surgery and midwifery) from French-language universities and *Aerts* (physician) from Dutch-speaking universities. Physicians must register with the provincial councils of the Ordre des Médecins, and their diplomas must be approved by the provincial medical board, which also has the power to authorize the license to practice to foreign medical graduates.

Belgium, as a member of the EU, cooperates with other countries in recognizing physicians qualified to practice in other EU countries, as specified by Directive 2005/36/EC of the European Parliament. This allows qualified professionals to practice their profession in other EU states on a temporary basis and requires that the host country automatically recognize qualifications for certain professions, including physicians, nurses, dentists, midwives, and pharmacists, if certain conditions have been met (for instance, facility in the language of the host country may be required). Belgium also has licensing agreements for physicians with Iceland, Liechtenstein, Norway, and South Africa.

In 2008, Belgium had 2.99 physicians per 1,000 population, 1.20 pharmaceutical personnel per 1,000, 0.73 dentistry personnel per 1,000, and 0.30 nurses and midwives per 1,000. In 2001, 7.8 percent of physicians practicing in Belgium were trained abroad, primarily in the Netherlands, Italy, the United Kingdom, and France.

Government Role in Health Care

According to WHO, in 2010, Belgium spent $50 billion on health care, or $4,618 per capita. Health care was funded entirely by domestic expenditures, with 75 percent representing government expenditures, 20 percent spending by households, and 5 percent other expenditures. In 2010, Belgium allocated 15 percent of government spending to health, and government expenditure on health represented 8 percent of GDP; both rank low in comparison to other high-income European countries. In 2001, the Belgian government created a reserve fund to provide for the increasing health care needs of an aging population.

Public Health Programs

The Scientific Institute of Public Health (IPH) is located in Brussels and headed by Johan Peeters. The IPH is a public service arm of the federal government and has more than 500 staff members; the function of the IPH is to provide expertise and service in the field of public health and to conduct research in support of health policy. Major activities include disease surveillance; inspection of products, including food, drugs, and vaccines, to see that they meet prescribed norms; risk assessment of chemical products, genetically modified organisms, and so on; research on the environment and health; and management of collections of microorganisms.

In 2010, essentially all of the Belgian population had access to improved sanitation facilities and access to improved sources of drinking water. According to the World Higher Education Database (WHED), seven universities in Belgium offer programs in epidemiology or public health: the Catholic University College of Bruges-Ostend, the KHKempen University College, the Institute of Tropical Medicine in Antwerp, the Catholic University of Louvain, the State University of Liege, the Free University of Brussels, and Ghent University.

BELIZE

Belize is a country in Central America, sharing borders with Guatemala and Mexico and having a coastline on the Caribbean Sea. The area of 8,867 square miles (22,966 square kilometers) is similar to that of Massachusetts, and the July 2012 population was estimated at 327,719. In 2010, 52 percent of the population lived in urban areas, and the 2010 to 2015 annual rate of urbanization was estimated at 2.7 percent. The capital and largest city is Belmopan (with a 2009 estimated population of 20,000). The population growth rate in 2012 was estimated as 2.0 percent, the birth rate 26.0 births per 1,000 population, the net migration rate 0.0 migrants per 1,000, and the total fertility rate 3.2 children per woman. The United Nations High Commissioner for Refugees (UNHCR) estimated that, in 2010,

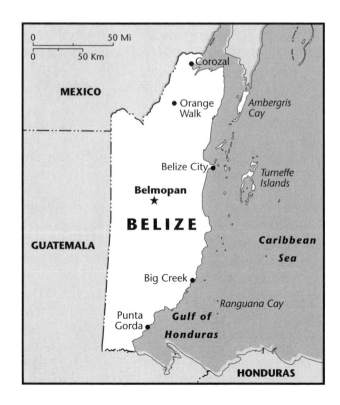

there were 134 refugees and persons in refugee-like situations in Belize.

Formerly the colony of British Honduras, Belize became independent in 1981; it is involved in an ongoing border dispute with Guatemala, which did not recognize Belize as a country until 1992. In 2011, Belize was classified as a country with high human development (the second-highest category) on the United Nations Development Programme's (UNDP's) Human Development Index (HDI), with a score of 0.699 (on a scale where 1 denotes high development and 0 low development). Life expectancy at birth in 2012 was estimated at 68.28 years, and per capita gross domestic product (GDP) in 2011 was estimated at $8,300. According to the World Economic Forum's *Global Gender Gap Index 2011*, Belize ranked 100th out of 135 countries on gender equality with a score of 0.649 (on a scale with a theoretical range of 1 for equality to 0 for inequality and an actual range in 2011 from 0.8530 to 0.4873).

Emergency Health Services

According to the World Health Organization (WHO), as of 2007, Belize had a formal and publicly available emergency care (prehospital care) system, accessible through a national universal access number. Accident and emergency care is provided at public hospitals.

Insurance

Belize has a social insurance system, as specified by the Social Security Act of 4 October, passed in 1979. The system covers employed people of ages 14 to 64; the self-employed and public servants are included, but military personnel, casual laborers, and persons employed fewer than eight hours a week are excluded. The system is funded by contributions from the employed and self-employed, based on income, and contributions from employers. There are no statutory medical benefits; instead, cash payments are provided for specified conditions. To receive cash maternity and sickness benefits or a cash maternity grant (a lump sum payment), the insured must have contributed to the system for at least 50 weeks; in the case of a maternity grant, it may be paid if the woman giving birth is not eligible but is married to a man who is eligible. Cash sickness benefits are 80 percent of covered wages for 234 days, with weekly minimum and maximum benefits, and with possible extensions. The maternity benefit is 80 percent of covered wages for up to 14 weeks, also with minimum and maximum benefits; the maternity grant is BZD 300 per child. The system is administered by the Social Security Board, with general supervision by the Ministry of Finance.

Costs of Hospitalization

The costs of hospitalization are included in the national public health system. Most hospital beds (357) are within the public system, while the private system provides 79 beds.

Access to Health Care

Universal access to health care is provided through the national public health system; this system includes hospital-based care organized through Belize's four health regions and primary care provided through a network of clinics, health centers, and health posts. In 2005, over half of all health personnel were located in Belize City. In rural areas, care is provided through mobile health services, rural health centers, community nursing aides, and traditional birth attendants. In 2005, the health care delivery network reported 720 outpatient visits per 1,000 population, 75 hospital discharges per 1,000, and almost 7,500 live births. All districts have mental health units providing outpatient and community services, while inpatient mental health services are provided at Rockview and Belmopan Hospitals. Belize has five private hospitals with a total of 79 beds and a private care delivery network of 54 outpatient clinics and facilities, some of which offer specialized services including dentistry, gastroenterology, and dermatology.

According to WHO, in 2007, 95 percent of births in Belize were attended by skilled personnel (for example, physicians, nurses, or midwives). The 2010 immunization rates for 1-year-olds were 96 percent for diphtheria and pertussis (DPT3), 98 percent for measles (MCV), and 96 percent for Hib (Hib3). In 2010, an estimated 53 percent of persons with advanced human immunodeficiency virus (HIV) infection were receiving antiretroviral therapy in accordance with the 2010 WHO guidelines. According to WHO, in 2010, Belize had 3.33 magnetic resonance imaging (MRI) machines per 1 million population and 13.30 computer tomography (CT) machines per 1 million.

Cost of Drugs

The costs of drugs listed on the Belize Drug Formulary are covered by the national public health system for treatment in the public sector. From 2004 to 2005, Belize spent $4.1 million on pharmaceutical procurement.

Health Care Facilities

Belize has eight hospitals and a network of about 75 health clinics, plus mobile clinics to serve the rural population. In 2009, Belize had 1.10 hospital beds per 1,000 population, and in 2010, 6.36 health centers per 100,000, 0.29 district or rural hospitals per 100,000, 0.06 provincial hospitals per 100,000, and 0.12 specialized hospitals per 100,000.

Major Health Issues

In 2008, WHO estimated that 28 percent of years of life lost in Belize were due to communicable diseases, 43 percent to noncommunicable diseases, and 30 percent to injuries. In 2008, the age-standardized estimate of cancer deaths was 111 per 100,000 for men and 91 per 100,000 for women; for cardiovascular disease and diabetes, 249 per 100,000 for men and 263 per 100,000 for women; and for chronic respiratory disease, 42 per 100,000 for men and 14 per 100,000 for women.

Belize's maternal mortality rate (death from any cause related to or aggravated by pregnancy) was estimated in 2008 as 94 maternal deaths per 100,000 live births. The infant mortality rate, defined as the number of deaths of infants younger than 1 year, was estimated at 21.37 per 1,000 live births as of 2012. In 2010, tuberculosis incidence was 40.0 per 100,000 population, tuberculosis prevalence 41.0 per 100,000, and deaths due to tuberculosis among HIV-negative people 4.90 per 100,000. As of 2009, an estimated 2.3 percent of adults age 15 to 49 were living with HIV or acquired immune deficiency syndrome (AIDS).

Health Care Personnel

Belize has one medical school, the Central American Health Sciences University Belize Medical College in Belize City, which began operation in 1996. The language of instruction is English, and the basic medical degree course lasts 4.5 years. The curriculum is patterned after that of U.S. medical schools, and graduates are allowed to sit for the medical boards and apply for residencies in the United States and the United Kingdom. Several other private medical schools have opened and closed in Belize in recent years, including St. Matthews University (1997–2002), the Medical University of the Americas (2002–2007), and the Grace University School of Medicine (2000–2004). In 2009, Belize had 0.83 physicians per 1,000 population,

0.39 pharmaceutical personnel per 1,000, 0.04 dentistry personnel per 1,000, 0.54 community and traditional health workers per 1,000, and 1.96 nurses and midwives per 1,000.

Government Role in Health Care

According to WHO, in 2010, Belize spent $74 million on health care, coming to $293 per capita. Most (94 percent) of this care was provided through domestic funding, with 6 percent provided by funding from abroad. Belize allocated 11 percent of total government expenditures to health care, and government spending on health care represented 3 percent of GDP; both figures are low in comparison with other low- and middle-income countries in the Americas region.

Public Health Programs

According to WHO, in 2009, Belize had 0.21 environmental and public health workers per 1,000 population. In 2010, 90 percent of the population had access to improved sanitation facilities, with access higher for the urban (93 percent) than for the rural population (90 percent). Access to improved sources of drinking water was nearly universal (98 percent). According to the World Higher Education Database (WHED), no universities in Belize offer programs in epidemiology or public health.

BENIN

Benin is a west African country sharing borders with Burkina Faso, Niger, Nigeria, and Togo and having a coastline on the Bight of Benin. The area is 43,484 square miles (112,622 square kilometers, similar to Pennsylvania), and the population in 2012 was estimated at 9.6 million. In 2010, 42 percent of the population lived in urban areas, and the 2010 to 2015 annual rate of urbanization was estimated at 4.0 percent. The capital is Porto-Novo, and the largest city is Cotonou, which is also the seat of government (with a 2009 estimated population of 815,000). The July 2012 population growth rate of 2.9 percent in 2012 was the 14th-highest in the world due to a high birth rate (37.55 births per 1,000 population, the 17th-highest in the world) and a high total fertility rate (5.22 children per woman, the 15th-highest in the world); the net migration rate was 0.0 migrants per 1,000 population. The United Nations

High Commissioner for Refugees (UNHCR) estimated that, in 2010, there were 7,139 refugees and persons in refugee-like situations in Benin.

A former French colony, Benin achieved independent in 1960. According to the Ibrahim Index, in 2011, Benin ranked 11th among 53 African countries in terms of governance performance, with a score of 60 (out of 100). Benin ranked tied for 100th among 183 countries on the *Corruption Perceptions Index 2011*, with a score of 3.0 (on a scale where 0 indicates highly corrupt and 10 very clean).

In 2011, Benin was classified as a country with low human development (the lowest of four categories) on the United Nations Development Programme's (UNDP's) Human Development Index (HDI), with a score of 0.427 (on a scale where 1 denotes high development and 0 low development). Life expectancy at birth in 2012 was estimated at 60.26 years, and estimated gross domestic product (GDP) per capita in 2011 was $1,500, among the 30 lowest in the world. In 2003, the Gini Index (a measure of dispersion, in which perfect equality is denoted by 0 and maximum inequality is denoted by 100) for family income was 36.5. According to the World Economic Forum's *Global Gender Gap Index 2011*, Benin ranked 128th out of 135 countries on gender equality with a score of 0.583 (on a scale with a theoretical range of 1 for equality to 0 for inequality and an actual range in 2011 from 0.8530 to 0.4873).

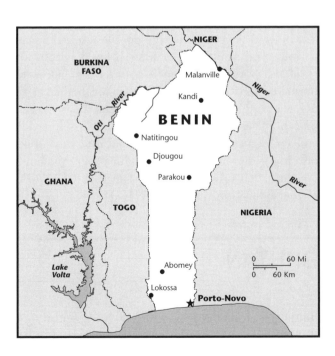

Emergency Health Services

According to the World Health Organization (WHO), as of 2007, Benin did not have a formal and publicly available system for providing prehospital care (emergency care).

Insurance

Benin has a social insurance system that provides only maternity benefits. Employed women are covered, with some exceptions, including agricultural workers, cooperative members, those working in the informal sector, apprentices and interns, and the self-employed. Civil servants are covered under a separate system. The system is funded by employers, who pay 0.2 percent of gross payroll. To receive benefits, the insured must have been covered for at least six months. The maternity benefit is 100 percent of earnings for six weeks before birth and eight weeks after; if there are complications from the birth, the benefit may be extended for an additional four weeks. Some maternity and child health services are provided under the system of Family Allowances, and the 1998 labor code requires employers to pay 60 percent of the costs of medical care for the dependents (children and the spouse) of employees. The National Social Security Fund administers the social insurance system, with general supervision from the Ministry of Labor and Public Administration.

Costs of Hospitalization

No data available.

Access to Health Care

According to WHO, in 2008, 78 percent of births in Benin were attended by skilled personnel (for example, physicians, nurses, or midwives). In 2006, 61 percent of pregnant women in Benin received at least four prenatal care visits. The 2010 immunization rates for 1-year-olds were 83 percent for diphtheria and pertussis (DPT3), 69 percent for measles (MCV), and 83 percent for Hib (Hib3). In 2010, an estimated 58 percent of persons with advanced human immunodeficiency virus (HIV) infection were receiving antiretroviral therapy in accordance with the 2010 WHO guidelines.

According to WHO, in 2010, Benin had 0.35 computer tomography (CT) machines per 1 million population.

Cost of Drugs

No data available.

Health Care Facilities

Benin has a public health care network of eight hospitals, about 80 health centers, more than 300 community health centers, and about 300 village units; in addition, there are about 600 private health clinics. Medical care is more readily available in urban areas than in the countryside. In 2005, Benin had 0.50 hospital beds per 1,000 population, one of the 20 lowest rates in the world.

Major Health Issues

In 2008, WHO estimated that 75 percent of years of life lost in Benin were due to communicable diseases, 18 percent to noncommunicable diseases, and 7 percent to injuries. In 2008, the age-standardized estimate of cancer deaths was 84 per 100,000 for men and 95 per 100,000 for women; for cardiovascular disease and diabetes, 472 per 100,000 for men and 437 per 100,000 for women; and for chronic respiratory disease, 131 per 100,000 for men and 65 per 100,000 for women.

Benin's maternal mortality rate (death from any cause related to or aggravated by pregnancy) is high by global standards, estimated at 410 maternal deaths per 100,000 live births in 2008. A 2006 survey estimated the prevalence of female genital mutilation at 12.9 percent. The infant mortality rate, defined as the number of deaths of infants younger than 1 year, is also high, at 60.03 per 1,000 live births as of 2012. In 2006, 20.2 percent of children under age 5 were underweight (defined as 2 kilograms [kg] below standard weight-for-age at age 1, 3 kg below for ages 2 to 3, and 4 kg below for ages 4 to 5). In 2010, tuberculosis incidence was 94.0 per 100,000 population, tuberculosis prevalence 149.0 per 100,000, and deaths due to tuberculosis among HIV-negative people 0.86 per 100,000. As of 2009, an estimated 16.0 percent of adults age 15 to 49 were living with HIV or acquired immune deficiency syndrome (AIDS). In 2008, the age-standardized death rate from malaria was 57.3 per 100,000 population.

Health Care Personnel

In 2006, WHO identified Benin as one of 57 countries with a critical deficit in the supply of skilled health workers. Benin has one medical school, the Faculté des Sciences de la Santé in the Université National du Benin, located in Cotonou, which began offering instruction in 1970. The course of study for the basic medical course lasts seven years, and the degree awarded is Docteur en Médecine (doctor of medicine). In 2008, Benin had 0.06 physicians per 1,000 population, 0.03 laboratory health workers per 1,000, 0.90 health management and support workers per 1,000, and 0.77 nurses and midwives per 1,000.

The global "brain drain" (international migration of skilled personnel) does play a role in the relative undersupply of medical personnel in Benin: Michael Clemens and Bunilla Petterson estimate that 36 percent of Benin-born physicians and 12 percent of Benin-born nurses are working in one of nine developed countries, primarily in France.

Government Role in Health Care

According to WHO, in 2010, Benin spent $275 million on health care, a total that comes to $31 per capita. About two-thirds (64 percent) of this health care was provided with domestic funding, with the remaining 36 percent paid for by funding from abroad. Expenditures for health care were almost evenly split between households (47 percent) and the government (49 percent), with 5 percent spent by other entities. Benin allocated 9 percent of government expenditures to health care spending, and government expenditures on health represented 2 percent of GDP; both figures rank Benin low as compared to other low-income African countries. In 2009, according to WHO, official development assistance (ODA) for health in Benin came to $9.58 per capita.

Public Health Programs

According to WHO, in 2008, Benin had 0.02 environmental and public health workers per 1,000 population. Access to improved sanitation facilities was very low in 2010: 13 percent of the population had access to improved sanitation facilities (only 5 percent in rural areas versus 25 percent in urban areas). Access to improved sources of drinking water was higher, at 75 percent nationally, 84 percent in urban areas, and 68 percent in rural areas. According to C. B. Ijsselmuiden and colleagues, in 2007, Benin had one institution offering postgraduate public health programs; however, no such university is listed in the 2012 World Higher Education Database (WHED).

BHUTAN

Bhutan is a landlocked, mountainous country in southern Asia, sharing borders with China and India.

The area is 14,824 square miles (38,394 square kilo-meters, about half the size of Indiana) and the population in 2012 was estimated at 716,896. In 2010, 35 percent of the population lived in urban areas, and the 2010 to 2015 annual rate of urbanization was estimated at 3.7 percent. Thimphu is the capital and largest city (with a 2009 population estimated at 89,000). The July 2012 population growth rate was 1.2 percent, the birth rate 18.8 births per 1,000 population, the net migration rate 0.0 migrants per 1,000, and the total fertility rate 2.1 children per woman.

Bhutan has been independent for centuries (perhaps for its entire existence), but its foreign affairs were directed by Great Britain from 1865 onward and by India from 1947 to 2007. Bhutan is a monarchy, but the king ratified the country's constitution in 2008, and democratic elections were also held for the country's first parliament in 2008.

Bhutan ranks in the upper third (38th among 183 countries) in terms of perceived public-sector corruption with a score of 5.7. In 2011, Bhutan was classified as a country with medium human development (the second from the lowest of four categories) on the United Nations Development Programme's (UNDP's) Human Development Index (HDI), with a score of 0.522 (on a scale where 1 denotes high development and 0 low development). Life expectancy at birth in 2012 was estimated at 67.88 years, and estimated gross domestic product (GDP) per capita in 2011 was $6,000.

Emergency Health Services

According to the World Health Organization (WHO), as of 2007, Bhutan did not have a formal and publicly available system for providing prehospital care (emergency care).

Insurance

Health care in Bhutan is primarily financed through government expenditures through the Ministry of Health. A high priority is placed on providing access to basic health services throughout the country; as a result, per capita health spending has more than doubled over the past decade, from BTN 1400 in 2000 and 2001, to BTN 2847 in 2009 and 2010. Private health insurance plays a relatively minor role in the country, although some employers offer it. User fees are collected for some services, including X-rays, dental care, and private hospital rooms. The system is paid for out of general tax revenues.

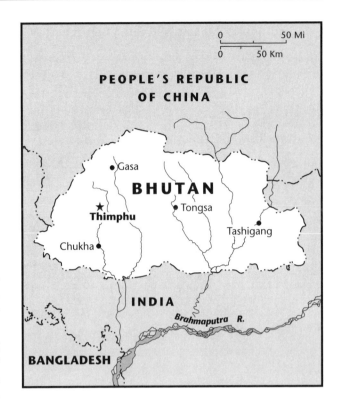

Costs of Hospitalization

No data available.

Access to Health Care

Although health care services are provided free in Bhutan, and the government has made a concerted effort to provide care in all regions of the country, the mountainous nature of Bhutan means that transportation to the nearest medical facility may still present a significant burden in time and money. Individuals may also incur out-of-pocket expenses for some types of hospital care, medicines, dental care, access to a private doctor or nurse, or fees for traditional practitioners. Of these types of expenses, extra hospital services were by far the greatest household medical expense, coming to BTN 299.3 million in 2009 and 2010, while expenditures for private physician and nursing services came to BTN 5.8 million, pharmacy expenses to BTN 4.1 million, and fees for traditional practitioners to BTN 6.2 million. Per capita household spending on medical expenses varies widely by district; from 2009 to 2010, Bumthang district had the lowest per capita household spending (BTN 124) and Wangdue Phodrang district the highest (BTN 1,633).

According to WHO, in 2007, 71.5 percent of births in Bhutan were attended by skilled personnel

Selected Health Indicators: Bhutan Compared With the Global Average (2010)

	Bhutan	Global Average
Male life expectancy at birth* (years)	62	66
Female life expectancy at birth* (years)	65	71
Under-5 mortality rate, both sexes (per 1,000 live births)	56	57
Adult mortality rate, both sexes* (probability of dying between 15 and 60 years per 1,000 population)	228	176
Maternal mortality ratio (per 100,000 live births)	180	210
HIV prevalence* (per 1,000 adults aged 15 to 49)	2	8
Tuberculosis prevalence (per 100,000 population)	181	178

Source: World Health Organization Global Health Observatory Data Repository.
*Data refers to 2009.

(for example, physicians, nurses, or midwives). The 2010 immunization rates for 1-year-olds were 91 percent for diphtheria and pertussis (DPT3) and 95 percent for measles (MCV). In 2010, an estimated 27 percent of persons with advanced human immunodeficiency virus (HIV) infection were receiving antiretroviral therapy in accordance with the 2010 WHO guidelines.

Cost of Drugs

From 2009 to 2010, Bhutan's total expenditures on medicines came to BTN 143.7 million, or BTN 206.5 per capita.

Health Care Facilities

In 2006, Bhutan had 1.70 hospital beds per 1,000 population. As of 2010, according to WHO, Bhutan had 26.45 health posts per 100,000 population, 1.65 health centers per 100,000, 1.38 district or rural hospitals per 100,000, 0.28 provincial hospitals per 100,000, and 0.14 specialized hospitals per 100,000.

Major Health Issues

In 2008, WHO estimated that 53 percent of years of life lost in Bhutan were due to communicable diseases, 33 percent to noncommunicable diseases, and 14 percent to injuries. In 2008, the age-standardized estimate of cancer deaths was 131 per 100,000 for men and 118 per 100,000 for women; for cardiovascular

disease and diabetes, 465 per 100,000 for men and 381 per 100,000 for women; and for chronic respiratory disease, 93 per 100,000 for men and 72 per 100,000 for women.

Compared to other countries at a similar level of development, Bhutan ranked sixth among 43 least-developed countries on the 2011 Mothers' Index, produced by the international nongovernmental organization (NGO) Save the Children, based on a number of health and social factors relating to women, children, and maternal and child care. Bhutan's maternal mortality rate (death from any cause related to or aggravated by pregnancy) was estimated in 2008 as 200 maternal deaths per 100,000 live births. The infant mortality rate, defined as the number of deaths of infants younger than 1 year, was estimated at 42.17 per 1,000 live births as of 2012. In 2008, 12.0 percent of children under age 5 were underweight (defined as 2 kilograms [kg] below standard weight-for-age at age 1, 3 kg below for ages 2 to 3, and 4 kg below for ages 4 to 5).

In 2010, tuberculosis incidence was 151.0 per 100,000 population, tuberculosis prevalence 181.0 per 100,000, and deaths due to tuberculosis among HIV-negative people 9.20 per 100,000. As of 2009, an estimated 0.2 percent of adults age 15 to 49 were living with HIV or acquired immune deficiency syndrome (AIDS). In 2008, the age-standardized death rate from malaria was 0.2 per 100,000 population.

Health Care Personnel

In 2006, WHO identified Bhutan as one of 57 countries with a critical deficit in the supply of skilled health workers. Bhutan has no medical schools. In 2007, Bhutan had 0.02 physicians per 1,000 population, 0.04 pharmaceutical personnel per 1,000, 0.55 health management and support workers per 1,000, 0.03 dentistry personnel per 1,000, 0.10 community and traditional health workers per 1,000, and 0.32 nurses and midwives per 1,000.

Government Role in Health Care

Health care in Bhutan is provided primarily through government services, and organization of the system is decentralized through a four-tier system of out-of-reach camps, basic health units, and district, national, and regional referral hospitals. According to WHO, in 2010, Bhutan spent $79 million on health care, an amount that comes to $108 per capita. Most (89 percent) of health care was funded by domestic sources, with the other 11 percent provided through funding from abroad. Most (87 percent) of the total spent on health care came from government expenditures, with 12 percent representing spending by households, and 1 percent spending by other entities. Bhutan allocated 10 percent of total government expenditures for health, and government expenditure on health represented 5 percent of GDP; both figures are lower than average among lower-middle-income southeast Asian region countries. In 2009, according to WHO, official development assistance (ODA) for health in Bhutan came to $6.84 per capita.

Public Health Programs

According to WHO, in 2007, Bhutan had 0.07 environmental and public health workers per 1,000 population. According to the World Higher Education Database (WHED), no university in Bhutan offers programs in epidemiology or public health.

BOLIVIA

Bolivia is a landlocked country in central South America, sharing borders with Peru, Chile, Argentina, Paraguay, and Brazil. The area is 424,164 square miles (1,098,581 square kilometers, about three times the size of Montana), and the 2012 population was estimated at 10.3 million. In 2010, 67 percent of the population lived in urban areas, and the 2010 to 2015 annual rate of urbanization was estimated at 2.2 percent. La Paz is the capital and largest city (with a 2009 population estimated at 1.6 million). The net migration rate is negative (negative 0.84 migrants per 1,000 population), and the July 2012 population growth rate was moderate at 1.66 percent. The United Nations High Commissioner for Refugees (UNHCR) estimated that, in 2010, there were 695 refugees and persons in refugee-like situations in Bolivia.

Bolivia became independent from Spain in 1825, and much of its subsequent political history has consisted of a series of coups. Democratic civilian rule was established in 1982, and the administration of Evo Morales addressed political and economic inequalities among different sectors of the population. Bolivia ranks near the bottom of the middle third (tied for 118th among 183 countries) in terms of perceived public-sector corruption with a score of 2.8.

In 2011, Bolivia was classified as a country with medium human development (the second from the lowest of four categories) on the United Nations Development Programme's (UNDP's) Human Development Index (HDI), with a score of 0.663 (on a scale where 1 denotes high development and 0 low development). Life expectancy at birth in 2012 was estimated at 67.90 years, and estimated gross domestic product (GDP) per capita in 2011 was $4,800. Income distribution in Bolivia is relatively unequal: In 2009, the Gini Index (a measure of dispersion, in which perfect equality is denoted by 0 and maximum inequality is denoted by 100) for family income was 58.2, among the highest in the world. According to the World Economic Forum's *Global Gender Gap Index 2011*, Bolivia ranked 62nd out of 135 countries on gender equality with a score of 0.6862 (on a scale with a theoretical range of 1 for equality to 0 for inequality and an actual range in 2011 from 0.8530 to 0.4873).

Emergency Health Services

Bolivia began upgrading its disaster response and emergency preparedness systems in 2003, and some municipalities and prefectures began organizing emergency operations centers. According to the World Health Organization (WHO), as of 2007, Bolivia had a formal and publicly available emergency care (prehospital care) system, accessible through a national universal access number. Doctors Without Borders (Médecins Sans Frontières, or MSF) began working in

Bolivia in 1986 and had 49 staff in the country at the end of 2010. The focus of MSF's work is combating Chagas disease, with particular emphasis on treating children (under age 15) and women in their childbearing years (under age 45), because the parasite carrying Chagas disease can be passed from mother to child. The MSF program includes raising awareness about the disease (an estimated 70 percent of women of childbearing age are infected), treating the infected, and educating people to recognize the vinchuca beetle that spreads the disease; the 2010 World Health Assembly resolution to control and eliminate Chagas disease incorporates many elements of this MSF program.

Insurance

Bolivia has a social insurance system providing cash and medical benefits to workers with coverage voluntary for the self-employed; persons older than 60 receive only medical benefits. The system is funded through employer contributions (10 percent of payroll), voluntary contributions from the self-employed, and contributions from pensioners (5 percent of pension). Medical benefits provided include preventive care, general and specialist care, hospitalization, surgery, diagnostic services, and medicine. Dependents are covered at the same level as the insured. The cash sickness benefit is 75 percent of earnings and continues for up to 26 weeks, with extension possible for up to 52 weeks. The maternity benefit is 95 percent of earnings for 45 days before and after the birth.

Under Bolivia's Family Benefits Program, unemployed women receive a mother and baby bonus during pregnancy and the first two years of the child's life; receipt of benefits is conditional on keeping regular medical appointments during this time. Uninsured mothers also receive a nursing allowance, paid for the first year of the child's life, and a grant at the child's birth. An insured mother receives payments for medical appointments before pregnancy and during the first two years of the child's life, a grant at the child's birth, and a nursing allowance for the first month of the child's life. The Family Benefits Program is administered through the National Secretariat of Pensions under the general supervision of the Ministry of Housing and Economic Development. The National Health Fund administers the social insurance system with supervision from the Ministry of Health and Sports.

As of 2005, 21 percent of the population was covered by the National Health Care Fund, an additional 5 percent by other national funds, and 5 to 10 percent

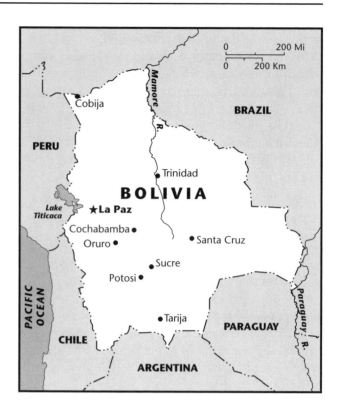

by private insurance. Theoretically, about 70 percent of the population is entitled to public-sector health services, but only about half are estimated to be able to access these services. Traditional medical techniques remain popular in rural Bolivia.

Costs of Hospitalization

Maternal and child care is provided free in hospitals as part of the public health system, but other hospital care must be paid for by the user.

Access to Health Care

According to Latinobarometer, an annual public opinion survey conducted in Latin America, 41 percent of citizens in Bolivia are satisfied with the level of health care available to them (the regional average is 51.9 percent). International donor agencies provide some services, including childhood vaccination programs. According to WHO, in 2008, 71 percent of births in Bolivia were attended by skilled personnel (for example, physicians, nurses, or midwives). In 2008, 72 percent of pregnant women in Bolivia received at least four prenatal care visits. The 2010 immunization rates for 1-year-olds were 80 percent for diphtheria and pertussis (DPT3), 79 percent for measles (MCV), and 80 percent for Hib (Hib3). In 2010, an estimated 20 percent of persons with advanced human immunodeficiency virus (HIV) infection were receiving antiretroviral therapy in accordance with the 2010 WHO guidelines.

Cost of Drugs

According to WHO, in 2008, the median availability of selected generic drugs in the public sector was 31.9 percent; in the private sector, the mean availability was 86.7 percent. The median price ratio (comparing the price in Bolivia to the international reference price) was 3.5 in the public sphere for selected generic medicines and 4.5 in the private sphere, meaning that prices were several times higher in Bolivia compared to the international reference prices.

Health Care Facilities

Health services in Bolivia are organized into four levels (national, departmental, municipal, and local), with 90 percent of health care establishments providing primary care, 6.6 percent secondary care, and 3.2 percent tertiary care. Most services are located in cities, with rural and marginal urban areas often without facilities. In 2004, 77.6 percent of health care facilities were in the public sector, 10.7 percent in the social security system, 5.5 percent run by nongovernmental organizations (NGOs), 3.2 percent by the Church, and 3 percent by the private sector. In 2009, Bolivia had 1.10 hospital beds per 1,000 population. As of 2010, according to WHO, Bolivia had 14.82 health posts per 100,000 population, 9.84 health centers per 100,000, 0.84 district or rural hospitals per 100,000, and 0.31 specialized hospitals per 100,000.

Major Health Issues

In 2008, WHO estimated that 55 percent of years of life lost in Bolivia were due to communicable diseases, 34 percent to noncommunicable diseases, and 11 percent to injuries. In 2008, the age-standardized estimate of cancer deaths was 77 per 100,000 for men and 83 per 100,000 for women; for cardiovascular disease and diabetes, 317 per 100,000 for men and 264 per 100,000 for women; and for chronic respiratory disease, 69 per 100,000 for men and 44 per 100,000 for women.

Bolivia's maternal mortality rate (death from any cause related to or aggravated by pregnancy) was estimated in 2008 as 180 maternal deaths per 100,000 live births. The infant mortality rate, defined as the number of deaths of infants younger than 1 year, was estimated at 40.94 per 1,000 live births as of 2012. In 2010,

tuberculosis incidence was 135.0 per 100,000 population, tuberculosis prevalence 209.0 per 100,000, and deaths due to tuberculosis among HIV-negative people 20.0 per 100,000. As of 2009, an estimated 0.2 percent of adults age 15 to 49 were living with HIV or acquired immune deficiency syndrome (AIDS).

Health Care Personnel

Bolivia has 10 medical schools, and 1 year of government service in a rural area is required after graduation. The basic medical training course lasts six years, and one year of supervised practice is also required. The degree granted is Médico y Cirujano (physician and surgeon). In 2001, Bolivia had 1.22 physicians per 1,000 population, 0.06 laboratory health workers per 1,000, 0.95 health management and support workers per 1,000, 0.71 dentistry personnel per 1,000, 0.19 community and traditional health workers per 1,000, and 2.13 nurses and midwives per 1,000.

Government Role in Health Care

According to WHO, in 2010, Bolivia spent $958 million on health care, a total that amounts to $97 per capita. Most (95 percent) of the funding for health care in Bolivia came from domestic sources, with 5 percent being funded from abroad. Government expenditures represent 63 percent of expenditures for health care, 29 percent represent spending by households, and 8 percent spending by other entities. Bolivia allocated 7 percent of government spending to health care, a low percentage in comparison to other low- and middle-income countries in the Americas, and government expenditure on health represented 3 percent of GDP, also when compared to other lower middle-income countries in the Americas region. In 2009, according to WHO, official development assistance (ODA) for health in Bolivia came to $6.28 per capita.

Public Health Programs

Bolivia's Ministry of Health and Sports targeted diabetes, cardiovascular and rheumatic disease, cancer, smoking, alcohol abuse, nutrition, sedentary lifestyles, and obesity as major issues for the 2005 to 2009 National Health Plan. Bolivia established a National Blood Program in 2002 and a National System of Health Laboratories in 2003. According to the World Higher Education Database (WHED), two universities in Bolivia offer programs in epidemiology or public health: the University of San Andres and the Technical University of Oruro.

BOSNIA AND HERZEGOVINA

Bosnia and Herzegovina is a country in southeastern Europe, sharing borders with Croatia, Montenegro, and Serbia, and having a small (12 mile or 20 km) coastline on the Adriatic Sea. The area is 19,767 square miles (51,197 square kilometers, similar to West Virginia), and the population in 2012 was estimated at 4.6 million. In 2010, 49 percent of the population lived in urban areas, and the 2010 to 2015 annual rate of urbanization was estimated at 1.1 percent. The capital and largest city is Sarajevo (with a 2009 population estimated at 392,000). The July 2012 population growth rate and net migration rate were both essentially 0, while the 2012 birth rate of 8.9 births per 1,000 population and the total fertility rate of 1.28 children per woman were both among the lowest in the world. The United Nations High Commissioner for Refugees (UNHCR) estimated that, in 2010, there were 7,016 refugees and persons in refugee-like situations in Bosnia and Herzegovina, and 113,365 internally displaced persons and persons in internally displaced-person-like situations.

Formerly part of Yugoslavia, Bosnia and Herzegovina declared its sovereignty in 1991 and its independence in 1992. Bosnia and Herzegovina was the site of extreme ethnic strife in the mid-1990s, and an international peacekeeping force led by the North Atlantic Treaty Organization (NATO) served in the country from 1995 to 1996. Bosnia and Herzegovina ranked tied for 91st among 183 countries on the *Corruption Perceptions Index 2011,* with a score of 3.2 (on a scale where 0 indicates highly corrupt and 10 very clean).

In 2011, Bosnia was classified as a country with high human development (the second-highest category) on the United Nations Development Programme's (UNDP's) Human Development Index (HDI), with a score of 0.733 (on a scale where 1 denotes high development and 0 low development). Life expectancy at birth in 2012 was estimated at 78.96 years, and per capita gross domestic product (GDP) in 2011 was estimated at $8,200. In 2007, the Gini Index (a measure of dispersion, in which perfect equality is denoted by 0 and maximum inequality is denoted by 100) for family income was 36.2. Unemployment in 2011 was estimated at 43.3 percent, among the highest rates in the world.

Emergency Health Services

According to the World Health Organization (WHO), as of 2007, Bosnia and Herzegovina had a formal and publicly available emergency care (prehospital care) system accessible through both a national universal access telephone number and a system of subnational numbers.

Insurance

A 2007 report by WHO estimated that 17 to 35 percent of the population was not covered for health care, depending on the region of the country.

Costs of Hospitalization

No data available.

Access to Health Care

A 2007 report by WHO found inequities in health services, with poor and people in rural areas being less able to access services. According to WHO, in 2006, 100 percent of births in Bosnia and Herzegovina were attended by skilled personnel (for example, physicians, nurses, or midwives). The 2010 immunization rates for 1-year-olds were 90 percent for diphtheria and pertussis (DPT3), 93 percent for measles (MCV), and 80 percent for Hib (Hib3). According to WHO, in 2010, Bosnia and Herzegovina had 0.80 magnetic

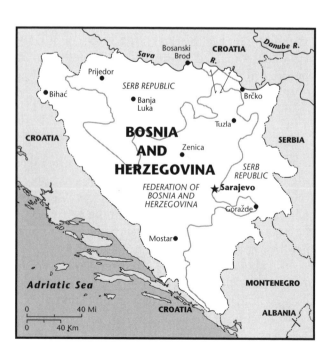

resonance imaging (MRI) machines per 1 million population and 2.39 computer tomography (CT) machines per 1 million.

Cost of Drugs

In 2009, total expenditures on pharmaceuticals represented 30.5 percent of total health expenditures in Bosnia and Herzegovina. Private expenditures on pharmaceuticals represented more than half (54.0 percent) of private expenditures on health.

Health Care Facilities

In 2005, Bosnia and Herzegovina had 3.04 hospital beds per 1,000 population. As of 2010, according to WHO, Bosnia and Herzegovina had 42.82 health posts per 100,000 population, less than 0.01 health centers per 100,000, 0.03 district or rural hospitals per 100,000, 0.88 provincial hospitals per 100,000, and 0.13 specialized hospitals per 100,000.

Major Health Issues

In 2008, WHO estimated that 5 percent of years of life lost in Bosnia and Herzegovina were due to communicable diseases, 86 percent to noncommunicable diseases, and 9 percent to injuries. In 2008, the age-standardized estimate of cancer deaths was 146 per 100,000 for men and 73 per 100,000 for women; for cardiovascular disease and diabetes, 425 per 100,000 for men and 373 per 100,000 for women; and for chronic respiratory disease, 21 per 100,000 for men and 13 per 100,000 for women. Unexploded ordinance and land mines remain a serious problem, with more than 15,000 people killed or injured annually.

Compared to other countries at a similar level of development, Bosnia and Herzegovina ranked third from last (41st out of 43 countries) on the 2011 Mothers' Index, produced by the international nongovernmental organization (NGO) Save the Children, based on a number of health and social factors relating to women, children, and maternal and child care. The maternal mortality rate (death from any cause related to or aggravated by pregnancy) in Bosnia and Herzegovina in 2008 was 9 maternal deaths per 100,000 live births. The infant mortality rate, defined as the number of deaths of infants younger than 1 year, was 8.47 per 1,000 live births as of 2012.

In 2010, tuberculosis incidence was 50.0 per 100,000 population, tuberculosis prevalence 60.0 per 100,000, and deaths due to tuberculosis among human immunodeficiency virus (HIV)-negative

people 3.00 per 100,000. As of 2009, an estimated 0.1 percent of adults age 15 to 49 were living with HIV or acquired immune deficiency syndrome (AIDS). In 2002, an estimated 21.7 percent of adults in Bosnia and Herzegovina were obese (defined as a body mass index, or BMI, of 30 or greater).

Health Care Personnel

Bosnia and Herzegovina has three medical schools, located in Tuzla, Banja Luka, and Sarajevo. In 2005, Bosnia and Herzegovina had 1.42 physicians per 1,000 population, 0.08 pharmaceutical personnel per 1,000, 0.16 dentistry personnel per 1,000, and 4.69 nurses and midwives per 1,000.

Government Role in Health Care

According to WHO, in 2010, Bosnia and Herzegovina spent $1.9 billion on health care, or $499 per capita. Most (98 percent) of the funding came from domestic sources, with 2 percent coming from abroad. Government expenditures represent 61 percent of expenditures for health care, with the other 39 percent coming from spending by households. Bosnia and Herzegovina allocated 17 percent of government spending to health care, a low percentage in comparison to other upper-middle-income European countries, and government expenditure on health represented 7 percent of gross domestic product (GDP), also low when compared to other upper-middle-income European countries. In 2009, according to WHO, official development assistance (ODA) for health in Bosnia and Herzegovina came to $8.76 per capita.

Public Health Programs

In 2010, access to improved sanitation facilities was close to universal in Bosnia and Herzegovina (95 percent), although lower in the rural (92 percent) than in the urban (99 percent) population. Access to improved sources of drinking water was nearly universal (99 percent). According to the World Higher Education Database (WHED), no university in Bosnia and Herzegovina offers programs in epidemiology or public health.

BOTSWANA

Botswana is a landlocked country in southern Africa, sharing borders with Namibia, Angola, Zambia,

Zimbabwe, and South Africa. The area is 224,607 square miles (581,730 square kilometers, similar to Texas), and the July 2012 population was estimated at 2.1 million. In 2010, 61 percent of the population lived in urban areas, and the 2010 to 2015 annual rate of urbanization was estimated at 2.3 percent. Gaborone is the capital and largest city (with an estimated 2009 population of 196,000). The population growth rate in 2012 was 1.5 percent, the birth rate 22.0 births per 1,000 population, the net migration rate 4.8 migrants per 1,000 (the 20th-highest in the world), and the total fertility rate 2.5 children per woman. The United Nations High Commissioner for Refugees (UNHCR) estimated that, in 2010, there were 2,986 refugees and persons in refugee-like situations in Botswana.

Formerly the British protectorate of Bechuanaland, Botswana became independent in 1966. According to the Ibrahim Index, in 2011, Botswana ranked third among 53 African countries in terms of governance performance, with a score of 76 (out of 100). Botswana's government is tied for 32nd among 183 countries on the *Corruption Perceptions Index 2011*, with a score of 6.1 (on a scale where 0 indicates highly corrupt and 10 very clean).

In 2011, Botswana was classified as a country with medium human development (the second from the lowest of four categories) on the United Nations Development Programme's (UNDP's) Human Development Index (HDI), with a score of 0.633 (on a scale where 1 denotes high development and 0 low development). Life expectancy at birth in 2012 was estimated at 55.71 years, among the 30 lowest in the world, and per capita gross domestic product (GDP) in 2011 was estimated at $16,300. According to the World Economic Forum's *Global Gender Gap Index 2011*, Botswana ranked 66th out of 135 countries on gender equality, with a score of 0.683 (on a scale with a theoretical range of 1 for equality to 0 for inequality and an actual range in 2011 from 0.8530 to 0.4873).

Emergency Health Services

According to the World Health Organization (WHO), as of 2007, Botswana had a formal and publicly available emergency care (prehospital care) system, accessible through a national universal access number.

Insurance

Botswana does not have a national social insurance program, and no statutory medical benefits are provided. The 2010 Employment Act requires some employers to

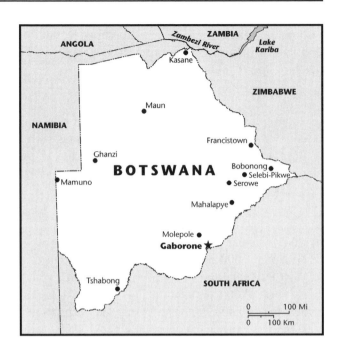

pay maternity benefits (at least 50 percent of pay and benefits) for six weeks before and after the birth and for employers to provide up to 20 days of paid sick leave per year. The 1982 Employment Act requires some employers to provide certain medical services to their employees and those employees' dependents, including transportation to a hospital. The Family Benefits system provides cash benefits and food rations to several classes of individuals, including those with a chronic health condition or disability. Old age and orphan care benefits are funded by the government.

Costs of Hospitalization

No data available.

Access to Health Care

According to WHO, in 2007, 94.6 percent of births in Botswana were attended by skilled personnel (for example, physicians, nurses, or midwives). In 2007, 73 percent of pregnant women in Botswana received at least four prenatal care visits. The 2010 immunization rates for 1-year-olds were 96 percent for diphtheria and pertussis (DPT3) and 94 percent for measles (MCV). In 2010, an estimated 93 percent of persons with advanced human immunodeficiency virus (HIV) infection were receiving antiretroviral therapy in accordance with the 2010 WHO guidelines. According to WHO, in 2010, Botswana had 1.56 magnetic resonance imaging (MRI) machines per 1 million population and 2.60 computer tomography (CT) machines per 1 million.

Cost of Drugs

No data available.

Health Care Facilities

In 2008, Botswana had 1.81 hospital beds per 1,000 population. As of 2010, according to WHO, Botswana had 0.80 district or rural hospitals per 100,000, 0.35 provincial hospitals per 100,000, and 0.15 specialized hospitals per 100,000.

Major Health Issues

In 2008, WHO estimated that 71 percent of years of life lost in Botswana were due to communicable diseases, 19 percent to noncommunicable diseases, and 10 percent to injuries. In 2008, the age-standardized estimate of cancer deaths was 69 per 100,000 for men and 74 per 100,000 for women; for cardiovascular disease and diabetes, 361 per 100,000 for men and 331 per 100,000 for women; and for chronic respiratory disease, 101 per 100,000 for men and 51 per 100,000 for women.

Botswana's maternal mortality rate (death from any cause related to or aggravated by pregnancy) was estimated in 2008 as 190 maternal deaths per 100,000 live births. The infant mortality rate, defined as the number of deaths of infants younger than 1 year, was 10.49 per 1,000 live births as of 2012. In 2000, 10.7 percent of children under age 5 were underweight (defined as 2 kilograms [kg] below standard weight-for-age at age 1, 3 kg below for ages 2 to 3, and 4 kg below for ages 4 to 5).

In 2010, tuberculosis incidence was 503.0 per 100,000 population, tuberculosis prevalence 380.0 per 100,000, and deaths due to tuberculosis among HIV-negative people 21.00 per 100,000. As of 2009, Botswana had the second-highest human immunodeficiency virus and acquired immune deficiency syndrome (HIV/AIDS) rates in the world; in that year, an estimated 24.8 percent of adults age 15 to 49 were living with HIV or AIDS. In 2010, more than 95 percent of pregnant women tested positive for HIV, one of the highest rates in the world. The mother-to-child transmission rate for HIV in 2010 was estimated at 33 percent, and 19 percent of deaths to children under age 5 were attributed to HIV. However, more than 95 percent of pregnant women who required maternal antiretroviral medicine were provided with it in 2010, and the 2009 mother-to-child transmission rate for HIV

was 3 percent. In 2008, the age-standardized death rate from malaria was 0.9 per 100,000 population.

Health Care Personnel

Botswana has no medical schools, but an agreement does exist with Norway. Physicians must register with the Botswana Medical Council in Gaborone, and foreigners must hold a work permit. In 2006, Botswana had 0.34 physicians per 1,000 population, 0.52 community and traditional health workers per 1,000, and 2.84 nurses and midwives per 1,000, and in 2004, there were 0.19 pharmaceutical personnel per 1,000 and 0.15 laboratory health workers per 1,000. The global "brain drain" (international migration of skilled personnel) plays a minor role in the relative undersupply of medical personnel in Botswana: Michael Clemens and Bunilla Petterson estimate that 11 percent of Botswana-born physicians and 2 percent of Botswana-born nurses are working in one of nine developed countries, primarily in the United Kingdom and South Africa.

Government Role in Health Care

According to WHO, in 2010, Botswana spent $1.2 billion on health care, a total that comes to $615 per capita. Most (82 percent) of this health care was provided with domestic funding, with the remaining 18 percent paid for by funding from abroad. Most funding for expenditures for health care represents government expenditures (73 percent), with 8 percent coming from spending by households and 19 percent expenditures by other entities. Botswana allocated 17 percent of government expenditures to health care spending, and government expenditures on health represented 6 percent of GDP; both figures rank Botswana low among other upper-middle-income African countries. In 2009, according to WHO, official development assistance (ODA) for health in Botswana came to $95.33 per capita.

Public Health Programs

According to WHO, in 2004, Botswana had 0.10 environmental and public health workers per 1,000 population. In 2010, access to improved sanitary facilities was relatively low, at 62 percent nationally (75 percent in urban areas, 41 percent in rural areas). Access to improved sources of drinking water was much higher, at 96 percent (99 percent in urban areas, 92 percent in rural areas). According to the World Higher Education Database (WHED), no university in Botswana offers programs in epidemiology or public health.

BRAZIL

Brazil is a country in eastern South America, sharing borders with 10 countries. It is fifth-largest country in the world and the largest in South America in terms of both area (3,287,612 square miles or 8,514,877 square kilometers, slightly smaller than the United States) and population (2012 estimate 205.7 million). In 2010, 87 percent of the population lived in urban areas, and the 2010 to 2015 annual rate of urbanization was estimated at 1.1 percent. The capital is Brasilia; the largest states are São Paolo (with a 2009 population estimated at 20.0 million, making São Paolo the largest metropolitan area in the Western Hemisphere) and Rio de Janeiro (with a 2009 population estimated at 11.8 million). The July 2012 population growth rate was 1.1 percent, the net migration rate negative 0.1 migrants per 1,000, the birth rate 17.5 births per 1,000 population, and the total fertility rate 2.2 children per woman. The United Nations High Commissioner for Refugees (UNHCR) estimated that, in 2010, there were 4,357 refugees and persons in refugee-like situations in Brazil.

Brazil became independent from Portugal in 1822. In the 20th century, it was ruled by a populist and military government until 1985, when the military regime ceded power to a civilian government. Brazil ranked tied for 63rd among 183 countries on the *Corruption Perceptions Index 2011* in terms of perceived public-sector corruption with a score of 3.8 (on a scale where 0 indicates highly corrupt and 10 very clean). In 2011, Brazil was classified as a country with high human development (the second-highest category) on the United Nations Development Programme's (UNDP's) Human Development Index (HDI), with a score of 0.718 (on a scale where 1 denotes high development and 0 low development). Life expectancy at birth in 2012 was estimated at 72.79 years, and per capita gross domestic product (GDP) in 2011 was estimated at $11,600. Income distribution in Brazil is relatively unequal: In 2012, the Gini Index (a measure of dispersion, in which perfect equality is denoted by 0 and maximum inequality is denoted by 100) for family income was 51.9, among the 20 highest in the world. According to the World Economic Forum's *Global Gender Gap Index 2011*, Brazil ranked 82nd out of 135 countries on gender equality with a score of 0.668 (on a scale with a theoretical range of 1 for equality to 0 for inequality and an actual range in 2011 from 0.8530 to 0.4873).

Emergency Health Services

According to the World Health Organization (WHO), as of 2007, Brazil had a formal and publicly available emergency care (prehospital care) system, accessible through a national universal access number. The United Health System (SUS) Mobile Emergency Care Service is the main component of the national Emergency Care Policy; 94 such services were in operation as of 2005. Doctors Without Borders (Médecins Sans Frontières, or MSF) began working in Brazil in 1991 and had 11 staff members in the country at the close of 2010. MSF provided emergency aid to people affected by the June 2010 flooding in northern Brazil, including provision of medical and psychological care; MSF trained local staff as well and handed authority for managing the project to Brazil in August 2010.

Insurance

According to Donald West and colleagues, as of 2010, Brazil had both a state-funded system providing universal care (SUS) and a private insurance market, which is primarily used by the middle and upper classes. Although everyone is entitled to SUS care, which is free, fewer than 60 percent of the population

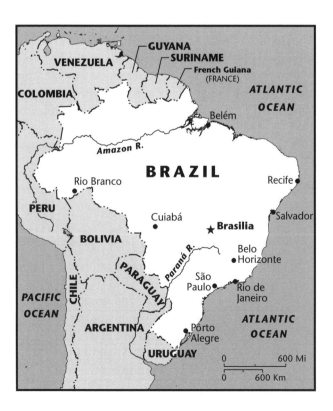

(primarily those with lower incomes) use it as their regular source of care; middle- and upper-income Brazilians with private insurance are more likely to use SUS services for procedures that are not covered by their own insurance or which are highly complex. SUS policy is set by the Ministry of Health, which also coordinates the system; service organization and delivery are provided by states and municipalities.

The Family Health Program (FHP), which is available in 95 percent of Brazil's cities (containing 55 percent of the population) and provides comprehensive primary care, has greatly increased access to care; the system is primarily funded through the federal government and managed at the municipal level. According to Ke Xu and colleagues, in 2003, 11.3 percent of households in Brazil experienced catastrophic health expenditures annually; "catastrophic" was defined as exceeding 40 percent of household income remaining after basic needs were met.

Costs of Hospitalization

According to Donald West and colleagues, Brazil has about 2,600 public hospitals (140,000 beds) and 4,800 private hospitals (330,000 beds). The hospital sphere is not managed efficiently in comparison to other Organisation for Economic Co-operation and Development (OECD) countries: In SUS hospitals, the mean occupancy rate is 45 percent, and 30 percent of admissions are for conditions that do not require inpatient care. Municipal hospitals are mostly small (with a mean size of 36 beds) and have particularly low occupancy rates (less than 30 percent). In addition, Brazilian hospitals on average have about 50 percent more staff than average OECD hospitals. Public hospitals are managed by municipal, state, or federal authorities, and most are publicly managed and financed. About 70 percent of private hospitals receive both public funding (through contracts with the SUS) and private funding; these are required to allocate 60 percent of their beds for SUS patients. About 20 percent of hospitals receive no SUS funding and are financed entirely through private funding.

Access to Health Care

According to Donald West and colleagues, Brazil provides comprehensive primary care services through the FHP, which is available in 95 percent of Brazil's cities (containing 55 percent of the population); the system is primarily funded through the federal government and managed at the municipal level. However, FHP faces several challenges, including variations in quality of care, slow adoption in areas where the middle classes are used to private care, poor integration with systems of secondary and tertiary care, and difficulties in recruiting and retaining physicians. According to Latinobarometer, an annual public opinion survey conducted in Latin America, 33 percent of citizens in Brazil are satisfied with the level of health care available to them (the regional average is 51.9 percent). In 2003, a survey found that 98 percent of Brazilians who sought health care were able to receive it, including 97 percent of those with incomes at or below the minimum wage.

According to WHO, in 2006, 98.4 percent of births in Brazil were attended by skilled personnel (for example, physicians, nurses, or midwives). In 2005, 87 percent of pregnant women in Brazil received at least four prenatal care visits. The 2010 immunization rates for 1-year-olds were 98 percent for diphtheria and pertussis (DPT3), 98 percent for measles (MCV), and 99 percent for Hib (Hib3). In 2010, an estimated 70 percent of persons with advanced human immunodeficiency virus (HIV) infection were receiving antiretroviral therapy in accordance with the 2010 WHO guidelines.

Cost of Drugs

In 2010, out-of-pocket medicines represented 2.0 percent of monthly family income in Brazil, and 31.5 percent of all health expenses (the largest single proportion of health expenses). Although more than half of the Brazilian population belongs to the SUS, which should in theory provide some medicines (those on the National List of Essential Medicines) for free, in reality, about half the population in a given public health catchment area receives free medicines, 10 percent receive them by donation or private insurance, and the remaining 40 percent purchase them out of pocket. Availability of medicine is a national problem: Some studies have found that 40 percent of the medicines prescribed in primary health care were not available at the time of prescription. To attempt to increase availability of medicines, in 2004, the Brazilian government began selling medicines at low prices through popular pharmacies that may be run by the government or in partnership with a private pharmacy; in the former, drugs are sold at cost, while in the latter, the government pays 90 percent of the price. In addition, many individuals have private insurance that does not cover the cost of medicines used

Health Expenditures: Brazil Compared With the Global Average (2009)

	Brazil	Global Average
Out-of-pocket expenditure as percent of private expenditure on health	57.2	50.2
Private prepaid plans as percent of private expenditure on health	41.0	38.9
Per capita total expenditure on health at average exchange rate (USD)	734	900
Per capita total expenditure on health (purchasing power parity, international dollars)	921	990
Per capita government expenditure on health at average exchange rate (USD)	320	549
Per capita government expenditure on health (purchasing power parity, international dollars)	401	584

Source: 2011 World Health Organization Global Health Expenditure Atlas.

in outpatient care. In 2007, out-of-pocket expenditures on medicines in Brazil came to BRL 44.8 billion ($19.3 billion); families spent 10 times as much money purchasing medicines as did the government.

A 2010 survey conducted in six cities in southern Brazil found varied availability among originator brands (65 percent), generic drugs (74 percent), and similar drugs (48 percent). The median price ratio (the median price in Brazil divided by the international reference price) showed that drugs were generally expensive in Brazil: The median price ratio was 18.7 for originator brands, 11.3 for generic drugs, and 8.6 for similar medicines. A different survey, conducted in 2009 in Brazil, found that bioequivalent generic drugs were less available in the public sector than brand names; for 71.4 percent of medicines, the availability of generics was under 10 percent. In the private sector, fewer types of bioequivalent generic drugs were available in Brazil than are available on the market.

Health Care Facilities

The majority (71 percent) of health care facilities in Brazil in 2002 provided only ambulatory care; most (76 percent) belonged to the public system. In 2002, Brazil had 7,397 hospitals, 4,809 of which were private, with most of these providing services to the SUS. Most (95 percent) diagnostic and treatment support facilities (for example, labs or radiology clinics) were also private, with 35 percent providing services to the SUS. About 88 percent of hospital beds in Brazil are in public facilities or in private facilities providing services to the SUS.

Major Health Issues

In 2008, WHO estimated that 20 percent of years of life lost in Brazil were due to communicable diseases, 56 percent to noncommunicable diseases, and 24 percent to injuries. In 2008, the age-standardized estimate of cancer deaths was 136 per 100,000 for men and 95 per 100,000 for women; for cardiovascular disease and diabetes, 304 per 100,000 for men and 226 per 100,000 for women; and for chronic respiratory disease, 54 per 100,000 for men and 32 per 100,000 for women.

Brazil's maternal mortality rate (death from any cause related to or aggravated by pregnancy) was estimated in 2008 as 58 maternal deaths per 100,000 live births. The infant mortality rate, defined as the number of deaths of infants younger than 1 year, was estimated at 20.50 per 1,000 live births as of 2012. Tuberculosis is a high priority for Brazilian public health authorities, particularly among the country's poor; in 2010, tuberculosis incidence was 43.0 per 100,000 population, tuberculosis prevalence 47.0 per 100,000, and deaths due to tuberculosis among HIV-negative people 2.60 per 100,000. WHO estimated that the case detection rate in 2010 was 88 percent.

The percent of adults age 15 to 49 living with human immunodeficiency virus and acquired immune deficiency syndrome (HIV/AIDS) was estimated in 2009 to be in the range of 0.3 to 0.6 percent. In 2010, 334,618 cases of malaria were reported. Malaria is endemic in the Brazilian Amazon region, and in 2008, the age-standardized death rate from malaria was 0.1 per 100,000 population. Leprosy remains a significant problem, with 4.9 cases per 10,000 population reported in 1998.

Health Care Personnel

Brazil has more than 80 medical schools. The basic course of medical education lasts six to nine years, and the degree awarded is Médico (doctor of medicine). Graduates must register with the university that awarded the degree or that is empowered to register degrees awarded from independent medical schools, and graduates of foreign medical schools must have their degrees accredited by a Brazilian university.

The license to practice medicine is granted by the regional medical council. In 2007, Brazil had 1.72 physicians per 1,000 population, 0.54 pharmaceutical personnel per 1,000, 1.15 dentistry personnel per 1,000, and 6.50 nurses and midwives per 1,000.

Government Role in Health Care

According to WHO, in 2010, Brazil spent $193 billion on health care, a total that comes to $990 per capita. Health care in Brazil was entirely paid for through domestic funding. The largest share (47 percent) was paid for by government expenditures, with the remainder (31 percent) provided by household spending and spending by other entities (22 percent). Brazil allocated 9.7 percent of government expenditures to health care spending, and government expenditures on health represented 4 percent of GDP; both figures rank Brazil low among other upper-middle-income countries in the Americas region. In 2009, according to WHO, official development assistance (ODA) for health in Brazil came to $0.16 per capita.

Public Health Programs

The Oswaldo Cruz Foundation (FIOCRUZ) in Rio de Janeiro, headed by Paulo Gadelha, promotes social development in Brazil. FIOCRUZ has over 7,500 employees and is the sentinel public entity within the Brazilian National Institute of Health. FIOCRUZ is involved with many scientific and applied activities, including research, education and training, quality control of medical products and services, and implementation of social programs. FIOCRUZ recently created five new units in impoverished areas of the country and is expanding its teaching and research programs. FIOCRUZ coordinates a National Network of Technical Schools in Health and a National Network of Health Government Schools and takes part in the National Network of Epidemiological Vigilance.

Under the leadership of FIOCRUZ, Brazil has established a network of 40 schools offering training in public health, with at least one course program offered in each of Brazil's 27 states. The training offered ranges from a six-month short course in public health to programs leading to the M.P.H., M.Sc., and Ph.D. degrees. As of 2007, Brazil had a ratio of 0.97 public health officers per 1,000 population. In 2010, access to improved sanitary facilities was much higher in urban areas (61 percent) than in rural areas (22 percent); the national average was 38 percent. Access to improved sources of drinking water was nearly universal in urban areas but only 85 percent in rural areas; the national average was 98 percent.

BRUNEI

Brunei is a southeast Asian country on the island of Borneo, sharing a border with Malaysia and a having a seacoast on the South China Sea. Total area is 2,226 square miles (5,765 square kilometers, similar to Delaware), and the July 2012 population was estimated at 408,786. In 2010, 76 percent of the population lived in urban areas, and the 2010 to 2015 annual rate of urbanization was estimated at 2.2 percent. Bandar Seri Begawan is the capital and largest city (with a 2009 population estimated at 22,000). The July 2012 population growth rate was 1.7 percent, fueled in part by a net migration rate of 2.55 migrants per 1,000 population (the 32nd-highest in the world).

Brunei became a British protectorate in 1888 and an independent country in 1984. Brunei ranked tied for 44th among 183 countries on the *Corruption Perceptions Index 2011,* with a score of 5.2 (on a scale where 0 indicates highly corrupt and 10 very clean). In 2011, Brunei was classified as a country with very high human development (the highest of four categories) on the United Nations Development

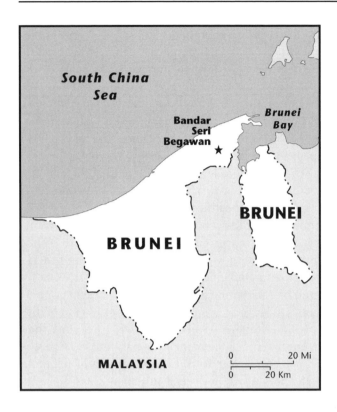

Costs of Hospitalization

No data available.

Access to Health Care

According to WHO, in 2009, 99.9 percent of births in Brunei were attended by skilled personnel (for example, physicians, nurses, or midwives). In 2009, 99 percent of pregnant women in Brunei received at least one prenatal care visit. The 2010 immunization rates for 1-year-olds were 94 percent for diphtheria and pertussis (DPT3), 95 percent for measles (MCV), and 94 percent for Hib (Hib3). According to WHO, in 2010, Brunei had 2.55 magnetic resonance imaging (MRI) machines per 1 million population and 7.65 computer tomography (CT) machines per 1 million.

Cost of Drugs

No data available.

Health Care Facilities

Brunei has four public hospitals, one private hospital, and a network of care centers including 15 regional health centers, 15 maternal health clinics, five medical centers, and mobile health clinics to serve citizens in isolated areas. In 2008, Brunei had 2.71 hospital beds per 1,000 population, and in 2010, 3.51 health posts per 100,000 population, 0.50 health centers per 100,000, 0.75 district or rural hospitals per 100,000, 0.50 provincial hospitals per 100,000, and 0.25 specialized hospitals per 100,000.

Major Health Issues

In 2008, WHO estimated that 13 percent of years of life lost in Brunei were due to communicable diseases, 71 percent to noncommunicable diseases, and 16 percent to injuries. In 2008, the age-standardized estimate of cancer deaths was 97 per 100,000 for men and 98 per 100,000 for women; for cardiovascular disease and diabetes, 293 per 100,000 for men and 275 per 100,000 for women; and for chronic respiratory disease, 69 per 100,000 for men and 44 per 100,000 for women.

The maternal mortality rate (death from any cause related to or aggravated by pregnancy) in Brunei in 2008 was 21 maternal deaths per 100,000 live births. The infant mortality rate, defined as the number of deaths of infants younger than 1 year, was 11.15 per 1,000 live births as if 2012. In 2010, tuberculosis incidence was 68.0 per 100,000 population, tuberculosis prevalence 91.0 per 100,000, and deaths due to tuberculosis among human immunodeficiency virus

Programme's (UNDP's) Human Development Index (HDI), with a score of 0.838 (on a scale where 1 denotes high development and 0 low development). Life expectancy at birth in 2012 was estimated at 76.37 years, and per capita gross domestic product (GDP) in 2011 was estimated at $49,400, among the highest in the world. According to the World Economic Forum's *Global Gender Gap Index 2011*, Brunei ranked 76th out of 135 countries on gender equality, with a score of 0.679 (on a scale with a theoretical range of 1 for equality to 0 for inequality and an actual range in 2011 from 0.8530 to 0.4873).

Emergency Health Services

According to the World Health Organization (WHO), as of 2007, Brunei had a formal and publicly available emergency care (prehospital care) system, accessible through a national universal access number.

Insurance

All residents of Brunei have access to medical benefits provided by the government, including inpatient and outpatient care by approved hospitals and providers. All residents of Brunei are covered by disability and old-age pensions, funded by contributions from wages and employers' payrolls.

(HIV)-negative people 2.70 per 100,000. As of 2009, an estimated 0.1 percent of adults age 15 to 49 were living with HIV or acquired immune deficiency syndrome (AIDS).

Health Care Personnel

Brunei has no medical schools. In 2008, Brunei had 1.42 physicians per 1,000 population, 0.11 pharmaceutical personnel per 1,000, 0.21 dentistry personnel per 1,000, and 4.88 nurses and midwives per 1,000. Many physicians and other health care personnel are foreign; in 2010, 388 foreign physicians were registered in Brunei (68.8 percent of the total), and 175 physicians were local. Among dentists, 42 were foreign (60 percent of the total) and 28 local. Among pharmacists, seven were foreign (16.3 percent of the total) and 36 local.

Government Role in Health Care

Health care in Brunei is provided by the government. According to WHO, in 2010, Brunei spent $352 million on health care, a total that comes to $882 per capita. Health care was paid for entirely through domestic funding, with the bulk (85 percent) representing government expenditures. Spending by households represented 15 percent of national expenditures on health care. Brunei allocated 8 percent of government expenditures to health care spending, and government expenditures on health represented 2 percent of GDP; both figures rank Brunei low among other high-income western Pacific region countries.

Public Health Programs

Brunei's National Health Care Plan 2000 to 2010 includes a number of public health goals, including reducing the prevalence of smoking and obesity, promoting oral and mental health, strengthening primary care, improving the quality of life for people with disabilities, and reducing sexually transmitted infections. According to the World Higher Education Database (WHED), no university in Brunei offers programs in epidemiology or public health.

BULGARIA

Bulgaria is a southeastern European country sharing borders with Greece, Macedonia, Romania, Serbia, and Turkey and having a coastline on the Black Sea. The area is 42,811 square miles (110,879 square kilometers, similar to Tennessee), and the July 2012 population was estimated at 7.0 million. In 2010, 71 percent of the population lived in urban areas, and the 2010 to 2015 annual rate of urbanization was estimated at negative 0.3 percent. Sofia is the capital and largest city (with a 2009 population estimated at 1.2 million). Bulgaria had a negative July 2012 population growth rate (negative 0.8 percent), fueled in part by a negative net migration rate (negative 2.84 migrants per 1,000 population), and a low birth rate (9.2 births per 1,000 population). The United Nations High Commissioner for Refugees (UNHCR) estimated that, in 2010, there were 5,530 refugees and persons in refugee-like situations in Bulgaria.

Bulgaria came within the Soviet sphere of influence after World War II, but Communist domination ended in 1990. Bulgaria ranked tied for 86th among 183 countries on the *Corruption Perceptions Index 2011*, with a score of 3.3 (on a scale where 0 indicates highly corrupt and 10 very clean). In 2011, Bulgaria was classified as a country with high human development (the second-highest category) on the United Nations Development Programme's (UNDP's) Human Development Index (HDI), with a score of 0.771 (on a scale where 1 denotes high development and 0 low development). Life expectancy at birth in 2012 was estimated at 73.84 years, and per capita gross domestic product (GDP) in 2011 was estimated at $13,500. In 2007, the Gini Index (a measure of dispersion, in which perfect equality is denoted by 0 and maximum inequality is denoted by 100) for family income was 45.3. According to the World Economic Forum's *Global Gender Gap Index 2011*, Bulgaria ranked 51st out of 135 countries on gender equality, with a score of 0.699 (on a scale with a theoretical range of 1 for equality to 0 for inequality and an actual range in 2011 from 0.8530 to 0.4873).

Emergency Health Services

Bulgaria's laws governing emergency health system date from the 1990s, as does Bulgarian recognition of emergency medicine as a medical specialty; by law, free access to hospitals for emergency care is provided for all persons, including the uninsured. Funding for the emergency system is provided entirely from the state budget for both in-hospital and out-of-hospital care. Bulgaria has two national telephone numbers for medical emergencies, 112 (the European Union, or EU, standard) and 150, and has 28 dispatch centers.

Insurance

Bulgaria has a social insurance system providing cash sickness and maternity benefits to employees and medical benefits to all residents. Both systems are funded by a combination of wage taxes, voluntary contributions from self-employed persons, and payroll taxes on employers. For workers, the rates are 1.4 percent of covered earnings for the cash benefit and 3.2 percent for medical benefits, with these percentages applied to earnings between BGN 240 and BGN 2,000 monthly. Self-employed people may make a voluntary contribution of 3.5 percent of declared covered earnings to be part of the social insurance system and pay 8 percent to the medical benefits system. For employers, the rate of contribution to the social insurance system is 2.1 percent, along with 4.8 percent for medical benefits.

Medical care is provided directly to patients and funded through contracts between the National Health Insurance Fund and medical institutions. Medical benefits include hospitalization, generalist and specialist care (which may be provided at home, at health care centers, or in the outpatient department of hospitals), prescription medications, dental care, and appliances. To be eligible for maternity benefits or cash sickness benefits, a person must have been covered for at least 12 months (maternity) or 6 months (sickness). The maternity benefit is 90 percent of earnings for 410 days; the sickness benefit is 80 percent of earnings for up to 90 days. Benefits are also provided for child care up to the age of 2 and for caring for a sick family member. The social insurance system is administered by the National Social Security Institute and medical benefits by the National Health Insurance Fund. According to Ke Xu and colleagues, in 2003, 2.0 percent of households in Bulgaria experienced catastrophic health expenditures annually; "catastrophic" was defined as exceeding 40 percent of household income remaining after basic needs were met.

Costs of Hospitalization

Although theoretically everyone is entitled to equal treatment within the health care system, in reality cash payments are frequently demanded in return for care, particularly for childbirth, surgery, and treatment for life-threatening conditions.

Access to Health Care

The government provides about half (54.5 percent) of the funding for health care services, with the private sector providing the remainder; almost all (98.4 percent) of private funding is out-of-pocket expenditures. The system of unofficial cash payments creates a barrier, particularly for more involved treatment, for those who cannot pay. According to the World Health Organization (WHO), in 2008, 99.6 percent of births in Bulgaria were attended by skilled personnel (for example, physicians, nurses, or midwives). The 2010 immunization rates for 1-year-olds were 94 percent for diphtheria and pertussis (DPT3), 97 percent for measles (MCV), and 91 percent for Hib (Hib3). In 2010, an estimated 24 percent of persons with advanced human immunodeficiency virus (HIV) infection were receiving antiretroviral therapy in accordance with the 2010 WHO guidelines.

Cost of Drugs

No data available.

Health Care Facilities

In 2008, Bulgaria had 6.49 hospital beds per 1,000 population, among the 30 highest ratios in the world.

Major Health Issues

In 2008, WHO estimated that 5 percent of years of life lost in Bulgaria were due to communicable diseases, 86 percent to noncommunicable diseases, and 9 percent to injuries. In 2008, the age-standardized estimate of cancer deaths was 179 per 100,000 for men and 101 per 100,000 for women; for cardiovascular disease and

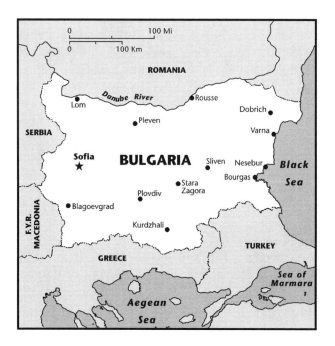

diabetes, 567 per 100,000 for men and 368 per 100,000 for women; and for chronic respiratory disease, 26 per 100,000 for men and 11 per 100,000 for women.

The maternal mortality rate (death from any cause related to or aggravated by pregnancy) in Bulgaria in 2008 was 13 maternal deaths per 100,000 live births. The infant mortality rate, defined as the number of deaths of infants younger than 1 year, was estimated at 16.13 per 1,000 live births as of 2012. In 2010, tuberculosis incidence was 40.0 per 100,000 population, tuberculosis prevalence 54.0 per 100,000, and deaths due to tuberculosis among HIV-negative people 4.20 per 100,000. An estimated 2.0 percent of new cases are multidrug resistant, as are 24 percent of retreatment cases. As of 2009, an estimated 0.1 percent of adults age 15 to 49 were living with HIV or acquired immune deficiency syndrome (AIDS).

Health Care Personnel

Bulgaria has five medical schools, located in Pleven, Sofia, Stara Zagora, Varna, and Plovdiv. The basic degree course lasts six or 6.5 years, and the degree awarded is Magister (physician). Two years of government service is required after graduation. License to practice medicine is granted to graduates of recognized medical schools (foreigners must also hold residence permits), and physicians must register with the Ministry of Health in Sofia. Bulgaria has agreements with all Newly Independent States (former members of the Soviet Union) and many other central and eastern European countries.

Bulgaria, as a member of the EU, cooperates with other countries in recognizing physicians qualified to practice in other EU countries, as specified by Directive 2005/36/EC of the European Parliament. This allows qualified professionals to practice their profession in other EU states on a temporary basis and requires that the host country automatically recognize qualifications for certain professions, including physicians, nurses, dentists, midwives, and pharmacists, if certain conditions have been met (for instance, facility in the language of the host country may be required). In 2008, Bulgaria had 3.64 physicians per 1,000 population, 0.83 dentistry personnel per 1,000, and 4.72 nurses and midwives per 1,000.

Government Role in Health Care

According to WHO, in 2010, Bulgaria spent $3.3 billion on health care, a total that comes to $435 per capita. Health care was entirely paid for through domestic funding, with the just over half (54 percent) representing government expenditures and the remainder of funding provided by spending by households (44 percent) and spending by other entities (1 percent). Bulgaria allocated 10 percent of government expenditures to health care spending, and government expenditures on health represented 4 percent of GDP; both figures rank Bulgaria low among middle- and upper-income European countries.

Public Health Programs

In 2010, access to improved sanitary facilities and improved sources of drinking water was essentially universal. According to the World Higher Education Database (WHED), two universities in Bulgaria offer programs in epidemiology or public health: the Medical University in Pleven and the Prof. Dr. Paraskev Stoyanov Medical University in Varna.

BURKINA FASO

Burkina Faso is a landlocked country in west Africa, sharing borders with Benin, Côte d'Ivoire, Ghana, Mali, Niger, and Togo. The area is 105,869 square miles (274,200 square kilometers, similar to Colorado), and the July 2012 population was estimated at 17.3 million. In 2010, 26 percent of the population lived in urban areas, and the 2010 to 2015 annual rate of urbanization was estimated at 6.2 percent. Ouagadougou is the capital and largest city, with the 2009 population estimated at 1.8 million. As of 2012, Burkina Faso had the fifth-highest birth rate in the world, at 43.20 births per 1,000 population, and the sixth-highest total fertility rate, at 6.07 children per woman; the July 2012 population growth rate was 3.1 percent, ninth-highest in the world, and the net migration rate was 0.0 migrants per 1,000 population. The United Nations High Commissioner for Refugees (UNHCR) estimated that, in 2010, there were 531 refugees and persons in refugee-like situations in Burkina Faso.

Formerly the French colony of Upper Volta, Burkina Faso became independent in 1960 and has experienced repeated military coups since then. According to the Ibrahim Index, in 2011, Burkina Faso ranked 18th among 53 African countries in terms of governance performance, with a score of 55 (out of 100). Burkina Faso ranked tied for 100th among 183

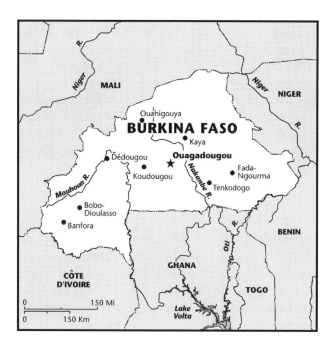

countries on the *Corruption Perceptions Index 2011,* with a score of 3.0 (on a scale where 0 indicates highly corrupt and 10 very clean).

In 2011, Burkina Faso was classified as a country with low human development (the lowest of four categories) on the United Nations Development Programme's (UNDP's) Human Development Index (HDI), with a score of 0.331 (on a scale where 1 denotes high development and 0 low development). Life expectancy at birth in 2012 was estimated at 54.07 years, among the 20 lowest in the world, and estimated gross domestic product (GDP) per capita in 2011 was $1,500, among the 30 lowest in the world. In 2007, the Gini Index (a measure of dispersion, in which perfect equality is denoted by 0 and maximum inequality is denoted by 100) for family income was 39.5. Unemployment in 2004 was estimated at 77.0 percent, among the highest rates in the world. According to the World Economic Forum's *Global Gender Gap Index 2011,* Burkina Faso ranked 115th out of 135 countries on gender equality with a score of 0.615 (on a scale with a theoretical range of 1 for equality to 0 for inequality and an actual range in 2011 from 0.8530 to 0.4873).

Emergency Health Services

According to the World Health Organization (WHO), as of 2007, Burkina Faso had a formal and publicly available emergency care (prehospital care) system, accessible through a national universal access telephone number.

Doctors Without Borders (Médecins Sans Frontières, or MSF) began working in Burkina Faso in 1995 and had 268 staff in the country at the end of 2010. One focus of MSF work is treating malaria; testing and treatment is offered to every patient at every MSF center in Burkina Faso. Childhood malnutrition is another focus: MSF operates programs aimed at children under the age of 5 in the towns of Yako and Titao and operates testing and treatment programs in 16 health centers; since 2007, 50,940 children have been treated by MSF for malnutrition.

Insurance

Burkina Faso has a social insurance program covering only maternity benefits. Only employed women are covered under the national program; the self-employed are excluded, and civil servants are covered under a separate system. The maternity benefit is 100 percent of earnings for 14 weeks; a woman must have at least three months of covered employment to receive the benefit. Insured women receive free prenatal medical care and free medical care for childbirth.

The social insurance system also provides a child supplement allowance for the first six children in a family, a constant attendant allowance if an individual requires constant care to perform the daily activities of living, and a disability pension (if an individual has lost at least two-thirds of earning capacity and has paid into the system for at least five years). Mothers and children receive some health care services under the Family Allowances law, and employers are required to provide some medical services under the labor code.

The social insurance system is managed by a board and a director, with financial supervision from the Ministry of Economy and Finance and technical supervision provided by the Ministry of Civil Service, Labor, and Social Security.

Costs of Hospitalization

No data available.

Access to Health Care

According to WHO, in 2006, 54 percent of births were attended by skilled personnel (for example, physicians, nurses, or midwives). In 2003, 18 percent of pregnant women in Burkina Faso received at least four prenatal care visits. The 2010 immunization rates for 1-year-olds were 95 percent for diphtheria and pertussis (DPT3), 94 percent for measles (MCV), and 95 percent for Hib (Hib3). In 2010, an estimated 49 percent of persons with advanced human immuno-deficiency virus (HIV) infection were receiving anti-retroviral therapy in accordance with the 2010 WHO guidelines. According to WHO, in 2010, Burkina Faso had fewer than 0.01 magnetic resonance imaging (MRI) machines per 1 million population and 0.20 computer tomography (CT) machines per 1 million.

Cost of Drugs

A 2009 survey found wide variation in the availability of drugs in Burkina Faso. In the public sector, the mean availability of generics was 73 percent, and availability of originator brands was 0.2 percent. In the private sector, the mean availability of generic medicines was 63 percent and, of originator brands, 44 percent. In the mission sector, the mean availability of generic medicines was 52 percent and, for originator brands, 2 percent. Drugs in the public sector are purchased by a procurement agency at prices close to international reference prices. However, in the private sector drugs are imported by private wholesalers at prices higher than international reference prices and then sold to pharmacies. In the public sector patients paid about 2.2 times the international reference prices for drugs, while in the private sector, the patient price was about three times the international reference price for the lowest-priced generic and 21 times the international price for originator brands. The lowest-priced generics were priced at about 2.8 times the international reference prices in the mission sector. Affordability varied widely depending on the drug required: The lowest-paid government worker would need from 0.2 to 9.7 days of wages to purchase generic medicines to treat common conditions and from 0.4 to 55.9 days of wages to purchase originator brands to treat common conditions. A 2007 study by WHO and the World Bank found that households may face catastrophic consequences due to the need to purchase medicines out of pocket.

Health Care Facilities

In 2006, Burkina Faso had 0.90 hospital beds per 1,000 population and, as of 2010, 10.35 health centers per 100,000, 0.98 district or rural hospitals per 100,000, 0.10 provincial hospitals per 100,000, and 0.02 specialized hospitals per 100,000.

Major Health Issues

In 2008, WHO estimated that 82 percent of years of life lost in Burkina Faso were due to communicable diseases, 12 percent to noncommunicable diseases, and 7 percent to injuries. In 2008, the age-standardized estimate of cancer deaths was 100 per 100,000 for men and 101 per 100,000 for women; for cardiovascular disease and diabetes, 500 per 100,000 for men and

Selected Health Indicators: Burkina Faso Compared With the Global Average (2010)

	Burkina Faso	Global Average
Male life expectancy at birth* (years)	49	66
Female life expectancy at birth* (years)	56	71
Under-5 mortality rate, both sexes (per 1,000 live births)	176	57
Adult mortality rate, both sexes* (probability of dying between 15 and 60 years per 1,000 population)	353	176
Maternal mortality ratio (per 100,000 live births)	300	210
HIV prevalence* (per 1,000 adults aged 15 to 49)	12	8
Tuberculosis prevalence (per 100,000 population)	82	178

Source: World Health Organization Global Health Observatory Data Repository.
*Data refers to 2009.

426 per 100,000 for women; and for chronic respiratory disease, 141 per 100,000 for men and 61 per 100,000 for women.

Burkina Faso's maternal mortality rate (death from any cause related to or aggravated by pregnancy) is quite high by global standards, estimated at 560 maternal deaths per 100,000 live births as of 2008. A 2006 survey estimated the prevalence of female genital mutilation at 72.5 percent. The combination of lack of skilled assistance at childbirth and child marriage leads to high rates of obstetric fistula. The infant mortality rate, defined as the number of deaths of infants younger than 1 year, is the ninth-highest in the world, at 79.84 per 1,000 live births as of 2012. Child malnutrition is a serious problem: In 2006, 37.4 percent of children under age 5 were underweight (defined as 2 kilograms [kg] below standard weight-for-age at age 1, 3 kg below for ages 2 to 3, and 4 kg below for ages 4 to 5), one of the highest rates in the world.

In 2008, the age-standardized death rate from malaria was 103.4 per 100,000 population, the fifth-highest in the world. In 2010, tuberculosis incidence was 55.0 per 100,000 population, tuberculosis prevalence 82.0 per 100,000, and deaths due to tuberculosis among HIV-negative people 8.10 per 100,000. As of 2009, an estimated 1.2 percent of adults age 15 to 49 were living with HIV or acquired immune deficiency syndrome (AIDS). As of December 2010, an estimated 60 percent of adults and 10 percent of children who needed antiretroviral therapy were receiving it.

Health Care Personnel

In 2006, WHO identified Burkina Faso as one of 57 countries with a critical deficit in the supply of skilled health workers. Burkina Faso has one medical school, the École Supérieure des Sciences de la Santé located in Ouagadougou, which began offering instruction in 1981. The basic training course lasts seven years, and the degree awarded is Doctorat d'État en Médecine (doctor of medicine). Ten years of government service is required after graduation.

Burkina Faso has agreements with France, countries from the former Soviet Union, and the member countries of the Conseil Africain et Malagache de l'Enseignement Supérieur (16 African countries who agree to recognize academic degrees granted by the other countries). The license to practice medicine is granted by the Ministry of Health, following the obligatory government service. Foreign physicians wishing to practice in Burkina Faso must hold a recognized degree and come from one of the countries with which the country has an agreement.

In 2008, Burkina Faso had 0.06 physicians per 1,000 population, 0.02 pharmaceutical personnel per 1,000, 0.04 laboratory health workers per 1,000, 0.85 health management and support workers per 1,000, and 0.73 nurses and midwives per 1,000. The global "brain drain" (international migration of skilled personnel) plays a role in the relative undersupply of medical personnel in Burkina Faso: Michael Clemens and Bunilla Petterson estimate that 20 percent of Burkina Faso-born physicians and 2 percent of Burkina Faso-born nurses are working in one of nine developed countries, primarily in France.

Government Role in Health Care

According to WHO, in 2010 Burkina Faso spent $655 million on health care, a total that comes to $40 per capita. Health care was primarily paid for through domestic funding (77 percent), with the remainder (23 percent) provided by funding from abroad. Just over half (51 percent) of spending on health care comes from government expenditure, with 36 percent representing spending by households and 13 percent spending by other entities.

Burkina Faso allocated 13 percent of government expenditures to health care spending, and government expenditures on health represented 3 percent of GDP; both figures rank Burkina Faso low among low-income African countries. In 2009, according to WHO, official development assistance (ODA) for health in Burkina Faso came to $7.33 per capita.

Public Health Programs

In 2010, 17 percent of the population of Burkina Faso had access to improved sanitary facilities, with access being higher among urban (50 percent) as opposed to rural (6 percent) populations. Access to improved sources of drinking water was much higher, with 79 percent of the population having such access (95 percent for the urban population, 73 percent for the rural). According to WHO, in 2006, Burkina Faso had fewer than 0.01 environmental and public health workers per 1,000 population. According to the World Higher Education Database (WHED), one university in Burkina Faso offers programs in epidemiology or public health: the International Centre for Research-Development of Animal Husbandry in Subhumid Zones, located in Bobo-Dioulasso.

BURUNDI

Burundi is a landlocked country in central Africa, sharing borders with Rwanda, Tanzania, and the Democratic Republic of the Congo. The area is 10,745 square miles (27,830 square kilometers, similar to Maryland), and the July 2012 population was estimated at 10.6 million. In 2010, 11 percent of the population lived in urban areas, and the 2010 to 2015 annual rate of urbanization was estimated at 4.9 percent. The capital and largest city is Bujumbura (estimated 2009 population of 455,000). The July 2012 population growth rate in Burundi was eighth-highest in the world, at 3.10 percent; the birth rate was also eighth-highest, at 40.58 per 1,000 population, and the total fertility rate was 6.08 children per women (the fifth-highest in the world). The United Nations High Commissioner for Refugees (UNHCR) estimated that, in 2010, there were 29,365 refugees and persons in refugee-like situations in Burundi and 157,167 internally displaced persons and persons in internally displaced-person-like situations.

Burundi was part of German East Africa, became a Belgian colony after World War I, and became independent in 1962. Ethnic violence between the Hutu and the Tutsi resulted two genocides and a civil war that lasted from 1993 to 2005. According to the Ibrahim Index, in 2011, Burundi ranked 36th among 53 African countries in terms of governance performance, with a score of 45 (out of 100). Corruption is perceived as a problem in Burundi: According to the *Corruption Perceptions Index 2011* Burundi ranked tied for 172nd among 183 countries in terms of perceived public-sector corruption, with a score of 1.9 (on a scale where 0 indicates highly corrupt and 10 very clean).

In 2011, Burundi was classified as a country with low human development (the lowest of four categories) on the United Nations Development Programme's (UNDP's) Human Development Index (HDI), with a score of 0.316 (on a scale where 1 denotes high development and 0 low development), the third lowest in the world. In 2011, the International Food Policy Research Institute (IFPRI) classified Burundi as a country with an "extremely alarming" hunger problem, with a Global Hunger Index (GHI) score of 37.9, the second highest in the world, and in March 2012, the World Food Programme estimated that 750,000 people in Burundi were food insecure due to weather, plant diseases, and high prices

for food. Life expectancy at birth in 2012 was estimated at 59.24 years, and estimated gross domestic product (GDP) per capita in 2011 was $400, among the 10 lowest in the world. In 1998, the Gini Index (a measure of dispersion, in which perfect equality is denoted by 0 and maximum inequality is denoted by 100) for family income was 42.4. According to the World Economic Forum's *Global Gender Gap Index 2011*, Burundi ranked 24th out of 135 countries on gender equality with a score of 0.727 (on a scale with a theoretical range of 1 for equality to 0 for inequality and an actual range in 2011 from 0.8530 to 0.4873).

Emergency Health Services

According to the World Health Organization (WHO), as of 2007, Burundi did not have a formal and publicly available system for providing prehospital care (emergency care). Doctors Without Borders (Médecins Sans Frontières, or MSF) began working in Burundi in 1992 and had 237 staff members in the country at the close of 2010. MSF operates a measles vaccination program in Burundi, supports reporting of outbreaks (including the 2010 cholera outbreak), runs malaria prevention programs, and provides free maternal and child care. MSF provides an ambulance service in Kabezi, where it also runs a medical center providing emergency obstetric and gynecological care.

Insurance

Several programs provide some medical assistance and health benefits to different populations within Burundi. A 1980 law provides medical benefits for the military and members of the civil service. A 1984 medical assistance program established a medical assistance program for the needy that provides health care, including maternity, medical, surgical, hospital, dental, and pharmaceutical services. Under the 1993 labor code, employers must provide medical care to their workers and the workers' dependents and pay sick leave at two-thirds of wages for up to three months per year. Under the same labor code, women are entitled to 12 weeks of maternity leave at 50 percent of wages, if they have been employed for at least six months.

Costs of Hospitalization

No data available.

Access to Health Care

Health workers are currently concentrated in Bujumbura, the national capital, with poor access for those

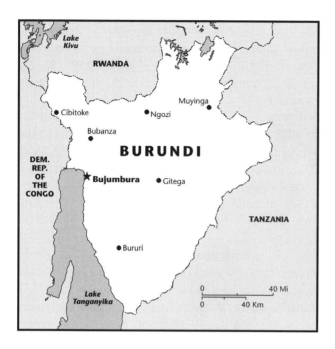

provided free of charge, including malaria, tuberculosis, sexually transmitted diseases (STDs), human immunodeficiency virus and acquired immune deficiency syndrome (HIV/AIDS), and some tropical diseases such as onchocerciasis (river blindness); vaccinations included on the WHO's Expanded Programme on Immunization (EPI) list are also provided free. Prices for drugs in Burundi are higher than international reference prices; for instance, prices for generic drugs in the public sector are 70 percent higher than international reference prices, and in the private sector, prices are more than twice as high for generics and 10 times as high as international reference prices.

Health Care Facilities
In 2006, Burundi had 0.73 hospital beds per 1,000 population, one of the 30 lowest rates in the world. As of 2010, according to WHO, Burundi had less than 0.01 health posts per 100,000 population, 6.07 health centers per 100,000, 0.39 district or rural hospitals per 100,000, 0.18 provincial hospitals per 100,000, and 0.04 specialized hospitals per 100,000.

Major Health Issues
In 2008, WHO estimated that 78 percent of years of life lost in Burundi were due to communicable diseases, 14 percent to noncommunicable diseases, and 8 percent to injuries. In 2008, the age-standardized estimate of cancer deaths was 105 per 100,000 for men and 109 per 100,000 for women; for cardiovascular disease and diabetes, 437 per 100,000 for men and 489 per 100,000 for women; and for chronic respiratory disease, 120 per 100,000 for men and 76 per 100,000 for women.

Burundi's maternal mortality rate (death from any cause related to or aggravated by pregnancy) is the sixth-highest in the world, estimated at 970 per 100,000 live births as of 2008. The infant mortality rate, defined as the number of deaths of infants younger than 1 year, has also been high, at 60.32 per 1,000 live births as of 2012. Child malnutrition is a serious problem: In 2000, 38.9 percent of children under age 5 were underweight (defined as 2 kilograms [kg] below standard weight-for-age at age 1, 3 kg below for ages 2 to 3, and 4 kg below for ages 4 to 5), one of the highest rates in the world. In 2010, tuberculosis incidence was 129.0 per 100,000 population, tuberculosis prevalence 162.0 per 100,000, and deaths due to tuberculosis among HIV-negative people 14.00 per 100,000. As of 2009, an estimated 3.3 percent of

in the hinterland; access is further hampered by poverty and an undeveloped infrastructure. Burundi's health care system also suffers from a lack of competent management staff and a poor supply system for drugs and other medical consumables. According to WHO, in 2005, 34 percent of births in Burundi were attended by skilled personnel (for example, physicians, nurses, or midwives). The 2010 immunization rates for 1-year-olds were 96 percent for diphtheria and pertussis (DPT3), 92 percent for measles (MCV), and 96 percent for Hib (Hib3). In 2010, an estimated 34 percent of persons with advanced human immunodeficiency virus (HIV) infection were receiving antiretroviral therapy in accordance with the 2010 WHO guidelines. According to WHO, in 2010, Burundi had fewer than 0.01 magnetic resonance imaging (MRI) machines per 1 million population and 0.25 computer tomography (CT) machines per 1 million.

Cost of Drugs
Burundi has a national health policy, Politique Nationale de Santé (PNS), but does not have a national drug policy, Politique Pharmaceutique Nationale (PPN). Burundi is a member of the World Trade Organization (WTO), but national law allows modifications to patent law for reasons of public health. Some individuals are eligible for free prescription medications, including children younger than 5 years, pregnant women, and the poor. Medications for some diseases are also

adults age 15 to 49 were living with HIV or AIDS. In 2010, 39 percent of pregnant women tested positive for HIV. The mother-to-child transmission rate for HIV in 2010 was estimated at 28 percent, and in 2009, 5.5 percent of deaths to children under age 5 were attributed to HIV. In 2008, the age-standardized death rate from malaria was 27.5 per 100,000 population.

Health Care Personnel

In 2006, WHO identified Burundi as one of 57 countries with a critical deficit in the supply of skilled health workers. Burundi has one medical school, the Faculté de Médecine de Bujumbura of the University of Burundi, located in Bujumbura. The language of instruction is French; the course of study is seven years, and the degree awarded is Docteur en Médecine (doctor of medicine). In 2004, Burundi had 0.03 physicians per 1,000 population, 0.01 pharmaceutical personnel per 1,000, 0.02 laboratory health workers per 1,000, 0.30 health management and support workers per 1,000, 0.09 community and traditional health workers per 1,000, and 0.19 nurses and midwives per 1.000. The global "brain drain" (international migration of skilled personnel) plays a role in the relative undersupply of medical personnel in Burundi: Michael Clemens and Bunilla Petterson estimate that 37 percent of Burundi-born physicians and 78 percent of Burundi-born nurses are working in one of nine developed countries, primarily in France, Belgium, and Canada.

Government Role in Health Care

Burundi has a National Health Development Plan (NHDP) and a long-term national health policy (for the years 2005 to 2015). The NHDP provides for a decentralized system, with community and family health services organized and funded at the district level. The NHDP addresses a number of issues, including training personnel, distributing resources throughout the country, and lowering financial barriers to care but is hampered by the poor quality of the country's infrastructure as well as its poverty.

According to WHO, in 2010, Burundi spent $174 million on health care, an amount that comes to $21 per capita. Nearly all (97 percent) of health care was funded by domestic sources, with the other 3 percent provided through funding from abroad. Most (82 percent) of the total spent on health care came from government expenditures, with the remaining 18 percent coming from spending by households. Burundi

allocated 7 percent of total government expenditures for health, and government expenditure on health represented 2 percent of GDP; both figures place Burundi in the median range of lower-middle-income African countries. In 2009, according to WHO, official development assistance (ODA) for health in Burundi came to $12.09 per capita.

Public Health Programs

In 2010, 46 percent of the population of Burundi had access to improved sanitary facilities, with access being nearly equal among urban (49 percent) and rural (46 percent) populations. Access to improved sources of drinking water was much higher, with 72 percent of the population having such access (83 percent for the urban population, 71 percent for the rural). According to the World Higher Education Database (WHED), one university in Burundi offers programs in epidemiology or public health: the University of Ngozi.

CAMBODIA

Cambodia is a southeast Asian country sharing borders with Laos, Thailand, and Vietnam and having a coastline on the Gulf of Thailand. The area is 68,153 square miles (176,515 square kilometers, similar to Oklahoma), and the July 2012 population was estimated as 15.0 million. In 2010, 20 percent of the population lived in urban areas, and the 2010 to 2015 annual rate of urbanization was estimated at 3.2 percent. The capital and largest city is Phnom Penh (with a 2009 estimated population of 1.5 million). Population growth in 2012 was 1.7 percent, the birth rate 25.2 births per 1,000 population, the net migration rate negative 0.3 migrants per 1,000, and the total fertility rate was 2.8 children per woman. The United Nations High Commissioner for Refugees (UNHCR) estimated that, in 2010, there were 129 refugees and persons in refugee-like situations in Cambodia.

Cambodia became part of French Indochina in 1887 and became independent in 1973. The country experienced much warfare from the 1970s onward, including rule by the Khmer Rouge (which killed an estimated 1.5 million Cambodians), occupation by Vietnam, and a civil war; sporadic violence continued even after the 1991 Paris Peace Accords. According to the *Corruption Perceptions Index 2011*, Cambodia ranked tied for 164th among 183 countries in terms of perceived public-sector corruption, with a score of 2.1 (on a scale where 0 indicates highly corrupt and 10 very clean).

In 2011, Cambodia was classified as a country with medium human development (the second from the lowest of four categories) on the United Nations Development Programme's (UNDP's) Human Development Index (HDI), with a score of 0.523 (on a scale where 1 denotes high development and 0 low development). However, Cambodia experienced severe flooding in September and October 2011, leaving about 60,000 households food insecure, according to the World Food Programme. Life expectancy at birth in 2012 was estimated at 63.04 years, and the estimated gross domestic (GDP) per capita in 2011 was $2,300. In 2007, the Gini Index (a measure of dispersion, in which perfect equality is denoted by 0 and maximum inequality is denoted by 100) for family income was estimated at 44.4. According to the World Economic Forum's *Global Gender Gap Index 2011*, Cambodia ranked 102nd out of 135 countries on gender equality with a score of 0.646 (on a scale with a theoretical range of 1 for equality to 0 for inequality and an actual range in 2011 from 0.8530 to 0.4873).

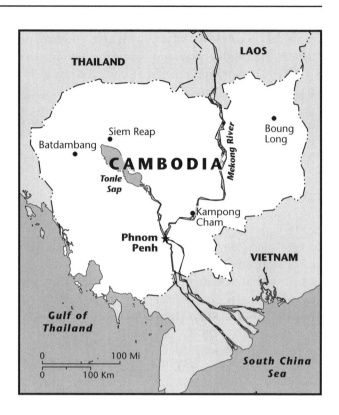

Emergency Health Services

According to the World Health Organization (WHO), as of 2007, Cambodia had a formal and publicly available emergency care (prehospital care) system, accessible through a national universal access telephone number. Doctors Without Borders (Médecins Sans Frontières, or MSF) began working in Cambodia in 1979 and had 145 staff members in the country at the close of 2010. MSF assisted in the cholera outbreaks of 2010 and helped improve the surveillance system for cholera and other infectious diseases. MSF provides human immunodeficiency virus and acquired immune deficiency syndrome (HIV/AIDS) and tuberculosis care in prisons, as well as general medical care, and is developing a comprehensive tuberculosis care program for Kampong Cham. In 2010, MSF handed over authority for general infectious disease treatment in the Khmer-Soviet Friendship Hospital to the local health care authorities.

Insurance

According to Ke Xu, in 2003, 5 percent of households in Cambodia experienced catastrophic health expenditures annually; "catastrophic" was defined as exceeding 40 percent of household income remaining after basic needs were met.

Costs of Hospitalization

No data available.

Access to Health Care

According to WHO, in 2005, 44 percent of births in Cambodia were attended by skilled personnel (for example, physicians, nurses, or midwives). In 2005, 27 percent of pregnant women in Cambodia received at least four prenatal care visits. The 2010 immunization rates for 1-year-olds were 92 percent for diphtheria and pertussis (DPT3), 93 percent for measles (MCV), and 92 percent for Hib (Hib3). In 2010, an estimated 92 percent of persons with advanced HIV infection were receiving antiretroviral therapy in accordance with the 2010 WHO guidelines. According to WHO, in 2010, Cambodia had 0.07 magnetic resonance imaging (MRI) machines per 1 million population, 1.24 computer tomography (CT) machines per 1 million, 0.07 telecolbalt units per 1 million, and 0.07 radiotherapy machines per 1 million.

Cost of Drugs

No data available.

Health Care Facilities

French colonists created a medical service in Cambodia in the mid-19th century to provide services for themselves; these services were centered in Phnom Penh. After independence, health care services were expanded, but the civil war and Vietnamese invasion damaged the infrastructure and resulted in the death or emigration of much of the trained medical corps. The health system has been improved since the signing of the Paris Peace Agreement in 1991, but as of 2004, Cambodia had 0.10 hospital beds per 1,000 population, one of the 10 lowest rates in the world. As of 2010, according to WHO, Cambodia had 0.80 health posts per 100,000 population, 7.02 health centers per 100,000, 0.43 district or rural hospitals per 100,000, 0.12 provincial hospitals per 100,000, and 0.06 specialized hospitals per 100,000.

Major Health Issues

In 2008, WHO estimated that 60 percent of years of life lost in Cambodia were due to communicable diseases, 30 percent to noncommunicable diseases, and 10 percent to injuries. In 2008, the age-standardized estimate of cancer deaths was 145 per 100,000 for men and 90 per 100,000 for women; for cardiovascular disease and diabetes, 480 per 100,000 for men and 339 per 100,000 for women; and for chronic respiratory disease, 129 per 100,000 for men and 60 per 100,000 for women.

Cambodia's maternal mortality rate (death from any cause related to or aggravated by pregnancy) was estimated in 2008 as 290 maternal deaths per 100,000 live births. The infant mortality rate, defined as the number of deaths of infants younger than 1 year, has been high, estimated at 54.08 per 1,000 live births in 2012. Child malnutrition is a serious problem: In 2008, 28.8 percent of children under age 5 were underweight (defined as 2 kilograms [kg] below standard weight-for-age at age 1, 3 kg below for ages 2 to 3, and 4 kg below for ages 4 to 5), one of the 20 highest rates in the world.

In 2010, tuberculosis incidence was 437.0 per 100,000 population, tuberculosis prevalence 660.0 per 100,000, and deaths due to tuberculosis among HIV-negative people 61.00 per 100,000. WHO estimated that the case detection rate in 2010 was 65 percent. As of 2009, an estimated 0.5 percent of adults age 15 to 49 were living with HIV or AIDS. In 2008, the age-standardized death rate from malaria was 3.3 per 100,000 population.

Health Care Personnel

In 2006, WHO identified Cambodia as one of 57 countries with a critical deficit in the supply of skilled health workers. Cambodia has two medical schools, the University of Health and Sciences in Phnom Penh, which began offering instruction in 1980, and the Faculty of Health Sciences of International University, also located in Phnom Penh, which began offering instruction in 2002. The basic training course lasts seven years, and the degree awarded is doctor of medicine. One year of government service is required after graduation. Physicians must register with the Ministry of Health in Phnom Penh. In 2008, Cambodia had 0.23 physicians per 1,000 population, 0.04 pharmaceutical personnel per 1,000, 0.02 dentistry personnel per 1,000, 0.11 community and traditional health workers per 1,000, and 0.79 nurses and midwives per 1,000.

Government Role in Health Care

According to WHO, in 2010, Cambodia spent $639 million on health care, an amount that comes to $45 per capita. Just over three-quarters (76 percent) of health care was funded from domestic sources, with the other 24 percent provided through funding from abroad. The largest share of spending on health care was provided by households (40 percent), followed by government expenditures (37 percent) and other expenditures (22 percent). Cambodia allocated 10 percent of total government expenditures for health, and government expenditure on health represented 2 percent of GDP; both figures place Cambodia in the median range of low-income western Pacific region countries. In 2009, according to WHO, official development assistance (ODA) for health in Cambodia came to $12.75 per capita.

Public Health Programs

Cambodia's National Institute of Public Health (NIPH) is located in Phnom Penh and is headed by Ung Sam An. NIPH is part of the Ministry of Health and conducts research as well as works with the provincial administrations. NIPH's activities include training key personnel in public health, analyzing health-related problems, developing interventions, and helping to implement reforms of the health care system. For instance, NIPH is currently developing a pilot project to improve maternal and child health in three underserved provinces by distributing vouchers good for medical care. NIPH also works cooperatively with many international organizations and foundations, including the U.S. Centers for

Disease Control and Prevention (CDC), the U.S. Rockefeller Foundation, and WHO. The National Public Health Laboratory (NPHL) acts as the national reference lab and also provides clinical lab services, supports epidemiology research, and performs quality assessment at the regional level.

In 2010, 31 percent of the population of Cambodia had access to improved sanitary facilities, with access higher among the urban (73 percent) as opposed to the rural (20 percent) population. Access to improved sources of drinking water was higher, although far from universal, with 64 percent of the population having such access (87 percent for the urban population, 58 percent for the rural). According to the World Higher Education Database (WHED), no university in Cambodia offers programs in epidemiology or public health.

CAMEROON

Cameroon is a west African country sharing borders with Nigeria, Chad, the Central African Republic, the Republic of the Congo, Gabon, and Equatorial Guinea. The area is 183,568 square miles (475,440 square kilometers, a bit larger than California), and the July 2012 population was estimated at 20.1 million. In 2010, 58 percent of the population lived in urban areas, and the 2010 to 2015 annual rate of urbanization was estimated at 3.3 percent. Yaoundé is the capital, and Douala the largest city (with a 2009 estimated population of 2.0 million). The July 2012 population growth rate was 2.1 percent; the birth rate was 32.5 births per 1,000 population, the net migration rate 0.0 migrants per 1,000, and the total fertility rate 4.1 children per woman. The United Nations High Commissioner for Refugees (UNHCR) estimated that, in 2010, there were 104,275 refugees and persons in refugee-like situations in Cameroon.

Cameroon was a French colony before becoming independent in 1960, and in 1961, it merged with the southern part of British Cameroon to become the Federal Republic of Cameroon. The country has generally enjoyed stability, allowing development of infrastructure and the economy, including a petroleum industry. According to the Ibrahim Index, in 2011, Cameroon ranked 36th among 53 African countries in terms of governance performance, with a score of 45 (out

of 100). Cameroon ranked tied for 134th among 183 countries on the *Corruption Perceptions Index 2011*, with a score of 2.5 (on a scale where 0 indicates highly corrupt and 10 very clean).

In 2011, Cameroon was classified as a country with low human development (the lowest of four categories) on the United Nations Development Programme's (UNDP's) Human Development Index (HDI), with a score of 0.482 (on a scale where 1 denotes high development and 0 low development). Life expectancy at birth in 2012 was estimated at 54.71 years, among the 30 lowest in the world, and estimated gross domestic product (GDP) per capita in 2011 was $2,300. In 2001, the Gini Index (a measure of dispersion, in which perfect equality is denoted by 0 and maximum inequality is denoted by 100) for family income was 44.6. Unemployment in 2001 was estimated at 30 percent. According to the World Economic Forum's *Global Gender Gap Index 2011*, Cameroon ranked 119th out of 135 countries on gender equality with a score of 0.607 (on a scale with a theoretical range of 1 for equality to 0 for inequality and an actual range in 2011 from 0.8530 to 0.4873).

Emergency Health Services

According to the World Health Organization (WHO), as of 2007, Cameroon had a formal and publicly available emergency care (prehospital care) system, accessible through a national universal access telephone number. Doctors Without Borders (Médecins Sans Frontières, or MSF) began working in Cameroon in 2000 and had 68 staff members in the country at the close of 2010. MSF runs a pilot program in Douala that helps people treated with antiretrovirals switch to second-line therapy, as a previous MSF study demonstrated that about 10 percent of patients become resistant to antiretrovirals after extended treatment with them. Since 2002, MSF has operated a program in Akonolinga, central Cameroon, to combat Buruli ulcer, and MSF also helped with cholera treatment during the severe epidemic that broke out in northern Cameroon in May 2010.

Insurance

Cameroon has social insurance that provides only maternity benefits and only for employed women. Insured women and the wives of insured men are provided with 100 percent of earnings for four weeks before and 10 weeks after birth; the latter period can be extended to 13 weeks if there are birth complications.

To receive this benefit, the insured person must have been employed for at least the prior six months. Employers are required to provide some medical services, and some free medical care is provided through government health facilities. The Family Allowances program provides some medical services to mothers and children. Both social insurance and the Family Allowances program are financed through employer payroll contributions. The National Social Insurance Fund is managed by a director general and council under the general supervision of the Ministry of Labor and Social Security.

Costs of Hospitalization
No data available.

Access to Health Care
According to the World Health Organization (WHO), in 2006, 59 percent of births in Cameroon were attended by skilled personnel (for example, physicians, nurses, or midwives). In 2004, 60 percent of pregnant women received at least four prenatal care visits. The 2010 immunization rates for 1-year-olds were 84 percent for diphtheria and pertussis (DPT3), 79 percent for measles (MCV), and 84 percent for Hib (Hib3). In 2010, an estimated 38 percent of persons with advanced human immunodeficiency virus (HIV) infection were receiving antiretroviral therapy in accordance with the 2010 WHO guidelines. According to WHO, in 2010, Cameroon had 0.05 magnetic resonance imaging (MRI) machines per 1 million population, 0.73 computer tomography (CT) machines per 1 million, 0.16 telecolbalt units per 1 million, and 0.16 radiotherapy machines per 1 million.

Cost of Drugs
According to WHO, in 2005, the median availability of selected generic drugs in the public sector in Cameroon was 58.3 percent; in the private sector, the mean availability was 52.5 percent. The median price ratio (comparing the price in Cameroon to the international reference price) was 2.2 in the public sphere for selected generic medicines and 13.6 in the private sphere, meaning that median prices in the public sphere were over twice as high, and in the private sphere, over 12 times as high as the international reference price.

Health Care Facilities
In 2006, Cameroon had 1.50 hospital beds per 1,000 population. As of 2010, according to WHO, Cameroon

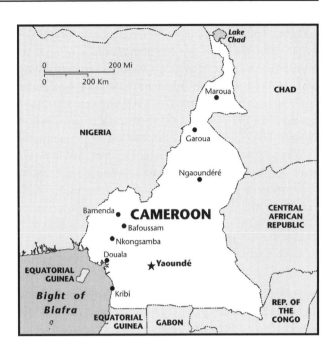

had 8.43 health posts per 100,000 population, 0.72 health centers per 100,000, 0.77 district or rural hospitals per 100,000, 0.09 provincial hospitals per 100,000, and 0.05 specialized hospitals per 100,000.

Major Health Issues
In 2008, WHO estimated that 77 percent of years of life lost in Cameroon were due to communicable diseases, 17 percent to noncommunicable diseases, and 7 percent to injuries. In 2008, the age-standardized estimate of cancer deaths was 84 per 100,000 for men and 77 per 100,000 for women; for cardiovascular disease and diabetes, 472 per 100,000 for men and 523 per 100,000 for women; and for chronic respiratory disease, 131 per 100,000 for men and 85 per 100,000 for women.

Cameroon's maternal mortality rate (death from any cause related to or aggravated by pregnancy) has been quite high by global standards, estimated at 600 maternal deaths per 100,000 live births in 2008. A 2004 survey estimated the prevalence of female genital mutilation at 1.4 percent. The infant mortality rate, defined as the number of deaths of infants younger than 1 year, also has been high, at 59.70 per 1,000 live births as of 2012. In 2006, 16.6 percent of children under age 5 were underweight (defined as 2 kilograms [kg] below standard weight-for-age at age 1, 3 kg below for ages 2 to 3, and 4 kg below for ages 4 to 5).

In 2010, tuberculosis incidence was 177.0 per 100,000 population, tuberculosis prevalence 185.0 per

100,000, and deaths due to tuberculosis among HIV-negative people 14.0 per 100,000. As of 2009, an estimated 5.3 percent of adults age 15 to 49 were living with HIV or acquired immune deficiency syndrome (AIDS). In 2010, 41 percent of pregnant women tested positive for HIV. The mother-to-child transmission rate for HIV in 2010 was estimated at 33 percent, and in 2009, 19 percent of deaths to children under age 5 were attributed to HIV. Malaria remains endemic in Cameroon, and in 2008, the age-standardized death rate from malaria was 73.0 per 100,000 population.

Health Care Personnel

In 2006, WHO identified Cameroon as one of 57 countries with a critical deficit in the supply of skilled health workers. Cameroon has one medical school, the Faculté de Médecine et des Sciences Biomédicales of the University of Yaoundé, which began offering instruction in 1969. The basic medical degree course lasts seven years, and the degree awarded is Docteur en Médecine. Physicians must register with the Ordre ational des Médecines in Yaoundé, and those who attended a foreign medical school must also provide a certificate of equivalence for their degrees. Cameroon has informal agreements with France and the United Kingdom (UK).

In 2004, Cameroon had 0.19 physicians per 1,000 population, 0.04 pharmaceutical personnel per 1,000, 0.11 laboratory health workers per 1,000, 0.36 dentistry personnel per 1,000, and 1.60 nurses and midwives per 1,000. The global "brain drain" (international migration of skilled personnel) plays a role in the relative undersupply of medical personnel in Cameroon: Michael Clemens and Bunilla Petterson estimate that 46 percent of Cameroon-born physicians and 19 percent of Cameroon-born nurses are working in one of nine developed countries, primarily in France, Belgium, the United States, and the UK.

Government Role in Health Care

Access to essential medicines is recognized as a right by national legislation. Cameroon has a list of essential medications (EMI), created in 2009, that includes about 400 medications. Cameroon also has a national pharmaceuticals policy, created in 2005; it covers a selection of EMI; financing, pricing, purchase, distribution, and regulation of drugs; pharmacovigilance; rational usage of medicines; human resource development; research; monitoring and evaluation; and traditional medicine. Cameroon is a member of the World Trade Organization (WTO) but allows

for several exceptions to patent regulation, including compulsory licensing for reasons of public health, the Bolar exception that allows manufacturers to perform research and testing to create generic drugs before a patent has expired, and parallel importing provisions (allowing import of drugs created for sale in a different country).

According to WHO, in 2010, Cameroon spent $1.2 billion on health care, an amount that comes to $61 per capita. Most (87 percent) of health care was funded from domestic sources, with the remaining 13 percent provided through funding from abroad. Household spending represented 66 percent of total health care spending, followed by government expenditures (30 percent) and other expenditures (4 percent). Cameroon allocated 9 percent of total government expenditures for health, and government expenditure on health represented 2 percent of GDP; both figures place Cameroon in the median range of lower-middle-income African countries. In 2009, according to WHO, official development assistance (ODA) for health in Cameroon came to $4.57 per capita.

Public Health Programs

In 2010, 49 percent of the population of Cameroon had access to improved sanitary facilities, with access being higher among the urban (58 percent) as opposed to the rural (36 percent) population. Access to improved sources of drinking water was higher, although far from universal, with 77 percent of the population having such access (95 percent for the urban population, 52 percent for the rural).

According to WHO, in 2004, Cameroon had fewer than 0.01 environmental and public health workers per 1,000 population. According to the World Higher Education Database (WHED), one university in Cameroon offers programs in epidemiology or public health: the University of Yaoundé.

CANADA

Canada is a North American country sharing a border with the United States (the world's longest unfortified land border). With an area of 3,855103 square miles (9,984,670 square kilometers), Canada is the second-largest country in the world; the population of 34.3 million is located primarily in the southern part of the country, within 99 mi. (160 km) of the U.S. border. In 2010, 81 percent of the population lived in urban areas, and the 2010 to 2015 annual rate of urbanization is estimated at 1.1 percent. Ottawa is the capital and Toronto the largest city (with a 2009 population estimated at 5.4 million). The July 2012 population growth rate was 0.8 percent, the birth rate 10.3 births per 1,000 population, the net migration rate 5.6 migrants per 1,000 (the 18th-highest in the world), and the total fertility rate 1.6 children per woman. The United Nations High Commissioner for Refugees (UNHCR) estimated that, in 2010, there were 165,549 refugees and persons in refugee-like situations in Canada.

Canada became a self-governing British dominion in 1867; among other provinces, it includes one with a French-speaking majority, Quebec. The Canadian government is noted for transparency and honesty: Canada ranked near the top (10th among 183 countries on the *Corruption Perceptions Index 2011,* with a score of 8.7 (on a scale where 0 indicates highly corrupt and 10 very clean). Canada ranked sixth (tied with Ireland) in 2011 on the United Nations Development Programme's (UNDP's) Human Development Index (HDI), with a score of 0.908 (on a scale where 1 denotes high development and 0 low development). Life expectancy at birth in 2012 was estimated at 81.48 years, among the highest in the world, and per capita gross domestic product (GDP) in 2011 was estimated at $40,300. In 2005, the Gini Index (a measure of dispersion, in which perfect equality is denoted by 0 and maximum inequality is denoted by 100) for family income was 32.1. According to the World Economic Forum's *Global Gender Gap Index 2011,* Canada ranked 18th out of 135 countries on gender equality with a score of 0.741 (on a scale with a theoretical range of 1 for equality to 0 for inequality and an actual range in 2011 from 0.8530 to 0.4873).

Emergency Health Services

Canada was one of the first countries to recognize emergency medicine as a specialty and to develop formal emergency medicine training programs; by 1982, there were six training programs for emergency medicine in Canada, and 27 by 2000, graduating about 100 physicians annually. In Canada, after-hours care is provided primarily in hospital emergency rooms and through walk-in clinics. Physicians are generally not required to provide after-hours care (although this is required in some group practices); a 2009 Commonwealth Fund Survey found that less than

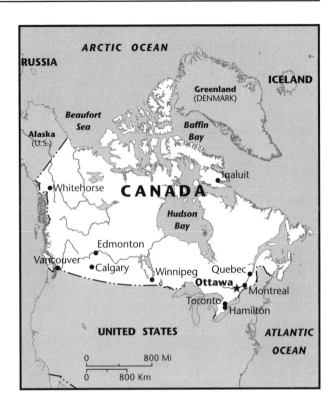

half (43 percent) of Canadian physician practices had an after-hours arrangement for their patients. Most walk-in, after-hours, and urgent care clinics are privately owned, and availability of after-hours care in 2009 ranged from 34 percent (Quebec) to 88 percent (Saskatchewan and Alberta). Most areas in Canada have Telehealth, a 24-hour free telephone service providing contact with a registered nurse for health advice. According to the World Health Organization (WHO), as of 2007, the emergency care (prehospital care) system in Canada included a national universal access telephone number.

Insurance

Canada has a universal public health program (called Medicare) that is administered at a regional level and financed through a combination of federal and provincial tax revenues. As a general rule, anyone residing in Canada is covered, although generally undocumented immigrants or those who have entered the country illegally are not covered; eligibility in such cases is determined at the provincial or territorial level. Canadians are allowed to purchase additional insurance that provides extra benefits, and approximately two-thirds do so. There are no caps on out-of-pocket spending; exemptions regarding cost sharing

Selected Health Indicators: Canada Compared With the Organisation for Economic Co-operation and Development (OECD) Country Average

	Canada	OECD average (2010 or nearest year)
Out-of-pocket expenditure on health (percent total expenditure on health), 2010	14.2	19.5
Out-of-pocket expenditure on health (per capita, USD purchasing power parity), 2010	630.8	558.4
Total expenditure on health (percent of GDP), 2010	11.4	9.5
Total expenditure on health (per capita, USD purchasing power parity), 2010	4,444.9	3,265
Public expenditure on health (per capita, USD purchasing power parity), 2010	3,158.2	2,377.8
Public expenditure on health (percent total expenditure on health), 2010	71.1	72.2
Hospital discharge rates, all causes (per 100,000 population), 2009	8,260.4	15,508
Average length of hospital stay, all causes (days), 2009	7.7	7.1

Source: OECD Health Data 2012 (Organisation for Economic Co-operation and Development, 2012).

(for example, for the elderly or low-income persons) are determined at the provincial level.

Primary care is paid for primarily on a fee-for-service basis, with some alternatives such as capitation and pay for performance also used. From 2007 to 2008, almost one-fourth (24 percent) of physician payments were made through arrangements other than fee for service. Some provinces offer pay-for-performance incentives; for instance, Ontario provides preventive care bonuses to physicians who surpass specified thresholds for screenings and immunizations. Hospital payments are handled through a combination of global budgets and, in some provinces, case-based payments; hospital payments do not include physician costs. Most patients are not required to register with a general practice physician, although this is required in some capitation models. However, most Canadians have family physicians that are the first contact with the health care system.

Medicare generally does not provide coverage for optometry or dental services, which are paid for primarily out of pocket or through private insurance; only 5 percent of dental costs in 2008 were paid for through public funds, as were 8 percent of vision care services.

Mental health care provided by a physician is universally covered, while allied health services are covered to varying degrees. Most social workers are salaried and work for government facilities or donation-supported agencies, although an increasing number are entering private practice. According to Ke Xu, in 2003, less than 0.1 percent of households in Canada experienced catastrophic health expenditures annually; "catastrophic" was defined as exceeding 40 percent of household income remaining after basic needs were met.

Costs of Hospitalization

According to Organisation for Economic Co-operation and Development (OECD) data, in 2009, hospital spending per capita in Canada was $1,223 (adjusted for differences in the cost of living), and hospital spending per discharge came to $13,483 in 2011. The average length of stay in acute care was 7.7 days (in 2009), and there were 84 hospital discharges per 1,000 population.

Access to Health Care

In 2009, according to OECD data, Canadians had an average of 6.5 physician visits. In 2010, almost half (45 percent) of Canadians reported that, when sick, they were able to get a medical appointment the same day or the next day. However, a higher proportion (65 percent) reported it was very or somewhat difficult to get medical care after usual office hours. For those who needed particular types of care, 41 percent reported they waited two or more months to see a specialist (of those who needed to see a specialist in the prior two years), 25 percent reported waiting four or more months for elective surgery (of those who required elective surgery in the prior two years), and 15 percent reported they had experienced an access barrier due to cost in the previous two years; an access barrier was defined as failing to fill or refill a prescription, failing to visit a physician, or failing to get recommended care. In 2010, 17 percent of Canadians reported experiencing a medical, medication, or lab test error in the previous two years, and 16 percent of those who needed to visit a specialist in the previous two years reported that the specialist did not have information about their medical history at the time of the appointment. However, 50 percent reported experiencing a gap in hospital discharge planning in the previous two years (either they did not receive a written plan for care, did not have arrangements made for follow-up visits, did not know whom to contact with questions, or did not receive instruction about when to seek further care).

Most acute care hospitals are not-for-profit and owned by governments, universities, religious organizations, and so on. Hospital annual budgets are usually negotiated with the regional health authority or the ministry of health for the province or territory, although recently some provinces have begun to provide activity-based funding as well, in some cases as part of an effort to reduce national wait times for services such as cataract surgery. According to WHO, in 2010, Canada had 6.67 magnetic resonance imaging (MRI) machines per 1 million population, 12.60 computer tomography (CT) machines per 1 million, and 0.93 positron emission tomography (PET) machines per 1,000,000.

A 2011 Commonwealth Fund Survey compared access to health care for sicker adults (those 18 and older in self-reported poor or fair health who had been treated for a serious illness or injury in the past year or been hospitalized in the past two years) in 11 OECD countries. This survey found that 20 percent of sicker Canadians surveyed reported having experienced access problems related to cost in the previous year; the most common result was failing to fill a prescription or skipping doses of a prescribed drug. Other problems reported include having serious problems paying their medical bills (8 percent), waiting six days or longer for needed care (22 percent), having difficulty getting after-hours care except in an emergency room (63 percent, the highest percentage of the 11 countries surveyed), and experiencing coordination gaps in care (40 percent).

According to WHO, in 2007, 100 percent of births in Canada were attended by skilled personnel (for example, physicians, nurses, or midwives). The 2010 immunization rates for 1-year-olds were 80 percent for diphtheria and pertussis (DPT3), 93 percent for measles (MCV), and 80 percent for Hib (Hib3).

Cost of Drugs

An independent body, the Patented Medicine Prices Review Board (PMPRB), regulates the factory gate prices of new medicines, but does not regulate the prices charged in pharmacies or by wholesalers. The PMPRB sets price levels based on the prices of comparable drugs in seven other countries, including the United States and the United Kingdom (UK). Prices for generic drugs are determined at the provincial level. In 2009, Canada established the Drug Safety and Effectiveness Network to inform decision making regarding prescription drugs by funding studies of the safety and effectiveness of pharmaceuticals already on the market. Real annual growth in pharmaceutical expenditures in Canada grew 7.3 percent in the years 1997 through 2005, faster than the 4.4 percent growth of total health expenditures (minus pharmaceutical expenditures) over those years.

Medicare covers the cost of prescription drugs used within hospitals, and coverage for drugs in other settings is determined at the provincial or territorial level. All provinces offer drug coverage for individuals receiving social assistances, and all provinces and territories offer drug coverage plans for people age 65 and over. Almost half (46 percent) of all spending on prescription drugs in Canada in 2009 was paid for through public expenditures. In 2009, according to OECD data, pharmaceutical spending per capita in Canada was $744 (adjusted for differences in the cost of living). According to Elizabeth Docteur, in 2004, generic drugs represented 16 percent of the market share by value and 41 percent of the market share by volume of the total pharmaceutical market.

As of 2011, Canada did not charge a value-added tax (VAT) for reimbursed medicines. The pharmacy dispensing fee varies depending on the specific drug plan and region of the country, as does the pharmacy markup. Wholesale markup is capped and averages 5 percent but depends on the specific drug plan and region of the country.

Health Care Facilities
In 2008, Canada had 3.40 hospital beds per 1,000 population. Canada has been relatively slow to implement electronic medical records, and the rate of uptake varies widely across the country. In 2009, about one-third (37 percent) of primary care physicians in Canada used electronic medical records. As of 2010, according to WHO, Canada had 0.88 district or rural hospitals per 100,000, 1.33 provincial hospitals per 100,000, and 0.14 specialized hospitals per 100,000.

Major Health Issues
In 2008, WHO estimated that 6 percent of years of life lost in Canada were due to communicable diseases, 79 percent to noncommunicable diseases, and 14 percent to injuries. In 2008, the age-standardized estimate of cancer deaths was 142 per 100,000 for men and 107 per 100,000 for women; for cardiovascular disease and diabetes, 152 per 100,000 for men and 90 per 100,000 for women; and for chronic respiratory disease, 27 per 100,000 for men and 16 per 100,000 for women.

The maternal mortality rate (death from any cause related to or aggravated by pregnancy) in Canada in 2008 was 12 maternal deaths per 100,000 live births. The infant mortality rate, defined as the number of deaths of infants younger than 1 year, was 4.85 per 1,000 live births in 2012. In 2010, tuberculosis incidence was 4.7 per 100,000 population, tuberculosis prevalence 5.6 per 100,000, and deaths due to tuberculosis among human immunodeficiency virus (HIV)-negative people 0.23 per 100,000. As of 2009, an estimated 0.3 percent of adults age 15-49 were living with HIV or acquired immune deficiency syndrome (AIDS). In 2004, an estimated 23.1 percent of adults in Canada were obese (defined as a body mass index, or BMI, of 30 or greater).

Health disparities are an issue in Canada: Certain groups, including the poor, the homeless, and aboriginal populations, suffer from a higher disease burden than other Canadians. In 2004, the Canadian government created the Public Health Agency of Canada to address population health issues, including disparities, and several provinces have also established agencies whose purposes include addressing health disparities.

In 2005, the federal government established the Aboriginal Health Transition Fund to improve access to health services for aboriginal Canadians.

Health Care Personnel
Canada has 16 medical schools that offer instruction in English or French. The basic medical training course lasts three to four years, and the degree awarded is doctor of medicine (M.D.) or Docteur en Médecine. Physicians must register with the Medical Council of Canada, while the license to practice is granted by the provincial licensing authorities after passage of a qualifying examination and completion of at least two years of postgraduate training. Canada and the United States have an agreement to mutually recognize medical degrees granted in either country. In 2006, Canada had 1.91 physicians per 1,000 population, 0.83 pharmaceutical personnel per 1,000, 1.12 laboratory health workers per 1,000, 0.10 health management and support workers per 1,000, 1.18 dentistry personnel per 1,000, and 10.05 nurses and midwives per 1,000. In 2000, 20.6 percent of practicing physicians in Canada were trained in another country, primarily the UK, South Africa, and India. However, in recent years more Canadian-trained physicians have emigrated from Canada than have immigrated to the country.

Government Role in Health Care
According to WHO, in 2010, Canada spent $178 million on health care, an amount that comes to $5,222 per capita. Canadian health care was entirely funded through domestic sources, with government expenditures providing 70 percent of total spending, followed by spending by households (15 percent) and other expenditures (15 percent). Household spending represented 66 percent of total health care spending, followed by government expenditures (30 percent) and other expenditures (4 percent). In 2009, Canada allocated 18.3 percent of total government expenditure to health, and in 2010, government expenditures on health came to 8 percent of GDP; the latter ranks high among high-income countries in the Americas region.

Public Health Programs
The Public Health Agency of Canada (PHAC) is located in Ottawa and is directed by David Butler-Jones. PHAC, created in 2004 in the wake of the severe acute respiratory syndrome (SARS) epidemic, is the leading public health institute in Canada and

has more than 2,400 members; its goals are to prevent disease and minimize avoidable injuries, build health capacity, and prepare for and respond to public health emergencies, such as infectious disease outbreaks and food-borne illness. PHAC conducts many campaigns to encourage good health practices among Canadians; for instance, it recently updated Canada's Physical Activity Guides for different age groups. According to the World Higher Education Database (WHED), 34 universities in Canada offer programs in epidemiology or public health. Access to improved sanitary facilities and improved sources of drinking water is essentially universal in Canada. According to WHO, in 2004, Canada had 0.04 environmental and public health workers per 1,000 population.

CAPE VERDE

Cape Verde is an island nation (consisting of 10 major islands and numerous smaller ones) in the North Atlantic off the western coast of Africa. The area is 1,557 square miles (4,033 square kilometers, a bit smaller than Rhode Island), and the July 2012 population was estimated as 523,568. Praia is the capital and largest city, with a 2009 population estimated at 125,000. The net migration rate in 2012 was negative 0.66 migrants per 1,000 people, the population growth rate 1.4 percent, the birth rate 21.2 births per 1,000 population, and the total fertility rate 2.4 children per woman.

Cape Verde was a Portuguese colony, serving as a trading center for slaves from Africa and a resupply stop for shipping; it became independent in 1975. Cape Verde has enjoyed one of Africa's most stable democratic governments, although the country has suffered economic hardship due to repeated drought, encouraging emigration and creating a large expatriate population. According to the Ibrahim Index, in 2011, Cape Verde ranked second among 53 African countries in terms of governance performance, with a score of 79 (out of 100). Cape Verde ranked tied for 41st among 183 countries on the *Corruption Perceptions Index 2011,* with a score of 5.5 (on a scale where 0 indicates highly corrupt and 10 very clean).

In 2011, Cape Verde was classified as a country with medium human development (the second from the lowest of four categories) on the United Nations Development Programme's (UNDP's) Human Development Index (HDI), with a score of 0.556 (on a scale where 1 denotes high development and 0 low development). Life expectancy at birth in 2012 was estimated at 71.0 years, and estimated gross domestic product (GDP) per capita in 2011 was $4,000. Unemployment in 2000 was estimated at 21.0 percent.

Emergency Health Services
According to the World Health Organization (WHO), as of 2007, Cape Verde did not have a formal and publicly available system for providing prehospital care (emergency care).

Insurance
Cape Verde has a social insurance system providing cash sickness and maternity benefits and covering employees in the public and private sectors; self-employed people, cooperative employees, and business owners can enroll voluntarily. Those in the social insurance program are also covered for medical benefits, as are a broad class of individuals, including pensioners and recipients of social insurance benefits. The system is funded through employee and employer contributions (4 percent of gross monthly earnings and 4 percent of gross monthly payroll, respectively). The maternity cash benefit is 90 percent of earnings for up to 60 days; the sickness cash benefit is 100 percent of earnings for the first three days (paid by the employer) and 70 percent of earnings for up to 1,095 days (paid by the National Social Insurance Institute). Medical benefits include medical and dental care, hospitalization, surgery, lab services, medications, home medical visits, and prostheses. Different levels of cost sharing apply to different services. The National Health Service administers the program, the National Social Insurance Institute pays the benefits, and the Ministry of Health provides general supervision.

Costs of Hospitalization
No data available.

Access to Health Care
According to WHO, in 2005, 78 percent of births in Cape Verde were attended by skilled personnel (for example, physicians, nurses, or midwives). In 2006, 72 percent of pregnant women in Cape Verde received at least four prenatal care visits. The 2010 immunization rates for 1-year-olds were 99 percent for diphtheria and pertussis (DPT3) and 96 percent for measles (MCV). In 2010, an estimated 43 percent of persons

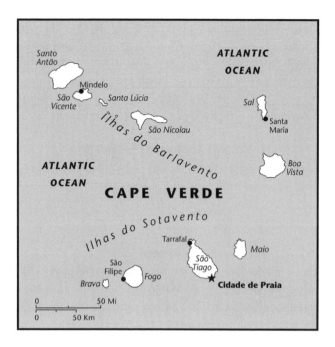

with advanced human immunodeficiency virus (HIV) infection were receiving antiretroviral therapy in accordance with the 2010 WHO guidelines. According to WHO, in 2010, Cape Verde had fewer than 0.01 magnetic resonance imaging (MRI) machines per 1 million population and 2.01 computer tomography (CT) machines per 1 million.

Cost of Drugs

A legal schedule specifies the share (15 to 50 percent) of the cost of medicines that is paid by individuals, with lower rates for pensioners; medicines are free to low-income pensioners.

Health Care Facilities

As of 2010, according to WHO, Cape Verde had 33.67 health posts per 100,000 population, 3.83 health centers per 100,000, 0.60 district or rural hospitals per 100,000, less than 0.01 provincial hospitals per 100,000, and 0.40 specialized hospitals per 100,000. In 2009, Cape Verde had 2.07 hospital beds per 1,000 population.

Major Health Issues

In 2008, WHO estimated that 43 percent of years of life lost in Cape Verde were due to communicable diseases, 40 percent to noncommunicable diseases, and 17 percent to injuries. In 2008, the age-standardized estimate of cancer deaths was 91 per 100,000 for men and 91

per 100,000 for women; for cardiovascular disease and diabetes, 341 per 100,000 for men and 260 per 100,000 for women; and for chronic respiratory disease, 92 per 100,000 for men and 36 per 100,000 for women.

In 2010, tuberculosis incidence was 147.0 per 100,000 population, tuberculosis prevalence 269.0 per 100,000, and deaths due to tuberculosis among HIV-negative people 28.00 per 100,000. In 2008, the age-standardized death rate from malaria was 0.1 per 100,000 population. Cape Verde's maternal mortality rate (death from any cause related to or aggravated by pregnancy) was estimated in 2008 as 94 maternal deaths per 100,000 live births. The infant mortality rate, defined as the number of deaths of infants younger than 1 year, was estimated at 26.02 per 1,000 live births in 2012.

Health Care Personnel

In 2008, Cape Verde had 0.57 physicians per 1,000 population, 1.89 health management and support workers per 1,000, 1.32 nurses and midwives per 1,000, and 0.14 community and traditional health workers per 1,000. The global "brain drain" (international migration of skilled personnel) plays a role in the relative undersupply of medical personnel in Cape Verde: Michael Clemens and Bunilla Petterson estimate that 51 percent of Cape Verde-born physicians and 41 percent of Cape Verde-born nurses are working in one of nine developed countries, primarily in Portugal.

Government Role in Health Care

According to WHO, in 2010, Cape Verde spent $77 million on health care, an amount that comes to $155 per capita. Cape Verde health care was funded primarily (88 percent) through domestic sources, with funding from abroad providing the remaining 12 percent. Government expenditures constitute 75 percent of health care spending, with spending by households providing the other 25 percent. In 2009, Cape Verde allocated 10 percent of total government expenditures to health, and in 2010, government expenditures on health came to 3 percent of GDP; both place Cape Verde in the medium range among low- and middle-income African countries. In 2009, according to WHO, official development assistance (ODA) for health in Cape Verde came to $17.21 per capita.

Public Health Programs

In 2010, 61 percent of the population of Cape Verde had access to improved sanitary facilities, with access being higher among the urban (73 percent) as opposed to the rural (43 percent) population. Access to improved sources of drinking water was higher, although not universal, with 88 percent of the population having such access (90 percent for the urban population, 85 percent for the rural). According to WHO, in 2004, Cape Verde had 0.02 environmental and public health workers per 1,000 population. According to the World Higher Education Database (WHED), one university in Cape Verde offers programs in epidemiology or public health: Jean Piaget University of Cape Verde, located in Praia.

CENTRAL AFRICAN REPUBLIC

The Central African Republic is a landlocked country in central Africa, sharing borders with Cameroon, Chad, the Democratic Republic of the Congo (DRC), the Republic of the Congo, South Sudan, and Sudan. The area is 240,535 square miles(622,984 square kilometers, a bit smaller than Texas), and the July 2012 population was estimated at 5.0 million. In 2010, 39 percent of the population lived in urban areas, and the 2010 to 2015 annual rate of urbanization was estimated at 2.5 percent. The capital and largest city is Bangui. Population growth was 2.1 percent in 2012 due to a high fertility rate (4.57 children per woman, the 28th-highest in the world) and birth rate (36.1 births per 1,000 population, the 25th-highest in the world); the net migration rate was 0.0 migrants per 1,000 population. The United Nations High Commissioner for Refugees (UNHCR) estimates that, in 2010, there were 21,574 refugees and persons in refugee-like situations in Central African Republic and 192,529 internally displaced persons and persons in internally displaced-person-like situations.

Formerly a French colony, the Central African Republic became independent in 1960. The Central African Republic's history since independence has been marked by periods of dictatorship, military rule, and corruption, and as of 2011, the country's stability was threatened by violent outbreaks, including some due to the activities of the militant group the Lord's Resistance Army. According to the Ibrahim Index, in 2011 the Central African Republic ranked near the bottom (48th out of 53) among African countries in terms of governance performance, with a score of 33 (out of 100). According to the *Corruption Perceptions Index 2011,* in the opinion of the business community, Central African Republic ranked tied for 152nd among 183 countries in terms of perceived public-sector corruption with a score of 2.2 (on a scale where 0 indicates highly corrupt and 10 very clean).

In 2011, the Central African Republic was classified as a country with low human development (the lowest of four categories) on the United Nations Development Programme's (UNDP's) Human Development Index (HDI), with a score of 0.343 (on a scale where 1 denotes high development and 0 low development). In 2011, the International Food Policy Research Institute (IFPRI) classified the Central African Republic as a country with an "alarming" hunger problem, and it received a Global Hunger Index (GHI) score of 27.0, the eighth-highest in the world. Life expectancy at birth in 2012 was estimated at 50.48 years, among the 10 lowest in the world, and the estimated gross domestic product (GDP) per capita in 2011 was $800, among the 10 lowest in the world. Income distribution in the Central African Republic is relatively unequal: In 1993, the Gini Index (a measure of dispersion, in which perfect equality is denoted by 0 and maximum inequality is denoted by 100) for family income was 61.3, among the highest in the world.

Emergency Health Services

According to the World Health Organization (WHO), as of 2007, the Central African Republic did not have a formal and publicly available system for providing prehospital care (emergency care).

Doctors Without Borders (Médecins Sans Frontières, or MSF) began working in the Central African Republic in 1997 and had 1,263 staff members in the country at the close of 2010. MSF currently has operations in six regions of the northern, southeastern, and southwestern areas of the country, focusing on providing medical care in areas beset by violence and providing emergency care. Since November 2009, MSF has provided medical care to approximately 15,000 refugees of violence in the Democratic Republic of the Congo (DRC). Since July 2010, MSF has provided approximately 28,700 medical consultations to people affected by the armed conflict in northern Central African Republic. MSF operates emergency programs to combat child malnutrition and offers pediatric care in southwestern Central

African Republic. In 2006, MSF opened a hospital in Paoua, caring for almost 7,000 patients and providing more than 35,000 consultations in 2010; MSF also runs a pediatric service at Bocaranga Hospital, providing approximately 1,000 consultations monthly. MSF established a referral hospital, which includes a maternal waiting house for women with high-risk pregnancies, in Ouham prefecture, a territory near the border of Chad controlled by rebel armies; in November, MSF set up a surgical camp in the hospital to repair obstetric fistulas.

Insurance

About two-thirds (65.2 percent) of the population of the Central African Republic was covered by public or private health insurance in 2000. The Central African Republic also has a social insurance system that pays only maternity benefits and only to employed women. The benefit is 50 percent of earnings for eight weeks before and six weeks after birth, with the period after birth extended to nine weeks if there are complications. Some health services are also provided to women during maternity leave. The system is funded by a 12 percent tax on employer payrolls; this money also funds a prenatal allowance, birth grants (for the first three births in a family), and a family allowance for up to six children younger than 15 (up to age 21 if disabled or still studying and up to age 18 if an apprentice) who attend school. To be eligible for Family Allowance benefits or maternity benefits, the insured person (a parent in the case of child benefits) must have at least six months of employment.

Costs of Hospitalization

No data available.

Access to Health Care

According to WHO, in 2006, 53 percent of births in Central African Republic were attended by skilled personnel (for example, physicians, nurses, or midwives). The 2010 immunization rates for 1-year-olds were 54 percent for diphtheria and pertussis (DPT3), 62 percent for measles (MCV), and 54 percent for Hib (Hib3). In 2010, an estimated 24 percent of persons with advanced human immunodeficiency virus (HIV) infection were receiving antiretroviral therapy in accordance with the 2010 WHO guidelines.

According to WHO, in 2010, the Central African Republic had fewer than 0.01 magnetic resonance imaging (MRI) machines per 1 million population and fewer than 0.01 computer tomography (CT) machines per 1 million.

Cost of Drugs

Expenditures for pharmaceuticals constituted about 5.2 percent of national total health expenditures, coming to more than $2.1 million. Per capita pharmaceutical expenditures came to $0.48. The Central African Republic is a member of the World Trade Organization (WTO) but allows for several exceptions to patent regulation, including compulsory licensing for reasons of public health, the Bolar exception that allows manufacturers to perform research and testing to create generic drugs before a patent has expired, and parallel importing provisions (allowing import of drugs created for sale in a different country). Drugs are provided free to children under 5 years, pregnant women, elderly persons, and the poor. Drugs to treat tuberculosis, human immunodeficiency virus and acquired immune deficiency syndrome (HIV/AIDS), trypanosomiasis, and filariasis are also free, as are those on WHO's Expanded Programme on Immunization (EPI) list.

Health Care Facilities

As of 2010, according to WHO, the Central African Republic had 12.77 health posts per 100,000 population, 2.09 health centers per 100,000, 0.30 district or rural hospitals per 100,000, 0.11 provincial hospitals per 100,000, and 0.09 specialized hospitals per 100,000. In 2006, the Central African Republic had 1.20 hospital beds per 1,000 population.

Major Health Issues

In 2008, WHO estimated that 78 percent of years of life lost in the Central African Republic were due to communicable diseases, 14 percent to noncommunicable diseases, and 7 percent to injuries. In 2008, the age-standardized estimate of cancer deaths was 83 per 100,000 for men and 76 per 100,000 for women; for cardiovascular disease and diabetes, 476 per 100,000 for men and 520 per 100,000 for women; and for chronic respiratory disease, 132 per 100,000 for men and 82 per 100,000 for women.

Central African Republic's maternal mortality rate (death from any cause related to or aggravated by pregnancy) is the eighth-highest in the world, estimated at 850 per 100,000 live births in 2008 data. A 2008 survey estimated the prevalence of female genital mutilation at 25.7 percent. The infant mortality rate, defined as the number of deaths of infants younger than 1 year, was fifth-highest in the world, at 97.17 per 1,000 live births, in 2012 data. In 2000, 21.8 percent of children under age 5 were underweight (defined as 2 kilograms [kg] below standard weight-for-age at age 1, 3 kg below for ages 2 to 3, and 4 kg below for ages 4 to 5). In 2010, tuberculosis incidence was 319.0 per 100,000 population, tuberculosis prevalence 376.0 per 100,000, and deaths due to tuberculosis among HIV-negative people 34.0 per 100,000. As of 2009, an estimated 4.7 percent of adults age 15 to 49 were living with HIV or AIDS. In 2008, the age-standardized death rate from malaria was 117.3 per 100,000 population, the third-highest in the world.

Health Care Personnel

In 2006, WHO identified the Central African Republic as one of 57 countries with a critical deficit in the supply of skilled health workers. The Central African Republic has one medical school, the Faculté des Sciences de la Santé of the University of Bangui, which began offering instruction in 1976. The basic course of training lasts six years, and the degree awarded is Docteur en Médecine (Diplôme d'État), or doctor of medicine (state diploma). In 2004, Central African Republic had 0.08 physicians per 1,000 population, 0.01 laboratory health workers per 1,000, 0.04 health management and support workers per 1,000, 0.05 community and traditional health workers per 1,000, and 0.41 nurses and midwives per 1,000. The global "brain drain" (international migration of skilled personnel) plays a role in the undersupply of medical personnel in Central African Republic: Michael Clemens and Bunilla Petterson estimate that 42 percent of Central African Republic-born physicians and 25 percent of Central African Republic-born nurses are working in one of nine developed countries, primarily in France.

Government Role in Health Care

The right to health, including the right to essential medicines and medical technology, is recognized by the 2004 national constitution. The Central African Republic has a National Health Policy (NHP) and a National Medicines Policy (NMP). The NMP includes selection of essential medicines; financing, pricing, purchase, distribution, and regulation of drugs; pharmacovigilance; rational usage of medicines; human resource development; research; and traditional medicine. According to WHO, in 2010, the Central African

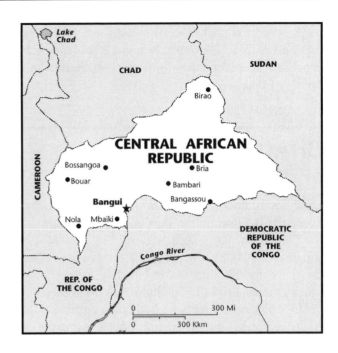

Republic spent $80 million on health care, an amount that comes to $18 per capita. Health care was funded primarily (87 percent) through domestic sources, with funding from abroad providing the remaining 13 percent. Most funding (61 percent) was provided by spending by households, with 35 percent coming from government expenditures, and 3 percent other expenditures. In 2010, the Central African Republic allocated 8 percent of total government expenditures to health, in the median range for low-income African countries, and government expenditures on health came to 1 percent of gross domestic product (GDP), ranking low when compared with other low-income African countries. In 2009, according to WHO, official development assistance (ODA) for health in Central African Republic came to $5.89 per capita.

Public Health Programs

In 2010, 34 percent of the population of the Central African Republic had access to improved sanitary facilities, with access being higher among the urban (43 percent) as opposed to the rural (28 percent) population. Access to improved sources of drinking water was higher, although far from universal, with 67 percent of the population having such access (92 percent for the urban population and 51 percent for the rural). According to WHO, in 2004, the Central African Republic had 0.01 environmental and public health workers per 1,000 population. According to the World Higher Education Database (WHED), one university in the Central African Republic offers programs in epidemiology or public health: the University of Bangui.

CHAD

Chad is a landlocked country in Central Africa sharing borders with Libya, Sudan, the Central African Republic, Cameroon, Niger, and Nigeria. The area of 496 square miles (1,284 square kilometers) is about three times the size of California, and the July 2012 population was estimated at 11.0 million. In 2010, 28 percent of the population lived in urban areas, and the 2010 to 2015 annual rate of urbanization is estimated at 4.6 percent. The capital and largest city is N'Djamena (with a 2009 population estimated at 808,000). The July 2012 population growth rate is 2.0 percent, despite a negative migration rate (negative 3.74 migrants per 1,000 population) and one of the highest death rates in the world (15.16 deaths per 1,000 population); the total fertility rate is 4.93 children per woman (the 21st-highest in the world), and the birth rate is 38.7 births per 1,000 (the 15th-highest in the world). The United Nations High Commissioner for Refugees (UNHCR) estimated that, in 2010, there were 347,939 refugees and persons in refugee-like situations in Chad and 131,000 internally displaced persons and persons in internally displaced-person-like situations.

Chad was a French colony until becoming independent in 1960; three decades of civil war and invasions from Libya followed. Peace was restored in 1990, and presidential elections were held in 1996 and 2001. However, Chad remains troubled by outbreaks of civil violence. According to the Ibrahim Index, in 2011, Chad ranked near the bottom (51st out of 53) among African countries in terms of governance performance, with a score of 31 (out of 100). Chad ranked tied for 168th among 183 countries on the *Corruption Perceptions Index 2011*, with a score of 2.0 (on a scale where 0 indicates highly corrupt and 10 very clean).

In 2011, Chad was classified as a country with low human development (the lowest of four categories) on the United Nations Development Programme's (UNDP's) Human Development Index (HDI), with a score of 0.328 (on a scale where 1 denotes high development and 0 low development). In 2011, the

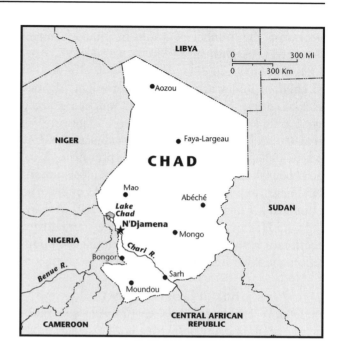

International Food Policy Research Institute (IFPRI) classified Chad as a country with an "extremely alarming" hunger problem, with a Global Hunger Index (GHI) score of 30.6, one of the highest in the world, and in 2012, the World Food Bank estimated that 1.2 million people in Chad required food assistance, due primarily to drought. Life expectancy at birth in 2012 was estimated at 48.69 years, the lowest in the world, and estimated gross domestic product (GDP) per capita in 2011 was $1,900. According to the World Economic Forum's *Global Gender Gap Index 2011*, Chad ranked 134th out of 135 countries on gender equality, with a score of 0.533 (on a scale with a theoretical range of 1 for equality to 0 for inequality and an actual range in 2011 from 0.8530 to 0.4873).

Emergency Health Services

According to the World Health Organization (WHO), as of 2007, Chad did not have a formal and publicly available system for providing prehospital care (emergency care). Doctors Without Borders (Médecins Sans Frontières, or MSF) began working in Chad in 1981 and had 773 staff members in the country at the close of 2010. In 2010, MSF operated programs in seven locations in southern and central Chad: N'Djamena, Bongor, Moissala, Am Timan, Kerfi, Abéché, and Dogdoré. Focus areas of MSF programs in Chad include providing medical care to displaced people; providing emergency nutritional programs;

treating malaria; and combating outbreaks of measles, cholera, and meningitis.

Insurance

Chad has a social insurance system that pays only maternity benefits, and only to employed women. The benefit is 50 percent of earnings for 6 weeks before and 8 weeks after birth, with the period after birth extended to 11 weeks if there are complications. To be eligible for maternity benefits, a woman must be employed for at least six months immediately prior to taking maternity leave. The system is funded by a 7.5 percent tax on employer payrolls; this money also provides birth grants (for the first three births in the insured's first marriage), a prenatal allowance, and a family allowance for children younger than 20 (up to age 21 if disabled or still studying and up to age 18 if an apprentice). To be eligible for Family Allowance benefits, the insured person (a parent in the case of child benefits) must work at least 20 days a month and have at least six months of employment. Some health and welfare services are provided to mothers and children as well, and employers are required to provide certain medical benefits to workers. The program is administered by the National Social Insurance Fund, with general supervision from the Ministry of Labor and Public Affairs.

Costs of Hospitalization

No data available.

Access to Health Care

According to WHO, in 2004, 20.7 percent of births in Chad were attended by skilled personnel (for example, physicians, nurses, or midwives). In 2004, 17 percent of pregnant women in Chad received at least four prenatal care visits. The 2010 immunization rates for 1-year-olds were 59 percent for diphtheria and pertussis (DPT3), 46 percent for measles (MCV), and 59 percent for Hib (Hib3). In 2010, an estimated 39 percent of persons with advanced human immunodeficiency virus (HIV) infection were receiving antiretroviral therapy in accordance with the 2010 WHO guidelines. According to WHO, in 2010, Chad had 0.09 computer tomography (CT) machines per 1 million population.

Cost of Drugs

Total pharmaceutical expenditures in Chad in 2011 came to $24.4 million, with per capita pharmaceutical expenditures at $2.24. Pharmaceutical expenses came to 6 percent of health spending, with about half the total (45.5 percent) coming from public expenditures. Chad's Essential Medicines List (EML) was revised in 2009 and included 287 medicines. Medicines on the EML are provided free of charge, including medications for malaria, tuberculosis, sexually transmitted disease (STD), and human immunodeficiency virus and acquired immune deficiency syndrome (HIV/AIDS). According to WHO, in 2004, the median availability of selected generic drugs in the public sector in Chad was 31.3 percent; in the private sector, the mean availability was 13.6 percent. The median price ratio (comparing the price in Chad to the international reference price) was 3.9 in the public sphere for selected generic medicines and 15.1 in the private sphere, indicating that median prices in the public sphere were almost four times as high and, in the private sphere, over 15 times as high as the international reference price.

Health Care Facilities

As of 2010, according to WHO, Chad had 6.72 health posts per 100,000 population, less than 0.01 health centers per 100,000, 0.57 district or rural hospitals per 100,000, 0.17 provincial hospitals per 100,000, and 0.01 specialized hospitals per 100,000. In 2005, Chad had 0.43 hospital beds per 1,000 population, one of the 20 lowest rates in the world.

Major Health Issues

In 2008, WHO estimated that 84 percent of years of life lost in Chad were due to communicable diseases, 11 percent to noncommunicable diseases, and 5 percent to injuries. In 2008, the age-standardized estimate of cancer deaths was 82 per 100,000 for men and 84 per 100,000 for women; for cardiovascular disease and diabetes, 483 per 100,000 for men and 517 per 100,000 for women; and for chronic respiratory disease, 134 per 100,000 for men and 80 per 100,000 for women.

Chad's maternal mortality rate (death from any cause related to or aggravated by pregnancy) is the third-highest in the world, estimated at 1,200 per 100,000 live births in 2008. A 2004 survey estimated the prevalence of female genital mutilation at 44.9 percent. The infant mortality rate, defined as the number of deaths of infants younger than 1 year, is the seventh-highest in the world, at 93.61 per 1,000 live births in 2012. Child malnutrition is a serious problem: In 2004, 33.9 percent of children under age 5 were underweight (defined as 2 kilograms [kg] below standard weight-for-age at age 1,

3 kg below for ages 2 to 3, and 4 kg below for ages 4 to 5), one of the 20 highest rates in the world.

In 2010, tuberculosis incidence was 276.0 per 100,000 population, tuberculosis prevalence 417.0 per 100,000, and deaths due to tuberculosis among HIV-negative people 47.00 per 100,000. As of 2009, an estimated 3.4 percent of adults age 15 to 49 were living with HIV or AIDS. In 2010, 7 percent of pregnant women tested positive for HIV. The mother-to-child transmission rate for HIV in 2010 was estimated at 33 percent, and in 2009, 2.7 percent of deaths to children under age 5 were attributed to HIV. In 2008, the age-standardized death rate from malaria was 119.3 per 100,000 population, the second-highest in the world. In 2008, the age-standardized death rate from child-hood-cluster diseases (pertussis, polio, diphtheria, measles, and tetanus) was 28.3 per 100,000 population, the fourth-highest in the world.

Health Care Personnel

In 2006, WHO identified Chad as one of 57 countries with a critical deficit in the supply of skilled health workers. Chad has one medical school, the Faculté des Sciences le la Santé in N'Djamena, which began offering instruction in 1975. The language of instruction is French, the course of training lasts seven years, and the degree awarded is Doctorat en Médecine (doctor of medicine). Physicians must register with the Ordre National des Médecins in N'Djamena. Chad has agreements with Algeria, Cameroon, the Central African Republic, the Republic of the Congo, and the Côte d'Ivoire. In 2004, Chad had 0.04 physicians per 1,000 population, 0.04 laboratory health workers per 1,000, 0.17 health management and support workers per 1,000, 0.03 community and traditional health workers per 1,000, and 0.28 nurses and midwives per 1,000. The global "brain drain" (international migration of skilled personnel) plays a role in the undersupply of medical personnel in Cameroon: Michael Clemens and Bunilla Petterson estimate that 22 percent of Chad-born physicians and 11 percent of Chad-born nurses are working in one of nine developed countries, primarily in France.

Government Role in Health Care

Chad has a national health policy and a plan to implement it, and a National Medicines Policy (NMP). Chad's NMP covers selection of essential medicines; financing, pricing, purchase, distribution, and regulation of drugs; pharmacovigilance; rational usage of medicines; human resource development; research; and traditional medicine. Chad is a member of the World Trade Organization (WTO) but allows for several exceptions to patent regulation, including compulsory licensing for reasons of public health, the Bolar exception that allows manufacturers to perform research and testing to create generic drugs before a patent has expired, and parallel importing provisions (allowing import of drugs created for sale in a different country). Direct advertising of prescription drugs to the public is banned.

According to WHO, in 2010, Chad spent $344 million on health care, an amount that comes to $31 per capita. Health care was funded primarily (92 percent) through domestic sources, with funding from abroad providing the remaining 8 percent. Most funding (73 percent) was provided by spending by households, with 26 percent coming from government expenditures and 2 percent from other expenditures. In 2010, Chad allocated 3 percent of total government expenditures to health, in the low range for low-income African countries, and government expenditures on health came to 1 percent of GDP, also low when compared with other low-income African countries. In 2009, according to WHO, official development assistance (ODA) for health in Chad came to $2.86 per capita.

Public Health Programs

In 2010, only 13 percent of the population of Chad had access to improved sanitary facilities, with access higher among the urban (30 percent) as opposed to the rural (6 percent) population. Access to improved sources of drinking water was higher, although far from universal, with 51 percent of the population having such access (70 percent for the urban population and 41 percent for the rural). According to WHO, in 2004, Chad had 0.03 environmental and public health workers per 1,000 population. According to the World Higher Education Database (WHED), one university in Chad offers programs in epidemiology or public health: the University of N'Djamena.

CHILE

Chile is a mountainous country in southwestern South America, sharing borders with Argentina, Bolivia, and Peru and having a lon, 3,999-mile (6,435-kilometer) Pacific coastline. The area of 291,933 square miles (756,102 square kilometers) is about twice that of Montana, and the July 2012 population was estimated at 17.1 million. In 2010, 89 percent of the population lived in urban areas, and the 2010 to 2015 annual rate of urbanization was estimated at 1.1 percent. The country is highly urbanized (89 percent); the 2012 population growth rate was 0.9 percent, the net migration rate 0.4 migrants per 1,000 population, the birth rate 14.3 births per 1,000, and the total fertility rate 1.9 children per woman. The United Nations High Commissioner for Refugees (UNHCR) estimated that, in 2010, there were 1,621 refugees and persons in refugee-like situations in Chile.

Chile was a Spanish colony before becoming independent in 1818. Augusto Pinochet took power by military coup in 1973, ruling until 1990, when a president was freely elected. The government has recently been considered honest and transparent: According to the *Corruption Perceptions Index 2011*, Chile ranked tied for 22nd among 183 with a score of 7.2 (on a scale where 0 indicates highly corrupt and 10 very clean). In 2011, Chile was classified as a country with very high human development (the highest of four categories) on the United Nations Development Programme's (UNDP's) Human Development Index (HDI), with a score of 0.805 (on a scale where 1 denotes high development and 0 low development). Life expectancy at birth in 2012 was estimated at 78.10 years, and per capita gross domestic product (GDP) in 2011 was estimated at $16,100. Income distribution in Chile is relatively unequal: In 2009, the Gini Index (a measure of dispersion, in which perfect equality is denoted by 0 and maximum inequality is denoted by 100) for family income was 52.1, among the 20 highest in the world. According to the World Economic Forum's *Global Gender Gap Index 2011*, Chile ranked 46th out of 135 countries on gender equality with a score of 0.703 (on a scale with a theoretical range of 1 for equality to 0 for inequality and an actual range in 2011 from 0.8530 to 0.4873).

Emergency Health Services

According to the World Health Organization (WHO), as of 2007, Chile had a formal and publicly available emergency care (prehospital care) system, accessible through a national universal access telephone number. Emergency services are provided primarily through the public health system through hospital and primary care emergency care services; from 2000 to 2005, 22 percent of consultations in the National Health Services System were for emergency care visits.

Insurance

Chile has a social insurance program (the National Health Fund; Fondo Nacional de Salud, or FONASA), but insured people may choose to opt out of the national system and contract with a private health institute; however, people must have some type of insurance. According to Donald West and colleagues, from 2010 to 2011, about 67 percent of the population was covered through FONASA. The unemployed, recipients of social benefits, and women during pregnancy and the six months after childbirth are included in the public system. The public system is funded by a 7 percent contribution of covered wages (for the employed), 7 percent of declared earnings (for the self-employed), or 7 percent of pension (for the retired); the minimum and maximum amounts used to calculate contributions are adjusted daily according to inflation. The government covers deficits and finances maternity benefits.

In the public system, benefits are provided through professionals and institutions registered with FONASA; benefits provided include hospitalization,

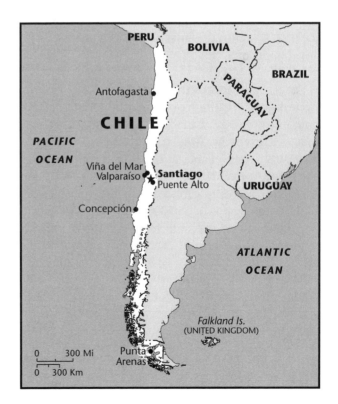

medical exams, general and specialist care, maternity care, dental care, and medicines. The minimum benefits provided under the public system are established under the General Scheme of Health Guarantees. The system includes some cost sharing, but not for primary assistance; in addition, the poor, persons older than 60, and beneficiaries of pensions or family allowances are exempt from cost sharing. In the public system, an individual signs a contract of at least 12 months with a private health institute. A variety of plans are available, including open and closed plans and preferred provider plans.

Benefits in private plans are required to be at least equal to the public system. Private insurance is managed by 13 Institutes of Public Health and Preventive Medicine (ISAPRES), which are regulated by the Ministry of Health. Those covered through the private system can choose to be treated by a provider in the public system, but this will require a copayment based on income.

Costs of Hospitalization

As of 2011, according to Donald West and colleagues, Chile had 2,017 public hospitals and 179 private hospitals. The public system is organized through 28 hospital and clinic service care regions; the government owns about two-thirds of inpatient capacity. Persons covered under a FONASA facility can choose to be treated in the public sector or can be treated in the private sector; the latter requires payment of a fee based on income.

Access to Health Care

According to Latinobarometer, an annual public opinion survey conducted in Latin America, 61 percent of citizens in Chile are satisfied with the level of health care available to them (the regional average is 51.9 percent). According to Donald West and colleagues, access to care is a significant problem in Chile, with more than 650,000 people on wait lists in the public system and a much higher ratio of patients to physicians in the public sector as compared to the private sector. However, reforms passed in 2003 and 2004 address these problems and are gradually being implemented. The most important reform is the creation of the Regime of Explicit Health Guarantees (AUGE), which prioritizes health problems, defines the appropriate medical response, defines a maximum waiting period for treatment, and specifies the maximum (based on income) a family can be required to pay for health care. The priority list was created by a team of health professionals who considered the years of healthy life lost by the condition as well as the frequency of the disease or condition and the cost of treatment. The number of diseases included under AUGE is increased each year.

According to WHO, in 2007, 99.8 percent of births in Chile were attended by skilled personnel (for example, physicians, nurses, or midwives). The 2010 immunization rates for 1-year-olds were 92 percent for diphtheria and pertussis (DPT3), 93 percent for measles (MCV), and 92 percent for Hib (Hib3). In 2010, an estimated 8 percent of persons with advanced human immunodeficiency virus (HIV) infection were receiving antiretroviral therapy in accordance with the 2010 WHO guidelines. In 2010 Chile had 4.98 magnetic resonance imaging (MRI) machines per 1 million population, 13.21 computer tomography (CT) machines per 1 million, 0.24 telecolbalt units per 1 million, and 0.24 radiotherapy machines per 1 million.

Cost of Drugs

Chile had about 1,500 community pharmacies in 2005, with about 90 percent owned by one of three franchises (Salco-Brand, Ahumada, or Cruz Verde). National drug policy is focused on ensuring a supply of drugs on the national essential drugs list; however, there are no price controls, and persons in the upper quintile of income spend 6.5 times as much on drugs as those in the lowest quintile. Use of generic drugs is common; in 2002, 38.5 percent of drugs sold in Chile were trademark generics, 39.3 percent generics, and 22.1 percent brand-name products.

Health Care Facilities

Most primary care facilities in Chile are administered by municipalities, while hospitals are gradually being granted autonomous rule. In 2005, Chile had 196 hospitals, including 99 rural hospitals and 60 high-complexity hospitals. The public outpatient network included 258 urban and 151 rural clinics, 70 family health centers, 115 primary care clinics attached to hospitals, and 40 outpatient mental health centers. As of 2010, according to WHO, Chile had 11.00 health posts per 100,000 population, 0.12 health centers per 100,000, 0.58 district or rural hospitals per 100,000, 0.13 provincial hospitals per 100,000, and 0.36 specialized hospitals per 100,000. In 2009, Chile had 2.10 hospital beds per 1,000 population.

Selected Health Indicators: Chile Compared With the Organisation for Economic Co-operation and Development (OECD) Country Average

	Chile	OECD average (2010 or nearest year)
Male life expectancy at birth, 2009	75.8	77
Female life expectancy at birth, 2009	81.8	82.5
Infant mortality (deaths per 1,000 live births), 2009	7.9	4.3
Doctor consultations (number per capita), 2009	3.2	6.4
Physicians licensed to practice (per 1,000 population), 2011	1.6	3.1
Nurses licensed to practice (per 1,000 population), 2011	1.5	8.6
Hospital beds (per 1,000 population), 2010	2.0	4.9

Source: OECD Health Data 2012 (Organisation for Economic Co-operation and Development, 2012).

Major Health Issues

In 2008, WHO estimated that 10 percent of years of life lost in Chile were due to communicable diseases, 71 percent to noncommunicable diseases, and 20 percent to injuries. In 2008, the age-standardized estimate of cancer deaths was 144 per 100,000 for men and 98 per 100,000 for women; for cardiovascular disease and diabetes, 196 per 100,000 for men and 117 per 100,000 for women; and for chronic respiratory disease, 39 per 100,000 for men and 21 per 100,000 for women. Chile's maternal mortality rate (death from any cause related to or aggravated by pregnancy) in 2008 was 26 maternal deaths per 100,000 live births. The infant mortality rate, defined as the number of deaths of infants younger than 1 year, was 7.36 per 1,000 live births as of 2012. In 2010, tuberculosis incidence was 19.0 per 100,000 population, tuberculosis prevalence 25.0 per 100,000, and deaths due to tuberculosis among HIV-negative people 1.60 per 100,000. As of 2009, an estimated 0.4 percent of adults age 15 to 49 were living with HIV or acquired immune deficiency syndrome (AIDS). Typhoid fever and paratyphoid fever are endemic, and the country experiences outbreaks of Hepatitis A every four to five years. In 2003, an estimated 21.9 percent of adults in Chile were obese (defined as a body mass index, or BMI, of 30 or greater).

Health Care Personnel

Chile has nine medical schools, three of which were founded in the 1990s. The basic medical training course lasts seven years, and the degree awarded is Médico Cirujano (physician and surgeon). In 2003, Chile had 1.09 physicians per 1,000 population, 0.43 dentistry personnel per 1,000, and 0.63 nurses and midwives per 1,000.

Government Role in Health Care

According to WHO, in 2010, Chile spent $16 billion on health care, an amount that comes to $947 per capita. Health care was funded entirely through domestic sources. About half (48 percent) of health care funding was provided by government expenditures, with 33 percent coming from household spending and 18 percent from other expenditures. In 2010, Chile allocated 16 percent of total government expenditures to health, in the high range for upper-middle-income countries of the Americas, and government expenditures on health came to 4 percent of GDP, placing Chile in the median range when compared with other upper-middle-income countries of the Americas region. In 2009, according to WHO, official development assistance (ODA) for health in Chile came to $0.13 per capita.

Public Health Programs

The Public Health Institute of Chile (ISP) is located in Santiago and directed by Maria Teresa Valenzuela. The ISP was created in 1979, although its history dates back to 1892, when Chile's Institute of Hygiene began developing a network of laboratories; it expanded its activities to include the development of vaccines, to help control communicable diseases, and to improve quality control activities, including standardizing methods of diagnosis and inspecting and testing of pharmaceutical products. ISP is organized into six departments, which together employ almost 700 people: the National Drug Agency, the National Biomedical and Reference Laboratory, Occupational Health, Environment Health, Administration and Finance, and Scientific Affairs.

Major current foci of the ISP include ensuring that all Chileans have access to safe medicines, ensuring the quality of analytical measurements, strengthening the body of epidemiological information in order to promote prevention, and improving internal management. In 2011, one department of the ISP, the National Biomedical and Reference Laboratory, helped manage outbreaks of cholera, hantavirus, salmonella, typhus, and pertussis.

The Ministry of Health operates a variety of preventive medicine programs, including immunization, control of respiratory diseases, prevention of traffic accidents, promotion of cancer screening, eradication of Chagas disease, and control of algal bloom (the red tide). In 2010, 96 percent of the population of Chile had access to improved sanitary facilities, with access being higher among the urban (96 percent) as opposed to the rural (83 percent) population. Access to improved sources of drinking water was higher, with 96 percent of the population having such access (99 percent for the urban population and 75 percent for the rural). According to the World Higher Education Database (WHED), seven universities in Chile offer programs in epidemiology or public health: the Catholic University of Chile, the Catholic University of Maule, the Catholic University of the North, the University of Chile, the University of the Frontier, the University of the Andes, and the Ibero-American University of Science and Technology.

CHINA

China is an east Asian country, sharing borders with 15 countries and having a Pacific coastline of 9,010 miles (14,500 kilometers). China includes Hong Kong (a former British colony) and Macau (a former Portuguese colony), both of which are special administrative regions granted some degree of autonomy; in

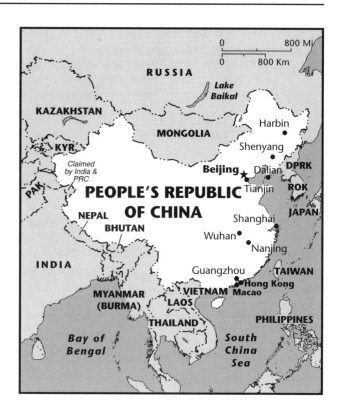

addition, the Chinese government considers Taiwan a province of China (while Taiwan considers itself to be an independent country). China is the most populous country in the world, with an estimated population (as of July 2012) of 1.3 billion people; it is also the fourth-largest country in the world by area, with an area of 3,705,375 square miles (9,596,877 square kilometers, slightly smaller than the United States). In 2010, 47 percent of the population lived in urban areas, and the 2010 to 2015 annual rate of urbanization was estimated at 2.3 percent. Beijing is the capital, while the largest city is Shanghai (with a 2009 population estimated at 16.6 million). The July 2012 population growth rate was 0.5 percent, low in part because government policies encourage small families; the birth rate was 12.3 births per 1,000 population, the net migration rate negative 0.3 migrants per 1,000, and the total fertility rate 1.6 children per woman. The United Nations High Commissioner for Refugees (UNHCR) estimated that, in 2010, there were 300,986 refugees and persons in refugee-like situations in China.

China was ruled by a communist system under Mao Zedong after World War II, but after 1978, the country became more focused on economic development, and China's economy expanded rapidly. China ranked tied for 75th among 183 countries in terms of perceived public-sector corruption on the *Corruption Perceptions Index 2011,* with a score of 3.6 (on a scale where 0 indicates highly corrupt and 10 very clean). In contrast, Hong Kong and Macau are perceived as less corrupt, with Hong Kong ranking 12th and Macau tied for 46th. In 2011, China was classified as a country with medium human development (the second from the lowest of four categories) on the United Nations Development Programme's (UNDP's) Human Development Index (HDI), with a score of 0.687 (on a scale where 1 denotes high development and 0 low development). Life expectancy at birth in 2012 was estimated at 74.84 years, and per capita gross domestic product (GDP) in 2011 in China was estimated at $8,400. According to the World Economic Forum's *Global Gender Gap Index 2011,* China ranked 61st out of 135 countries on gender equality, with a score of 0.687 (on a scale with a theoretical range of 1 for equality to 0 for inequality and an actual range in 2011 from 0.8530 to 0.4873).

Standards of living were considerably higher in China's two special administrative regions. Per capita GDP in 2011 in Hong Kong was estimated at $49,300, among the highest in the world, and per capita GDP in Macau was estimated at $33,000 in 2009. Life expectancy at birth is among the highest in the world in both Hong Kong and Macau, at 82.12 years in Hong Kong and 84.43 years in Macau. In 2011, Hong Kong was classified as having very high human development (the highest of four categories) on the United Nations Development Programme's (UNDP's) Human Development Index (HDI), with a score of 0.898 (on a scale where 1 denotes high development and 0 low development).

Emergency Health Services

According to the World Health Organization (WHO), as of 2007, China had a formal and publicly available emergency care (prehospital care) system, accessible through a national universal access telephone number. Doctors Without Borders (Médecins Sans Frontières, or MSF) began working in China in 1988 and had 24 staff members in the country at the close of 2010. MSF had provided human immunodeficiency virus and acquired immune deficiency syndrome (HIV/AIDS) care in Nanning (southern China) since 2003, targeting high-risk groups; this program was transferred to local authorities in 2010. MSF provided emergency assistance in the April 2010 earthquake in Qinghai province.

Insurance

China has a social insurance and mandatory individual account health care system; the first national law on social insurance was adopted in October 2010 and implemented in July 2011. Several different programs cover different individuals, depending on their locations and types of employment. Employees in state-owned enterprises are covered by the maternity insurance program; employees in urban areas working in nonprofit organizations, enterprises, social groups, and government organizations are covered by the urban medical insurance program; a separate urban resident medical insurance program covers nonsalaried urban employees, and farmers receive basic coverage through a rural cooperative medicare program. Rates of contribution to an individual's medical savings account are determined by local governments but are in the range of 2 percent and cover medical benefits only. The rural medicare program for farmers is funded through a flat rate contribution by individual farmers of CNY 20 a year, and the local government contributes about CNY 80, with the latter amount varying by province. Those covered by the nonsalaried urban resident plan contributed CNY 200 to CNY 300 annually for adults and about CNY 100 for children. Employers pay about 6 percent of payroll for medical benefits, split so 70 percent goes to the social insurance fund and 30 percent to the individual account of each insured individual.

The maternity benefit pays 100 percent of wages for up to 90 days, while the sickness benefits pays 60 to 100 percent (depending on length of employment) of wages for up to six months, then 40 to 60 percent of wages. Medical benefits are calculated according to the local average annual wage. The medical account pays benefits up to 10 percent of this wage; the social insurance fund for 10 percent to 600 percent of this wage; above 600 percent, costs are covered by public supplementary systems or private insurance. The maximum benefit for the rural cooperative medicare program and for nonsalaried urban residents varies by province. Several agencies and state-run enterprises administer different aspects of the program at the local level, with the Ministry of Human Resources and Social Security and the Ministry of Public Health providing guidance and supervision.

According to T. R. Reid, Hong Kong has a Beveridge system of health insurance dating back to its days as a British colony; in this type of system, health care is available through a government-financed system, but a private system of health care is also permitted.

Costs of Hospitalization

As of 2005, China had approximately 1,141 private hospitals, according to Donald West and colleagues; a plan to construct about 2,000 community hospitals in the years 2010 to 2013 was made. Patients pay most of the cost for care received in hospitals; this care includes services that would ordinarily be provided in an outpatient setting.

Access to Health Care

According to Donald West and colleagues, as of 2011, China had huge disparities in access to care, a problem dating back in part to the dismantling of the rural primary care system created prior to 1980. Most people receive all types of care from hospitals, although there are many local variations in organizing and financing services; some estimate that only one-third of the population has a secure source of health care. Hospitals receive about 90 percent of their funding through fees charged for services, so it is generally necessary to pay in order to receive care; the remaining 10 percent comes from the government and is based on the number of beds and size of the staff, a system that encouraged overconstruction and overstaffing.

In 2006, China saw nearly 10,000 protests against the quality of care or the lack of care provided in public hospitals; since then, the central government has made improving quality of, and access to, health care a priority. The central budget for health care was increased 87 percent between 2006 and 2007, and a major health care plan of reform was approved in 2009. In the years 2000 to 2013, about $124 billion was scheduled to be spent to improve local health care facilities, improve hospital management, and increase insurance coverage to 90 percent of the population. In addition, a program begun in 2006 aims to restore access to primary care through construction of community health centers offering Western and Chinese medicine, outpatient care, rehabilitation, birth control, preventive services, and case management for chronic illness.

According to WHO, in 2009, 96.3 percent of births in China were attended by skilled personnel (for example, physicians, nurses, or midwives). In 2009, 92 percent of pregnant women in China received at least one prenatal care visit. The 2010 immunization rates for 1-year-olds were 99 percent for diphtheria and pertussis (DPT3) and 99 percent for measles (MCV). In 2010, an estimated 32 percent of persons with advanced human immunodeficiency virus (HIV) infection were receiving antiretroviral therapy in accordance with the 2010 WHO guidelines.

Cost of Drugs

According to Ibis Sanchez-Serrano, in 2009, the pharmaceutical market in China was valued at $25.5 billion and was projected to reach $35.3 billion by 2014. Healthy China 2020, as phased in, was designed to greatly expand access to health care, including prescription drugs, with the final goal of universal coverage. According to WHO, in 2006, the median availability of selected generic drugs in the public sector in several regions of China (Shaanxi, Shandong, and Shanghai provinces) was 18.1 percent; in the private sector, the mean availability was 21.5 percent. The median price ratio (comparing the price in China to the international reference price) was 1.3 in both the public and private sectors for selected generic medicines, indicating that the price for these drugs in China was on average 30 percent higher than the international reference price.

According to Donald West and colleagues, medicine use in China is distorted by financial incentives to prescribe and to overprescribe expensive drugs because hospitals receive most of their revenues through fees charged for services, and physicians' salaries are low, encouraging them to seek bonus payments based on the revenues they bring in to the hospitals by charging for services and prescription drugs. For instance, antibiotics are prescribed to 75 percent of patients with common colds and 79 percent of hospital patients, a practice that not only drives up costs but also increases antibiotic resistance. One aspect of a health care reform plan introduced in the years 2010 to 2013 is to separate drug sales from hospital operations and to focus on essential drugs.

A 2006 survey of the availability of a market basket of medicines was conducted in Shanghai, a city of 16 million people in eastern China. Shanghai was one of the first cities in China to institute a policy of bulk purchasing for medicines; about 80 percent of pharmaceuticals used in hospitals and 75 percent used by health insurance companies were purchased in bulk from 2002 to 2006. In addition, in 2004, Shanghai adopted budgetary controls limiting the purchase of expensive medicines to 30 percent of total medicine expenditures in tertiary hospitals; in community hospitals, the limit is 5 percent, and in secondary

Selected Health Indicators: China Compared With the Global Average (2010)

	China	Global Average
Male life expectancy at birth* (years)	72	66
Female life expectancy at birth* (years)	76	71
Under-5 mortality rate, both sexes (per 1,000 live births)	18	57
Adult mortality rate, both sexes* (probability of dying between 15 and 60 years per 1,000 population)	116	176
Maternal mortality ratio (per 100,000 live births)	37	210
HIV prevalence* (per 1,000 adults aged 15 to 49)	1	8
Tuberculosis prevalence (per 100,000 population)	108	178

Source: World Health Organization Global Health Observatory Data Repository.
*Data refers to 2009.

hospitals, 20 percent. Most medicines are purchased from hospitals and public-sector facilities rather than private pharmacies.

Despite bulk purchasing, procurement prices in the public sector were generally higher than the international reference price, with a median price ratio of 1.52 (52 percent higher than the international reference price) for the lowest-priced generic drugs and 5.48 (more than five times as high) for originator brands. Patient prices in the public sector had a median price ratio of 2.03 for the lowest-priced generics and 5.64 for originator brands. Availability was poor in the public sector, with a median availability of 33.3 percent for the lowest-priced generics and 13.3 percent for originator brands. Prices were higher in the private sector, with a median price ratio of 1.77 for the lowest-priced generics and 8.76 for originator brands. Availability was also low in the private sector, with a median availability of 15 percent for the lowest-priced generic drugs and 10 percent for originator brands.

Most medicines to treat common chronic diseases were not affordable, or barely affordable, given the standard that a course of treatment should not cost more than 1 day's wages for the lowest-paid government worker. To treat diabetes for 30 days would require 1.1 days' wages for metformin or 2.3 days' wages for gliclazide, if the lowest-priced generics were purchased through the public sector; originator brands were much more expensive (requiring 5.9 and 4.7 days' wages, respectively), while the lowest-priced generic purchased in the private sector would cost 1.7 days' wages (for gliclazide; generic metformin was not available) and originator brands 5.1 days' wages (for metformin) and 4.4 (for gliclazide). Treatment of acute conditions was much more affordable, generally costing less than 1 day's wages to treat.

According to a 2011 report by Ye Lu and colleagues, most (95 percent) health care facilities in China are hospitals managed by the government, and most of the revenue in these hospitals is generated through fees; physicians as well as the hospital itself depend on fees for procedures and drug sales, creating an unfortunate incentive to prescribe more expensive medicines and medicines that may not be necessary. In 2006, almost half (42.7) of total health expenditures in China were spent on medicines. In the period of 1997 to 2007, the Chinese government introduced several measures intended to lower drug prices, but recent surveys have shown that medicines in China are higher than the international reference price and that affordability was a problem for some common chronic diseases, including diabetes and hypertension. In 2009, the Health Care Reform Plan announced a plan to establish a national list of essential medicines and to institute several other services intended to increase access to essential health care and medicines across the country.

Health Care Facilities

The Chinese health care system is based around hospitals, and there are few opportunities to receive care in any other setting. In 2009, China had 4.06 hospital beds per 1,000 population, among the 50 highest rates in the world. However, access to care is much better in large cities, where hospitals have advanced equipment and highly trained personnel, while in isolated, rural areas, hospitals may have little to offer in terms of modern care. In general, physicians are paid poorly and are trained in a variety of programs ranging from courses lasting only two years to programs similar to those offered in the West.

Major Health Issues

In 2008, WHO estimated that 15 percent of years of life lost in China were due to communicable diseases, 65 percent to noncommunicable diseases, and 19 percent to injuries. In 2008, the age-standardized estimate of cancer deaths was 182 per 100,000 for men and 105 per 100,000 for women; for cardiovascular disease and diabetes, 312 per 100,000 for men and 260 per 100,000 for women; and for chronic respiratory disease, 118 per 100,000 for men and 89 per 100,000 for women.

China's maternal mortality rate (death from any cause related to or aggravated by pregnancy) was estimated in 2008 as 38 maternal deaths per 100,000 live births. The infant mortality rate, defined as the number of deaths of infants younger than 1 year, was estimated at 15.62 per 1,000 live births as of 2012. By comparison, the infant mortality rate in Macau was 3.17 per 1,000 live births in 2012, tied for seventh-lowest in the world, and the infant mortality rate in Hong Kong was 2.90 per 1,000 live births (in 2012 data), also seventh-lowest in the world.

In 2010, tuberculosis incidence in China was 78.0 per 100,000 population, tuberculosis prevalence 108.0 per 100,000, and deaths due to tuberculosis among HIV-negative people 4.10 per 100,000. WHO estimated that the case detection rate in 2010 was 87 percent. An estimated 5.7 percent of new cases are multidrug resistant, as are 26 percent of retreatment cases. In Hong Kong, tuberculosis incidence was 80.0 per 100,000 population, tuberculosis prevalence 100.0 per 100,000, and deaths due to tuberculosis among HIV-negative people 6.10 per 100,000. In Macao, tuberculosis incidence was 76.0 per 100,000 population, tuberculosis prevalence 106.0 per 100,000, and deaths due to tuberculosis among HIV-negative people 6.10 per 100,000. As of 2009, an estimated 0.1 percent of adults age 15 to 49 in China were living with HIV or acquired immune deficiency syndrome (AIDS); the same rate of infection was estimated for Hong Kong.

Health Care Personnel

China has over 150 medical schools with instruction provided in Chinese, English, or both. The basic degree course lasts from three to eight years, and the degree awarded is bachelor of medicine. Graduates must complete a one-year internship before receiving a degree. Graduates of foreign medical schools must have their degrees approved by the National Education Department. Foreigners require special authorization to practice in China and must be registered with a Chinese medical institution. In 2009, China had 1.42 physicians per 1,000 population, 0.25 pharmaceutical personnel per 1,000, 0.16 laboratory health workers per 1,000, 0.68 health management and support workers per 1,000, 0.83 community and traditional health workers per 1,000, and 1.38 nurses and midwives per 1,000.

Government Role in Health Care

According to WHO, in 2010, China spent $298 billion on health care, an amount that comes to $221 per capita. Health care was funded entirely through domestic sources. Just over half (54 percent) of health care funding was provided by government expenditures, with 37 percent coming from household spending and 10 percent from other expenditures. In 2010, China allocated 12 percent of total government expenditures to health, placing it in the median range among other upper-middle-income countries in the western Pacific region, and government expenditures on health came to 3 percent of gross domestic product (GDP), placing China in the low range when compared with other upper-middle-income countries in the western Pacific region. In 2009, according to WHO, official development assistance (ODA) for health in China came to $0.26 per capita.

Public Health Programs

China's Center for Disease Control and Prevention (CDC) is located in Beijing and directed by Wang Yu. The CDC, with more than 2,100 employees organized into 22 departments, is China's leading public health agency; it focuses primarily on infectious diseases but plans to expand its work in chronic diseases, food safety, and cancer as well. The CDC launched a massive immunization effort during the H1N1 pandemic in 2009 and also instituted quarantines and border screenings to help contain the disease. Priorities for the CDC include research into disease control and prevention, implementation of disease control programs, conducting applied scientific research, providing technical training and assistance for local and regional public health services, managing public health issues such as food safety and environmental health, and constructing a public health information system.

The Centre for Health Protection (CHP) in Hong Kong, headed by Thomas Tsang, focuses on expanding the disease surveillance network, creating an epidemiology training program, optimizing the capacity of health care providers, developing applied research, and creating response plans for emergencies. The CHP includes five departments: Emergency Response and Information, Infection Control, Programme Management and Professional Development, Public Health Laboratory Services, and Surveillance and Epidemiology. In 2010, 64 percent of the population of China had access to improved sanitary facilities, with access being higher among the urban (74 percent) as opposed to the rural (56 percent) population. Access to improved sources of drinking water was higher, although far from universal, with 91 percent of the population having such access (98 percent for the urban population and 85 percent for the rural). According to the World Higher Education Database (WHED), 19 universities in China offer programs in epidemiology or public health, including one in Hong Kong (the Chinese University of Hong Kong).

COLOMBIA

Colombia is a country in northern South America sharing borders Panama, Peru, Venezuela, Ecuador, and Brazil and having coastlines on both the Caribbean Sea and the North Pacific Ocean. The area of 439,732 square miles (1,138,901 square kilometers) is about twice the size of Texas, and the July 2012 population was estimated at 45.3 million. In 2010, 75 percent of the population lived in urban areas, and the 2010 to 2015 annual rate of urbanization was estimated at 1.7 percent. Bogota is the capital and largest city (with a 2009 population estimated at 8.3 million). The 2012 population growth rate was 1.1 percent, the net migration rate negative 0.7 migrants per 1,000 population, the birth rate 17.2 births per 1,000, and the total fertility rate 2.1

children per woman. The United Nations High Commissioner for Refugees (UNHCR) estimated that, in 2010, there were 212 refugees and persons in refugee-like situations in Colombia, and 3,672,054 internally displaced persons and persons in internally displaced-person-like situations.

A former Spanish colony, Colombia became independent in 1830. Colombia has experienced periods of internal violence in the late 20th and early 21st centuries, caused by both insurgent groups and the drug trade (Colombia is the world's leading cultivator of coca). Colombia ranked tied for 80th among 183 countries on the *Corruption Perceptions Index 2011,* with a score of 3.4 (on a scale where 0 indicates highly corrupt and 10 very clean). In 2011, Colombia was classified as a country with high human development (the second-highest category) on the United Nations Development Programme's (UNDP's) Human Development Index (HDI), with a score of 0.710 (on a scale where 1 denotes high development and 0 low development). Life expectancy at birth in 2012 was estimated at 74.79 years, and per capita gross domestic product (GDP) in 2011 was estimated at $10,100. Income distribution in Colombia is relatively unequal: In 2010, the Gini Index (a measure of dispersion, in which perfect equality is denoted by 0 and maximum inequality is denoted by 100) for family income was 56.0, among the highest in the world. According to the World Economic Forum's *Global Gender Gap Index 2011,* Colombia ranked 80th out of 135 countries on gender equality, with a score of 0.671 (on a scale with a theoretical range of 1 for equality to 0 for inequality and an actual range in 2011 from 0.8530 to 0.4873).

Emergency Health Services

According to the World Health Organization (WHO), as of 2007, Colombia had a formal and publicly available emergency care (prehospital care) system. As of 2005, 72.2 percent of districts and departments in Colombia had staff trained in emergency and disaster care. Doctors Without Borders (Médecins Sans Frontières, or MSF) began working in Colombia in 1985 and had 306 staff members in the country at the close of 2010. In northern Colombia, MSF carried out more than 13,000 consultations in areas affected by violence and provided almost 9,000 consultations through a mobile clinic in Norte de Santander. MSF provided more than 12,000 mental health consultations in several regions of Colombia and published

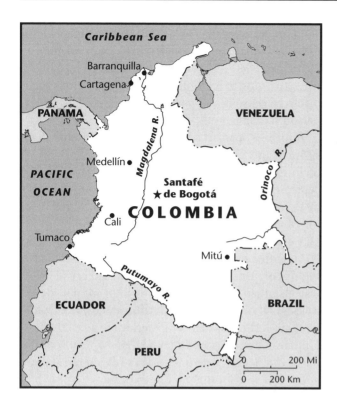

a report, *Three Times Victims: Victims of Violence, Silence, and Neglect, Armed Conflict and Mental Health in the Department of Caquetá, Colombia,* based on its work in Caquetá. MSF has provided maternity and reproductive care, including treatment for victims of sexual violence in Quibdó; this program was transferred to a local provider in 2010. MSF provides diagnosis and care of multidrug-resistant tuberculosis in the port city of Buenaventura, runs a program to diagnose and treat Chagas disease in Arauca, and provided emergency care after the 2010 floods.

Insurance

Colombia has a social insurance system covering all employees residing in Colombia, plus students, pensioners, and apprentices; in the future, it is planned to extend coverage to all. Police and military personnel are covered by special systems. The system is funded by wage contributions (4 percent) and employer payroll contributions (12.5 percent); the government finances the program for people with low incomes. Medical benefits are provided through either public or private health care at the choice of the insured; covered benefits include medical care, hospitalization, surgery, maternity care, drugs, and dental care. Cash sickness benefits are two-thirds of earnings for

180 days; the maternity benefit is 100 percent of earnings for 84 days; the paternity benefit is 100 percent of earnings for 4 days. The Mandatory Health Plan, subsidized by the government, provides care for the poor. According to Ke Xu and colleagues, in 2003, 6.3 percent of households in Colombia experienced catastrophic health expenditures annually; "catastrophic" was defined as exceeding 40 percent of household income remaining after basic needs were met.

Costs of Hospitalization

No data available.

Access to Health Care

According to Latinobarometer, an annual public opinion survey conducted in Latin America, 61 percent of citizens in Colombia are satisfied with the level of health care available to them (the regional average is 51.9 percent). According to WHO, in 2005, 96 percent of births in Colombia were attended by skilled personnel (for example, physicians, nurses, or midwives). In 2005, 83 percent of pregnant women in Colombia received at least four prenatal care visits. The 2010 immunization rates for 1-year-olds were 88 percent for diphtheria and pertussis (DPT3), 88 percent for measles (MCV), and 88 percent for Hib (Hib3). In 2010, an estimated 34 percent of persons with advanced human immunodeficiency virus (HIV) infection were receiving antiretroviral therapy in accordance with the 2010 WHO guidelines.

Cost of Drugs

Colombia has had a National Pharmaceutical Policy since December 2003, and the Ministry of Social Protection oversees the pharmaceutical system. According to WHO, in 2008, the median availability of selected generic drugs in the public sector in Colombia was 86.7 percent; in the private sector, the mean availability was 87.9 percent. The median price ratio (comparing the price in Colombia to the international reference price) was 3.1 in the private sphere for selected generic medicines, indicating that median prices in the public sphere were more than three times as high as the international reference price.

Health Care Facilities

In 2006, Colombia had 58,010 health care sites, including 872 public hospitals. Health care is decentralized and implemented at the district, department, and municipality levels. There are more than 6,000 health laboratories throughout the country, including 33 public health laboratories located in the departmental capitals and 110 blood banks located throughout the country. In 2007, Colombia had 1.00 hospital beds per 1,000 population.

Major Health Issues

In 2008, WHO estimated that 21 percent of years of life lost in Colombia were due to communicable diseases, 43 percent to noncommunicable diseases, and 36 percent to injuries. In 2008, the age-standardized estimate of cancer deaths was 113 per 100,000 for men and 92 per 100,000 for women; for cardiovascular disease and diabetes, 206 per 100,000 for men and 167 per 100,000 for women; and for chronic respiratory disease, 43 per 100,000 for men and 30 per 100,000 for women.

Colombia's maternal mortality rate (death from any cause related to or aggravated by pregnancy) was estimated in 2008 as 84 maternal deaths per 100,000 live births. The infant mortality rate, defined as the number of deaths of infants younger than 1 year, was estimated at 15.92 per 1,000 live births as of 2012. In 2010, tuberculosis incidence was 34.0 per 100,000 population, tuberculosis prevalence 48.0 per 100,000, and deaths due to tuberculosis among HIV-negative people 2.80 per 100,000. As of 2009, an estimated 0.5 percent of adults age 15 to 49 were living with HIV or acquired immune deficiency syndrome (AIDS). In 2008, the age-standardized death rate from malaria was 0.3 per 100,000 population.

Health Care Personnel

Colombia has 28 medical schools with instruction offered in Spanish and sometimes English or French as well. The basic degree course lasts six to seven years, and the degree awarded is Médico or Médico Cirujano (physician or physician and surgeon). One year of government service is required after graduation. The license to practice medicine is granted by the Ministry of Health in Bogotá, and foreign medical graduates must have their degrees validated. In 2002, Colombia had 1.35 physicians per 1,000 population, 0.78 dentistry personnel per 1,000, and 0.55 nurses and midwives per 1,000.

Government Role in Health Care

According to WHO, in 2010, Colombia spent $22 billion on health care, an amount that comes to $472 per capita. Health care was funded entirely through domestic sources. Almost three-quarters (73 percent)

of health care funding was provided by government expenditures, with 20 percent coming from household spending and 8 percent from other expenditures. In 2010, Colombia allocated 20 percent of total government expenditures to health, placing it in the high range compared with other upper-middle-income countries in the Americas region, and government expenditures on health came to 6 percent of GDP, also high when compared with other upper-middle-income countries in the Americas region. In 2009, according to WHO, official development assistance (ODA) for health in Colombia came to $70.20 per capita.

Public Health Programs

Colombia's National Institute of Health (INS) is located in Bogatá and directed by Juan Gonzalo Lopez Casas. INS is a member of the Health System and the National System of Science and Technology and has administrative and financial autonomy within the Ministry of Social Protection. INS functions include coordinating and conducting scientific research; advising, implementing, and managing health-related programs; advising the national government and local authorities; developing a system of epidemiological surveillance; acting as a national reference lab and overseeing other labs in the national network; and training personnel in scientific and technical areas.

In 2010, 77 percent of the population of Colombia had access to improved sanitary facilities, with access being higher among the urban (82 percent) as opposed to the rural (63 percent) population. Access to improved sources of drinking water was higher, although not universal, with 92 percent of the population having such access (99 percent for the urban population and 72 percent for the rural). According to the World Higher Education Database (WHED), six universities in Colombia offer programs in epidemiology or public health: the Universidad Pontificia Bolivariana, the Pontificia Universidad Javeriana, the Autonomous University of Manizales, the University of Antioquia, the University of Valle, and the Fundación Universitaria Juan N. Corpas.

COMOROS

Comoros is an island nation in the Indian Ocean, located between Madagascar and the southeast coast

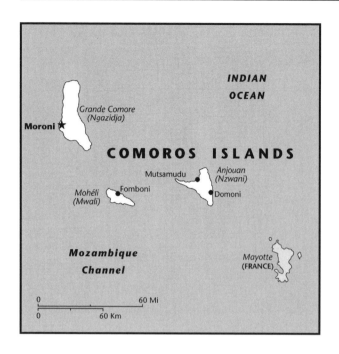

of Africa; Comoros consists of four major islands and many smaller islands. Comoros claims the island of Mayotte as well (it is officially an overseas department of France). The area of 864 square miles (2,235 square kilometers) is about 12 times that of Washington, D.C., and the July 2012 population was estimated at 737,284. In 2010, 28 percent of the population lived in urban areas, and the 2010 to 2015 annual rate of urbanization was estimated at 2.8 percent. The capital is Moroni, located on the island of Grand Comoros. The July 2012 population growth rate was 2.1 percent, despite a negative net migration rate (negative 2.68 migrants per 1,000 population); the total fertility rate is 4.1 children per woman (the 38th-highest in the world), and the birth rate is 31.5 births per 1,000 population (the 41st-highest in the world).

Comoros became independent from France in 1975 and has experienced more than 20 attempted or successful coups since then. In 2011, Comoros ranked 31st among 53 African countries on the Ibrahim Index (evaluating governance performance), with a score of 47 (out of 100) and also ranked tied for 143rd among 183 countries on the *Corruption Perceptions Index 2011,* with a score of 2.4 (on a scale where 0 indicates highly corrupt and 10 very clean). In 2011, Comoros was classified as a country with low human development (the lowest of four categories) on the United Nations Development Programme's (UNDP's) Human Development Index (HDI), with

a score of 0.433 (on a scale where 1 denotes high development and 0 low development). In 2011, the International Food Policy Research Institute (IFPRI) classified Comoros as a country with an "alarming" hunger problem, with a Global Hunger Index (GHI) score of 26.2, the ninth-highest in the world.

Life expectancy at birth in 2012 was estimated at 62.74 years, and the estimated gross domestic product (GDP) per capita in 2011 was $1,200, among the 20 lowest in the world.

Emergency Health Services
According to the World Health Organization (WHO), as of 2007, Comoros did not have a formal and publicly available system for providing prehospital care (emergency care).

Insurance
No data available.

Costs of Hospitalization
No data available.

Access to Health Care
Each major island in Comoros has a hospital, but most are poorly staffed and supplied, and people who need advanced care seek it outside the country if they can afford to do so. According to WHO, in 2000 (the most recent year for which data was available), 62 percent of births in Comoros were attended by skilled personnel (for example, physicians, nurses, or midwives). The 2010 immunization rates for 1-year-olds were 72 percent for diphtheria and pertussis (DPT3), 74 percent for measles (MCV), and 81 percent for Hib (Hib3). In 2010, it was estimated that more than 95 percent of persons with advanced human immunodeficiency virus (HIV) infection were receiving antiretroviral therapy in accordance with the 2010 WHO guidelines. According to WHO, in 2010, Comoros had fewer than 0.01 magnetic resonance imaging (MRI) machines per 1 million population and 1.51 computer tomography (CT) machines per 1 million population.

Cost of Drugs
In Comoros, medicines for a few diseases are provided free: These include antimalarials, antitubercular medications, medications for human immunodeficiency virus and acquired immune deficiency syndrome (HIV/AIDS), and vaccines included on the WHO Expanded Programme on Immunization (EPI) list.

Health Care Facilities

As of 2010, according to WHO, Comoros had 7.08 health posts per 100,000 population, 1.63 health centers per 100,000, 0.27 district or rural hospitals per 100,000, 0.27 provincial hospitals per 100,000, and 0.14 specialized hospitals per 100,000. In 2006, Comoros had 2.20 hospital beds per 1,000 population.

Major Health Issues

In 2008, WHO estimated that 68 percent of years of life lost in Comoros were due to communicable diseases, 24 percent to noncommunicable diseases, and 8 percent to injuries. In 2008, the age-standardized estimate of cancer deaths was 88 per 100,000 for men and 93 per 100,000 for women; for cardiovascular disease and diabetes, 433 per 100,000 for men and 468 per 100,000 for women; and for chronic respiratory disease, 116 per 100,000 for men and 72 per 100,000 for women.

In 2010, tuberculosis incidence was 37.0 per 100,000 population, tuberculosis prevalence 68.0 per 100,000, and deaths due to tuberculosis among HIV-negative people 7.30 per 100,000. As of 2009, an estimated 0.1 percent of adults age 15 to 49 were living with HIV or AIDS. In 2010, 36,538 cases of malaria were reported. In 2008, the age-standardized death rate from malaria was 38.9 per 100,000 population.

Compared to other countries at a similar level of development, Comoros ranked ninth (tied with the Solomon Islands) among the 43 least-developed countries on the 2011 Mothers' Index, produced by the international nongovernmental organization (NGO) Save the Children, based on a number of health and social factors relating to women, children, and maternal and child care. The maternal mortality rate in Comoros (death from any cause related to or aggravated by pregnancy) is high by global standards, estimated at 340 maternal deaths per 100,000 live births as of 2008. The infant mortality rate, defined as the number of deaths of infants younger than 1 year, is also high, at 68.97 per 1,000 live births as of 2012. In 2000, 25.0 percent of children under age 5 were underweight (defined as 2 kilograms [kg] below standard weight-for-age at age 1, 3 kg below for ages 2 to 3, and 4 kg below for ages 4 to 5).

Health Care Personnel

In 2006, WHO identified Comoros as one of 57 countries with a critical deficit in the supply of skilled health workers. In 2004, Comoros had 0.15 physicians per 1,000 population, 0.05 pharmaceutical personnel per 1,000, 0.08 laboratory health workers per 1,000, 0.34 health management and support workers per 1,000, 0.04 dentistry personnel per 1,000, 0.05 community and traditional health workers per 1,000, and 0.74 nurses and midwives per 1,000. The global "brain drain" (international migration of skilled personnel) plays a role in the undersupply of medical personnel in Comoros: Michael Clemens and Bunilla Petterson estimate that 32 percent of Comoros-born physicians and 23 percent of Comoros-born nurses are working in one of nine developed countries, primarily in France, Belgium, and the United States.

Government Role in Health Care

Comoros has a National Health Policy (NHP) and a National Medicines Policy (NMP). The NMP covers selection of essential medicines; purchase, distribution, and regulation of drugs; pharmacovigilance; rational usage of medicines; human resource development; and traditional medicine. Direct advertising of prescription drugs to the public is banned. According to WHO, in 2010, Comoros spent $24 million on health care, an amount that comes to $33 per capita. Health care was funded primarily (81 percent) through domestic sources, with the remaining 19 percent funded by resources from abroad. Two-thirds (67 percent) of health care funding was provided by government expenditures, with the remaining 33 percent coming from household spending. In 2010, Comoros allocated 13 percent of total government expenditures to health, placing it in the high range as compared with other low-income African countries, and government expenditures on health came to 3 percent of GDP, in the median range for low-income African countries. In 2009, according to WHO, official development assistance (ODA) for health in Comoros came to $11.17 per capita.

Public Health Programs

In 2010, 36 percent of the population of Comoros had access to improved sanitary facilities, with access being higher among the urban (50 percent) as opposed to the rural (30 percent) population. Access to improved sources of drinking water was higher, although not universal, with 95 percent of the population having such access (91 percent for the urban population and 97 percent for the rural). According to WHO, in 2004, Comoros had 0.02 environmental and public health workers per 1,000 population. According to the World

Higher Education Database (WHED), no university in Comoros offers programs in epidemiology or public health.

CONGO, DEMOCRATIC REPUBLIC OF THE

The Democratic Republic of the Congo (DRC) is a country in Central Africa sharing borders with nine countries and having a small (23 mile or 37 km) coastline on the Atlantic Ocean. The area of 905,355 square miles (2,344,858 square kilometers) makes the DRC the 11th-largest country in the world and the largest in sub-Saharan Africa, and the July 2012 population of 73.6 million was the 19th-largest in the world. In 2010, 35 percent of the population lived in urban areas, and the 2010 to 2015 annual rate of urbanization was estimated at 4.5 percent. Kinshasa is the capital and largest city (with a 2009 population estimated at 8.4 million). The July 2012 population growth rate was 2.6 percent (the 25th-highest in the world) despite a negative net migration rate (negative 0.5 migrants per 1,000 population); the total fertility rate of 5.09 children per woman is one of the 20 highest in the world, as is the birth rate of 37.0 births per 1,000 population. The United Nations High Commissioner for Refugees (UNHCR) estimated that, in 2010, there were 107,580 refugees and persons in refugee-like situations in the DRC and 460,754 internally displaced persons and persons in internally displaced-person-like situations.

The DRC, a former Belgian colony, became independent in 1960 and has suffered a long history of dictatorship, civil war, and ethnic strife. According to the Ibrahim Index, in 2011, the DRC ranked near the bottom (50th out of 53) among African countries in terms of governance performance, with a score of 32 (out of 100). Government corruption is perceived as a serious problem: The DRC ranked tied for 164th among 183 countries on the *Corruption Perceptions Index 2011,* with a score of 2.1 (on a scale where 0 indicates highly corrupt and 10 very clean).

In 2011, the DRC was classified as a country with low human development (the lowest of four categories) on the United Nations Development Programme's (UNDP's) Human Development Index (HDI), with a score of 0.286 (on a scale where 1 denotes high development and 0 low development). In 2011, the International Food Policy Research Institute (IFPRI) classified the DRC as a country with an "extremely alarming" hunger problem, with a Global Hunger Index (GHI) score of 39.0, one of the highest in the world. Life expectancy at birth in 2012 was estimated at 55.74 years, among the 30 lowest in the world, and estimated gross domestic product (GDP) per capita in 2011 was $300, the lowest in the world. According to the World Food Programme, in October 2011, about 4.5 million people in the DRC were facing acute food crises.

Emergency Health Services

According to the World Health Organization (WHO), as of 2007, the DRC did not have a formal and publicly available system for providing prehospital care (emergency care). Doctors Without Borders (Médecins Sans Frontières, or MSF) began working in the DRC in 1981 and had 2,766 staff members in the country at the close of 2010. Programs in the DRC represent MSF's largest investment in terms of staff, budget, and number of programs; services are provided in Kinshasa and much of the northern, eastern, and southern regions of the country. MSF teams in Kinshasa, Kisangani, Lubumbashi, and Mbandaka work with the Ministry of Health to monitor and respond to outbreaks of infectious disease; in 2010, these teams responded to 10 outbreaks, including measles and yellow fever. In the conflict zones of the DRC, MSF provided more than 1 million consultations, assisted in over 19,000 births, and carried out more than 10,000 surgeries. After a fuel tanker explosion in South Kivu in July 2010, MSF provided medical and mental health care, including skin grafting.

Insurance

The insurance industry is poorly developed in the DRC. However, some associations have created mutual insurance programs; for instance Bwamanda covers teachers. Medical care is provided for the disabled and pensioners and their dependents in government hospitals and clinics. The labor code requires employers to provide medical care for workers and their dependents and to provide sickness and maternity leave. The disabled may also be eligible for home health care if they require constant assistance to perform daily activities.

Costs of Hospitalization

No data available.

Access to Health Care

According to WHO, in 2010, 74 percent of births in the DRC were attended by skilled personnel (for example, physicians, nurses, or midwives). In 2007, 47 percent of pregnant women received at least four prenatal care visits. The 2010 immunization rates for 1-year-olds were 63 percent for diphtheria and pertussis (DPT3) and 68 percent for measles (MCV). In 2010, an estimated 14 percent of persons with advanced human immunodeficiency virus (HIV) infection were receiving antiretroviral therapy in accordance with the 2010 WHO guidelines. According to WHO, in 2010, the DRC had fewer than 0.01 magnetic resonance imaging (MRI) machines per 1 million population and 0.08 computer tomography (CT) machines per 1 million.

Cost of Drugs

Most drugs in the DRC are paid for by out-of-pocket expenses, except for vaccines on WHO's Expanded Programme on Immunization (EPI) list, drugs to treat tuberculosis, drugs for human immunodeficiency virus and acquired immune deficiency syndrome (HIV/AIDS), some antiparasitic drugs, and bed nets impregnated with insecticide. The Ministry of the National Economy regulates profit margins for drugs, which are set at 20 percent for wholesalers and 33 percent for pharmacies. According to WHO, in 2007, the median availability of selected generic drugs in the public sector in the DRC was 55.6 percent; in the private sector, the mean availability was 65.4 percent. The median price ratio (comparing the price in the DRC to the international reference price) was 2.0 in the public sphere for selected generic medicines and 2.3 in the private sphere, indicating that median prices in the public and private spheres were twice as high as the international reference price.

Health Care Facilities

As of 2010, according to WHO, the DRC had 0.44 district or rural hospitals per 100,000 population and 0.02 provincial hospitals per 100,000. In 2006, the DRC had 0.80 hospital beds per 1,000 population, one of the 30 lowest rates in the world.

Major Health Issues

In 2008, WHO estimated that 82 percent of years of life lost in the DRC were due to communicable diseases, 11 percent to noncommunicable diseases, and 7 percent to injuries. In 2008, the age-standardized estimate of cancer deaths was 89 per 100,000 for men

and 86 per 100,000 for women; for cardiovascular disease and diabetes, 462 per 100,000 for men and 492 per 100,000 for women; and for chronic respiratory disease, 127 per 100,000 for men and 74 per 100,000 for women.

In 2008, the age-standardized death rate from malaria was 96.4 per 100,000 population, the seventh-highest in the world. In 2010, tuberculosis incidence was 327.0 per 100,000 population, tuberculosis prevalence 535.0 per 100,000, and deaths due to tuberculosis among HIV-negative people 54.00 per 100,000. WHO estimates that the case detection rate in 2010 was 53 percent. An estimated 2.2 percent of new cases are multidrug resistant, as are 9.4 percent of retreatment cases. In 2010, 11 percent of pregnant women tested positive for HIV. The mother-to-child transmission rate for HIV in 2010 was estimated at 37 percent, and in 2009, 1.1 percent of deaths to children under age 5 were attributed to HIV. In 2010, over 24.1 million cases of malaria were reported.

The DRC's maternal mortality rate (death from any cause related to or aggravated by pregnancy) is quite high by global standards, estimated at 670 maternal deaths per 100,000 live births as of 2008. The infant mortality rate, defined as the number of deaths of infants younger than 1 year, is also high, at 76.63 per 1,000 live births as of 2012. In 2007, 28.2 percent of children under age 5 were underweight (defined as 2 kilograms [kg] below standard

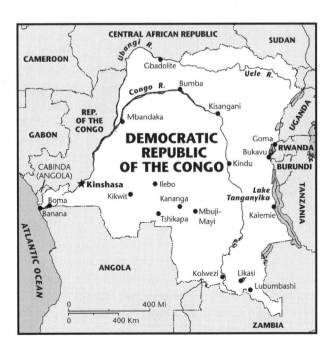

weight-for-age at age 1, 3 kg below for ages 2 to 3, and 4 kg below for ages 4 to 5).

Health Care Personnel

In 2006, WHO identified the DRC as one of 57 countries with a critical deficit in the supply of skilled health workers. The DRC has three medical schools, located in Kinshasa, Kisangani, and Lubumbashi. The basic course of training lasts six to seven years, and the degree awarded is Docteur en Medécine, Chirurgie et Accouchement (doctor of medicine, surgery, and midwifery). In 2004, the DRC had 0.11 physicians per 1,000 population, 0.02 pharmaceutical personnel per 1,000, 0.01 laboratory health workers per 1,000, 0.28 health management and support workers per 1,000, and 0.53 nurses and midwives per 1,000. The global "brain drain" (international migration of skilled personnel) plays a role in the undersupply of medical personnel in the DRC: Michael Clemens and Bunilla Petterson estimate that 9 percent of DRC-born physicians and 12 percent of DRC-born nurses are working in one of nine developed countries, primarily in France, Belgium, the United States, and South Africa.

Government Role in Health Care

Health care in the DRC has three levels of organization: central, provincial, and peripheral. The central or national level is responsible for setting policies, standards, and guidelines; providing tertiary care; and monitoring care provision in the provinces. The provincial level includes 65 health districts and 11 provinces and provides supervision and guidance to care at the local level. Primary health care is provided at the peripheral or local level. The DRC has a National Medicines Policy (NMP) developed in 1987 and revised in 2008; the goal is to supply an adequate and affordable supply of drugs to the population. The national list of essential medicines was revised in 2010 and includes 671 drugs. More than 3,500 branded pharmaceuticals and 1,680 generic drugs are registered with the patent office.

According to WHO, in 2010, the DRC spent $1.0 billion on health care, an amount that comes to $16 per capita. About two-thirds (67 percent) of health care funding was provided from domestic sources, the remaining third (33 percent) from funding from abroad. The largest share of spending (43 percent) for health care came from government expenditures, followed by household spending (36 percent) and other sources (22 percent). In 2010, the DRC allocated 9 percent of total government expenditures to health, and government expenditures on health came to 3 percent of GDP; on both measures, the DRC ranks in the median range when compared with other low-income African countries. In 2009, according to WHO, official development assistance for health in the DRC came to $4.81 per capita.

Public Health Programs

In 2010, 24 percent of the population of the DRC had access to improved sanitation facilities (the access was reported as equal for both urban and rural populations), and 45 percent had access to improved sources of drinking water (27 percent in rural areas and 79 percent in urban). According to the World Higher Education Database (WHED), three universities in the DRC offer programs in epidemiology or public health: the University of Kinshasa Binza, the University of Lubumbashi, and the Protestant University of the Congo.

CONGO, REPUBLIC OF THE

The Republic of the Congo (Congo) is a central African country, sharing borders with Angola, Cameroon, the Central African Republic, the Democratic Republic of the Congo, and Gabon and having a coastline on the south Atlantic Ocean. The area of 132,047 square miles(342,000 square kilometers) makes Congo about the size of Montana, and the July 2012 population was estimated at 4.4 million. In 2010, 62 percent of the population lived in urban areas, and the 2010 to 2015 annual rate of urbanization was estimated at 3.0 percent. Brazzaville is the capital and largest city (with a 2009 population estimated at 1.3 million). The population growth rate in 2012 was 2.9 percent (the 15th-highest in the world), the net migration rate negative 0.4 migrants per 1,000 population, the birth rate 40.1 births per 1,000 (the 10th-highest in the world), and the total fertility rate 5.6 children per woman (the 10th-highest in the world). The United Nations High Commissioner for Refugees (UNHCR) estimated that, in 2010, there were 133,112 refugees and persons in refugee-like situations in Congo.

A former French colony, Congo became independent in 1960. The first democratically elected government took office in 1992; in 1997, a period of ethnic and political unrest began, with accord being reached in 2003. According to the Ibrahim Index, in 2011, Congo ranked 40th among 53 African countries in terms of governance performance, with a score of 42 (out of 100). Congo ranked tied for 152nd among 183 countries on the *Corruption Perceptions Index 2011,* with a score of 2.2 (on a scale where 0 indicates highly corrupt and 10 very clean). In 2011, Congo was classified as a country with medium human development (the second from the lowest of four categories) on the United Nations Development Programme's (UNDP's) Human Development Index (HDI), with a score of 0.533 (on a scale where 1 denotes high development and 0 low development). Life expectancy at birth in 2012 was estimated at 55.27 years, among the 30 lowest in the world, and the estimated gross domestic product (GDP) per capita in 2011 was $4,600.

Emergency Health Services

According to the World Health Organization (WHO), as of 2007, Congo did not have a formal and publicly available system for providing prehospital care (emergency care). Doctors Without Borders (Médecins Sans Frontières, or MSF) began working in Congo in 1997 and had 384 staff members in the country at the close of 2010. MSF operated in the extreme south (Pointe-Noire) and northern (Impfondo, Bolembé, and Bétou) regions of Congo in 2010. MSF also provided medical

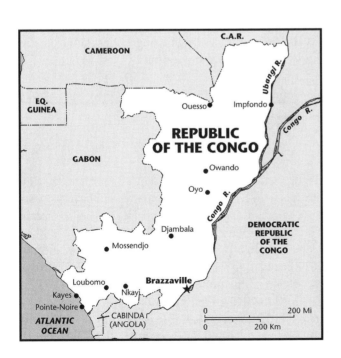

care in Impfondo, offering about 3,600 consultations monthly; in July, this operation was moved to Bolembé. In the rapidly growing province of Likouala in northern Congo, MSF established a hospital in Bétou in 2003, treating about 3,000 patients monthly; MSF has since established six health centers in the district as well as mobile medical teams who provide about 10,000 consultations per month. MSF responded to the 2010 polio epidemic in southern Congo, treating patients and assisting in a polio vaccination campaign.

Insurance

Congo has a social insurance system covering only maternity benefits and only for employed women. The system is funded by employer contributions (10.03 percent of covered payroll); the same system funds Congo's Family Allowances program. The maternal benefit is 50 percent of daily covered earnings for 15 weeks, with a possible three-week extension if there are birth complications. The woman giving birth is reimbursed for medical maternity expenses, and some maternal and child benefits are also provided under the Family Allowances system. These include a prenatal allowance of XAF 2,000 per month for up to nine months, a birth grant of XAF 1,000 (for up to three births), and a family allowance of XAF 2,000 per month per child, up to age 16 (17 if the child is an apprentice and 20 if he or she is disabled or a student). To receive the prenatal allowance, the woman must undergo required physical exams. The system is administered by the National Social Security Fund under the supervision of the Ministry of Labor, Employment, and Social Security.

Costs of Hospitalization
No data available.

Access to Health Care
In 2006, 75 percent of pregnant women in Congo received at least four prenatal care visits. In 2010, an estimated 42 percent of persons with advanced human immunodeficiency virus (HIV) infection were receiving antiretroviral therapy in accordance with the 2010 WHO guidelines.

Cost of Drugs
According to WHO, in 2007, the median availability of selected generic drugs in the public sector in Congo was 21.2 percent; in the private sector, the mean availability was 31.3 percent. The median price ratio (comparing the price in Congo to the international reference price)

was 6.5 in the public sphere for selected generic medicines and 11.5 in the private sphere, indicating that median prices in the public sphere were more than six times as high and, in the private sphere, more than 11 times as high as the international reference price.

Health Care Facilities

In 2005, Congo had 1.60 hospital beds per 1,000 population.

Major Health Issues

In 2008, WHO estimated that 73 percent of years of life lost in Congo were due to communicable diseases, 17 percent to noncommunicable diseases, and 10 percent to injuries. In 2008, the age-standardized estimate of cancer deaths was 83 per 100,000 for men and 76 per 100,000 for women; for cardiovascular disease and diabetes, 482 per 100,000 for men and 444 per 100,000 for women; and for chronic respiratory disease, 133 per 100,000 for men and 64 per 100,000 for women.

In 2010, tuberculosis incidence was 372.0 per 100,000 population, tuberculosis prevalence 545.0 per 100,000, and deaths due to tuberculosis among HIV-negative people 49.00 per 100,000. As of 2009, an estimated 3.4 percent of adults age 15 to 49 were living with HIV or acquired immune deficiency syndrome (AIDS). Congo's maternal mortality rate (death from any cause related to or aggravated by pregnancy) has been quite high by global standards, estimated at 580 maternal deaths per 100,000 live births as of 2008. The infant mortality rate, defined as the number of deaths of infants younger than 1 year, also has been high, at 74.22 per 1,000 live births as of 2012. In 2005, 11.8 percent of children under age 5 were underweight (defined as 2 kilograms [kg] below standard weight-for-age at age 1, 3 kg below for ages 2 to 3, and 4 kg below for ages 4 to 5).

Health Care Personnel

In 2006, WHO identified Congo as one of 57 countries with a critical deficit in the supply of skilled health workers. In 2007, Republic of the Congo had 0.10 physicians per 1,000 population, 0.02 pharmaceutical personnel per 1,000, 0.09 laboratory health workers per 1,000, 1.10 health management and support workers per 1,000, 0.03 community and traditional health workers per 1,000, and 0.82 nurses and midwives per 1,000. Michael Clemens and Bunilla Petterson estimate that 53 percent of Republic of the Congo-born physicians and 12 percent of Republic of the Congo-born

nurses are working in one of nine developed countries, primarily in France and South Africa (physicians) and France, Belgium, and the United States (nurses).

Government Role in Health Care

According to WHO, in 2010, Congo spent $292 million on health care, an amount that comes to $72 per capita. Most health care funding (96 percent) came from domestic sources, with 4 percent coming from abroad. Health care purchasing was almost evenly split between government expenditures (47 percent) and household expenditures (53 percent). In 2010, Congo allocated 5 percent of its total government expenditures to health, and government expenditures on health came to 1 percent of GDP; both figures are in the low range for lower-middle-income African countries. In 2009, according to WHO, official development assistance (ODA) for health in Congo came to $9.56 per capita.

Public Health Programs

In 2010, 18 percent of the population of Congo had access to improved sanitary facilities, with access being slightly higher among the urban (20 percent) as opposed to the rural (15 percent) population. Access to improved sources of drinking water was higher, although not universal, and with a wide urban versus rural discrepancy, with 71 percent of the population having such access (95 percent for the urban population and 32 percent for rural). According to WHO, in 2007, Congo had fewer than 0.01 environmental and public health workers per 1,000 population. According to the World Higher Education Database (WHED), no university in Congo offers programs in epidemiology or public health.

COSTA RICA

Costa Rica is a country in Central America, sharing borders with Nicaragua and Panama and having coastlines on the Caribbean Sea and North Pacific Ocean. The area of 19,730 square miles (51,100 square kilometers) is slightly smaller than West Virginia, and the 2012 population was estimated at 4.6 million. In 2010, 64 percent of the population lived in urban areas, and the 2010 to 2015 annual rate of urbanization was estimated at 2.1 percent. San Jose is the capital and largest city (with a 2009 population estimated at 1.4 million).

The July 2012 population growth rate was 1.3 percent, the birth rate 16.4 births per 1,000 population, the net migration rate 0.9 migrants per 1,000, and the total fertility rate 1.9 children per woman. The United Nations High Commissioner for Refugees (UNHCR) estimated that, in 2010, there were 26,218 refugees and persons in refugee-like situations in Costa Rica.

Costa Rica became independent from Spain in 1821; it has enjoyed a relatively peaceful and democratic existence. Costa Rica ranked tied for 50th among 183 countries on the *Corruption Perceptions Index 2011,* with a score of 4.8 (on a scale where 0 indicates highly corrupt and 10 very clean). In 2011, Costa Rica was classified as a country with high human development (the second-highest category) on the United Nations Development Programme's (UNDP's) Human Development Index (HDI), with a score of 0.744 (on a scale where 1 denotes high development and 0 low development). Life expectancy at birth in 2012 was estimated at 77.89 years, and per capita gross domestic product (GDP) in 2011 was estimated at $11,500. Income distribution in Costa Rica is relatively unequal: In 2009, the Gini Index (a measure of dispersion, in which perfect equality is denoted by 0 and maximum inequality is denoted by 100) for family income was 50.3. According to the World Economic Forum's *Global Gender Gap Index 2011*, Costa Rica ranked 25th out of 135 countries on gender equality, with a score of 0.727 (on a scale with a theoretical range of 1 for equality to 0 for inequality and an actual range in 2011 from 0.8530 to 0.4873).

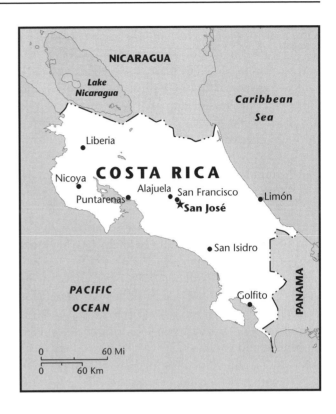

Emergency Health Services

According to the World Health Organization (WHO), as of 2007, Costa Rica had a formal and publicly available emergency care (prehospital care) system, accessible through a national universal access telephone number. In case of emergency, patients may seek care from any hospital or clinic offering the needed care, bypassing the usual method of access through the primary care system.

Insurance

Costa Rica has a social insurance program, with medical benefits provided to all residents; visitors may be covered for emergency care through international agreements. Employed people, the poor, pensioners, and prisoners are also eligible for cash maternity and sickness benefits. The program is funded through wage contributions (5.5 percent of gross earnings), pensioner contributions (5 percent of pensions), contributions from the self-employed (4.75 to 7.75 percent of declared earnings), and payroll contributions from employers (9.25 percent). Maternity benefits are funded half by employer contributions and half through the Social Insurance Fund. Medical care is provided directly to patients in the medical facilities of the Social Insurance Fund. Benefits include hospitalization; medicines; general, specialist, and maternity care; dental care; auditory services; limited optometry services; and appliances. The program is administered by the Costa Rican Social Insurance Fund, which owns and operates 152 clinics and 29 hospitals. According to Ke Xu and colleagues, in 2003, 0.1 percent of households in Costa Rica experienced catastrophic health expenditures annually; "catastrophic" was defined as exceeding 40 percent of household income remaining after basic needs were met.

Costs of Hospitalization

No data available.

Access to Health Care

Health is identified as a basic human right in the constitution, and the entire population of Costa

Rica is entitled to use the public services provided by the Costa Rican Social Security Fund (CRSS). Primary care is provided by basic comprehensive health care teams, consisting of a physician, a nurse, and a primary care technician; each team is responsible for about 4,000 people. Secondary care is provided through a network of 10 health centers and 20 hospitals, while tertiary care is provided at five specialized hospitals and three national general hospitals. According to Latinobarometer, an annual public opinion survey conducted in Latin America, 66 percent of citizens in Costa Rica are satisfied with the level of health care available to them (the regional average is 51.9 percent).

According to WHO, in 2007, 98.7 percent of births in Costa Rica were attended by skilled personnel (for example, physicians, nurses, or midwives). The 2010 immunization rates for 1-year-olds were 88 percent for diphtheria and pertussis (DPT3), 83 percent for measles (MCV), and 90 percent for Hib (Hib3). In 2010, an estimated 65 percent of persons with advanced human immunodeficiency virus (HIV) infection were receiving antiretroviral therapy in accordance with the 2010 WHO guidelines. According to WHO, in 2010, Costa Rica had 0.6 magnetic resonance imaging (MRI) machines per 1 million population, 3.10 computer tomography (CT) machines per 1 million, 0.66 telecolbalt units per 1 million, and 0.66 radiotherapy machines per 1 million.

Cost of Drugs

Costa Rica does not regulate the price of drugs, so prices are determined through the processes of supply and demand.

Health Care Facilities

Primary care is provided by basic comprehensive health care teams located throughout the country, and each of Costa Rica's 104 health areas has a clinic providing lab services, X-ray services, and so on. Costa Rica has 28 hospitals, including three national general hospitals, and specialized hospitals dedicated to rehabilitation, psychiatric care, geriatric care, children's health, and women's health. As of 2010, according to WHO, Costa Rica had 2.21 health posts per 100,000 population, 0.69 health centers per 100,000, 0.28 district or rural hospitals per 100,000, 0.24 provincial hospitals per 100,000, and 0.30 specialized hospitals per 100,000. In 2008, Costa Rica had 1.20 hospital beds per 1,000 population.

Major Health Issues

In 2008, WHO estimated that 13 percent of years of life lost in Costa Rica were due to communicable diseases, 62 percent to noncommunicable diseases, and 25 percent to injuries. In 2008, the age-standardized estimate of cancer deaths was 120 per 100,000 for men and 93 per 100,000 for women; for cardiovascular disease and diabetes, 181 per 100,000 for men and 137 per 100,000 for women; and for chronic respiratory disease, 33 per 100,000 for men and 22 per 100,000 for women.

Costa Rica's maternal mortality rate (death from any cause related to or aggravated by pregnancy) was estimated in 2008 as 44 maternal deaths per 100,000 live births. The infant mortality rate, defined as the number of deaths of infants younger than 1 year, was 9.20 per 1,000 live births as of 2012. In 2010, tuberculosis incidence was 13.0 per 100,000 population, tuberculosis prevalence 18.0 per 100,000, and deaths due to tuberculosis among HIV-negative people 1.10 per 100,000. As of 2009, an estimated 0.3 percent of adults age 15 to 49 were living with HIV or acquired immune deficiency syndrome (AIDS).

Health Care Personnel

Costa Rica has five medical schools, all located in San José. The basic course of training lasts five to six years, followed by a year of supervised medical practice, and the degree granted is Licenciado en Medicina (bachelor of medicine). One year of government service after graduation is required. Physicians must register with the Colegio de Médicos y Cirujanos de Costa Rica, and foreign medical graduates must have their degrees validated. Foreigners must live in Costa Rica for five years before becoming eligible for a medical license. In 2000, Costa Rica had 1.32 physicians per 1,000 population, 0.53 pharmaceutical personnel per 1,000, 4.68 health management and support workers per 1,000, 0.48 dentistry personnel per 1,000, 1.29 community and traditional health workers per 1,000, and 0.93 nurses and midwives per 1,000.

Government Role in Health Care

According to WHO, in 2010, Costa Rica spent $3.8 billion on health care, an amount that comes to $811 per capita. Health care was funded almost entirely (99 percent) through domestic sources, with the remaining 1 percent funded by resources from abroad. Two-thirds (68 percent) of health care funding was provided by government expenditures, with 28 percent coming from household spending and 4 percent from other sources. In 2010, Costa Rica allocated 29 percent of total government expenditures to health, placing it in the high range as compared with other upper-middle-income countries in the Americas region, and government expenditures on health came to 7 percent of GDP, also ranking high in comparison with other upper-middle-income countries in the Americas region. In 2009, according to WHO, official development assistance (ODA) for health in Costa Rica came to $0.50 per capita.

Public Health Programs

Costa Rica's National Institute for Research on Nutrition and Health (INCIENSA), located in Tres Rios, is directed by Dr. Lissette Navas and managed under the auspices of the Ministry of Health. It is responsible for public health education, research, and the development of a national network of labs and surveillance systems. The National References (CNR) coordinate surveillance, do quality control for lab work, conduct research, and train individuals in public health practices.

In 2010, access to improved sources of drinking water in Costa Rica was essentially universal, and 95 percent of the population had access to improved sanitary facilities. According to WHO, in 2000, Costa Rica had 0.32 environmental and public health workers per 1,000 population. According to the World Higher Education Database (WHED), three universities in Costa Rica offer programs in epidemiology or public health: the University of Costa Rica, the University of Ibero-America, and Santa Lucia University, all three located in San Jose.

CÔTE D'IVOIRE

Côte d'Ivoire is a west African country sharing borders with Burkina Faso, Ghana, Guinea, Liberia, and Mali. The area of 124,504 square miles (322,463 square kilometers), is somewhat larger than New Mexico, and the July 2012 population was estimated at 22.0 million. In 2010, 51 percent of the population lived in urban areas, and the 2010 to 2015 annual rate of urbanization was estimated at 3.7 percent. The capital is Yamoussoukro, while Abidjan is the seat of government and largest city (with a 2009 population estimated at 4.0 million). The population growth rate in 2012 was 2.0 percent,

the birth rate 30.4 births per 1,000 population, the net migration rate 0.0 migrants per 1,000, and the total fertility rate 3.8 children per woman. The United Nations High Commissioner for Refugees (UNHCR) estimated that, in 2010, there were 26,218 refugees and persons in refugee-like situations in Côte d'Ivoire and 22,625 internally displaced persons and persons in internally displaced-person-like situations.

Côte d'Ivoire became independent from France in 1960; its history since 1999 has been marked by a military coup, a civil war, and repeated outbreaks of internal violence. According to the Ibrahim Index, in 2011, Côte d'Ivoire ranked near the bottom (46th out of 53) among African countries in terms of governance performance, with a score of 36 (out of 100). Government corruption is perceived as a problem: Côte d'Ivoire ranked tied for 152nd among 183 countries on the *Corruption Perceptions Index 2011*, with a score of 2.2 (on a scale where 0 indicates highly corrupt and 10 very clean).

In 2011, Côte d'Ivoire was classified as a country with low human development (the lowest of four categories) on the United Nations Development Programme's (UNDP's) Human Development Index (HDI), with a score of 0.40 (on a scale where 1 denotes high development and 0 low development). Life expectancy at birth in 2012 was estimated at 57.25 years, among the 30 lowest in the world, and estimated gross domestic product (GDP) per capita

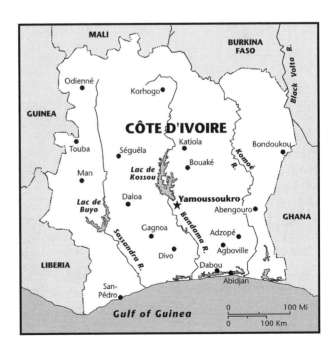

in 2011 was $1,600, among the 30 lowest in the world. In 2008, the Gini Index (a measure of dispersion, in which perfect equality is denoted by 0 and maximum inequality is denoted by 100) for family income was 41.5. According to the World Economic Forum's *Global Gender Gap Index 2011*, Côte d'Ivoire ranked 130th out of 135 countries on gender equality, with a score of 0.577 (on a scale with a theoretical range of 1 for equality to 0 for inequality and an actual range in 2011 from 0.8530 to 0.4873).

Emergency Health Services

In 2011, the World Health Organization (WHO) was actively involved in providing health services in the parts of Côte d'Ivoire most affected by civil unrest; current activities include building camps for displaced people, rebuilding health facilities damaged in the fighting, supplying medical staff and supplies, implementing emergency vaccination campaigns, and conducting disease surveillance, particularly for polio, meningitis, measles, cholera, and hemorrhagic fever.

Insurance

Côte d'Ivoire has a social insurance system covering cash and medical benefits for maternity only. Employed women are covered, including day laborers and temporary workers. Civil servants are covered under a separate system. The system is funded through employer contributions (0.75 percent of payroll). The cash maternity benefit is 100 percent of wages for six weeks before birth and eight weeks after, with an additional three weeks of coverage after birth possible if there are complications. Medical care is provided from the third month of pregnancy, and dependents are provided care through the National Social Insurance Fund. Family benefits are provided through employment-related insurance; these include birth grants for up to three children in a first marriage, a prenatal allowance provided a woman attends three medical examinations during that time, and family allowances for each child aged 2 to 13 years (up to age 18 if the child is an apprentice and up to age 21 if a student or disabled).

The National Social Insurance Fund is governed by a board, and the Ministry of Economy and Finance provides financial supervision.

Costs of Hospitalization

No data available.

Access to Health Care

According to WHO, in 2006, 57 percent of births in Côte d'Ivoire were attended by skilled personnel (for example, physicians, nurses, or midwives). In 2005, 45 percent of pregnant women received at least four prenatal care visits. The 2010 immunization rates for 1-year-olds were 85 percent for diphtheria and pertussis (DPT3), 70 percent for measles (MCV), and

Selected Health Indicators: Côte d'Ivoire Compared With the Global Average (2010)

	Côte d'Ivoire	Global Average
Male life expectancy at birth* (years)	49	66
Female life expectancy at birth* (years)	52	71
Under-5 mortality rate, both sexes (per 1,000 live births)	123	57
Adult mortality rate, both sexes* (probability of dying between 15 and 60 years per 1,000 population)	495	176
Maternal mortality ratio (per 100,000 live births)	400	210
HIV prevalence* (per 1,000 adults aged 15 to 49)	34	8
Tuberculosis prevalence (per 100,000 population)	156	178

Source: World Health Organization Global Health Observatory Data Repository.
*Data refers to 2009.

85 percent for Hib (Hib3). In 2010, an estimated 37 percent of persons with advanced human immunodeficiency virus (HIV) infection were receiving antiretroviral therapy in accordance with the 2010 WHO guidelines. According to WHO, in 2010, Côte d'Ivoire had 0.15 magnetic resonance imaging (MRI) machines per 1 million population and 0.68 computer tomography (CT) machines per 1 million.

Cost of Drugs

Total pharmaceutical expenses in 2007 in Côte d'Ivoire came to $338.2 million, or $16.90 per capita. Pharmaceutical expenses came to 1.5 percent of GDP and 27.3 percent of total health expenses. Some medications are provided for free, including those for malaria, tuberculosis, human immunodeficiency virus and acquired immune deficiency syndrome (HIV/AIDS), and the vaccinations on WHO's Expanded Programme on Immunization (EPI) list.

Health Care Facilities

As of 2010, according to WHO, Côte d'Ivoire had 12.18 health centers per 100,000 population, 1.19 district or rural hospitals per 100,000, 0.47 provincial hospitals per 100,000, and 0.10 specialized hospitals per 100,000. In 2006, Côte d'Ivoire had 0.40 hospital beds per 1,000 population, one of the 10 lowest rates in the world.

Major Health Issues

In 2008, WHO estimated that 71 percent of years of life lost in Côte d'Ivoire were due to communicable diseases, 19 percent to noncommunicable diseases, and 11 percent to injuries. In 2008, the age-standardized estimate of cancer deaths was 80 per 100,000 for men and 79 per 100,000 for women; for cardiovascular disease and diabetes, 548 per 100,000 for men and 524 per 100,000 for women; and for chronic respiratory disease, 155 per 100,000 for men and 84 per 100,000 for women. In 2008, the age-standardized death rate from malaria was 69.1 per 100,000 population. In 2010, tuberculosis incidence was 139.0 per 100,000 population, tuberculosis prevalence 156.0 per 100,000, and deaths due to tuberculosis among HIV-negative people 11.0 per 100,000. As of 2009, an estimated 63.4 percent of adults age 15 to 49 were living with HIV or AIDS. In 2010, 59 percent of pregnant women tested positive for HIV. The mother-to-child transmission rate for HIV in 2010 was estimated at 27 percent, and in 2009, 4.4 percent of deaths to children

under age 5 were attributed to HIV. In 2010, 62,726 cases of malaria were reported.

Compared to other countries at a similar level of development, Côte d'Ivoire ranked last among 80 less-developed countries on the 2011 Mothers' Index, produced by the international nongovernmental organization (NGO) Save the Children, based on a number of health and social factors relating to women, children, and maternal and child care. Côte d'Ivoire's maternal mortality rate (death from any cause related to or aggravated by pregnancy) is high by global standards, estimated at 470 maternal deaths per 100,000 live births as of 2008. A 2006 survey estimated the prevalence of female genital mutilation at 36.4 percent. The infant mortality rate, defined as the number of deaths of infants younger than 1 year, is high, at 63.20 per 1,000 live births as of 2012. In 2006, 16.7 percent of children under age 5 were underweight (defined as 2 kilograms [kg] below standard weight-for-age at age 1, 3 kg below for ages 2 to 3, and 4 kg below for ages 4 to 5).

Health Care Personnel

In 2006, WHO identified Côte d'Ivoire as one of 57 countries with a critical deficit in the supply of skilled health workers. Côte d'Ivoire has one medical school, the Faculté de Médecine of the University of Abidjan, which began offering instruction in 1966. The basic course of training lasts eight years, and the degree awarded is the Doctorat d'État en Médecine (doctor of medicine). Physicians must register with the Conseil National de l'Ordre des Médecines, and the license to practice medicine is granted to citizens who have graduated from a recognized medical school, while foreigners require special authorization.

In 2008, Côte d'Ivoire had 0.14 physicians per 1,000 population, 0.02 pharmaceutical personnel per 1,000, 0.90 health management and support workers per 1,000, 0.01 dentistry personnel per 1.000, and 0.48 nurses and midwives per 1,000. The global "brain drain" (international migration of skilled personnel) plays a role in the undersupply of medical personnel in Côte d'Ivoire: Michael Clemens and Bunilla Petterson estimate that 14 percent of Côte d'Ivoire–born physicians and 7 percent of Côte d'Ivoire–born nurses are working in one of nine developed countries, primarily in France (and the United States in the case of nurses).

Government Role in Health Care

Access to essential medications is considered part of the right to health in Côte d'Ivoire, as specified in the national constitution. The National Medicines Policy (NMP) of Côte d'Ivoire includes selection of essential medicines; financing, pricing, purchase, distribution, and regulation of drugs; pharmacovigilance; rational usage of medicines; human resource development; research; and traditional medicine. Côte d'Ivoire is a member of the World Trade Organization (WTO) but allows for several exceptions to patent regulation, including compulsory licensing for reasons of public health, the Bolar exception that allows manufacturers to perform research and testing to create generic drugs before a patent has expired, and parallel importing provisions (allowing import of drugs created for sale in a different country).

According to WHO, in 2010 Côte d'Ivoire spent $1.2 billion on health care, an amount that comes to $60 per capita. Health care was funded primarily (90 percent) through domestic sources, with the remaining 10 percent funded by resources from abroad. More than three-quarters (77 percent) of health care funding was provided by household spending, with 22 percent coming from government spending and 1 percent from other sources. In 2010, Côte d'Ivoire allocated 5 percent of total government expenditures to health, and government expenditures on health came to 1 percent of GDP; on both measures, Côte d'Ivoire ranks low among low- and middle-income African countries. In 2009, according to WHO, official development assistance for health in Côte d'Ivoire came to $8.88 per capita.

Public Health Programs

The National Institute of Public Health for Côte d'Ivoire, located in Abidjan and directed by Dinard Kouassi, was founded in 1970 and conducted more than 400 projects in its first 25 years. The National Institute of Public Health has trained many public health specialists through teaching at universities and graduate schools, conducted research, and contributed to public policy. Activities of the National Institute of Public Health were curtailed due to civil war, but the institute is currently working to return to full capacity and is developing a strategic plan to improve public health in Côte d'Ivoire.

In 2010, only 24 percent of the population of Côte d'Ivoire had access to improved sanitary facilities, with access being higher among the urban (36 percent) as opposed to the rural (11 percent) population. Access to improved sources of drinking water was higher, although not universal, with 80 percent of the population having such access (91 percent for the urban population and 68 percent for the rural). According to C. B. Ijsselmuiden and colleagues, in 2007, Côte d'Ivoire had one institution offering postgraduate public health programs. According to WHO, in 2008, Côte d'Ivoire had 0.07 environmental and public health workers per 1,000 population.

CROATIA

Croatia is a country in southeastern Europe, sharing borders with Bosnia and Herzegovina, Hungary, Serbia, Montenegro, and Slovenia and having a coastline on the Adriatic Sea. The area of 21,851 square miles (56,594 square kilometers) makes Croatia slightly smaller than West Virginia, and the July 2012 population was estimated at 4.5 million. In 2010, 58 percent of the population lived in urban areas, and the 2010 to 2015 annual rate of urbanization was estimated at 0.4 percent. The capital and largest city is Zagreb. The July 2012 population growth rate was negative 0.1 percent, despite a positive net migration rate (1.51 migrants per 1,000 population); the total fertility rate was 1.44 children per woman and the birth rate 9.57 births per 1,000 population. The United Nations High Commissioner for Refugees (UNHCR) estimated that, in 2010, there

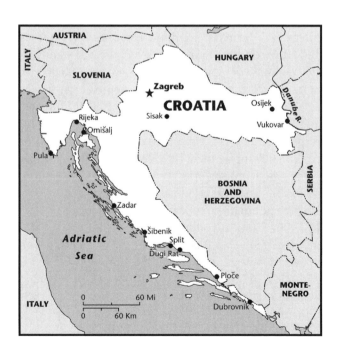

were 936 refugees and persons in refugee-like situations in Croatia and 160 internally displaced persons and persons in internally displaced-person-like situations.

Croatia declared its independence from Yugoslavia in 1991 and was the scene of a bitter conflict with Serbia through much of the 1990s. Croatia ranked tied for 66th among 183 on the *Corruption Perceptions Index 2011,* with a score of 4.0 (on a scale where 0 indicates highly corrupt and 10 very clean). In 2011, Croatia was classified as a country with very high human development (the highest of four categories) on the United Nations Development Programme's (UNDP's) Human Development Index (HDI), with a score of 0.796 (on a scale where 1 denotes high development and 0 low development). Life expectancy at birth in 2012 was estimated at 75.99 years, and per capita gross domestic product (GDP) in 2011 was estimated at $18,300. Income distribution is among the most equal in the world: In 2009, the Gini Index (a measure of dispersion, in which perfect equality is denoted by 0 and maximum inequality is denoted by 100) for family income was 29.0. According to the World Economic Forum's *Global Gender Gap Index 2011,* Croatia ranked 50th out of 135 countries on gender equality with a score of 0.701 (on a scale with a theoretical range of 1 for equality to 0 for inequality and an actual range in 2011 from 0.8530 to 0.4873).

Emergency Health Services

According to the World Health Organization (WHO), as of 2007, the emergency care (prehospital care) system in Croatia included a national universal access telephone number.

Insurance

Croatia has a social insurance system providing medical benefits to large sectors of the population, including employed persons (including civil servants and public-sector employees), the self-employed, salaried apprentices working full time, military personnel, temporary contract workers, persons working for a foreign employer (if not covered by a plan in the employer's country), farmers, unemployed persons, pensioners, children under age 18 (under age 26 if students), and dependents of the insured. Cash sickness benefits are limited primarily to the employed, excluding farmers, but maternity benefits are available to both the employed and the unemployed. The system is financed by employer payroll contributions

(15 percent of covered payroll), contributions from the self-employed (15 percent of income), and nontaxpaying farmers (7.5 percent). The government covers the costs for maternity benefits for the unemployed, parental leave, and newborn child assistance.

Medical care is provided through institutions that contract with the Croatian Institute for Health Insurance; both public and private institutions are included. Care provided includes hospitalization, primary and specialist care, dental care, some medicines, lab services, maternity care, preventive care, some medical technology, emergency aid, rehabilitation services, and transportation. Coinsurance is 20 percent for people without complementary insurance, but care is free for children younger than 18 and some other classes of people, including the disabled, the unemployed, some voluntary blood donors, and persons with low incomes.

The maternity benefit is 100 percent of earnings from 28 days before the due date until the child is 6 months old; maternal leave is mandatory from 28 days before until 42 days after the due date. Either the mother or the father can use parental leave, and for the third child and subsequent children, this is extended until the child is 2 years old. Unemployed parents receive financial assistance for 12 months (36 months for the third and subsequent children). The Croatian Institute for Health Insurance administers the program, with general supervision from the Ministry of Health and Social Services. According to Ke Xu and colleagues, in 2003, 0.2 percent of households in Croatia experienced catastrophic health expenditures annually; "catastrophic" was defined as exceeding 40 percent of household income remaining after basic needs were met.

Costs of Hospitalization

All hospitals in Croatia are state run, although a person may enter them from a private clinic or with the referral of a private medical practitioner. Hospitals are paid by a combination of day rates (adjusted according to the level of hospital: general, regional, or university), physician payments, and reimbursement for inputs such as goods and drugs. Physician payments are based on a medical points system specifying more than 90,000 procedures and their point values. This system encourages overuse of hospitals, and rising costs (more than 70 percent from 1994 to 1998 alone) led the government to impose caps on inpatient spending.

Access to Health Care

Croatia has both public and private health care systems, although all hospitals are public. Local health facilities, including health center and home-care agencies, are managed by county governments. Access to advanced care tends to be limited to large cities, and those in other areas must travel to get this type of care. However, access to basic services is very good: According to WHO, in 2008, 99.9 percent of births in Croatia were attended by skilled personnel (for example, physicians, nurses, or midwives). The 2010 immunization rates for 1-year-olds were 96 percent for diphtheria and pertussis (DPT3), 95 percent for measles (MCV), and 96 percent for Hib (Hib3). In 2010, an estimated 89 percent of persons with advanced human immunodeficiency virus (HIV) infection were receiving antiretroviral therapy in accordance with the 2010 WHO guidelines.

According to WHO, in 2010, Croatia had 7.01 magnetic resonance imaging (MRI) machines per 1 million population, 14.47 computer tomography (CT) machines per 1 million, 0.45 positron emission tomography (PET) machines per 1 million, 0.68 telecolbalt units per 1 million, and 0.68 radiotherapy machines per 1 million.

Cost of Drugs

Total pharmaceutical expenditures in Croatia in 2008 came to 3.392 million HRK ($690.8 million); the per capita pharmaceutical expenditure was 766 HRK ($156). Total pharmaceutical expenditures amounted to 13 percent of total health expenditures, and 1.1 percent of the GDP. Croatia is a member of the World Trade Organization (WTO) but allows for several exceptions to patent regulation, including compulsory licensing for reasons of public health and the Bolar exception. Drugs sold in Croatia must be registered, with exceptions made for urgent medical need. In 2011, the Croatia registration list included 3,773 pharmaceutical products. Advertising and promotion of prescription medications is regulated by law, and direct advertising to the public is prohibited.

Some individuals are entitled to medications for free, including pregnant women, children under the age of 5, elderly people, and the poor. In addition, medications on the essential medications list are provided for free, as are drugs to treat malaria, tuberculosis, sexually transmitted diseases (STDs), and human immunodeficiency virus and acquired immune deficiency syndrome (HIV/AIDS); vaccinations on WHO's Expanded Programme on Immunization (EPI) list are also provided for free.

The Croatian Institute for Health Institute publishes two lists of medications, one for those considered essential, and that are covered by mandatory insurance, and a second complementary list of medications that are partially covered by mandatory insurance. Price markup on medications is regulated by the Croatian government; a 2009 survey found that medications in the public sector in Croatia were sold for an average markup of 8.5 percent and more than 40 percent in the private sector.

Health Care Facilities

As of 2010, according to WHO, Croatia had 0.82 health posts per 100,000 population, 0.30 health centers per 100,000, 0.50 district or rural hospitals per 100,000, 0.66 provincial hospitals per 100,000, and 0.34 specialized hospitals per 100,000. In 2008, Croatia had 5.49 hospital beds per 1,000 population, among the 50 highest rates in the world.

Major Health Issues

In 2008, WHO estimated that 3 percent of years of life lost in Croatia were due to communicable diseases, 85 percent to noncommunicable diseases, and 11 percent to injuries. In 2008, the age-standardized estimate of cancer deaths was 225 per 100,000 for men and 115 per 100,000 for women; for cardiovascular disease and diabetes, 352 per 100,000 for men and 240 per 100,000 for women; and for chronic respiratory disease, 26 per 100,000 for men and eight per 100,000 for women.

The maternal mortality rate (death from any cause related to or aggravated by pregnancy) in Croatia in 2008 was 14 maternal deaths per 100,000 live births. The infant mortality rate, defined as the number of deaths of infants younger than 1 year, was 6.06 per 1,000 live births as of 2012. In 2010, tuberculosis incidence was 21.0 per 100,000 population, tuberculosis prevalence 27.0 per 100,000, and deaths due to tuberculosis among HIV-negative people 2.30 per 100,000. As of 2009, an estimated 0.1 percent of adults age 15 to 49 were living with HIV or AIDS. In 2003, an estimated 22.3 percent of adults in Croatia were obese (defined as a body mass index, or BMI, of 30 or greater).

Health Care Personnel

Croatia has four medical schools, two of which began operation in the 1990s. The basic course for a medical degree lasts six years. In 2007, Croatia had 2.59 physicians per 1,000 population, 0.57 pharmaceutical personnel per 1,000, 0.72 dentistry personnel per 1,000, and 5.58 nurses and midwives per 1,000.

Government Role in Health Care

Croatia has a National Health Policy (NHP), updated in 2006, and various policies regulating pharmaceuticals. Croatia has several national policies regulating pharmaceuticals, including selection of essential medications (in 2011, 770 medicines were determined to be essential); financing, pricing, purchase, distribution, and regulation of drugs; pharmacovigilance; rational usage of medicines; human resource development; research; and traditional medicine.

According to WHO, in 2010, Croatia spent $4.7 billion on health care, an amount that comes to $1,067 per capita. Health care was funded entirely through domestic sources. Most (85 percent) of health care funding was provided by government expenditures, with 15 percent coming from household spending and 1 percent from other sources. In 2010, Croatia allocated 18 percent of total government expenditures to health, relatively high when compared to other high-income European countries, and government expenditures on health came to 7 percent of GDP on both measures, putting Croatia in the median range among high-income European countries. In 2009, according to WHO, official development assistance for health in Croatia came to $0.81 per capita.

Public Health Programs

The Croatian National Institute of Public Health, which is located in Zagreb and directed by Zeljko Baklaic, was established in 1923. It currently has a staff of approximately 100, organized into five branches: Microbiology, Addiction Prevention, Social Medicine, Health Studies, and the Epidemiology of Infectious and Chronic Diseases. The institute conducts lab diagnostics and analysis and monitors factors affecting the health of the Croatian people, including food and water safety and acute and chronic diseases.

Access to improved sanitary facilities was nearly universal in 2010, as was access to improved sources of drinking water. According to the World Higher Education Database (WHED), one university in Croatia offers programs in epidemiology or public health: the University of Rijeka.

CUBA

Cuba is an island nation in the Caribbean, consisting of one main island and many smaller islands. The area of 43,189 square miles (111,860 square kilometers) makes Cuba slightly smaller than Pennsylvania, and the July 2012 population was estimated at 11.1 million, making it the most populous Caribbean nation. In 2010, 75 percent of the population lived in urban areas, and the 2010 to 2015 annual rate of urbanization was estimated at 0.0 percent. Havana is the capital and largest city (with a 2009 population estimated at 2.1 million). Population growth in 2012 was negative 0.1 percent due in part to a negative net migration rate (negative 3.6 migrants per 1,000 population), a low birth rate (10.0 births per 1,000 population) and a low total fertility rate (1.45 children per woman). The United Nations High Commissioner for Refugees (UNHCR) estimated that, in 2010, there were 377 refugees and persons in refugee-like situations in Cuba.

Cuba was a Spanish colony, then a possession of the United States; it became independent in 1902. Fidel Castro came to power in 1959, and the country became communist; the United States has had an economic embargo against Cuba since 1961. Cuba ranked tied for 61st among 183 countries on the *Corruption Perceptions Index 2011*, with a score of 4.2 (on a scale where 0 indicates highly corrupt and 10 very clean). In 2011, Cuba was classified as a country with high human development (the second-highest category) on the United Nations Development Programme's (UNDP's) Human Development Index (HDI), with a score of 0.776 (on a scale where 1 denotes high development and 0 low development). Life expectancy at birth in 2012 was estimated at 77.87 years, and per capita gross domestic product (GDP) in 2011 was estimated at $9,900. According to the World Economic Forum's *Global Gender Gap Index 2011*, Cuba ranked 20th out of 135 countries on gender equality with a score of 0.739 (on a scale with a theoretical range of 1 for equality to 0 for inequality and an actual range in 2011 from 0.8530 to 0.4873).

Emergency Health Services

According to the World Health Organization (WHO), as of 2007, Cuba had a formal and publicly available emergency care (prehospital care) system, accessible through both a national universal access telephone

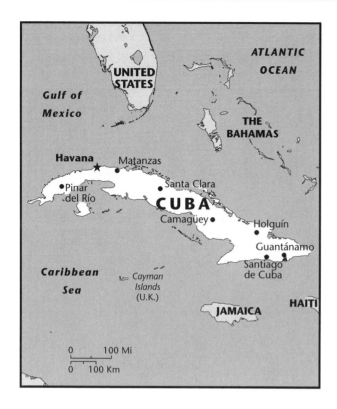

individual cash maternity benefits are available to the self-employed and artists. The cash sickness benefit is 60 percent of average daily earnings for six months, with the possibility to extend another six months; medical review is required on a regular basis for the benefits to continue to be paid. The maternity benefit is 100 percent of average earnings for 6 weeks prior to and 12 weeks after the due date; if the mother chooses to stay home to care for the child, the benefit continues until the child is 1 year old. The program is administered by the Ministry of Labor and Social Security.

Costs of Hospitalization

In 2006, Cuba allocated 1.66 billion pesos, or 52.0 percent of its health budget, to hospital care.

Access to Health Care

Health policy is established by the Ministry of Public Health, and all health care is provided in public facilities. According to WHO, in 2007, 100 percent of births in Cuba were attended by skilled personnel (for example, physicians, nurses, or midwives). The 2010 immunization rates for 1-year-olds were 96 percent for diphtheria and pertussis (DPT3), 99 percent for measles (MCV), and 96 percent for Hib (Hib3). In 2010, an estimated 95 percent of persons with advanced human immunodeficiency virus (HIV) infection were receiving antiretroviral therapy in accordance with the 2010 WHO guidelines. According to WHO, in 2010, Cuba had 0.80 magnetic resonance imaging (MRI) machines per 1 million population and 4.82 computer tomography (CT) machines per 1 million.

Cost of Drugs

Many drugs and biological products are produced locally in Cuba, and manufacturing is in compliance with WHO standards. In 2005, Cuba's expenditures for drugs and related supplies were 308.0 million pesos.

Health Care Facilities

Cuba has a network of health care facilities including 248 hospitals, 470 laboratories in polyclinics and 248 laboratories in secondary care facilities, 1,228 oral health care facilities, and numerous polyclinics delivering primary care services. The National Blood and Transfusion Medicine Program includes 27 provincial blood banks, 35 municipal blood banks, and 121 permanent blood collection centers. As of 2010, according to WHO, Cuba had 7.53 health posts per 100,000 population, 0.64 health centers per 100,000,

number and regional access numbers. The Integrated Emergency Medical System provides emergency services, urgent care, and critical care. In 2004, a system of municipal intensive care units was established to provide round-the-clock urgent and emergency services in 121 municipalities; in 2005, they provided care to more than 50,000 patients.

Insurance

Cuba has a social insurance system with universal medical benefits for all citizens and residents, and cash benefits are also available to some classes of people. The program is funded by taxes of 1 to 5 percent on earnings, 5 percent of sales from agricultural cooperatives, 25 percent of declared income for the self-employed, and payroll taxes paid by the employer (12.5 percent of gross for public-sector employers and 14.5 percent for private-sector employers); the government covers deficits. Free medical benefits are provided at public medical centers. Benefits provided include hospitalization (including medicine and food during hospitalization), medical care, maternity care, dental care, and rehabilitation.

Cash sickness benefits are available to employed people, the military, interior ministry staff, and members of agricultural cooperatives; besides these,

Selected Health Indicators: Cuba Compared With the Global Average (2010)

	Cuba	Global Average
Male life expectancy at birth* (years)	76	66
Female life expectancy at birth* (years)	80	71
Under-5 mortality rate, both sexes (per 1,000 live births)	6	57
Adult mortality rate, both sexes* (probability of dying between 15 and 60 years per 1,000 population)	99	176
Maternal mortality ratio (per 100,000 live births)	73	210
HIV prevalence* (per 1,000 adults aged 15 to 49)	1	8
Tuberculosis prevalence (per 100,000 population)	13	178

Source: World Health Organization Global Health Observatory Data Repository.
*Data refers to 2009.

0.15 district or rural hospitals per 100,000, 1.47 provincial hospitals per 100,000, and 0.43 specialized hospitals per 100,000. In 2009, Cuba had 5.90 hospital beds per 1,000 population, one of the 30 highest ratios in the world.

Major Health Issues

In 2008, WHO estimated that 8 percent of years of life lost in Cuba were due to communicable diseases, 78 percent to noncommunicable diseases, and 13 percent to injuries. In 2008, the age-standardized estimate of cancer deaths was 160 per 100,000 for men and 114 per 100,000 for women; for cardiovascular disease and diabetes, 236 per 100,000 for men and 194 per 100,000 for women; and for chronic respiratory disease, 23 per 100,000 for men and 18 per 100,000 for women.

Compared to other countries at a similar level of development, Cuba ranked first among 80 less-developed countries on the 2011 Mothers' Index, produced by the international nongovernmental organization (NGO) Save the Children, based on a number of health and social factors relating to women, children, and maternal and child care. Cuba's maternal mortality rate (death from any cause related to or aggravated by pregnancy) was estimated in 2008 as 53 maternal deaths per 100,000 live births. The infant mortality rate, defined as the number of deaths of infants younger than 1 year, was 4.83 per 1,000 live births as of 2012. In 2010, tuberculosis incidence was 9.3 per 100,000 population, tuberculosis prevalence 13.0 per 100,000, and deaths due to tuberculosis among HIV-negative people 0.29 per 100,000. As of 2009, an estimated 0.1 percent of adults age 15 to 49 were living with HIV or acquired immune deficiency syndrome (AIDS).

Health Care Personnel

Cuba has 14 medical schools. The basic course of training lasts six years, and the degree awarded is Doctor en Medicina (doctor of medicine). Government service is obligatory after graduation. Physicians must register with the Ministerio de Salud Pública in Havana, and graduates of foreign medical schools must have their degrees validated. In 2007, Cuba had 6.40 physicians per 1,000 population, 0.62 pharmaceutical workers per 1,000, 0.95 laboratory health workers per 1,000, 1.78 dentistry personnel per 1,000, and 8.64 nurses and midwives per 1,000. Cuba also provides free premedical and medical education for citizens of other countries at the Latin American School of Medicine in Havana, which draws students from Africa, Latin America, North America, and the Middle East.

Government Role in Health Care

According to WHO, in 2010, Cuba spent $6.8 billion on health care, an amount that comes to $607 per capita. Health care was funded entirely through domestic sources. Most (91 percent) of health care funding was provided by government expenditures, with 9 percent coming from household spending. In 2010, Cuba allocated 17 percent of total government expenditures to health, placing it in the median range when compared with other upper-middle-income countries in the Americas, and government expenditures on health came to 10 percent of GDP, placing it in the high range when compared with other upper-middle-income countries in the Americas region. In 2009, according to WHO, official development assistance for health in Cuba came to $1.03 per capita.

Public Health Programs

The Institute of Tropical Medicine "Pedro Kouri" (IPK), located in Havana and directed by Jorge Pérez Avila, is Cuba's leading public health institute. IPK has a staff of 700 organized into five departments: microbiology, parasitology, medical care, epidemiology, and teaching. The primary goals of IPK are to prevent the spread of disease, collaborate with international health institutes, and facilitate biomedical training and research. Recent areas of activity include conducting a study of HIV transmission and developing community strategies to control mosquitoes and prevent the spread of dengue fever.

The National Occupational Safety and Health Program monitors exposure to chemicals and other hazards. All provinces and municipalities have health trend and analysis units to gather and interpret information about health and disease trends. In 2010, 91 percent of the population of Cuba had access to improved sanitary facilities, with access being higher among the urban (94 percent) as opposed to the rural (81 percent) population. Access to improved sources of drinking water was higher, although not universal, with 94 percent of the population having such access (96 percent for the urban population and 89 percent for the rural). According to WHO, in 2010, Cuba had 0.25 environmental and public health workers per 1,000 population.

CYPRUS

Cyprus is an island nation in the Mediterranean Sea, south of Turkey. The area of 3,572 square miles (9,251 square kilometers) is about three-fifths the

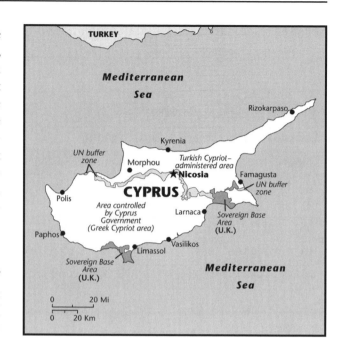

size of Connecticut, and the July 2012 population was estimated at 1.1 million. In 2010, 70 percent of the population lived in urban areas, and the 2010 to 2015 annual rate of urbanization was estimated at 1.3 percent. Nicosia is the capital and largest city (with a 2009 population estimated at 240,000). The July 2012 population growth rate is 1.6 percent due in large part to one of the highest net migration rates in the world (10.8 migrants per 1,000 population); the total fertility rate is 1.5 children per woman, and the birth rate 11.4 births per 1,000 population.

Cyprus was a British colony and became independent in 1963; violence between Greek and Turkish people has been a recurrent feature of its existence; a buffer zone (the Green Line) controlled by the United Nations (UN) separates the northern (Turkish) region from the southern (Cypriot) region. The government has a reputation for honesty and transparency: Cyprus ranked 30th among 183 countries on the *Corruption Perceptions Index 2011*, with a score of 6.3 (on a scale where 0 indicates highly corrupt and 10 very clean).

In 2011, Cyprus was classified as a country with very high human development (the highest of four categories) on the United Nations Development Programme's (UNDP's) Human Development Index (HDI), with a score of 0.840 (on a scale where 1 denotes high development and 0 low development). Life expectancy at birth in 2012 was estimated at 78.00 years, and per capita gross domestic product (GDP) in 2011 was estimated at $29,100. Income distribution is among the most equal in the world: In 2005, the Gini Index (a measure of dispersion, in which perfect equality is denoted by 0 and maximum inequality is denoted by 100) for family income was 29.0. According to the World Economic Forum's *Global Gender Gap Index 2011*, Cyprus ranked 93rd out of 135 countries on gender equality with a score of 0.657 (on a scale with a theoretical range of 1 for equality to 0 for inequality and an actual range in 2011 from 0.8530 to 0.4873).

Emergency Health Services

The laws governing the emergency health system in Cyprus date from the 2000s; by law, free access to hospitals for emergency care is provided for all persons, including the uninsured. Funding for the emergency system is provided from several sources. Cyprus uses only one telephone number for medical emergencies, 112 (the European Union, or EU, standard); the country has 25 dispatch centers, with interconnectivity among centers.

Insurance

Cyprus has a social insurance system that provides cash benefits to employed and self-employed people (those working for their families are excluded) and medical benefits for certain population groups, including the military and police forces, civil servants, the poor, and people with certain chronic diseases. The system is funded by taxes on wages (6.8 percent of covered earnings) and incomes of self-employed people (12.6 percent of covered earnings) and employer contributions (6.8 percent of covered payroll). Voluntary contributors pay 11 percent of covered earnings if working in Cyprus and 13.6 percent if working abroad. Medical benefits, including treatment, hospitalization, prescription drugs, and maternity care, are provided in government hospitals. Medical services are provided through the Ministry of Health, and administration is provided by the Social Insurance Service of the Ministry of Labor and Social Insurance.

Costs of Hospitalization

No data available.

Access to Health Care

According to the World Health Organization (WHO), in 2007, 100 percent of births in Cyprus were attended by skilled personnel (for example, physicians, nurses, or midwives). The 2010 immunization rates for 1-year-olds were 99 percent for diphtheria and pertussis (DPT3), 87 percent for measles (MCV), and 96 percent for Hib (Hib3).

According to WHO, in 2010, Cyprus had 19.06 magnetic resonance imaging (MRI) machines per 1 million population and 30.50 computer tomography (CT) machines per 1 million.

Cost of Drugs

No data available.

Health Care Facilities

Public health services are provided at low cost in Cyprus, and rural citizens are served through a system of mobile health units and weekly visits from district physicians. As of 2010, according to WHO, Cyprus had 3.44 health centers per 100,000 population, 7.16 provincial hospitals per 100,000, and 0.63 specialized hospitals per 100,000. In 2006, Cyprus had 3.72 hospital beds per 1,000 population.

Major Health Issues

In 2008, WHO estimated that 4 percent of years of life lost in Cyprus were due to communicable diseases, 81 percent to noncommunicable diseases, and 15 percent to injuries. In 2008, the age-standardized estimate of cancer deaths was 101 per 100,000 for men and 65 per 100,000 for women; for cardiovascular disease and diabetes, 225 per 100,000 for men and 150 per 100,000 for women; and for chronic respiratory disease, 26 per 100,000 for men and 14 per 100,000 for women.

Compared to other countries at a similar level of development, Cyprus ranked third among 80 less-developed countries on the 2011 Mothers' Index, produced by the international nongovernmental organization (NGO) Save the Children, based on a number of health and social factors relating to women, children, and maternal and child care. The maternal mortality rate (death from any cause related to or aggravated by pregnancy) in Cyprus in 2008 was 10 maternal deaths per 100,000 live births. The infant mortality rate, defined as the number of deaths of infants younger than 1 year, was 9.05 per 1,000 live births as of 2012. In 2010, tuberculosis incidence was 4.4 per 100,000 population, tuberculosis prevalence 5.5 per 100,000, and deaths due to tuberculosis among human immunodeficiency virus (HIV)-negative people 0.25 per 100,000. As of 2009, an estimated 0.1 percent of adults age 15 to 49 were living with HIV or acquired immune deficiency syndrome (AIDS).

Health Care Personnel

Cyprus, as a member of the EU, cooperates with other countries in recognizing physicians qualified to practice in other EU countries, as specified by Directive 2005/36/EC of the European Parliament. This allows qualified professionals to practice their profession in other EU states on a temporary basis and requires that the host country automatically recognize qualifications for certain professions, including physicians, nurses, dentists, midwives, and pharmacists, if certain conditions have been met (for instance, facility in the language of the host country may be required). In 2006, Cyprus had 2.30 physicians per 1,000 population, 0.19 pharmaceutical personnel per 1,000, 0.85 dentistry personnel per 1,000, and 3.98 nurses and midwives per 1,000.

Government Role in Health Care

According to WHO, in 2010, Cyprus spent $1.4 billion on health care, an amount that comes to $1,705 per capita. Health care was funded entirely through domestic sources. Almost half (49 percent) of health care funding was provided by household spending, with 42 percent coming from government expenditures and 10 percent from other sources. In 2010, Cyprus allocated 5 percent of total government expenditures to health, and government expenditures on health came to 2 percent of gross domestic product (GDP); on both measures, Cyprus ranks in the low range when compared with other high-income European countries.

Public Health Programs

In 2010, access to improved sanitary facilities and improved sources of drinking water was essentially universal in Cyrus. According to WHO, in 2008, Cyprus had 0.11 environmental and public health workers per 1,000 population. According to the World Higher Education Database (WHED), no university in Cyprus offers programs in epidemiology or public health.

CZECH REPUBLIC

The Czech Republic is a landlocked country in central Europe, sharing borders with Germany, Poland,

Slovakia, and Austria. The area is 30,450 square miles (78,867 square kilometers, comparable to South Carolina), and the July 2012 population was estimated at 10.2 million. In 2010, 74 percent of the population lived in urban areas, and the 2010 to 2015 annual rate of urbanization was estimated at 0.3 percent. Prague is the capital and largest city (with a 2009 population estimated at 1.2 million). The July 2012 population growth rate was negative 0.1 percent despite a positive net migration rate of 1.0 migrants per 1,000 population; the total fertility rate of 1.27 children per woman is one of the lowest in the world, as is the birth rate of 8.6 births per 1,000 population.

The Czech Republic was part of Czechoslovakia, a country created after World War I that became part of the Soviet sphere of influence after World War II. In 1989, Czechoslovakia became a democratic country and peaceably separated from Slovakia in 1993. The Czech Republic ranked tied for 57th among 183 countries in terms on the *Corruption Perceptions Index 2011*, with a score of 4.0 (on a scale where 0 indicates highly corrupt and 10 very clean). In 2011, the Czech Republic was classified as a country with very high human development (the highest of four categories) on the United Nations Development Programme's (UNDP's) Human Development Index (HDI), with a score of 0.865 (on a scale where 1 denotes high development and 0 low development). Life expectancy at birth in 2012 was estimated at 77.38 years, and per capita gross domestic product (GDP) in 2011 was estimated at $25,900. In 2009, the Gini Index (a measure of dispersion, in which perfect equality is denoted by 0 and maximum inequality is denoted by 100) for family income was 31.0. According to the World Economic Forum's *Global Gender Gap Index 2011*, the Czech Republic ranked 75th out of 135 countries on gender equality, with a score of 0.679 (on a scale with a theoretical range of 1 for equality to 0 for inequality and an actual range in 2011 from 0.8530 to 0.4873).

Emergency Health Services

The Czech Republic's laws governing the emergency health system date from the 1990s, as does Czech recognition of emergency medicine as a medical specialty; by law, free access to hospitals for emergency care is provided for all persons, including the uninsured. Funding for the emergency system is provided from multiple sources. The Czech Republic uses only one national telephone number for medical emergencies, 155; the country has 40 dispatch centers.

Insurance

The Czech Republic provides universal medical benefits for everyone residing in the country and for employees of companies resident in the country. A social insurance system provides cash benefits as well to some population sectors. The system is funded through contributions from wages (4.5 percent of monthly covered earnings), contributions from the income of self-employed persons (14.9 percent, with a lower flat fee for those with low incomes), and employer payroll contributions (11.3 percent). The government makes up deficits and provides medical benefits for certain classes of people. Medical benefits covered include inpatient and outpatient care, preventive care, emergency and rescue services, spa treatments, medical assessments, autopsy and transportation of the deceased, treatment for stomatologic diseases (diseases of the mouth), emergency and rescue services, and transportation. Cost sharing is required for some services, including medical visits, hospitalization, and prescription drugs, but some population sectors pay nothing. The sickness benefit is 60 percent of average income, paid for one year, with a possible extension for a second year. The maternity benefit is 60 percent of income for 28 weeks. The system is administered by the Czech Social Security Administration, with the Ministry of Labor and Social Affairs supervising the administration of sickness insurance and the Ministry of Health supervising medical services. According to

Ke Xu and colleagues, in 2003, less than 0.1 percent of households in the Czech Republic experienced catastrophic health expenditures annually; "catastrophic" was defined as exceeding 40 percent of household income remaining after basic needs were met.

Costs of Hospitalization

In 2008, according to the Organisation for Economic Co-operation and Development (OECD), hospital spending represented 45.8 percent of total spending on health and $796 per capita; 75 percent of payments were based on the prospective global budget, 15 percent on per-case payments, and 8 percent on per-procedure payments.

Access to Health Care

According to the World Health Organization (WHO), in 2008, 99.9 percent of births in the Czech Republic were attended by skilled personnel (for example, physicians, nurses, or midwives). The 2010 immunization rates for 1-year-olds were 99 percent for diphtheria and pertussis (DPT3), 98 percent for measles (MCV), and 99 percent for Hib (Hib3). According to WHO, in 2010, the Czech Republic had 5.04 magnetic resonance imaging (MRI) machines per 1 million population, 13.47 computer tomography (CT) machines per 1 million, 0.58 positron emission tomography (PET) machines per 1 million, 1.45 telecolbalt units per 1 million, and 1.45 radiotherapy machines per 1 million.

Cost of Drugs

As of 2011, the Czech Republic charged a reduced value-added tax (5 percent, as opposed to the standard 19 percent) for medicines, levied at the wholesale level, and charged 10 percent for over-the-counter medicines. The wholesale markup averages 5 to 7 percent, and the retail markup averages 22 to 24 percent; the total margin is set at 29 percent. Real annual growth in pharmaceutical expenditures in the Czech Republic grew 3.9 percent from 1997 to 2005, about the same as the 3.7 percent growth of total health expenditures (minus pharmaceutical expenditures) over those years.

Health Care Facilities

As of 2010, according to WHO, the Czech Republic had 229.33 health posts per 100,000 population, 0.16 health centers per 100,000, 0.41 district or rural hospitals per 100,000, 0.65 provincial hospitals per

100,000, and 0.26 specialized hospitals per 100,000. In 2008, the Czech Republic had 7.18 hospital beds per 1,000 population, among the 20 highest ratios in the world.

Major Health Issues

In 2008, WHO estimated that 8 percent of years of life lost in the Czech Republic were due to communicable diseases, 83 percent to noncommunicable diseases, and 13 percent to injuries. In 2008, the age-standardized estimate of cancer deaths was 202 per 100,000 for men and 116 per 100,000 for women; for cardiovascular disease and diabetes, 315 per 100,000 for men and 203 per 100,000 for women; and for chronic respiratory disease, 21 per 100,000 for men and nine per 100,000 for women.

The maternal mortality rate (death from any cause related to or aggravated by pregnancy) in the Czech Republic in 2008 was eight maternal deaths per 100,000 live births, among the lowest in the world. The infant mortality rate, defined as the number of deaths of infants younger than 1 year, was 3.70 per 1,000 live births as of 2012. In 2010, tuberculosis incidence was 6.8 per 100,000 population, tuberculosis prevalence 8.4 per 100,000, and deaths due to tuberculosis among human immunodeficiency virus (HIV)-negative people 0.43 per 100,000. As of 2009, an estimated 0.1 percent of adults age 15 to 49 were living with HIV or acquired immune deficiency syndrome (AIDS).

Health Care Personnel

The Czech Republic has seven medical schools, located in Brno, Hradec Kralove, Olomouc, Plzen, and Prague. The basic course of training lasts six-years, and the degree awarded is Doktor Vseobecné Medicíny Zkratka (M.U.Dr., general practitioner). Two years of government service is required after graduation. The Czech Medical Chamber grants the license to practice medicine to graduates who have passed the postgraduate professional examination. Graduates of foreign medical schools must have their degrees validated and may also have to pass further examinations, including a language exam, although Czech Republic has multilateral and bilateral agreements with many countries.

Czech Republic, as a member of the European Union (EU), cooperates with other countries in recognizing physicians qualified to practice in other EU countries, as specified by Directive 2005/36/EC of the European Parliament. This allows qualified professionals to practice their profession in other EU states on a temporary basis and requires that the host country automatically recognize qualifications for certain professions, including physicians, nurses, dentists, midwives, and pharmacists, if certain conditions have been met (for instance, facility in the language of the host country may be required). In 2008, the Czech Republic had 3.63 physicians per 1,000 population, 0.58 pharmaceutical personnel per 1,000, 0.69 dentistry personnel per 1,000, and 8.55 nurses and midwives per 1,000.

Government Role in Health Care

According to WHO, in 2010, the Czech Republic spent $16 billion on health care, an amount that comes to $1,480 per capita. Health care was funded entirely through domestic sources. Most (84 percent) health care funding was provided by government expenditures, with 15 percent coming from household spending and 2 percent from other sources. In 2010, the Czech Republic allocated 15 percent of total government expenditures to health, and government expenditures on health came to 7 percent of gross domestic product (GDP); on both measures, the Czech Republic ranks in the median range when compared with other high-income European countries.

Public Health Programs

The National Institute of Public Health (NIPH) for the Czech Republic is located in Prague and directed by Jitka Sosnovcová. The primary tasks of the NIPH are promoting and protecting health, preventing disease, and studying the impact of environmental factors on health; principal activities include scientific research, environmental monitoring, preparation of legislation in accordance with the norms of the EU, providing scientific and methodological advice, and offering expert opinions on matters of public health. NIPH concentrates on major health problems, including outbreaks of severe infections such as AIDS and hepatitis, and promotion of good health behaviors. NIPH also provides consultations to working professionals and helps train physicians and other health care workers. In 2010, access to improved sanitary facilities in the Czech Republic was nearly universal (98 percent overall, with 99 percent for the urban population and 97 percent for the rural), and access to improved sources of drinking water was essentially universal.

According to the World Higher Education Database (WHED), eight universities in the Czech Republic offer programs in epidemiology or public health: the University of South Bohemia in Ceske Budejovice, the University of Ostrava, Charles University in Prague, the University of Pardubice, Tomas Bata University in Zlín, the University of Veterinary and Pharmaceutical Sciences in Brno, the University of Economics in Prague, and the University of West Bohemia.

DENMARK

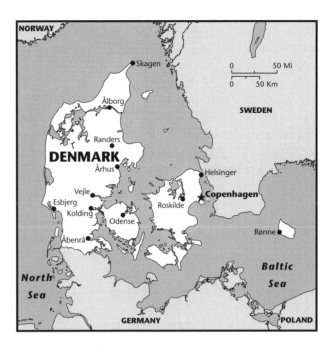

Denmark is a northern European country sharing a border with Germany; the country consists of a peninsula and numerous islands; Greenland and the Faroe Islands are part of Denmark but have political autonomy. The area (excluding Greenland and the Faroe Islands) is 16,639 square miles (43,094 square kilometers, about twice the size of Massachusetts), and the coastline on the North Sea covers 4,545 miles (7,314 kilometers). The Danish population of 5.5 million is highly urbanized: In 2010, 87 percent of the population lived in urban areas, including those who lived in the Copenhagen metropolitan area; the 2010 to 2015 annual rate of urbanization was estimated at 0.4 percent. Copenhagen is the capital and largest city (with a 2009 estimated population of 1.2 million). The net migration rate in 2012 was 2.4 migrants per 1,000 population, the 33rd-highest in the world; the population growth rate was 0.2 percent, the total fertility rate 1.74 children per woman, and the birth rate 10.22 births per 1,000 population.

Denmark was the dominant force in much of Scandinavia from the 15th through the early 19th century and also established colonies in the Caribbean and North Atlantic in the 18th century. In 1849, Denmark became a constitutional monarchy, and the Danish government has a reputation for transparency and honesty, ranking tied for second among 183 countries on the *Corruption Perceptions Index 2011,* with a score of 9.4 (on a scale where 0 indicates highly corrupt and 10 very clean). In 2011, Denmark was classified as a country with very high human development (the highest of four categories) on the United Nations Development Programme's (UNDP's) Human Development Index (HDI), with a score of 0.895 (on a scale where 1 denotes high development and 0 low

development). Life expectancy at birth in 2012 was estimated at 78.78 years, and the per capita gross domestic product (GDP) in 2011 was estimated at $40,200. Income distribution is among the most equal in the world: In 2011, the Gini Index (a measure of dispersion, in which perfect equality is denoted by 0 and maximum inequality is denoted by 100) for family income was estimated at 24.8. Gender equality is also high in Denmark: According to the World Economic Forum's *Global Gender Gap Index 2011,* Denmark ranked seventh out of 135 countries on gender equality, with a score of 0.778 (on a scale with a theoretical range of 1 for equality to 0 for inequality and an actual range in 2011 from 0.8530 to 0.4873).

Emergency Health Services

Denmark's laws governing its emergency health system date from the 2000s; by law, free access to hospitals for emergency care is provided for all persons, including the uninsured. Funding for the emergency system is provided entirely from public sources for both in-hospital and out-of-hospital care. Denmark uses only one national telephone number for medical emergencies, 112 (the European Union, or EU, standard); the country has eight dispatch centers, which are interconnected. General practice physicians provide after-hours care on a voluntary basis; they are paid higher fees than those paid during regular operating hours. After-hours care is organized at the regional level and is provided mainly through clinics that are often located in or near hospital emergency departments.

Insurance

Denmark has a national health service that is financed through an earmarked income tax, and all registered residents of Denmark are entitled to largely free health care. The health services cover all primary and hospital services as well as long-term care, mental health services, and preventive services. Cost sharing applies primarily to adult dental care, corrective lenses, and outpatient drugs. Danes are allowed to purchase additional insurance that provides extra benefits, including access to private facilities; complementary private health insurance has been available in Denmark since the 1970s, and currently, about 40 percent of Danes use it.

Out-of-pocket copayments decrease as the total out-of-pocket spending increases, and there is a cap on out-of-pocket spending for drugs for the chronically ill. Financial assistance for out-of-pocket expenses is also available for the terminally ill and for people with low incomes. Primary care is paid for through a mix of fee-for-service and capitation models. Hospital payments are handled through a combination of global budgets and case-based payments; hospital payments do not include physician costs. Most patients (98 percent) are required to register with a general practice physician.

A 2004 study by the World Health Organization (WHO) found that none of the Danish population had substitutive voluntary health insurance (covering services that would otherwise be available from the state), and 28 percent had complementary voluntary health insurance (covering services not covered or those not fully covered by the state) or had supplementary health insurance (providing increased choice or faster access to services). Many voluntary policies are provided as a perk of employment and are seen by some as introducing inequality into the health care system (because many groups are essentially excluded from this type of policy, including students, the elderly, the unemployed, and those with chronic illnesses). According to Ke Xu and colleagues, in 2003, less than 0.1 percent of households in Denmark experienced catastrophic health expenditures annually; "catastrophic" was defined as exceeding 40 percent of household income remaining after basic needs were met.

Costs of Hospitalization

Denmark is divided into five administrative regions that have the authority to run hospitals, provide hospital care, and pay for physicians, dentists, physiotherapists, and pharmaceuticals. Other services, including nursing homes, health visitors, home nurses, municipal dentists, and drug and alcohol

Selected Health Indicators: Denmark Compared With the Organisation for Economic Co-operation and Development (OECD) Country Average

	Denmark	OECD average (2010 or nearest year)
Male life expectancy at birth, 2010	77.2	77
Female life expectancy at birth, 2010	81.4	82.5
Tobacco consumption (percent of population 15+ who are daily smokers), 2010	20	21.1
Alcohol consumption (liters per capita [age 15+]), 2010	10.3	9.4
Obesity (percent of female population with a BMI>30 kg/m2, self-reported), 2010	13.1	14.8
Obesity (percent of male population with a BMI>30 kg/m2, self-reported), 2010	13.7	15.1

Source: OECD Health Data 2012 (Organisation for Economic Co-operation and Development, 2012).

addiction treatment, are the responsibility of Denmark's 98 municipalities.

According to Organisation for Economic Co-operation and Development (OECD) data, in 2009, hospital spending per capita in Denmark was $1,893 (adjusted for differences in the cost of living), and hospital spending per discharge came to $11,112 in 2011. There were 170 hospital discharges per 1,000 population. In 2008, according to the OECD, 80 percent of hospital spending was provided as part of a prospective global budget, and 20 percent on payment per case and diagnosis-related group (DRG).

Access to Health Care

Health care is organized in Denmark under the basis of universal access, which includes universal coverage and subsidies and caps to reduce the financial burden for copayments on those least able to afford them. Almost all hospital beds (97 percent) are located in publicly owned hospitals, and patients are able to choose which public hospital they prefer. If waiting time for a procedure exceeds one month, patients are allowed to use private facilities.

In 2009, according to OECD data, people in Denmark had an average of 4.6 physician visits. The 2010 immunization rates for 1-year-olds were 90 percent for diphtheria and pertussis (DPT3), 85 percent for measles (MCV), and 90 percent for Hib (Hib3). According to the World Health Organization (WHO), in 2010, Denmark had 14.11 magnetic resonance imaging (MRI) machines per 1 million population, 24.55 computer tomography (CT) machines per 1 million, and 6.05 positron emission tomography (PET) machines per 1 million.

Cost of Drugs

Pharmaceutical companies are required to report their prices on a monthly basis to the federal government, and a price list is provided to pharmacies. As a general rule, pharmacies must provide the cheapest among several drugs with the same active ingredients unless a physician has specifically stated that a particular drug should be provided. If patients choose a more expensive drug, they pay the price out of pocket. In hospitals, prices are controlled through coordinated purchasing.

In 2009, according to OECD data, pharmaceutical spending per capita in Denmark was $319 (adjusted for differences in the cost of living). Real annual growth in pharmaceutical expenditures in Denmark grew 3.1 percent from 1997 to 2005, about the same as the 3.3 percent growth of total health expenditures (minus pharmaceutical expenditures) over those years. According to Elizabeth Docteur, in 2004, generic drugs represented 32 percent of the market share by value and 65 percent of the market share by volume of the total pharmaceutical market. As of 2011, Denmark charged its standard value-added tax (VAT) rate (25 percent) for medicines. The pharmacy dispensing fee for prescribed medications was fixed at DKK 9.25 (1.24 euros). Wholesale markups are unregulated and average 4 percent; retail markups were set (as of 2007) at a flat fee plus 8.8 percent of the purchase price.

Health Care Facilities

Denmark has a national strategy for applying information technology to health care, and all primary care clinics use electronic medical records. The country has a national health portal with differential aspects for citizens and health personnel; it includes medical records and histories for individuals, treatment guidelines and scientific information for practitioners, and information about hospitals (for example, waiting times or treatments offered); physicians may use the system to access test results and other records for their own patients. There is a national standard for hospital electronic patient records (EPRs), although each region has developed its own record system. As of 2010, according to WHO, Denmark had 69.93 health posts per 100,000 population, 4.52 health centers per 100,000, 0.52 district or rural hospitals per 100,000, 0.41 provincial hospitals per 100,000, and 0.09 specialized hospitals per 100,000. In 2008, Denmark had 3.57 hospital beds per 1,000 population.

Major Health Issues

In 2008, WHO estimated that 5 percent of years of life lost in Denmark were due to communicable diseases, 85 percent to noncommunicable diseases, and 10 percent to injuries. In 2008, the age-standardized estimate of cancer deaths was 177 per 100,000 for men and 133 per 100,000 for women; for cardiovascular disease and diabetes, 180 per 100,000 for men and 107 per 100,000 for women; and for chronic respiratory disease, 34 per 100,000 for men and 28 per 100,000 for women.

Denmark ranked fifth among more developed countries in the 2011 Mothers' Index, produced by the international nongovernmental organization (NGO) Save the Children, based on a number of health and social factors relating to women, children, and maternal and child care. The maternal mortality rate (death from any cause related to or aggravated by pregnancy) in Denmark in 2008 was five maternal deaths per 100,000 live births, among the lowest in the world. The infant mortality rate, defined as the number of deaths of infants younger than 1 year, was 4.19 per 1,000 live births as of 2012 data. In 2010, tuberculosis incidence was 6.0 per 100,000 population, tuberculosis prevalence 7.4 per 100,000, and deaths due to tuberculosis among human immunodeficiency virus (HIV)-negative people 0.28 per 100,000. As of 2009, an estimated 0.2 percent of adults age 15 to 49 were living with HIV or acquired immune deficiency syndrome (AIDS).

Health Care Personnel

Denmark has three medical schools, located in Aarhus, Copenhagen, and Odense. The basic training course lasts 6.5 years, and the degree awarded is Candidatus medicinae (doctor of medicine). Denmark, as a member of the European Union (EU), cooperates with other countries in recognizing physicians qualified to practice in other EU countries, as specified by Directive 2005/36/EC of the European Parliament. This allows qualified professionals to practice their profession in other EU states on a temporary basis and requires that the host country automatically recognize qualifications for certain professions, including physicians, nurses, dentists, midwives, and pharmacists if certain conditions have been met (for instance, facility in the language of the host country may be required). In 2007, Denmark had 3.42 physicians per 1,000 population, 0.48 pharmaceutical personnel per 1,000, 0.84 dentistry personnel per 1,000, and 14.54 nurses and midwives per 1,000. In 2001, 7.8 percent of physicians practicing in Denmark were trained abroad, primarily in Norway, Spain, and Germany.

Government Role in Health Care

According to WHO, in 2010, Denmark spent $36.0 billion on health care, an amount that comes to $6,422 per capita. Health care funding was provided entirely from domestic sources. Most (85 percent) spending on health care was provided by government expenditure, with 13 percent provided by household spending and 2 percent from other sources. In 2010, Denmark allocated 17 percent of total government expenditures to health, and government expenditures on health came to 10 percent of GDP; on both measures, Denmark

ranks in the high range when compared with other high-income European countries.

Public Health Programs

Denmark's national institute of public health, the Staten Institut for Folkesundhed, is a research institute within the Faculty of Health Sciences of the University of Southern Denmark. The institute employs about 100 people and focuses its activities on research into health and disease, training of physicians and public health officials, and research into the functioning of the Danish health care system. The institute has six primary areas of focus: alcohol; child health; the National Health Interview System (SUSY), and health behaviors, lifestyles, and living conditions; the KRAM survey covering diet, tobacco and alcohol use, and physical activity; public health in Greenland; and registry-based research. Access to improved sources of drinking water and improved sanitary facilities was essentially universal in 2010. According to the World Higher Education Database (WHED), one university in Denmark offers programs in epidemiology or public health: Aarhus University.

DJIBOUTI

Djibouti is a country in east Africa, sharing borders with Eritrea, Ethiopia, and Somali, and having a coastline on the Gulf of Aden. The area of 8,958 square miles (23,200 square kilometers) makes Djibouti slightly smaller than Massachusetts, and the July 2012 population was estimated at 774,389. In 2010, 76 percent of the population lived in urban areas, and the 2010 to 2015 annual rate of urbanization was estimated at 1.8 percent. The capital is Djibouti City. The country's population growth is 2.3 percent, the 36th-highest in the world; the net migration rate is 6.0 migrants per 1,000 population (the 16th-highest in the world); the birth rate 24.9 births per 1,000; and the total fertility rate 2.6 children per woman. The United Nations High Commissioner for Refugees (UNHCR) estimated that, in 2010, there were 15,104 refugees and persons in refugee-like situations in Djibouti.

Djibouti is a former French colony that became independent in 1977 but retains close ties with France. According to the Ibrahim Index, in 2011, Djibouti ranked 29th among 53 African countries in terms of governance performance, with a score of 49 (out of 100). Djibouti ranked tied for 100th among 183 countries on the *Corruption Perceptions Index 2011,* with a score of 3.0 (on a scale where 0 indicates highly corrupt and 10 very clean). In 2011, Djibouti was classified as a country with low human development (the lowest of four categories) on the United Nations Development Programme's (UNDP's) Human Development Index (HDI), with a score of 0.430 (on a scale where 1 denotes high development and 0 low development).

In 2011, the International Food Policy Research Institute (IFPRI) classified Djibouti as a country with an "alarming" hunger problem, with a Global Hunger Index (GHI) score of 22.5 (where 0 reflects no hunger and higher scores more hunger), and in 2012, the World Food Programme reported that Djibouti was experiencing water shortages and high food prices (much of Djibouti's food is imported from Ethiopia). Life expectancy at birth in 2012 was estimated at 61.57 years, and estimated gross domestic product (GDP) per capita in 2011 was $2,600. Unemployment in 2007 was estimated at 59.0 percent, among the highest rates in the world.

Emergency Health Services

Doctors Without Borders (Médecins Sans Frontières, or MSF) began working in Djibouti in 2008 and had 128 staff members in the country at the close of 2010.

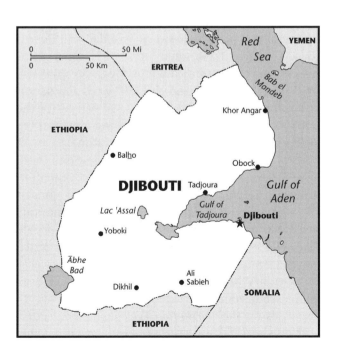

MSF efforts are concentrated in the capital of Djibouti City, where the focus is on treating malnutrition in children, providing measles vaccinations, and testing and treating children for tuberculosis. In 2010, more than 3,620 children in Djibouti received care from MSF, and more than 1,000 malnourished children were provided hospital care.

Insurance

According to Ke Xu and colleagues, in 2003, 0.3 percent of households in Djibouti experienced catastrophic health expenditures annually; "catastrophic" was defined as exceeding 40 percent of household income remaining after basic needs were met.

Costs of Hospitalization

No data available.

Access to Health Care

According to the World Health Organization (WHO), in 2006, 93 percent of births in Djibouti were attended by skilled personnel (for example, physicians, nurses, or midwives). In 2002, 7 percent of pregnant women received at least four prenatal care visits. The 2010 immunization rates for 1-year-olds were 88 percent for diphtheria and pertussis (DPT3), 85 percent for measles (MCV), and 88 percent for Hib (Hib3).

Cost of Drugs

No data available.

Health Care Facilities

Medical facilities in Djibouti are largely limited to Djibouti City and the surrounding towns, and in 2004, WHO reported only 129 physicians and 257 nurses working in the country.

Major Health Issues

In 2008, WHO estimated that 65 percent of years of life lost in Djibouti were due to communicable diseases, 24 percent to noncommunicable diseases, and 10 percent to injuries. In 2008, the age-standardized estimate of cancer deaths was 95 per 100,000 population for men and 80 per 100,000 for women; for cardiovascular disease and diabetes, 526 per 100,000 for men and 453 per 100,000 for women; and for chronic respiratory disease, 56 per 100,000 for men and 44 per 100,000 for women.

In 2008, the age-standardized death rate from malaria was 1.1 per 100,000 population.

Djibouti's maternal mortality rate (death from any cause related to or aggravated by pregnancy) was estimated in 2008 as 300 maternal deaths per 100,000 live births. A 2006 survey estimated the prevalence of female genital mutilation at 93.1 percent. The infant mortality rate, defined as the number of deaths of infants younger than 1 year, was estimated at 53.31 per 1,000 live births as of 2012. Child malnutrition is a serious problem: In 2006, 29.6 percent of children under age 5 were underweight (defined as 2 kilograms [kg] below standard weight-for-age at age 1, 3 kg below for ages 2 to 3, and 4 kg below for ages 4 to 5), one of the 20 highest rates in the world. In 2010, tuberculosis incidence was 620.0 per 100,000 population, tuberculosis prevalence 839.0 per 100,000, and deaths due to tuberculosis among human immunodeficiency virus (HIV)-negative people 71.00 per 100,000. As of 2009, an estimated 2.5 percent of adults age 15 to 49 were living with HIV or acquired immune deficiency syndrome (AIDS).

Health Care Personnel

In 2006, WHO identified Djibouti as one of 57 countries with a critical deficit in the supply of skilled health workers. Djibouti has no medical schools. Physicians wishing to practice in Djibouti must register with the Ordre des Médecins. Graduates of recognized medical schools are granted a license by the Ministère de la Santé Publique et des Affaires Sociales, but foreigners must receive authorization in order to practice. In 2006, Djibouti had 0.23 physicians per 1,000 population, and in 2008 had 0.80 nurses and midwives per 1,000 and 0.12 dentistry personnel per 1,000. The global "brain drain" (international migration of skilled personnel) plays a minor role in the relative undersupply of medical personnel in Djibouti: Michael Clemens and Bunilla Petterson estimate that 23 percent of Djibouti-born physicians and 2 percent of Djibouti-born nurses are working in one of nine developed countries, primarily in France.

Government Role in Health Care

According to WHO, in 2010, Djibouti spent $81.0 million on health care, an amount that comes to $92 per capita. About three-quarters (76 percent) of health care funding was provided from domestic sources, with the remaining 24 percent funded by sources from abroad. About two-thirds (65 percent) of spending on health care was provided by government expenditures, with 34 percent provided

by household spending (36 percent) and less than 1 percent from other sources. In 2010, Djibouti allocated 14 percent of total government expenditures to health, and government expenditures on health came to 5 percent of GDP; on both measures, Djibouti ranks in the high range when compared with other lower-middle-income eastern Mediterranean region countries. In 2009, according to WHO, official development assistance (ODA) for health in Djibouti came to $15.32 per capita.

Public Health Programs

According to WHO, in 2005, Djibouti had 0.03 environmental and public health workers per 1,000 population. In 2010, 50 percent of the population had access to improved sanitation facilities, with access much higher for urban (63 percent) than rural (10 percent) populations. A similar pattern was observed in access to improved sources of drinking water; overall, 88 percent of the population had such access, with a much higher proportion of urban (99 percent) than rural (54 percent) dwellers. According to the World Higher Education Database (WHED), no university in Djibouti offers programs in epidemiology or public health.

DOMINICA

Dominica is an island country in the Caribbean Sea, located about halfway between Trinidad and Puerto Rico. The area of 290 square miles (751 square kilometers) makes Dominica about four times the size of Washington, D.C., and the July 2012 population was estimated at 73,126. In 2010, 67 percent of the population lived in urban areas, and the 2010 to 2015 annual rate of urbanization is estimated at 0.3 percent. Roseau is the capital and largest city (with a 2009 estimated population of 14,000). Population growth is 0.2 percent; the net migration rate is one of the highest in Latin America (negative 5.4 migrants per 1,000 population), while the total fertility rate (2.1 children per woman) and birth rate (15.6 births per 1,000 population) are both moderate.

Dominica became independent from Great Britain in 1980. Dominica ranks tied for 44th among 183 countries on the *Corruption Perceptions Index 2011*, with a score of 5.2 (on a scale where 0 indicates highly

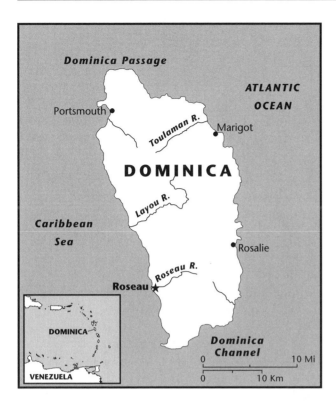

corrupt and 10 very clean). In 2011, Dominica was classified as a country with high human development (the second-highest category) on the United Nations Development Programme's (UNDP's) Human Development Index (HDI), with a score of 0.724 (on a scale where 1 denotes high development and 0 low development). Life expectancy at birth in 2012 was estimated at 76.18 years, and per capita gross domestic product (GDP) in 2011 was estimated at $13,600. Unemployment in 2000 was estimated at 23.0 percent.

Emergency Health Services

The ambulance service in Dominica is part of the Fire Department and includes personnel trained as emergency medical technicians. The major trauma facility for the country is in the Princess Margaret Hospital.

Insurance

Dominica has a social insurance system covering the employed, self-employed, and apprentices aged 16 to 60. The system is funded through wage contributions (4 percent of covered earnings), contributions from the self-employed (10 percent of declared net earnings), and employers' contributions (6.75 percent of covered payroll). There are no statutory medical benefits for the insured or their dependents; only cash

benefits are provided. Maternity benefits are 60 percent of average earnings 6 weeks before and after the due date, or a lump sum maternity benefit of XCD 500. The sickness benefit is 60 percent of average earnings for up to 26 weeks.

Costs of Hospitalization

Primary care provided at district hospitals is free; however, secondary care services, provided at the Princess Margaret Hospital, require payment of fees according to a schedule, including technical procedures, specialist visits, and hospitalization. Special government programs exist to reduce or waive fees for some individuals, including handicapped children and low-income people.

Access to Health Care

Primary care in Dominica is administered at the district level: There are seven districts grouped into two administrative regions. Each district has four to seven Type I health clinics providing primary care services free of charge. According to the World Health Organization (WHO), in 2008, 100 percent of births in Dominica were attended by skilled personnel (for example, physicians, nurses, or midwives). The 2010 immunization rates for 1-year-olds were 98 percent for diphtheria and pertussis (DPT3), 99 percent for measles (MCV), and 98 percent for Hib (Hib3). Lab services are provided for free in government labs for residents who have been referred from district clinics or from the accident and emergency department.

Two district hospitals (Marigot and Portsmouth Hospitals) are also part of the primary care network and offer limited inpatient services. Secondary care services are provided at the Princess Margaret Hospital, the only referral hospital in the country, and these services require payment (although mechanisms are in place to reduce or waive fees in some cases). Tertiary care services are provided outside the country or by visiting specialists, and these costs are borne by the patient. According to WHO, in 2010, Dominica had fewer than 0.01 magnetic resonance imaging (MRI) machines per 1 million population and 14.97 computer tomography (CT) machines per 1 million.

Cost of Drugs

Dominica participates in the Pharmaceuticals Procurement Service of the Organization of Eastern Caribbean States (OECS), and essential medicines are provided free at district pharmacies.

Health Care Facilities

As of 2010, according to WHO, Dominica had 90.03 health posts per 100,000 population, less than 0.01 health centers per 100,000, 2.95 district or rural hospitals per 100,000, 2.95 provincial hospitals per 100,000, and less than 0.01 specialized hospitals per 100,000. In 2009, Dominica had 3.80 hospital beds per 1,000 population.

Major Health Issues

In 2008, WHO estimated that 16 percent of years of life lost in Dominica were due to communicable diseases, 74 percent to noncommunicable diseases, and 11 percent to injuries. In 2008, the age-standardized estimate of cancer deaths was 191 per 100,000 for men and 116 per 100,000 for women; for cardiovascular disease and diabetes, 315 per 100,000 for men and 301 per 100,000 for women; and for chronic respiratory disease, 54 per 100,000 for men and 24 per 100,000 for women. Malaria was eradicated in 1962, although occasionally an imported case is identified, and dengue fever remains a problem. The infant mortality rate, defined as the number of deaths of infants younger than 1 year, was 12.38 per 1,000 live births as of 2012. No information is available from WHO on the maternal mortality rate in Dominica. In 2010, tuberculosis incidence was 13.0 per 100,000 population, tuberculosis prevalence 20.0 per 100,000, and deaths due to tuberculosis among human immunodeficiency virus (HIV)-negative people 3.40 per 100,000.

Health Care Personnel

One medical school is located in Dominica, the School of Medicine of Ross University in Roseau, which began offering instruction in 1978. The language of instruction is English, and many students are from other countries, including the United States. Physicians wishing to practice must register with the Dominica Medical Board and must have completed an 18-month internship after graduation. Foreigners must have an offer of employment in order to be licensed. In 1997, Dominica had 0.50 physicians per 1,000 population, 0.50 dentistry personnel per 1,000, and 4.17 nurses and midwives per 1,000. Despite having a medical school in Dominica, the country has a relative undersupply of physicians because most of the students are foreigners who do not stay to practice in Dominica. Alok Bhargava and colleagues placed Dominica first among countries most affected by medical "brain drain" (international migration of skilled personnel) in 2004.

Government Role in Health Care

According to WHO, in 2010, Dominica spent $28.0 million on health care, an amount that comes to $419 per capita. Almost all (98 percent) of health care funding was provided from domestic sources, with the remaining 2 percent funded by sources from abroad. Over two-thirds (70 percent) of spending on health care was provided by government expenditures, with 26 percent provided by household spending and 4 percent from other sources. In 2010, Dominica allocated 11 percent of its total government expenditures to health, placing it in the median range when compared to other upper- to middle-income countries in the Americas region, and government expenditures on health came to 5 percent of GDP, placing Dominica in the high range when compared with other upper- to middle-income countries in the Americas region.

Public Health Programs

Dominica's Health Information Unit is responsible for disease surveillance; it is led by the national epidemiologist and includes a National Public Health Surveillance and Response Team. The public water system is managed by the Dominica Water and Sewerage Company. In 2010, 81 percent of the population of Dominica had access to improved sanitation facilities (84 percent in rural areas and 80 percent in urban), and 95 percent had access to improved sources of drinking water (92 percent in rural areas and 96 percent in urban).

DOMINICAN REPUBLIC

The Dominican Republic is a Caribbean country occupying the eastern two-thirds of the island of Hispaniola and sharing a border with Haiti. The area of 18,792 square miles (48,670 square kilometers) makes the Dominican Republic about twice the size of New Hampshire, and the July 2012 population was estimated at 10.1 million. In 2010, 69 percent of the population lived in urban areas, and the 2010 to 2015 annual rate of urbanization was estimated at 2.1 percent. The July 2012 population growth rate was 1.3 percent despite a negative net migration rate (negative 2.0 migrants per 1,000 population); the total fertility rate is 2.4 children per woman and the birth rate 19.4 births per 1,000 population. The United Nations High Commissioner for Refugees (UNHCR) estimated that, in 2010, there were 154 refugees and persons in refugee-like situations in the Dominican Republic.

The Dominican Republic was a colony of both France and Spain and became independent in 1865; the country has had numerous periods of dictatorship and civil unrest since. The Dominican Republic ranked tied for 129th among 183 countries on the *Corruption Perceptions Index 2011*, with a score of 2.6 (on a scale where 0 indicates highly corrupt and 10 very clean). In 2011, the Dominican Republic was classified as a country with medium human development (the second from the lowest of four categories) on the United Nations Development Programme's (UNDP's) Human Development Index (HDI), with a score of 0.689 (on a scale where 1 denotes high development and 0 low development). Life expectancy at birth in 2012 was estimated at 77.44 years, and per capita gross domestic product (GDP) in 2011 was estimated at $9,300. Income distribution in the Dominican Republic is relatively unequal: In 2007, the Gini Index (a measure of dispersion, in which perfect equality is denoted by 0 and maximum inequality is denoted by 100) for family income was 48.4. According to the World Economic Forum's *Global Gender Gap Index 2011*, the Dominican Republic ranked 81st out of 135 countries on gender equality, with a score of 0.668 (on a scale with a theoretical range of 1 for equality to 0 for inequality and an actual range in 2011 from 0.8530 to 0.4873).

Emergency Health Services

According to the World Health Organization (WHO), as of 2007, the Dominican Republic had a formal and publicly available emergency care (prehospital care) system accessible through a national universal access telephone number. Public hospitals provide emergency services through doctors on 24-hour call.

Insurance

The Dominican Republic has a universal medical benefits system and a social insurance system providing cash benefits to the employed and pensioners. The system is funded by a wage tax (3.04 percent of covered earnings) and an employer payroll tax (7.09 percent of covered earnings). Medical care covered includes inpatient and outpatient care, preventive care, maternity care, surgery, emergency care, medicines, and prostheses for the disabled. Medicines are covered at 70 percent and are provided free to those on social

assistance. Pediatric health care is provided until age 5 and includes child development programs, health care, and nutrition programs. The maternity benefit is equivalent to three months' earnings for the insured, paid for six weeks prior to and after the due date. For low-income people, a nursing allowance is also paid for the first year of the child's life. The sickness benefit is 60 percent of earnings for up to 26 weeks; if the patient is hospitalized, the benefit is 40 percent of earnings. In 2002, 21.1 percent of the population had private health insurance (44.4 percent in the highest-income quintile and 21.1 percent in the lowest).

Costs of Hospitalization

No data available.

Access to Health Care

Primary care is organized by interdisciplinary teams consisting of a physician, a nursing assistant, a community health agent, and several health promoters; these teams are responsible for about 500 families each. Hospital care is provided through the Secretariat of Public Health and the Dominican Social Security Institute, which operate more than 60 hospitals between them. According to Latinobarometer, an annual public opinion survey conducted in Latin

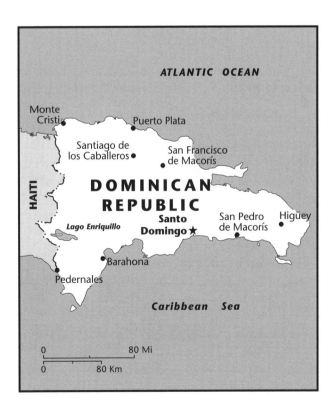

America, 67 percent of citizens in the Dominican Republic are satisfied with the level of health care available to them (the regional average is 51.9 percent). The number of health services facilities has been dramatically increased since the 1980s, and there are now health clinics and pharmacies throughout the country.

According to WHO, in 2007, 98 percent of births in the Dominican Republic were attended by skilled personnel (for example, physicians, nurses, or midwives). In 2007, 95 percent of pregnant women received at least four prenatal care visits. The 2010 immunization rates for 1-year-olds were 88 percent for diphtheria and pertussis (DPT3), 79 percent for measles (MCV), and 81 percent for Hib (Hib3). In 2010, an estimated 72 percent of persons with advanced human immunodeficiency virus (HIV) infection were receiving antiretroviral therapy in accordance with the 2010 WHO guidelines.

Cost of Drugs

In 2005, the Dominican Republic's list of essential drugs included 871 pharmaceutical formulations and 468 drugs. Drugs for the public sector are procured through the Essential Drugs Program; this program supplies drugs to hospitals and medical centers at subsidized prices that were on average 250 percent below the cost of purchasing the same products directly. Drug assistance is also provided free or at reduced cost for those enrolled in the Dominican Social Security System. In private pharmacies, drug prices are not controlled, and there are sometimes large differences between the international reference price of a drug and the price charged by a particular pharmacy.

Health Care Facilities

The Secretariat of Public Health operates a network including six specialized hospitals, eight regional hospitals, 107 municipal hospitals, and 22 provincial hospitals, while the Dominican Social Security Institute operates a network including three national and specialized hospitals, 15 general hospitals, and two regional hospitals. In 2009, the Dominican Republic had 1.00 hospital beds per 1,000 population.

Major Health Issues

In 2008, WHO estimated that 42 percent of years of life lost in the Dominican Republic were due to communicable diseases, 42 percent to noncommunicable diseases, and 17 percent to injuries. In 2008, the age-standardized estimate of cancer deaths was 109 per 100,000 for men and 96 per 100,000 for women; for cardiovascular disease and diabetes, 312 per 100,000 for men and 329 per 100,000 for women; and for chronic respiratory disease, 36 per 100,000 for men and 36 per 100,000 for women. In 2008, the age-standardized death rate from malaria was 0.1 per 100,000 population, and bilharzia remains a threat.

Selected Health Indicators: Dominican Republic Compared With the Global Average (2010)

	Dominican Republic	Global Average
Male life expectancy at birth* (years)	71	66
Female life expectancy at birth* (years)	72	71
Under-5 mortality rate, both sexes (per 1,000 live births)	27	57
Adult mortality rate, both sexes* (probability of dying between 15 and 60 years per 1,000 population)	160	176
Maternal mortality ratio (per 100,000 live births)	150	210
HIV prevalence* (per 1,000 adults aged 15 to 49)	9	8
Tuberculosis prevalence (per 100,000 population)	90	178

Source: World Health Organization Global Health Observatory Data Repository.
*Data refers to 2009.

The Dominican Republic's maternal mortality rate (death from any cause related to or aggravated by pregnancy) was estimated in 2008 as 100 maternal deaths per 100,000 live births. The infant mortality rate, defined as the number of deaths of infants younger than 1 year, was estimated at 21.30 per 1,000 live births as of 2012.

In 2010, tuberculosis incidence was 67.0 per 100,000 population, tuberculosis prevalence 90.0 per 100,000, and deaths due to tuberculosis among HIV-negative people 8.20 per 100,000. As of 2009, an estimated 0.9 percent of adults age 15 to 49 were living with HIV or acquired immune deficiency syndrome (AIDS). Dengue fever is endemic in the Dominican Republic, and malaria is primarily an issue in rural areas.

Health Care Personnel

The Dominican Republic has 10 medical schools, which offer a basic medical training course lasting four to seven years. An additional two years of supervised clinical practice are also required before granting the degree Doctor en Medicina (doctor of medicine). One year of government service work in a rural area is required after graduation. The Secretaria de Estado de Salud Pública in Santo Domingo grants the license to practice medicine. In 2000, the Dominican Republic had 1.88 physicians per 1,000 population, 0.40 pharmaceutical personnel per 1,000, 0.84 dentistry personnel per 1,000, and 1.84 nurses and midwives per 1,000.

Government Role in Health Care

According to WHO, in 2010, the Dominican Republic spent $3.2 billion on health care, an amount that comes to $323 per capita. Almost all (99 percent) of health care funding was provided from domestic sources, with the remaining 1 percent funded by sources from abroad. The largest share (43 percent) of spending on health care was provided by government expenditures, with 37 percent provided by household spending and 19 percent from other sources. In 2010, the Dominican Republic allocated 14 percent of its total government expenditures to health, placing it in the median range when compared to other upper- to middle-income countries in the Americas region; government expenditures on health came to 3 percent of GDP, placing the Dominican Republic in the low range when compared with other upper- to middle-income countries in the Americas region. In 2009, according to WHO, official development assistance (ODA) for health in the Dominican Republic came to $6.71 per capita.

Public Health Programs

In 2005, 83 percent of the population of the Dominican Republic had access to improved sanitation facilities (75 percent in rural areas and 87 percent in urban), and 86 percent had access to improved sources of drinking water (84 percent in rural areas and 87 percent in urban). According to the World Higher Education Database (WHED), no university in the Dominican Republic offers programs in epidemiology or public health.

ECUADOR

Ecuador is a country in northwest South America, sharing borders with Colombia and Peru and having a coastline on the Pacific Ocean; Ecuador includes the Galapagos Islands. The area of 109,484 square miles (283,561 square kilometers) makes Ecuador slightly smaller than Nevada, and the July 2012 population was estimated at 15.2 percent. In 2010, 67 percent of the population lived in urban areas, and the 2010 to 2015 annual rate of urbanization was estimated at 2.0 percent. Quito is the capital and Guyaquil the largest city (with a 2009 population estimated at 2.6 million). The July 2012 population growth rate was 1.4 percent; the net migration rate is negative 0.4 migrants per 1,000 population, the birth rate 19.6 births per 1,000, and the total fertility rate 2.4 children per woman. The United Nations High Commissioner for Refugees (UNHCR) estimated that, in 2010, there were 52,905 refugees and persons in refugee-like situations in Ecuador.

Ecuador became independent from Spain in 1830. Ecuador ranked tied for 120th among 183 countries on the *Corruption Perceptions Index 2011*, with a score of 2.7 (on a scale where 0 indicates highly corrupt and 10 very clean). In 2011, Ecuador was classified as a country with high human development (the second-highest category) on the United Nations Development Programme's (UNDP's) Human Development Index (HDI), with a score of 0.720 (on a scale where 1 denotes high development and 0 low development). Life expectancy at birth in 2012 was estimated at 75.94 years, and per capita gross domestic product (GDP) in 2011 was estimated at $8,300. Income distribution in Ecuador is relatively unequal: In 2011, the Gini Index (a measure of dispersion, in which perfect equality is denoted by 0 and maximum

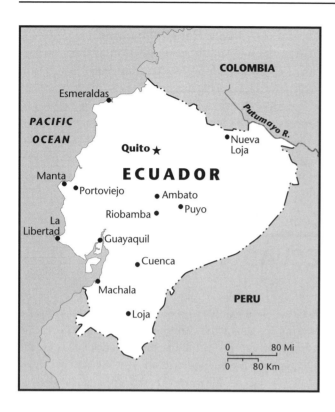

inequality is denoted by 100) for family income was 47.3. According to the World Economic Forum's *Global Gender Gap Index 2011*, Ecuador ranked 45th out of 135 countries on gender equality with a score of 0.704 (on a scale with a theoretical range of 1 for equality to 0 for inequality and an actual range in 2011 from 0.8530 to 0.4873).

Emergency Health Services

According to the World Health Organization (WHO), as of 2007, Ecuador did not have a formal and publicly available system for providing prehospital care (emergency care).

Insurance

Ecuador has social insurance with mandatory coverage for the employed, recipients of public benefits (old age, disability, survivor, or work injury), and voluntary coverage for those who wish it. Agricultural workers and small-scale fishermen are covered under a separate system. The system is funded through employer payroll taxes (5.71 percent), contributions from voluntary members (5.71 percent of gross earnings), contributions from the self-employed (5.71 percent of gross declared earnings), and contributions for recipients of survivor pensions (4.15 percent of

pension). The government pays the total cost for beneficiaries of work injury, disability, and old-age pensions. Medical benefits are provided through medical facilities of the Social Security Institute, including hospitalization, surgery, general and specialist care, lab services, dental care, and medicine.

The maternity benefit is 75 percent of earnings for 2 weeks before and 10 weeks after the due date. The sickness cash benefit is 75 percent of earnings for up to 70 days and then 66 percent for 182 days. The system is administered and operated through the Social Security Institute.

Costs of Hospitalization

In 2002, 34.4 percent of health care spending in Ecuador went for hospital services.

Access to Health Care

According to Latinobarometer, an annual public opinion survey conducted in Latin America, 48 percent of citizens in Ecuador are satisfied with the level of health care available to them (the regional average is 51.9 percent). According to the U.S. State Department, medical care is far more available in large cities in Ecuador than in the countryside; while pharmacies are readily available in cities, the supply of medications may be limited. According to the World Health Organization (WHO), in 2005, 80 percent of births in Ecuador were attended by skilled personnel (for example, physicians, nurses, or midwives). In 2004, 58 percent of pregnant women received at least four prenatal care visits. The 2010 immunization rates for 1-year-olds were 99 percent for diphtheria and pertussis (DPT3), 98 percent for measles (MCV), and 99 percent for Hib (Hib3). In 2010, an estimated 63 percent of persons with advanced human immunodeficiency virus (HIV) infection were receiving antiretroviral therapy in accordance with the 2010 WHO guidelines.

Cost of Drugs

In 2002, 29.6 percent of public expenditures on health in Ecuador went to purchase medicines. According to WHO, in 2008, the median availability of selected generic drugs in the public sector in Ecuador was 41.7 percent; in the private sector, the mean availability was 71.7 percent. The median price ratio (comparing the price in Ecuador to the international reference price) was 5.0 in the private sphere, indicating that median prices in the public sphere were five times as high as the international reference price.

Health Care Facilities

As of 2010, according to WHO, Ecuador had 3.17 health posts per 100,000 population, 0.39 health centers per 100,000, 0.06 district or rural hospitals per 100,000, 0.20 provincial hospitals per 100,000, and 0.10 specialized hospitals per 100,000. In 2008, Ecuador had 1.50 hospital beds per 1,000 population.

Major Health Issues

In 2008, WHO estimated that 30 percent of years of life lost in Ecuador were due to communicable diseases, 45 percent to noncommunicable diseases, and 25 percent to injuries. In 2008, the age-standardized estimate of cancer deaths was 122 per 100,000 for men and 116 per 100,000 for women; for cardiovascular disease and diabetes, 190 per 100,000 for men and 143 per 100,000 for women; and for chronic respiratory disease, 23 per 100,000 for men and 14 per 100,000 for women.

Ecuador's maternal mortality rate (death from any cause related to or aggravated by pregnancy) was estimated in 2008 as 110 maternal deaths per 100,000 live births. The infant mortality rate, defined as the number of deaths of infants younger than 1 year, was estimated at 19.06 per 1,000 live births as of 2012. In 2010, tuberculosis incidence was 65.0 per 100,000 population, tuberculosis prevalence 103.0 per 100,000, and deaths due to tuberculosis among human immunodeficiency virus (HIV)-negative people 6.70 per 100,000. As of 2009, an estimated 0.4 percent of adults age 15 to 49 were living with HIV or acquired immune deficiency syndrome (AIDS).

Health Care Personnel

Ecuador has 11 medical schools offering a course of training lasting six to eight years and awarding the degree Doctor en Medicine y Cirugía (doctor of medicine and surgery). One year of government service in a rural area is required after graduation. Physicians must register with the Colegio Médico de Pichincha, and the license to practice is granted by the Ministry of Public Health in Quito following completion of the obligatory year of service. Graduates of foreign medical schools must have their degrees validated by an Ecuadorian university. In 2000, Ecuador had 1.48 physicians per 1,000 population, 0.17 dentistry personnel per 1,000, and 1.66 nurses and midwives per 1,000.

Government Role in Health Care

According to WHO, in 2010, Ecuador spent $4.7 billion on health care, an amount that comes to $328 per capita. Almost half (49 percent) of spending on health care was provided by household spending, with 37 percent provided by government expenditures and 14 percent from other sources. In 2010, Ecuador allocated 7 percent of its total government expenditures to health, placing it in the low range when compared to other upper- to middle-income countries in the Americas region; government expenditures on health came to 3 percent of GDP, also placing Ecuador in the low range when compared with other upper- to middle-income countries in the Americas region. In 2009, according to WHO, official development assistance (ODA) for health in Ecuador came to $1.53 per capita.

Public Health Programs

Ecuador's National Institute for Hygiene and Tropical Medicine "Leopoldo Izquieta Perez" was founded in 1941; it is located in Guyaquil and directed by Marcelo Aguilar Velazco. The national institute is part of the Ministry of Public Health and has as its mission to improve population health. It acts as the central health registry for Ecuador and is responsible for a number of other activities, including training personnel; conducting scientific research into the prevention, diagnosis, and control of disease; developing technologies and products used to safeguard human and animal health; and regulating drugs, food, cosmetics, biological products, and similar products.

In 2010, 92 percent of the Ecuadoran population had access to improved sanitation facilities (84 percent in rural areas and 96 percent in urban), and 94 percent had access to improved sources of drinking water (89 percent in rural areas and 96 percent in urban). According to the World Higher Education Database (WHED), three universities in Ecuador offer programs in epidemiology or public health: the Institute of Technology in Chimborazo, the National University of Loja, and San Francisco University in Quito.

EGYPT

Egypt is a north African country, sharing borders with Libya, Sudan, and Israel and having coastlines on the Mediterranean Sea and Red Sea (1,522 miles or 2,450 kilometers total). The area of 386,662 square miles (1,001,450 square kilometers, the 30th-largest in the

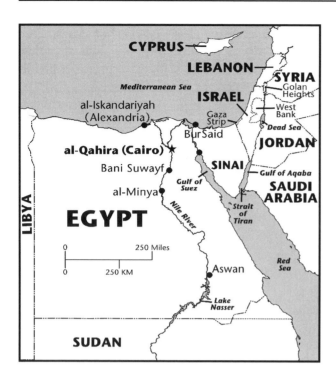

In 2011, Egypt was classified as a country with medium human development (the second from the lowest of four categories) on the United Nations Development Programme's (UNDP's) Human Development Index (HDI), with a score of 0.644 (on a scale where 1 denotes high development and 0 low development). A February 2012 survey by the World Food Programme found that about half of households in Egypt relied on charity, government assistance, and family assistance to meet their basic needs. Life expectancy at birth in 2012 was estimated at 72.93 years, and the estimated gross domestic product (GDP) per capita in 2011 was $6,500. In 2001, the Gini Index (a measure of dispersion, in which perfect equality is denoted by 0 and maximum inequality is denoted by 100) for family income was 34.4. According to the World Economic Forum's *Global Gender Gap Index 2011*, Egypt ranked 123rd out of 135 countries on gender equality, with a score of 0.593 (on a scale with a theoretical range of 1 for equality to 0 for inequality and an actual range in 2011 from 0.8530 to 0.4873).

Emergency Health Services

According to the World Health Organization (WHO), as of 2007, Egypt had a formal and publicly available emergency care (prehospital care) system accessible through a national universal access telephone number. Doctors Without Borders (Médecins Sans Frontières, or MSF) began working in Egypt in 2010 and had 19 staff members in the country at the close of 2010. MSF provides maternal and child health care in Ezbet el Haggana, part of Cairo, and assists the Egyptian staff working in this area.

Insurance

Egypt has a social insurance system covering employed persons, with coverage gradually being extended to students; the self-employed, household workers, small-scale artisans, and temporary agricultural workers are excluded. The system is funded by an earnings tax (1 percent of covered earnings), pensioner contributions (1 percent of pension; 2 percent of survivor pensions), and employer payroll contributions (4 percent of covered payroll or 3 percent of the employers providing cash sickness benefits). The maternity benefit is paid for a maximum of three pregnancies and is 75 percent of wages for up to 90 days. The sickness benefit is 75 percent of wages for up to 90 days and then 85 percent for up to 180 days;

world) makes Egypt about three times as large as New Mexico, and the July 2012 population of 83.7 million was the largest in the Arab world. In 2010, 43.4 percent of the population lived in urban areas, and the 2010 to 2015 annual rate of urbanization was estimated at 2.1 percent. Cairo is the capital and largest city (with a 2009 population estimated at 10.9 million). The July 2012 population growth rate was 1.9 percent despite a negative net migration rate (negative 0.2 migrants per 1,000 population); the birth rate was 24.2 births per 1,000 population, and the total fertility rate was 2.9 children per woman. The United Nations High Commissioner for Refugees (UNHCR) estimated that, in 2010, there were 25,096 refugees and persons in refugee-like situations in Egypt.

Egypt became partially independent from Great Britain in 1922 and achieved full independence in 1952. In 2011, massive demonstrations prompted the resignation of President Hosni Mubarak, the suspension of the constitution, and the dissolution of the national parliament. According to the Ibrahim Index, in 2011 Egypt ranked 10th among 53 African countries in terms of governance performance, with a score of 61 (out of 100). Egypt ranked tied for 112th among 183 countries on the *Corruption Perceptions Index 2011,* with a score of 2.9 (on a scale where 0 indicates highly corrupt and 10 very clean).

for some conditions, the benefit is 100 percent of wages. The Health Insurance Organization administers medical benefits, the national Organization for Social Insurance administers contributions and cash benefits, and the Ministry of Health and Population provides general supervision. According to Ke Xu and colleagues, in 2003, 2.8 percent of households in Egypt experienced catastrophic health expenditures annually; "catastrophic" was defined as exceeding 40 percent of household income remaining after basic needs were met.

Costs of Hospitalization
No data available.

Access to Health Care
More than half of health care expenditures come from the private sector, and many Egyptians cannot afford care; in contrast, well-off Egyptians often have private insurance and can afford to pay for care. According to WHO, in 2008, 79 percent of births were attended by skilled personnel (for example, physicians, nurses, or midwives). In 2008, 66 percent of pregnant women received at least four prenatal care visits. The 2010 immunization rates for 1-year-olds were 97 percent for diphtheria and pertussis (DPT3) and 96 percent for measles (MCV). In 2010, an estimated 10 percent of persons with advanced human immunodeficiency virus (HIV) infection were receiving antiretroviral therapy in accordance with the 2010 WHO guidelines.

Cost of Drugs
No data available.

Health Care Facilities
As of 2010, according to WHO, Egypt had 0.39 health posts per 100,000 population, 0.26 health centers per 100,000, 0.50 district or rural hospitals per 100,000, and 0.12 specialized hospitals per 100,000. In 2009, Egypt had 1.70 hospital beds per 1,000 population.

Major Health Issues
In 2008, WHO estimated that 24 percent of years of life lost in Egypt were due to communicable diseases, 65 percent to noncommunicable diseases, and 11 percent to injuries. In 2008, the age-standardized estimate of cancer deaths was 107 per 100,000 for men and 76 per 100,000 for women; for cardiovascular disease and diabetes, 427 per 100,000 for men and 384

per 100,000 for women; and for chronic respiratory disease, 33 per 100,000 for men and 24 per 100,000 for women. Egypt has one of the highest adult obesity rates in the world, estimated at 28.8 percent in 2000; obesity is defined as a body mass index (BMI) of 30 or above.

Egypt's maternal mortality rate (death from any cause related to or aggravated by pregnancy) was estimated in 2008 as 82 maternal deaths per 100,000 live births. A 2008 survey estimated the prevalence of female genital mutilation at 91.1 percent. The infant mortality rate, defined as the number of deaths of infants younger than 1 year, was estimated at 24.23 per 1,000 live births as of 2012. In 2010, tuberculosis incidence was 18.0 per 100,000 population, tuberculosis prevalence 28.0 per 100,000, and deaths due to tuberculosis among HIV-negative people 0.82 per 100,000. As of 2009, an estimated 0.1 percent of adults age 15 to 49 were living with HIV or acquired immune deficiency syndrome (AIDS). In 2008, the age-standardized death rate from malaria was 0.1 per 100,000 population. Trachoma remains a problem, particularly in rural areas; in some communities, more than 30 percent of children are infected.

Health Care Personnel
Egypt has 16 medical schools. The basic degree course lasts six to seven years and a year of supervised clinical practice is also required after completion of studies. The degree granted is the bachelor of medicine and surgery. Two years of work in government service is required after graduation. Physicians must register with the General Medical Association and the Ministry of Health and Population, with licensure granted to each graduate with a diploma or master's degree in a specialization. Graduates of overseas medical schools must have their degrees validated. Egypt has agreements with a number of Arabic, European, and African countries.

In 2009, Egypt had 2.83 physicians per 1,000 population, 1.67 pharmaceutical personnel per 1,000, 0.42 dentistry personnel per 1,000, and 3.52 nurses and midwives per 1,000. The global "brain drain" (international migration of skilled personnel) plays a minor role in the supply of medical personnel in Egypt: Michael Clemens and Bunilla Petterson estimate that 5 percent of Egypt-born physicians and 1 percent of Egypt-born nurses are working in one of nine developed countries, primarily in the United States and the United Kingdom.

Government Role in Health Care

According to WHO, in 2010, Egypt spent $10.0 billion on health care, an amount that comes to $123 per capita. Almost all health care funding (99 percent) was provided from domestic sources, with the remaining 1 percent provided by funds from abroad. Over half (61 percent) of spending on health care was provided by household spending, with 37 percent provided by government expenditures and 1 percent from other sources. In 2010, Egypt allocated 6 percent of its total government expenditures to health, and government expenditures on health came to 2 percent of GDP; both figures place Egypt in the median range when compared with other lower middle-income countries in the eastern Mediterranean region. In 2009, according to WHO, official development assistance (ODA) for health in Egypt came to $1.41 per capita.

Public Health Programs

In 2010, 95 percent of the population had access to improved sanitation facilities (93 percent in rural areas and 97 percent in urban), and access to improved sources of drinking water was close to universal (99 percent in rural areas and 100 percent in urban). According to WHO, in 2004, Egypt had 0.13 environmental and public health workers per 1,000 population. According to the World Higher Education Database (WHED), eight universities in Egypt offer programs in epidemiology or public health: Ain Shams University in Cairo, Al-Ahram Canadian University in Giza, Al-Azhar University in Cairo, Assiut University, Cairo University, Fayoum University, Alexandria University, and two campuses of the Suez Canal University in Port Said and Ismailia.

EL SALVADOR

El Salvador is a country in Central America, sharing borders with Guatemala and Honduras and having a coastline on the Pacific Ocean. The area is 8,124 square miles (21,041 square kilometers), similar to Massachusetts), and the July 2012 population was estimated at 6.1 million. In 2010, 64 percent of the population lived in urban areas, and the 2010 to 2015 annual rate of urbanization was estimated at 1.4 percent. San Salvador is the capital and largest city (with a 2009 estimated population at 1.5 million). The population growth rate

in 2012 was 0.3 percent; the net migration rate, negative 8.8 migrants per 1,000 population, was one of the 15 highest emigration rates in the world; the birth rate was 17.4 births per 1,000 population; and the total fertility rate was 2.0 children per woman. The United Nations High Commissioner for Refugees (UNHCR) estimated that, in 2010, there were seven refugees and persons in refugee-like situations in El Salvador.

El Salvador became independent from Spain in 1839. Its modern history was marked by a civil war from 1880 to 1992, which cost an estimated 75,000 lives. El Salvador ranked tied for 80th among 183 countries on the *Corruption Perceptions Index 2011,* with a score of 3.4 (on a scale where 0 indicates highly corrupt and 10 very clean). In 2011, El Salvador was classified as a country with medium human development (the second from the lowest of four categories) on the United Nations Development Programme's (UNDP's) Human Development Index (HDI), with a score of 0.674 (on a scale where 1 denotes high development and 0 low development). Life expectancy at birth in 2012 was estimated at 73.69 years, and estimated gross domestic product (GDP) per capita in 2011 was $7,600. Income distribution in El Salvador is relatively unequal: In 2007, the Gini Index (a measure of dispersion, in which perfect

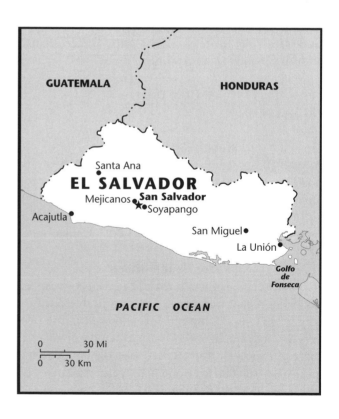

equality is denoted by 0 and maximum inequality is denoted by 100) for family income was 46.9. According to the World Economic Forum's *Global Gender Gap Index 2011*, El Salvador ranked 94th out of 135 countries on gender equality with a score of 0.657 (on a scale with a theoretical range of 1 for equality to 0 for inequality and an actual range in 2011 from 0.8530 to 0.4873).

Emergency Health Services

According to the World Health Organization (WHO), as of 2007, El Salvador did not have a formal and publicly available system for providing prehospital care (emergency care). However, El Salvador is in the process of establishing emergency medical services around the country and, as of 2005, had created 66 health units providing round-the-clock care; there are also two emergency care centers in the country.

Insurance

El Salvador has a social insurance system covering employed and self-employed workers in commerce and industry, pensioners, and household workers; teachers, casual workers, and agricultural workers are excluded. The system is funded through wage taxes (3 percent of covered earnings), pension contributions (6 percent of survivor and work injury pensions and 7.8 percent of disability or old-age pensions), contributions from the self-employed (10.5 percent of

declared income), and employer payroll contributions (7.5 percent of covered payroll). The maternity benefit is 100 percent of average earnings for 12 weeks; a layette and milk are also provided. The sickness benefit is 75 percent of average earnings for 26 weeks and may be extended for another 26 weeks. Medical benefits for insured persons include most medical care, hospitalization, medicine, maternity care, and dental care. Unemployed people can receive medical benefits for one year; children of insured people receive medical care up to age 12, and wives of insured persons receive medical, dental, and maternity care. The Social Insurance system operates its own clinics and hospitals and administers the program.

Costs of Hospitalization

No data available.

Access to Health Care

Although theoretically the Ministry of Public Health provides services to 80 percent of the Salvadoran population, in practice this number is closer to 50 percent. In order to provide more care to the underserved, El Salvador created the Health Assistance Fund (FOSALUD) in 2005 to provide free basic health services and emergency care; 3.8 million people were served by this fund in 2007. According to Latinobarometer, an annual public opinion survey conducted in Latin America, 64 percent of citizens in El Salvador are satisfied with

Selected Health Indicators: El Salvador Compared With the Global Average (2010)

	El Salvador	Global Average
Male life expectancy at birth* (years)	68	66
Female life expectancy at birth* (years)	76	71
Under-5 mortality rate, both sexes (per 1,000 live births)	16	57
Adult mortality rate, both sexes* (probability of dying between 15 and 60 years per 1,000 population)	200	176
Maternal mortality ratio (per 100,000 live births)	81	210
HIV prevalence* (per 1,000 adults aged 15 to 49)	8	8
Tuberculosis prevalence (per 100,000 population)	31	178

Source: World Health Organization Global Health Observatory Data Repository.
*Data refers to 2009.

the level of health care available to them (the regional average is 51.9 percent).

According to WHO, in 2008, 84 percent of births were attended by skilled personnel (for example, physicians, nurses, or midwives). In 2008, 78 percent of pregnant women received at least four prenatal care visits. The 2010 immunization rates for 1-year-olds were 92 percent for diphtheria and pertussis (DPT3), 92 percent for measles (MCV), and 92 percent for Hib (Hib3). In 2010, an estimated 59 percent of persons with advanced human immunodeficiency virus (HIV) infection were receiving antiretroviral therapy in accordance with the 2010 WHO guidelines. According to WHO, in 2010, El Salvador had 0.65 magnetic resonance imaging (MRI) machines per 1 million population, 3.75 computer tomography (CT) machines per 1 million, 0.49 telecolbalt units per 1 million, and 0.49 radiotherapy machines per 1 million.

Cost of Drugs

According to WHO, in 2006, the median availability of selected generic drugs in the public sector in El Salvador was 53.8 percent; in the private sector, the mean availability was 69.2 percent. The median price ratio (comparing the price in El Salvador to the international reference price) was 28.3 in the private sphere for selected generic medicines, indicating that median prices in the public sphere were more than 28 times the international reference prices.

Health Care Facilities

As of 2010, according to WHO, El Salvador had 9.46 health posts per 100,000 population, 0.05 health centers per 100,000, 0.40 district or rural hospitals per 100,000, 0.03 provincial hospitals per 100,000, and 0.05 specialized hospitals per 100,000. In 2009, El Salvador had 1.10 hospital beds per 1,000 population.

Major Health Issues

In 2008, WHO estimated that 22 percent of years of life lost in El Salvador were due to communicable diseases, 46 percent to noncommunicable diseases, and 32 percent to injuries. In 2008, the age-standardized estimate of cancer deaths was 78 per 100,000 for men and 113 per 100,000 for women; for cardiovascular disease and diabetes, 201 per 100,000 for men and 304 per 100,000 for women; and for chronic respiratory disease, 29 per 100,000 for men and 27 per 100,000 for women.

El Salvador's maternal mortality rate (death from any cause related to or aggravated by pregnancy) was estimated in 2008 as 110 maternal deaths per 100,000 live births. The infant mortality rate, defined as the number of deaths of infants younger than 1 year, was estimated at 19.66 per 1,000 live births as of 2012. In 2010, tuberculosis incidence was 28.0 per 100,000 population, tuberculosis prevalence 31.0 per 100,000, and deaths due to tuberculosis among HIV-negative people 0.92 per 100,000. As of 2009, an estimated 0.8 percent of adults age 15 to 49 were living with HIV or acquired immune deficiency syndrome (AIDS). Dengue fever is endemic to El Salvador, and more than 7,000 cases were reported in 2004 and 2005.

Health Care Personnel

In 2006, WHO identified El Salvador as one of 57 countries with a critical deficit in the supply of skilled health workers. El Salvador has six medical schools, located in San Salvador, Santa Ana, and Santa Tecla. The basic medical degree course requires seven to eight years, with an additional year of supervised clinical practice also required. One year of government service is obligatory after graduation. The license to practice medicine is granted by the Junta de Vigilancia de la Profesión Médica in San Salvador. In 2008, El Salvador had 1.60 physicians per 1,000 population, 0.32 pharmaceutical personnel per 1,000, 0.30 laboratory health workers per 1,000, 0.65 dentistry personnel per 1,000, and 0.41 nurses and midwives per 1,000.

Government Role in Health Care

According to WHO, in 2010, El Salvador spent $1.5 billion on health care, an amount that comes to $327 per capita. Almost all health care funding (98 percent) was provided from domestic sources, with the remaining 2 percent provided by funds from abroad. Over half (62 percent) of spending on health care was provided by government expenditures, with 34 percent provided by household spending and 4 percent from other sources. In 2010, El Salvador allocated 13 percent of its total government expenditures to health, and government expenditures on health came to 4 percent of GDP; both figures place El Salvador in the median range when compared with other lower-middle-income countries in the Americas region. In 2009, according to WHO, official development assistance (ODA) for health in El Salvador came to $3.90 per capita.

Public Health Programs

The Ministry of Public Health and Social Assistance, located in San Salvador and directed by María Isabel

Rodríguez, is charged with providing scientific and technical information to guide national health policy and improve knowledge and practice in medicine and public health. Strategic objectives of the ministry include health communication; training and development of personnel in public health; surveillance, monitoring, evaluation, and analysis of threats to public health; and research into health and the determinants of risks to public health. In 2010, 87 percent of the population of El Salvador had access to improved sanitation facilities (87 percent in rural areas and 83 percent in urban), and 88 percent had access to improved sources of drinking water (76 percent in rural areas and 94 percent in urban). According to the World Higher Education Database (WHED), no university in El Salvador offers programs in epidemiology or public health.

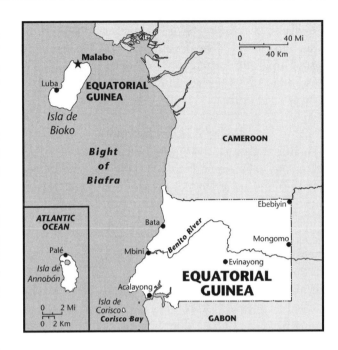

EQUATORIAL GUINEA

Equatorial Guinea is a west-central African country, sharing borders with Cameroon and Gabon and having a coastline on the Gulf of Guinea; the country consists of territory on the African mainland, one large island (Bioko), and a number of smaller islands. The area is 10,831 square miles (28,051 square kilometers, similar to Maryland), making it one of the smallest countries in Africa; the July 2012 population was estimated at 685,991. In 2010, 40 percent of the population lived in urban areas, and the 2010 to 2015 annual rate of urbanization was estimated at 3.1 percent. The capital and largest city is Malabo (with a 2009 population estimated at 128,000). The July 2012 population growth rate was 2.6 percent, the 24th-highest in the world; the birth rate was 34.8 births per 1,000 population, the net migration rate 0.0 migrants per 1,000, and the total fertility rate 4.8 children per woman, the 23rd-highest in the world.

Formerly a Spanish colony, Equatorial Guinea became independent in 1968. Although the country has large oil reserves, human development has been hampered since 1979 by the dictatorship of President Teodoro Obiang. According to the Ibrahim Index, in 2011, Equatorial Guinea ranked 44th among 53 African countries in terms of governance performance, with a score of 37 (out of 100). Equatorial Guinea's government is ranked among the most corrupt in the world (172nd among 183 countries) with a score of 1.9 on the *Corruption Perceptions Index 2011*(on a scale where 0 indicates highly corrupt and 10 very clean). In 2011, Equatorial Guinea was classified as a country with medium human development (the second from the lowest of four categories) on the United Nations Development Programme's (UNDP's) Human Development Index (HDI), with a score of 0.537 (on a scale where 1 denotes high development and 0 low development). Life expectancy at birth in 2012 was estimated at 62.75 years, and per capita gross domestic product (GDP) in 2011 was estimated at $19,300. Unemployment in 2009 was estimated at 22.3 percent.

Emergency Health Services
No data available.

Insurance
Equatorial Guinea has a social insurance system covering the employed, pensioners, the disabled, and family members of the insured. Self-employed people are not included in the system. The system is funded by wage contributions (4.5 percent of gross earnings) and employer contributions (21.5 percent of gross payroll). Medical care is provided for up to 26 weeks, with a 25 percent copayment for care and 50 percent for medications; medicine during pregnancy, the postnatal period, and hospitalization is provided free. The cash benefit is 50 percent of wages for up to

26 weeks, and the maternity benefit is 75 percent of wages for six weeks before and after the due date. The program is administered by the Social Security Institute under the supervision of the Ministry of Labor and Social Security.

Costs of Hospitalization

Equatorial Guinea has limited facilities for hospital care, and payment in cash is usually required before services will be provided; in addition, patients may need to bring their own medical supplies.

Access to Health Care

According to the World Health Organization (WHO), in 2000 (the most recent data available), 65 percent of births in Equatorial Guinea were attended by skilled personnel (for example, physicians, nurses, or midwives). In 2001, 37 percent of pregnant women received at least four prenatal care visits. The 2010 immunization rates for 1-year-olds were 33 percent for diphtheria and pertussis (DPT3) and 51 percent for measles (MCV). In 2010, an estimated 24 percent of persons with advanced human immunodeficiency virus (HIV) infection were receiving antiretroviral therapy in accordance with the 2010 WHO guidelines.

Cost of Drugs

No data available.

Health Care Facilities

In 2009, Equatorial Guinea had 1.92 hospital beds per 1,000 population.

Major Health Issues

In 2008, WHO estimated that 74 percent of years of life lost in Equatorial Guinea were due to communicable diseases, 18 percent to noncommunicable diseases, and 8 percent to injuries. In 2008, the age-standardized estimate of cancer deaths was 85 per 100,000 for men and 81 per 100,000 for women; for cardiovascular disease and diabetes, 476 per 100,000 for men and 492 per 100,000 for women; and for chronic respiratory disease, 132 per 100,000 for men and 77 per 100,000 for women. Malaria, yellow fever, and cholera remain serious problems in Equatorial Guinea; in 2008, the age-standardized death rate from malaria was 55.6 per 100,000 population. In 2010, tuberculosis incidence was 135.0 per 100,000 population, tuberculosis prevalence 121.0 per 100,000, and deaths due to tuberculosis among HIV-negative

people 5.50 per 100,000. As of 2009, an estimated 5.0 percent of adults age 15 to 49 were living with HIV or acquired immune deficiency syndrome (AIDS).

Death from vaccine-preventable childhood diseases is also common by world standards: In 2008, the age-standardized death rate from childhood-cluster diseases (pertussis, polio, diphtheria, measles, and tetanus) was 45.1 per 100,000 population, the second-highest in the world. Equatorial Guinea's maternal mortality rate (death from any cause related to or aggravated by pregnancy) was estimated in 2008 as 280 maternal deaths per 100,000 live births. The infant mortality rate, defined as the number of deaths of infants younger than 1 year, was also high, at 75.18 per 1,000 live births as if 2012. In 2004, 10.6 percent of children under age 5 were underweight (defined as 2 kilograms [kg] below standard weight-for-age at age 1, 3 kg below for ages 2 to 3, and 4 kg below for ages 4 to 5).

Health Care Personnel

In 2006, WHO identified Equatorial Guinea as one of 57 countries with a critical deficit in the supply of skilled health workers. In 2004, Equatorial Guinea had 0.30 physicians per 1,000 population, 0.24 pharmaceutical personnel per 1,000, 0.17 laboratory health workers per 1,000, 0.15 health management and support workers per 1,000, 0.65 dentistry personnel per 1,000, 2.51 community and traditional health workers per 1,000, and 0.53 nurses and midwives per 1,000. The global "brain drain" (international migration of skilled personnel) plays a role in the relative under-supply of medical personnel in Equatorial Guinea: Michael Clemens and Bunilla Petterson estimate that 63 percent of Equatorial Guinea-born physicians and 38 percent of Equatorial Guinea-born nurses are working in one of nine developed countries, primarily in Spain.

Government Role in Health Care

According to WHO, in 2010, Equatorial Guinea spent $628 million on health care, an amount that comes to $896 per capita. Almost all health care funding (98 percent) was provided from domestic sources, with the remaining 2 percent provided by funds from abroad. More than three-quarters (76 percent) of spending on health care was provided by government expenditures, with 22 percent provided by household spending and 2 percent from other sources. In 2010, Equatorial Guinea allocated 7 percent of its total government expenditures to health, and government expenditures on health came to 3 percent of GDP; both figures place Equatorial Guinea in the median range when compared with other high-income African countries. In 2009, according to WHO, official development assistance (ODA) for health in Equatorial Guinea came to $17.71 per capita.

Public Health Programs

According to WHO, in 2004, Equatorial Guinea had 0.04 environmental and public health workers per 1,000 population. In 2010, 89 percent of the population of Equatorial Guinea had access to improved sanitation facilities (87 percent in rural areas and 92 percent in urban), and 51 percent had access to improved sources of drinking water (42 percent in rural areas and 66 percent in urban). According to the World Higher Education Database (WHED), no university in Equatorial Guinea offers programs in epidemiology or public health.

ERITREA

Eritrea is a country in northeastern Africa, sharing borders with Ethiopia, Sudan, and Djibouti and having a coastline (1,388 miles or 2,234 kilometers) on the Red

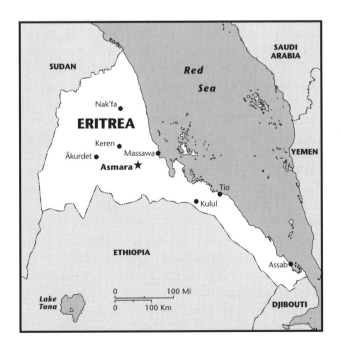

Sea. The area of 45,406 square miles (117,600 square kilometers) makes Eritrea slightly larger than Pennsylvania, and the July 2012 population was estimated at 6.1 million. In 2010, 22 percent of the population lived in urban areas, and the 2010 to 2015 annual rate of urbanization was estimated at 5.2 percent. Asmara is the capital and largest city (with a 2009 population estimated at 649,000). The population growth rate in 2012 was 2.4 percent (the 32nd-highest in the world), the birth rate 32.1 births per 1,000 population (the 36th highest in the world), the net migration rate 0.0 migrants per 1,000, and the total fertility rate 4.4 children per woman (the 32nd-highest in the world). The United Nations High Commissioner for Refugees (UNHCR) estimated that, in 2010, there were 4,809 refugees and persons in refugee-like situations in Eritrea.

After World War II, Eritrea was part of the African region ruled by Great Britain and was federated with Ethiopia in 1950. In 1961, an Eritrean independence movement started a 30-year struggle; in 1993, Eritrea became independent, although boundary disputes between the two countries continued.

According to the Ibrahim Index, in 2011, Eritrea ranked near the bottom (47th out of 53) among African countries in terms of governance performance, with a score of 35 (out of 100). Eritrea ranked tied for 134th among 183 countries in terms of perceived public-sector corruption with a score of 2.5 on the *Corruption Perceptions Index 2011* (on a scale where 0 indicates highly corrupt and 10 very clean).

In 2011, Eritrea was classified as a country with low human development (the lowest of four categories) on the United Nations Development Programme's (UNDP's) Human Development Index (HDI), with a score of 0.349 (on a scale where 1 denotes high development and 0 low development). In 2011, the International Food Policy Research Institute (IFPRI) classified Eritrea as a country with an "extremely alarming" hunger problem, with a Global Hunger Index (GHI) score of 33.9, the third-highest in the world. Life expectancy at birth in 2012 was estimated at 62.46 years, and estimated gross domestic product (GDP) per capita in 2011 was $700, among the 10 lowest in the world.

Emergency Health Services

According to the World Health Organization (WHO), as of 2007, Eritrea did not have a formal and publicly available system for providing prehospital care (emergency care).

Insurance

Eritrea does not have a national health program or national insurance system, but some services are provided for free to those who cannot afford them.

Costs of Hospitalization

No data available.

Access to Health Care

According to WHO, in 2002, 28 percent of births were attended by skilled personnel (for example, physicians, nurses, or midwives). In 2005, 45 percent of pregnant women received at least four prenatal care visits. The 2010 immunization rates for 1-year-olds were 99 percent for diphtheria and pertussis (DPT3), 99 percent for measles (MCV), and 9 percent for Hib (Hib3). In 2010, an estimated 42 percent of persons with advanced human immunodeficiency virus (HIV) infection were receiving antiretroviral therapy in accordance with the 2010 WHO guidelines. According to WHO, in 2010, Eritrea had 0.20 magnetic resonance imaging (MRI) machines per 1 million population and 0.41 computer tomography (CT) machines per 1 million.

Cost of Drugs

Eritrea's National Medicines Policy (NMP) includes the selection of essential medicines, pricing and financing of medicines, and procurement, distribution, and regulation of medicines. The promotion and advertising of prescription medications is controlled by law, and direct marketing to the public is prohibited. Medications are provided free of charge to pregnant women and to the poor, and medications on the Essential Medicines List (EML) are also provided free, including drugs to treat malaria, tuberculosis, sexually transmitted diseases (STDs), and human immunodeficiency virus and acquired immune deficiency syndrome (HIV/AIDS); the vaccines on the Expanded Programme on Immunization (EPI) list, provided by WHO, are also provided for free. Medicine prices are regulated by the Ministry of Health, and retail prices are monitored. Almost all (99 percent) medications prescribed in public clinics are on the national EML, and generic substitution is allowed in both public- and private-sector dispensing facilities.

Health Care Facilities

As of 2010, according to WHO, Eritrea had 3.52 health posts per 100,000 population, 1.07 health centers per 100,000, 0.30 district or rural hospitals per 100,000, 0.11 provincial hospitals per 100,000, and 0.02 specialized hospitals per 100,000. In 2006, Eritrea had 1.15 hospital beds per 1,000 population.

Major Health Issues

In 2008, WHO estimated that 64 percent of years of life lost in Eritrea were due to communicable diseases, 23 percent to noncommunicable diseases, and 14 percent to injuries. In 2008, the age-standardized estimate of cancer deaths was 92 per 100,000 for men and 80 per 100,000 for women; for cardiovascular disease and diabetes, 403 per 100,000 for men and 363 per 100,000 for women; and for chronic respiratory disease, 110 per 100,000 for men and 52 per 100,000 for women.

Eritrea's maternal mortality rate (death from any cause related to or aggravated by pregnancy) was estimated in 2008 as 280 maternal deaths per 100,000 live births. A 2002 survey estimated the prevalence of female genital mutilation at 88.7 percent. A 1997 survey found that about 90 percent of women had undergone genital mutilation. The infant mortality rate, defined as the number of deaths of infants younger than 1 year, was estimated at 40.34 per 1,000 live births as of 2012. Child malnutrition is a serious problem: In 2002, 34.5 percent of children under age 5 were underweight (defined as 2 kilograms [kg] below standard weight-for-age at age 1, 3 kg below for ages 2 to 3, and 4 kg below for ages 4 to 5), one of the 20 highest rates in the world.

In 2010, tuberculosis incidence was 100.0 per 100,000 population, tuberculosis prevalence 128.0 per 100,000, and deaths due to tuberculosis among HIV-negative people 12.00 per 100,000. As of 2009, an estimated 0.8 percent of adults age 15 to 49 were living with HIV or AIDS. In 2008, the age-standardized death rate from malaria was 0.5 per 100,000 population.

Health Care Personnel

In 2006, WHO identified Eritrea as one of 57 countries with a critical deficit in the supply of skilled health workers. In 2004, Eritrea had 0.05 physicians per 1,000 personnel, 0.02 pharmaceutical personnel per 1,000, 0.06 laboratory health workers per 1,000, 0.18 health management and support workers per 1,000, and 0.58 nurses and midwives per 1,000. The global "brain drain" (international migration of skilled personnel) plays a role in the relative undersupply of medical personnel in Eritrea: Michael Clemens and Bunilla Petterson estimate that 36 percent of Eritrea-born physicians and 38 percent of Eritrea-born nurses are working in one of nine developed countries, primarily in the United States

Government Role in Health Care

The right to health, including access to essential medicines and medical technology, is recognized by national legislation. Eritrea has a National Health Policy (NHP) and a National Medicines Policy (NMP), both created by the Ministry of Health. The NMP covers selection of essential medicines; financing, pricing, purchase, distribution, and regulation of drugs; pharmacovigilance; rational usage of medicines; human resource development; research; and traditional medicine. According to WHO, in 2010, Eritrea spent $63 million on health care, an amount that comes to $12 per capita. About two-thirds (62 percent) of health care funding was provided from domestic sources, with the remaining 38 percent provided by funds from abroad. Spending on health care was almost evenly split between government expenditures (48 percent) and spending by households (52 percent). In 2010, Eritrea allocated 4 percent of its total government expenditures to health, and government expenditures on health came to 1 percent of gross domestic product (GDP); both figures place Eritrea in the low range when compared with other low-income African countries. In 2009, according to WHO, official development assistance (ODA) for health in Eritrea came to $5.65 per capita.

Public Health Programs

According to WHO, in 2002, Eritrea had 0.02 environmental and public health workers per 1,000 population. In 2005, 13 percent of the population of Eritrea had access to improved sanitation facilities (4 percent in rural areas and 52 percent in urban), and 60 percent had access to improved sources of drinking water (57 percent in rural areas and 74 percent in urban). According to the World Higher Education Database (WHED), no university in Eritrea offers programs in epidemiology or public health.

ESTONIA

Estonia is a northern European country, sharing borders with Latvia and Russia and having a coastline on the Baltic Sea; the country includes a mainland portion, two large islands, and many smaller islands. The

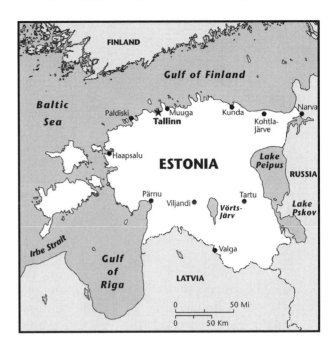

area of 17,463 square miles (45,228 square kilometers) is comparable to that of New Hampshire and Vermont combined, and the July 2012 population was estimated at 1.3 million. In 2010, 69 percent of the population lived in urban areas, and the 2010 to 2015 annual rate of urbanization was estimated at 0.1 percent. Tallinn is the capital and largest city (with a 2009 population estimated at 399,000). The net migration rate is among the lowest in Europe (negative 3.3 migrants per 1,000 population), and the July 2012 population growth rate is negative (negative 0.65 percent, among the 10 lowest in the world).

Estonia became independent in 1918 but was forced to become part of the Soviet Union in 1940; it became independent once again in 1991. The government has a reputation for transparency and honesty, ranking 29th among 183 countries in terms of perceived public-sector corruption on the *Corruption Perceptions Index 2011,* with a score of 6.4 (on a scale where 0 indicates highly corrupt and 10 very clean). In 2011, Estonia was classified as a country with very high human development (the highest of four categories) on the United Nations Development Programme's (UNDP's) Human Development Index (HDI), with a score of 0.835 (on a scale where 1 denotes high development and 0 low development). Life expectancy at birth in 2012 was estimated at 73.58 years, and per capita gross domestic product (GDP) in 2011 was estimated at $20,200. In 2010, the Gini Index (a measure of dispersion, in which perfect equality is denoted by 0 and maximum inequality is denoted by 100) for family income was 31.3. According to the World Economic Forum's *Global Gender Gap Index 2011*, Estonia ranked 52nd out of 135 countries on gender equality with a score of 0.698 (on a scale with a theoretical range of 1 for equality to 0 for inequality and an actual range in 2011 from 0.8530 to 0.4873).

Emergency Health Services

Estonia's laws governing the emergency health system date from the 1990s, as does Estonian recognition of emergency medicine as a medical specialty; by law, free access to hospitals for emergency care is provided for all persons, including the uninsured. Funding for the emergency system is provided entirely from public funds. Estonia has two national telephone numbers for medical emergencies, 112 (the European Union, or EU, standard) and 150, and one dispatch center.

Insurance

Estonia has a social insurance system paid for by a social tax. Insured people include those working on an employment contract; public servants; managers and supervisors; military conscripts; those receiving unemployement benefits, state pensions, or child care or social allowances; nonworking spouses of public servants and diplomats; those caring for disabled people; those who worked in nuclear waste elimination; people younger than 19; and students. The system is funded by employer contributions (13 percent of payroll) and contributions from self-employed people (13 percent of declared earnings); those outside the covered categories who join the system voluntarily pay a flat fee of EEK 1,679.

Medical benefits are provided through national and local health care institutions. Cost sharing is required for some medications, according to a set schedule, with lower rates for children and those receiving pensions and for some types of care. Dental care is free for children age 18 and younger. The maternity benefit is 100 percent of the reference wage (the insured's average gross daily wage for the previous year) for up to 140 days; an adoption allowance is paid for up to 70 days. The cash sickness benefit is paid by the employer for the fourth to eighth day of illness; after that, the Health Insurance Fund pays the benefit as a percentage of the reference wage (for example, 80 percent for hospitalization or 100 percent for a work injury). Wage compensation is also provided if the individual must change jobs due to incapacity. According to Ke Xu and colleagues, in 2003, 0.3 percent of households in Estonia experienced catastrophic health expenditures annually; "catastrophic" was defined as exceeding 40 percent of household income remaining after basic needs were met.

Costs of Hospitalization

In 2008, according to the Organisation for Economic Co-operation and Development (OECD), hospital spending represented 46.5 percent of total spending on health, and $563 per capita; hospitals were paid through case-based payments. As of 2002, there was an overall cap on inpatient services.

Access to Health Care

Household surveys have determined that, in a two-week recall period, more than one-third (38 percent) of adults in Estonia reported that they did not take one or more medicines prescribed due to cost. For adults from poor households, more than half (52 percent) reported not taking all prescribed medications due to cost. A similar pattern prevailed for adults with chronic conditions; overall, 74 percent of adults with chronic conditions took all prescribed medicines as opposed to 68 percent of adults from poor households. Compliance was higher for people with acute conditions: Only 4.2 percent reported not taking all prescribed medicines. According to the World Health Organization (WHO), in 2010, Estonia had 8.20 magnetic resonance imaging (MRI) machines per 1 million population, 14.91 computer tomography (CT) machines per 1 million, and 0.75 positron emission tomography (PET) machines per 1 million. According to WHO, in 2006, 10 percent of births were attended by skilled personnel (for example, physicians, nurses, or midwives). The 2010 immunization rates for 1-year-olds were 94 percent for diphtheria and pertussis (DPT3), 95 percent for measles (MCV), and 94 percent for Hib (Hib3).

Cost of Drugs

In 2005, total pharmaceutical expenditure in Estonia came to EEK 2,345 million ($199.9 million), or EEK 1,750 ($149.18) per capita. Pharmaceutical expenditures accounted for 16 percent of total health expenditures and 1 percent of GDP. Estonia is a member of the World Trade Organization (WTO) and honors patents but also has national legislation that implements the Trade-Related Aspects of Intellectual Property Rights (TRIPS) agreement, including compulsory

Selected Health Indicators: Estonia Compared With the Organisation for Economic Co-operation and Development (OECD) Country Average

	Estonia	OECD average (2010 or nearest year)
Male life expectancy at birth, 2010	70.6	77
Female life expectancy at birth, 2010	80.5	82.5
Infant mortality (deaths per 1,000 live births), 2010	3.3	4.3
Potential years of life lost, all causes, female population (per 100,000, aged 0–69 years), 2010	2,879	2,457
Potential years of life lost, all causes, male population (per 100,000, aged 0–69 years), 2010	8,720	4,798
Alcohol consumption (liters per capita [age 15+]), 2010	11.4	9.4
Tobacco consumption (percent of population 15+ who are daily smokers), 2010	26.2	21.1
Hospital beds (per 1,000 population), 2010	5.3	4.9

Source: OECD Health Data 2012 (Organisation for Economic Co-operation and Development, 2012).

licensing in the service of public health, Bolar exceptions (allowing procedures so a generic equivalent can be approved before the patent on the drug expires), and parallel importing of pharmaceuticals.

Pharmaceutical products must be registered in Estonia before they can be sold, although there are exceptions and waivers as well; in 2007, 3,112 pharmaceutical products were registered in Estonia. Advertising and promotion of prescription medicine is controlled by the State Agency of Medicines, and direct advertising to the public is prohibited. No population groups are entitled to free drugs, but drugs for certain conditions are provided for free under the public health system or social insurance schemes; diseases covered include tuberculosis, and human immunodeficiency virus and acquired immune deficiency syndrome (HIV/AIDS), as are vaccines listed on the Expanded Programme on Immunization (EPI) list, published by WHO.

Partial coverage for prescription drugs is provided through most insurance on an outpatient basis, with drugs provided in the hospital covered 100 percent. The national Essential Medicines List (EML) includes 444 medicines; drugs on this list prescribed on an outpatient basis are reimbursed at a 50 percent rate by most insurance schemes. Drugs for serious epidemic diseases are reimbursed at 100 percent, and drugs for chronic diseases at 75 percent or 90 percent. No recent surveys on medication prices have been conducted in Estonia, but the median wholesale markup for a basket of key medicines is 9 percent, and the median pharmacist markup is 18 percent. Prescription by International Nonproprietary Names (generics) is mandatory.

Health Care Facilities

As of 2010, according to WHO, Estonia had 36.16 health posts per 100,000 population, 1.34 district or rural hospitals per 100,000, 0.30 provincial hospitals per 100,000, and 0.22 specialized hospitals per 100,000. In 2008, Estonia had 5.71 hospital beds per 1,000 population, among the 30 highest ratios in the world, reflecting the influence of the Soviet method of organizing health care.

Major Health Issues

In 2008, WHO estimated that 4 percent of years of life lost in Estonia were due to communicable diseases, 77 percent to noncommunicable diseases, and 19 percent to injuries. In 2008, the age-standardized estimate of cancer deaths was 220 per 100,000 for men and 103 per 100,000 for women; for cardiovascular disease and diabetes, 469 per 100,000 for men and 233 per 100,000 for women; and for chronic respiratory disease, 28 per 100,000 for men and six per 100,000 for women.

The maternal mortality rate (death from any cause related to or aggravated by pregnancy) in Estonia in 2008 was 12 maternal deaths per 100,000 live births. The infant mortality rate, defined as the number of deaths of infants younger than 1 year, was 6.94 per 1,000 live births as of 2012. In 2010, tuberculosis incidence was 25.0 per 100,000 population, tuberculosis prevalence 26.0 per 100,000, and deaths due to tuberculosis among HIV-negative people 2.90 per 100,000. An estimated 18 percent of new tuberculosis cases, and 44 percent of retreatment cases, are multidrug resistant. As of 2009, an estimated 1.2 percent of adults age 15 to 49 were living with HIV or AIDS.

Health Care Personnel

Estonia has one medical school, the Tartu Ülikool Arstiteaduskond in Tartu. The basic course for the medical degree requires six years of training. Estonia, as a member of the EU, cooperates with other countries in recognizing physicians qualified to practice in other EU countries, as specified by Directive 2005/36/EC of the European Parliament. This allows qualified professionals to practice their profession in other EU states on a temporary basis and requires that the host country automatically recognize qualifications for certain professions, including physicians, nurses, dentists, midwives, and pharmacists, if certain conditions have been met (for instance, facility in the language of the host country may be required). In 2008, Estonia had 3.41 physicians per 1,000 population, 0.66 pharmaceutical personnel per 1,000, 0.94 dentistry personnel per 1,000, and 6.82 nurses and midwives per 1,000.

Government Role in Health Care

The right to health, including access to essential medicines and medical technologies, is recognized in Estonian national legislation. Estonia has a National Health Policy (NHP), updated in 2009, and a National Health Policy Implementation Plan, written in 2011. Estonia also has a National Medicines Policy (NMP), written in 2002, that covers selection of essential medicines; financing, pricing, purchase, distribution, and regulation of drugs; pharmacovigilance; and rational usage of medicines; however, pharmaceutical policy implementation is not regularly monitored.

According to WHO, in 2010, Estonia spent $1.1 billion on health care, an amount that comes to $853 per capita. About two-thirds (61 percent) of health care funding was provided by sources from abroad, with the remaining 39 percent provided by domestic funding. Government expenditures provided most (79 percent) of spending on health care, with 20 percent provided by household spending and 2 percent by other sources. In 2010, Estonia allocated 12 percent of its total government expenditures to health, and government expenditures on health came to 5 percent of GDP; both figures place Estonia in the low range when compared with other high-income European countries.

Public Health Programs

Estonia's National Institute for Health and Development (NIHD), located in Tallinn, was established in 2003 to raise the quality of life and promote the health of the Estonia population through research and knowledge-based development. Among the ongoing programs of the NIHD are the National Children's Rights Strategy, the National Tuberculosis Prevention Programme (2004 to 2007), the National Strategy for the Prevention of Cardiovascular Diseases (2005 to 2020), the National Strategy on Prevention for Drug Abuse (2005 to 2012), the National HIV/AIDS Prevention Strategy (2006 to 2015), and the National Cancer Prevention Strategy (2007 to 2015). The NIHD also works on projects involving capacity building and health promotion and projects funded by WHO, the Global Fund, and EU.

According to WHO, in 2000, Estonia had 0.08 environmental and public health workers per 1,000 population. In 2010, 95 percent of the population of Estonia had access to improved sanitation facilities (94 percent in rural areas and 96 percent in urban), and 88 percent had access to improved sources of drinking water (97 percent in rural areas and 99 percent in urban). According to the World Higher Education Database (WHED), no university in Estonia offers programs in epidemiology or public health.

ETHIOPIA

Ethiopia is a landlocked country in east Africa, sharing borders with Somalia, Kenya, Sudan, and Eritrea. The area is 426,373 square miles (1,104,300 square kilometers), making Ethiopia the 27th-largest country in the world and about twice the size of Texas; the July 2012 population was 93.8 million (the 13th-largest in the world). In 2010, 17 percent of the population lived in urban areas, and the 2010 to 2015 annual rate of urbanization was estimated at 3.8 percent. Addis Ababa is the capital and largest city (with a 2009 population estimated at 2.9 million). As of July 2012, Ethiopia had the fifth-highest population growth rate in the world, at 3.18 percent, the sixth-highest birth rate in the world, at 42.59 per 1,000 population, and the seventh-highest total fertility rate, at 5.97 children per woman. The United Nations High Commissioner for Refugees (UNHCR) estimates that, in 2010, there were 154,295 refugees and persons in refugee-like situations in Ethiopia.

Ethiopia is the only African country to have largely avoided becoming a colony for most of its history (with the exception of occupation by Italy in the years 1936 to 1941). Emperor Haile Selassie ruled the country from 1930 to 1974, when he was deposed in a coup. The country suffered repeated coups and rebellions over the next 20 years; this, plus repeated periods of drought, created a massive number of refugees. Eritrea separated from Ethiopia 1993, although the two countries continued to dispute their boundaries. According to the Ibrahim Index, in 2011, Ethiopia ranked 34th among 53 African countries in terms of governance performance, with a score of 46 (out of 100). Ethiopia ranked tied for 120th among 183 countries on the *Corruption Perceptions Index 2011,* with a score of 2.7 (on a scale where 0 indicates highly corrupt and 10 very clean).

In 2011, Ethiopia was classified as a country with low human development (the lowest of four categories) on the United Nations Development Programme's (UNDP's) Human Development Index (HDI), with a score of 0.363 (on a scale where 1 denotes high development and 0 low development). In 2011, the International Food Policy Research Institute (IFPRI) classified Ethiopia as a country with an "alarming" hunger problem, with a Global Hunger Index (GHI) score of 28.7, the fifth-highest in the world. Life expectancy at birth in 2012 was estimated at 56.56 years, among the 30 lowest in the world, and estimated gross domestic product (GDP) per capita in 2011 was $1,100, among the 20 lowest in the world. In 2000, the Gini Index (a measure of dispersion, in which perfect equality is denoted by 0 and maximum inequality is denoted by 100) for family income was 30.0. According to the

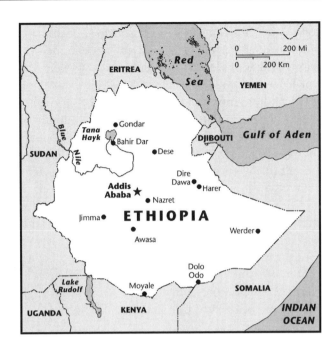

World Economic Forum's *Global Gender Gap Index 2011,* Ethiopia ranked 116th out of 135 countries on gender equality with a score of 0.614 (on a scale with a theoretical range of 1 for equality to 0 for inequality and an actual range in 2011 from 0.8530 to 0.4873).

Emergency Health Services

According to the World Health Organization (WHO), as of 2007, Ethiopia did not have a formal and publicly available system for providing prehospital care (emergency care). Some infrastructure for providing emergency medicine has developed in the past 10 years, thanks largely to the work of Dr. Tesafaye Mekonnen Bayleygne at Black Lion Hospital in Addis Ababa. Black Lion Hospital now has a residency program in emergency medicine, and Addis Ababa has a first responder service organized through the Fire and Emergency Services system. Various international efforts have also provided training and equipment for emergency medicine, but many challenges remain in developing a comprehensive system.

Doctors Without Borders (Médecins Sans Frontières, or MSF) began working in Ethiopia in 1984 and had 1,049 staff members in the country at the close of 2010. MSF currently has projects in the Somali Regional State (eastern Ethiopia), Amhara (north), Gambela (west), and Oromia (south central). In the Somali region, an insecure area prone to violent confrontations, MSF provides health services through hospitals, clinics, and mobile medical teams and provides care in refugee camps near the border with Ethiopia. In Oramia, MSF's focus is on child malnutrition, and the organization also provides food rations to women who are pregnant or breast-feeding. In the Amhara region, MSF focuses on treating *kala azar* (visceral leishmaniasis), human immunodeficiency virus and acquired immune deficiency syndrome (HIV/AIDS), and malnutrition; in addition, an MSF project treating malnutrition in the wake of an emergency food situation in Telemt was transferred in 2010 to the Ethiopian Ministry of Health. In the Gambela region, MSF runs a health center, treating many refugees of the violence in southern Sudan and providing health care through mobile medical teams to isolated populations.

Insurance

Ethiopia provides no statutory benefits for medical care. Employers are required to pay sick leave for at least three months (100 percent of earnings for the first month and 50 percent for the second and third) and maternity leave for up to 45 days after giving birth.

Costs of Hospitalization

No data available.

Access to Health Care

According to the U.S. Department of State, medical facilities in Addis Ababa are limited, and access to modern health care anywhere else in the country is even harder to obtain, with chronic shortages of equipment and drugs. According to WHO, in 2005, 6 percent of births were attended by skilled personnel (for example, physicians, nurses, or midwives), one of the lowest percentages in the world. In 2005, 12 percent of pregnant women received at least four prenatal care visits. The 2010 immunization rates for 1-year-olds were 86 percent for diphtheria and pertussis (DPT3), 81 percent for measles (MCV), and 86 percent for Hib (Hib3).

Cost of Drugs

In 2006, total pharmaceutical expenditures in Ethiopia came to 2.44 billion birr ($289.70) and per capita pharmaceutical expenditures 29.35 birr ($3.49). Pharmaceutical expenditures were almost one-third (32.9 percent) of total health expenditures, and 1.0 percent of gross domestic product (GDP). Most pharmaceutical expenditures were paid for privately, with public expenditures constituting only 9.5 percent of the total. Patients in public health facilities were prescribed a mean of 2.0 drugs, almost all (98.3) on the national Essential Medicines List (EML).

Drugs in Ethiopia are distributed by the public sector, the private sector, city councils, and the Ethiopian Red Cross. There is no price regulation on drugs and no ceiling on markups; a wholesale markup of 20 to 40 percent is common on imported drugs and 5 to 10 percent on those manufactured in the country. Public health service pharmacies charge a 25 percent markup, and municipal pharmacies charge 20 percent. Generic substitution is allowed in both public- and private-sector dispensing facilities. Some drugs are provided free to those who cannot afford them, and for certain illnesses, including malaria, tuberculosis, and HIV/AIDS; vaccines included on WHO's Expanded Programme on Immunization (EPI) list are also free.

A 2006 survey found that the price of drugs constituted a barrier to access for many in Ethiopia, particularly those needing medicines to treat chronic conditions. In the public sector, generic drugs were procured for 31 percent less than the international reference prices, but for the most common generics, the price was several times higher; for instance, Ethiopia paid more than twice the international market price for penicillin and metronidazole and more than 40 times the international reference price for hydrochlorothiazide. The median price for the lowest-priced generic drugs was 1.35 of the international reference price (that is, on average, these drugs were sold for 35 percent more than the international reference price); the median availability of the lowest-priced generic at public facilities was 59.6 percent.

Innovator brands are not used in the public sector, and only a limited number of innovator brands are found in the private sector (eight of 26 medicines surveyed, in this case). In the private sector, the median price for the lowest-priced generics was 2.25 of the international reference price, and the median for innovator brands was 11.55 of the international reference price. The median availability of the lowest-priced generics was 96 percent, while the median availability of innovator brands was very low. In special pharmacies and Ethiopian Red Cross outlets, availability of the lowest-priced generics was 78.6 percent, and the median price was 1.70 of the international reference prices.

Health Care Facilities

As of 2010, according to WHO, Ethiopia had 17.18 health posts per 100,000 population, less than 0.01 health centers per 100,000, 0.22 district or rural hospitals per 100,000, and 0.03 specialized hospitals per 100,000. In 2008, Ethiopia had 0.18 hospital beds per 1,000 population, one of the 10 lowest rates in the world. According to WHO, in 2010, Ethiopia had 0.04 magnetic resonance imaging (MRI) machines per 1 million population, 0.26 computer tomography (CT) machines per 1 million, 0.02 telecolbalt units per 1 million, and 0.02 radiotherapy machines per 1 million.

Major Health Issues

In 2008, WHO estimated that 70 percent of years of life lost in Ethiopia were due to communicable diseases, 20 percent to noncommunicable diseases, and 9 percent to injuries. In 2008, the age-standardized estimate of cancer deaths was 97 per 100,000 for men and 87 per 100,000 for women; for cardiovascular disease and diabetes, 486 per 100,000 for men and 530 per 100,000 for women; and for chronic respiratory disease, 135 per 100,000 for men and 85 per 100,000 for women. In 2008, the age-standardized death rate from malaria was 7.2 per 100,000 population.

Ethiopia's maternal mortality rate (death from any cause related to or aggravated by pregnancy) was high by global standards, estimated at 470 maternal deaths per 100,000 live births as of 2008. A 2005 survey estimated the prevalence of female genital mutilation at 74.3 percent. The infant mortality rate, defined as the number of deaths of infants younger than 1 year, also has been high, at 75.29 per 1,000 live births as of 2012. Child malnutrition is a serious problem: In 2005, 34.6 percent of children under age 5 were underweight (defined as 2 kilograms [kg] below standard weight-for-age at age 1, 3 kg below for ages 2 to 3, and 4 kg below for ages 4 to 5), one of the highest rates in the world.

In 2010, tuberculosis incidence was 261.0 per 100,000 population, tuberculosis prevalence 394.0 per 100,000, and deaths due to tuberculosis among human immunodeficiency virus (HIV)-negative people 35.00 per 100,000. An estimated 1.6 percent of new tuberculosis cases, and 12 percent of retreatment cases, are multidrug resistant. WHO estimated that the case detection rate in 2010 was 72 percent. In 2010, 26 percent of pregnant women tested positive for HIV. In 2010, almost 1.2 million cases of malaria were reported.

Health Care Personnel

In 2006, WHO identified Ethiopia as one of 57 countries with a critical deficit in the supply of skilled health workers. Ethiopia has four medical schools, located in Addis Ababa, Gondar, Jimma, and Awassa. The basic training course for a medical degree requires six years of study, with an additional year of supervised clinical practice also required. The degree awarded is doctor of medicine. Work in government service after graduation is obligatory. Physicians must register with the Ministry of Health. In 2007, Ethiopia had 0.02 physicians per 1,000, 0.02 pharmaceutical personnel per 1,000, 0.02 laboratory health workers per 1,000, 0.30 community and traditional health workers per 1,000, and 0.24 nurses and midwives per 1,000. The global "brain drain" (international migration of skilled personnel) plays a role in the relative undersupply of medical personnel in Ethiopia: Michael Clemens and Bunilla Petterson estimate that 30 percent of Ethiopia-born physicians and 17 percent of Ethiopia-born nurses are working in one of nine developed countries, primarily in the United States.

Government Role in Health Care

The right to health, including access to essential medications and technologies, is recognized in Ethiopian national health policy. Ethiopia has a National Health Policy (NHP), enacted in 1993; a National Health Policy Implementation Plan, enacted in 1995; and a National Medicines Policy (NMP), enacted in 2007. Ethiopia also has a national program to monitor medicine and promote its rational use and a national policy to combat antimicrobial resistance. Ethiopia's NMP includes the selection of essential medicines; financing, pricing, purchase, distribution, and regulation of drugs; rational usage of medicines; human resource development; research; and traditional medicine. Ethiopia applied for membership in the World Trade Organization (WTO) in 2003, but it had not been granted as of December 2011. Ethiopian laws allow for relaxation of licensing provisions in the interest of public health and parallel importing of drugs. Promotion and advertising of prescription drugs are regulated by the government, and direct marketing to the public is forbidden.

According to WHO, in 2010, Ethiopia spent $1.3 billion on health care, an amount that comes to $16 per capita. About two-thirds (61 percent) of health care funding was provided from domestic sources, with the remaining 39 percent provided by funds from abroad. The largest share (54 percent) of health care spending was provided by government expenditures, with 37 percent coming from spending by households and 9 percent by other sources. In 2010, Ethiopia allocated 13 percent of its total government expenditures to health, placing it in the high range among low-income African countries; government expenditures on health came to 3 percent of GDP, placing Ethiopia in the low range when compared with other low-income African countries. In 2009, according to WHO, official development assistance (ODA) for health in Ethiopia came to $10.39 per capita.

Public Health Programs

The Ethiopian Health & Nutrition Research Institute (EHNRI), located in Addis Ababa and headed by Amha Kebede, was founded in 1996 to facilitate the use of health research to inform national policy. Priorities of the EHNRI include controlling communicable diseases and diseases related to poor living conditions and malnutrition; conducting research on traditional medicine and integrating its practice into modern medicine; conducting applied health research on major health problems; and strengthening the nation's research capabilities, including the development of national public health lab services.

According to WHO, in 2007, Ethiopia had 0.01 environmental and public health workers per 1,000 population. In 2010, 21 percent of the population of Ethiopia had access to improved sanitation facilities (19 percent in rural areas and 29 percent in urban), and 44 percent had access to improved sources of drinking water (34 percent in rural areas and 97 percent in urban). According to the World Higher Education Database (WHED), five universities in Ethiopia offer programs in epidemiology or public health: Addis Ababa University, Haramaya University, Hawassa University, Jimma University, and the University of Gondar.

FIJI

Fiji is an island nation in the south Pacific Ocean, consisting of two main islands (Viti Levu and Vanua Levu) and numerous smaller islands. The area of 7,056 square miles (18,274 square kilometers) makes Fiji about the size of New Jersey, and the 2012 population

was estimated at 890,057. In 2010, 52 percent of the population lived in urban areas, and the 2010 to 2015 annual rate of urbanization was estimated at 1.3 percent. Suva is the capital. Fiji's net migration rate was negative 7.11 migrants per 1,000 population as of 2012; the July 2012 population growth rate was 0.8 percent, the birth rate was 20.7 births per 1,000 population, and the total fertility rate was 2.6 children per woman. Formerly a British colony, Fiji became independent in 1970. Democratic rule has been interrupted by several coups, in 1987, 2000, and 2006; political unrest, plus a constitution favoring the native Fijian population, has led to high emigration by Fiji's Indian citizens.

In 2011, Fiji was classified as a country with medium human development (the second from the lowest of four categories) on the United Nations Development Programme's (UNDP's) Human Development Index (HDI), with a score of 0.688 (on a scale where 1 denotes high development and 0 low development). Life expectancy at birth in 2012 was estimated at 71.59 years, and the estimated gross domestic product (GDP) per capita in 2011 was $4,600. According to the World Economic Forum's *Global Gender Gap Index 2011*, Fiji ranked 109th out of 135 countries on gender equality, with a score of 0.625 (on a scale with a theoretical range of 1 for equality to 0 for inequality and an actual range in 2011 from 0.8530 to 0.4873).

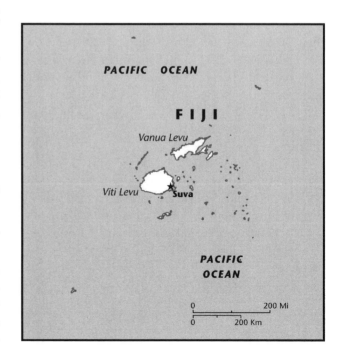

Emergency Health Services

According to the World Health Organization (WHO), as of 2007, Fiji had a formal and publicly available emergency care (prehospital care) system, accessible through a national universal access telephone number.

Insurance

Fiji's current health care system is based on the system in place during the British colonial period, in which health services were provided by the government. User fees have always been part of the system but fell from 10.5 percent of all health expenditures in 1970 to between 2.5 and 3.5 percent as of 2011.

Costs of Hospitalization

Hospital care is heavily subsidized by the government, although a user-pays system for those who could afford private rooms was instituted in 1978.

Access to Health Care

Fiji spends less of its GDP on health than any other Pacific Island nation, and health infrastructure remains limited; facilities include 24 hospitals and 74 clinics. According to WHO, in 2007, 98.5 percent of births were attended by skilled personnel (for example, physicians, nurses, or midwives). The 2010 immunization rates for 1-year-olds were 99 percent for diphtheria and pertussis (DPT3), 91 percent for measles (MCV), and 99 percent for Hib (Hib3). In 2010, an estimated 33 percent of persons with advanced human immunodeficiency virus (HIV) infection were receiving antiretroviral therapy in accordance with the 2010 WHO guidelines. According to WHO, in 2010, Fiji had fewer than 0.01 magnetic resonance imaging (MRI) machines per 1 million population and 3.55 computer tomography (CT) machines per 1 million.

Cost of Drugs

Fiji has a national Essential Medicines List (EML); in the public sector, prescriptions are generally written for generics, while in the private sector, both generic and brand-name drugs are prescribed. Pharmacists are required by law to dispense the prescribed drug but, in practice, may discuss alternative generics with the patients. Drugs are purchased for the public sector through international competitive tender from WHO-approved suppliers, but in the private sector, physicians and pharmacists may import any medicine (with the exception of restricted substances, including narcotics) meeting either the U.S. Pharmacopeia or British Pharmacopeia standards. Some pharmacists also purchase drugs in bulk from Fiji Pharmaceutical Services at a 20 percent markup.

A 2004 survey of private pharmacies found that generic drugs were more widely available than innovator brand drugs: Almost two-thirds (63.3 percent) of outlets had at least one generic version of the drugs surveyed, while about one-third (36.7 percent) had the innovator brand. The median price ratio for the lowest-price generic in relation to the international reference price was 2.73 (meaning that the drug sold for almost three times the international reference price); for the most popular generic, the median price ratio was 2.49 and, for the innovator brand, 9.21. Sometimes the differences were more extreme: For instance, for 500 milligrams of ciprofloxacin, the median price ratio for the lowest-priced generic was 4.06, while for the innovator brand, it was 79.01. Medicines in the private sector were generally affordable, at least to the employed: For instance, the lowest-paid government worker would have to work 48 minutes to earn enough to pay for a course of treatment with amoxicillin or atenolol and 1 hour and 36 minutes to pay for a course of treatment with amitriptyline, diclofenac, or ranitidine.

Health Care Facilities

Fiji has two national hospitals (St. Giles Hospital and Tamavua/Twomey Hospital), three divisional hospitals (Colonial War Memorial Hospital, Lautoka Hospital, and Labasa Hospital), and numerous health centers and nursing stations providing more basic services. In 2000, Fiji had 2.08 hospital beds per 1,000 population.

Major Health Issues

In 2008, WHO estimated that 23 percent of years of life lost in Fiji were due to communicable diseases, 67 percent to noncommunicable diseases, and 10 percent to injuries. In 2008, the age-standardized estimate of cancer deaths was 106 per 100,000 for men and 122 per 100,000 for women; for cardiovascular disease and diabetes, 580 per 100,000 for men and 328 per 100,000 for women; and for chronic respiratory disease, 91 per 100,000 for men and 44 per 100,000 for women.

In 2010, tuberculosis incidence was 27.0 per 100,000 population, tuberculosis prevalence 40.0 per 100,000, and deaths due to tuberculosis among HIV-negative people 3.60 per 100,000. As of 2009, an estimated 0.1

percent of adults age 15 to 49 were living with HIV or acquired immune deficiency syndrome (AIDS). In 2004, an estimated 23.9 percent of adults in Fiji were obese (defined as a body mass index, or BMI, of 30 or greater). Fiji's maternal mortality rate (death from any cause related to or aggravated by pregnancy) in 2008 was 26 maternal deaths per 100,000 live births. The infant mortality rate, defined as the number of deaths of infants younger than 1 year, was 10.73 per 1,000 live births as of 2012.

Health Care Personnel

Fiji has one medical school, the Fiji School of Medicine in Suva, which began offering instruction in 1885 as the Suva Medical School. The basic medical degree course requires six years of training, and completion of a one-year internship is required before a medical license is awarded. Government service is obligatory after graduation. Graduates of foreign medical schools must hold a contract with a government. In 2003, Fiji had 0.45 physicians per 1,000 population, 0.11 pharmaceutical personnel per 1,000, 0.07 dentistry personnel per 1,000, and 1.98 nurses and midwives per 1,000. Alok Bhargava and colleagues place Fiji 10th among countries most affected by the medical "brain drain" (international migration of skilled personnel) in 2004.

Government Role in Health Care

Fiji's health care system is based on the system in place when the country became independent from Great Britain, although it has been modified numerous times since 1970. Fiji's most recent National Health Policy (NHP) dates from 1994 and has been gradually implemented since then; it also has an Essential Medicines List (EML). According to WHO, in 2010, Fiji spent $133 million on health care, an amount that comes to $154 per capita. Most (91 percent) of health care funding was provided from domestic sources, with the remaining 9 percent provided by funds from abroad. More than two-thirds (70 percent) of health care spending was provided by government expenditures, with 20 percent coming from spending by households and 10 percent from other sources. In 2010, Fiji allocated 9 percent of its total government expenditures to health, and government expenditures on health came to 3 percent of GDP; both figures place Fiji in the low range when compared to other low-income western Pacific region countries. In 2009, according to WHO, official development assistance (ODA) for health in Fiji came to $6.56 per capita.

Public Health Programs

Fiji's Division of Public Health is responsible for providing primary care to the public as well as for developing public health policies and evaluating the effectiveness of programs in areas such as health promotion, food and nutrition, environmental health, control of communicable diseases, and noncommunicable diseases. According to WHO, in 2009, Fiji had 0.14 environmental and public health workers per 1,000 population. In 2010, 83 percent of the population had access to improved sanitation facilities (71 percent in rural areas and 94 percent in urban), and 98 percent had access to improved sources of drinking water (95 percent in rural areas and 10 percent in urban). According to the World Higher Education Database (WHED), one university in Fiji offers programs in epidemiology or public health: Fiji National University, located in Suva.

FINLAND

Finland is a northern European country, sharing borders with Norway, Sweden, and Russia and a coastline on the Baltic Sea. The area of 130,559 square miles (338,145 square kilometers) is similar to Montana, and the July 2012 population was estimated at 5.3 million. In 2010, 85 percent of the population lived in urban areas, and the 2010 to 2015 annual rate of urbanization was estimated at 0.6 percent. The capital and largest city is Helsinki. The July 2012 population growth rate was less than 0.1 percent; the net migration rate is 0.6 migrants per 1,000 population, the birth rate 10.4 per 1,000, and the total fertility rate 1.7 children per woman.

Formerly a duchy of Sweden, then Russia, Finland became independent in 1917. Finland's government has a reputation for transparency and honesty: Finland ranked tied for second among 183 countries on the *Corruption Perceptions Index 2011* with a score of 9.4 (on a scale where 0 indicates highly corrupt and 10 very clean). In 2011, Finland was classified as a country with very high human development (the highest of four categories) on the United Nations Development Programme's (UNDP's) Human Development Index (HDI), with a score of 0.882 (on a scale where 1 denotes high development and 0 low development). Life expectancy at birth in 2012 was estimated at 79.41 years, and per capita gross domestic product (GDP) in 2011 was

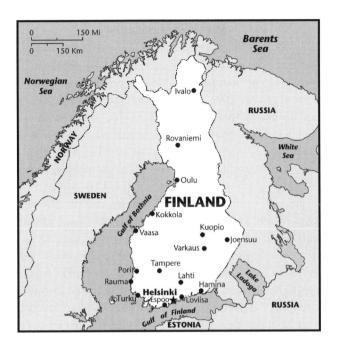

estimated at $38,300. Income distribution is among the most equal in the world: In 2008 the Gini Index (a measure of dispersion, in which perfect equality is denoted by 0 and maximum inequality is denoted by 100) for family income was 26.8. Finland has achieved a high level of gender equality: According to the World Economic Forum's *Global Gender Gap Index 2011*, Finland ranked third out of 135 countries on gender equality with a score of 0.838 (on a scale with a theoretical range of 1 for equality to 0 for inequality and an actual range in 2011 from 0.8530 to 0.4873).

Emergency Health Services

Finland's laws governing the emergency health system date from the 1990s; by law, free access to hospitals for emergency care is provided for all persons, including the uninsured. Funding for the emergency system is from multiple sources. Finland has only one national telephone number for medical emergencies, 112 (the European Union standard); the country has 15 dispatch centers that are interconnected.

Insurance

Finland has a social insurance system that includes both a public-sector health services program and a private-sector insurance program; everyone residing in Finland is covered by both the health services program and the maternity and sickness cash benefit program. Both systems are funded by contributions from wages

(1.7 percent of gross monthly earnings for the medical benefits, 0.93 percent for cash sickness and maternity benefits, and 1.64 percent for pensions and other benefits), contributions from the self-employed (1.47 percent of net monthly earnings for medical benefits and 0.95 or 1.05 percent of gross monthly earnings for cash sickness and maternity benefits), and employer payroll contributions (2.23 percent of monthly payroll for medical, cash sickness, and maternity benefits). The government provides subsidies as required for cash sickness and maternity benefits and covers 50 percent of the cost of medical benefits. Most services provided by municipal health services are free or carry low charges (for example, 13.70 euros for a physician's visit), and the medical benefit system provides cash refunds for certain medical expenses (for example, 75 percent for prescription medication once a limit is reached, and 60 percent of private physician fees). Prenatal and postnatal maternity care at medical centers is free.

The maternity benefit is a percentage of average earnings on a sliding scale (for example, 70 percent for the lowest incomes and 25 percent for the highest) for up to 105 days; a paternity allowance is also paid for up to 18 days, and a parent's allowance for 158 days (paid to either parent) after maternity benefits cease. The sickness benefit is a percentage of daily earnings, paid on a sliding scale (for example, 70 percent for the lowest incomes to 25 percent for the highest) for up to 300 days; for the first 9 days of sickness, the employer pays 100 percent of daily earnings. A special sickness benefit based on a percentage of earnings is paid for up to 60 days in the hospital and 60 days at home. The Social Insurance Institution administers the program, with general supervision from the Ministry of Social Affairs and Health.

A 2004 study by the World Health Organization (WHO) found that none of the Finnish population had substitutive voluntary health insurance (covering services that would otherwise be available from the state), while varying percentages had supplementary health insurance (providing increased choice or faster access to services), mainly young children: More than one-third (34.8 percent) of children under age 7 had supplementary voluntary health insurance, as compared to 25.7 percent of children ages 7 to 18 and 6.7 percent of adults. According to Ke Xu and colleagues, in 2003, 0.4 percent of households in Finland experienced catastrophic health expenditures annually; "catastrophic" was defined as exceeding 40 percent of household income remaining after basic needs were met.

Costs of Hospitalization

In 2008, according to the Organisation for Economic Co-operation and Development (OECD), hospital spending in Finland represented 35.3 percent of the country's total spending on health and $1,010 per capita; hospitals were paid per case and diagnosis-related group (DRG).

Access to Health Care

Access to good-quality, prompt health care is considered the right of anyone residing in Finland. Primary health care is provided through municipal health centers, whose services include physical exams, medical care, ambulance services, maternal and child health, oral health, and school health care. Specialized medical care is provided by hospital districts. Private health care is also available, and physicians' and dentists' fees are partially subsidized. According to WHO, in 2009, 100 percent of births were attended by skilled personnel (for example, physicians, nurses, or midwives). The 2010 immunization rates for 1-year-olds were 99 percent for diphtheria and pertussis (DPT3), 98 percent for measles (MCV), and 99 percent for Hib (Hib3).

Cost of Drugs

As of 2011, Finland charged a reduced value-added tax (VAT) rate (8 percent versus the standard of 22 percent) for medicines. The pharmacy dispensing fee is fixed at 0.42 euros per item. The wholesale markup is unregulated but averages 2 to 4 percent; it is regulated indirectly through the reimbursement system. The retail markup is based on purchase price. Real annual growth in pharmaceutical expenditures in Finland grew 5.1 percent from 1997 to 2005, faster than the 3.6 percent growth of total health expenditure (minus pharmaceutical expenditures) over those years. According to Elizabeth Docteur, in 2004, generic drugs represented 8 percent of the market share by value and 13 percent of the market share by volume of the total pharmaceutical market.

Health Care Facilities

As of 2010, according to WHO, Finland had 41.01 health posts per 100,000 population, 3.62 health centers per 100,000, 0.43 district or rural hospitals per 100,000, 0.88 provincial hospitals per 100,000, and 0.09 specialized hospitals per 100,000. In 2008, Finland had 6.52 hospital beds per 1,000 population, among the 20 highest ratios in the world.

Major Health Issues

In 2008, WHO estimated that 3 percent of years of life lost in Finland were due to communicable diseases, 77 percent to noncommunicable diseases, and 20 percent to injuries. In 2008, the age-standardized estimate of cancer deaths was 127 per 100,000 for men and 85 per 100,000 for women; for cardiovascular disease and diabetes, 211 per 100,000 for men and 106 per 100,000 for women; and for chronic respiratory disease, 20 per 100,000 for men and seven per 100,000 for women.

In 2010, tuberculosis incidence was 6.7 per 100,000 population, tuberculosis prevalence 8.5 per 100,000, and deaths due to tuberculosis among human immunodeficiency virus (HIV)-negative people 0.67 per 100,000. As of 2009, an estimated 0.1 percent of adults age 15 to 49 were living with HIV or acquired immune deficiency syndrome (AIDS). Finland ranked seventh among more developed countries in the 2011 Mothers' Index, produced by the international nongovernmental organization (NGO) Save the Children, based on a number of health and social factors relating to women, children, and maternal and child care. The maternal mortality rate (death from any cause related to or aggravated by pregnancy) in Finland in 2008 was eight maternal deaths per 100,000 live births, among the lowest in the world. The infant mortality rate, defined as the number of deaths of infants younger than 1 year, was 3.40 per 1,000 live births as of 2012, also among the lowest in the world.

Health Care Personnel

Finland has five medical schools, located in Helsinki, Kuopio, Oulu, Tampere, and Turku. The basic degree course lasts six years, and two years of practical training is also required before the license to practice medicine is granted. The degree awarded is the Lääketieteen lisensiaatti (licentiate in medicine). Physicians must register with the National Board of Medicolegal Affairs in Helsinki. Graduates of foreign medical schools must complete an additional six months of training and pass three examinations. Finland has agreements with other European Union (EU) countries and the other Nordic countries.

Finland, as a member of the EU, cooperates with other countries in recognizing physicians qualified to practice in other EU countries, as specified by Directive 2005/36/EC of the European Parliament. This allows qualified professionals to practice their profession in other EU states on a temporary basis and requires that the host country automatically recognize qualifications for certain professions, including physicians, nurses, dentists, midwives, and pharmacists, if certain conditions have been met (for instance, facility in the language of the host country may be required). In 2008, Finland had 2.74 physicians per 1,000 population and, in 2007, had 1.07 pharmaceutical personnel per 1,000, 0.78 dentistry personnel per 1,000, and 15.52 nurses and midwives per 1,000.

Government Role in Health Care
According to WHO, in 2010, Finland spent $21 billion on health care, an amount that comes to $3,984 per capita. All of health care funding was provided from domestic sources. Three-quarters (75 percent) of health care spending was provided by government expenditures, with 19 percent coming from spending by households, and 6 percent from other sources. In 2010, Finland allocated 12 percent of its total government expenditures to health, and government expenditures on health came to 7 percent of GDP; both figures place Finland in the low range when compared to other high-income European countries.

Public Health Programs
The National Institute for Health and Welfare (THL), located in Helsinki and headed by Pekka Puska, was created in 2009 through the merger of the National Public Health Institute and the National Research and Development Center for Welfare and Health. The THL has a staff of more than 1,400 and works to improve the health and welfare of the Finnish population, prevent diseases and social problems, and help develop local social and health services. The THL is also responsible for monitoring health services throughout the country and has satellite offices in Jyvaskyla, Kuopio, Oulu, Tampere, Turku, and Vaasa. In 2010, access to improved sanitation facilities and improved sources of drinking water was essentially universal in Finland. According to the World Higher Education Database (WHED), 20 universities in Finland offer programs in epidemiology or public health.

FRANCE

France is a western European country, sharing borders with eight countries, and having coastlines on the Mediterranean Sea and the North Atlantic Ocean.

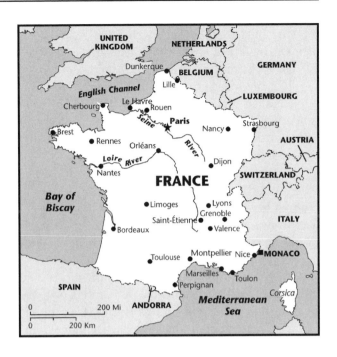

The area of 248,573 square miles (643,801 square kilometers) makes France slightly smaller than Texas, and the July 2012 population of 65.6 million was the 21st-largest in the world. In 2010, 85 percent of the population lived in urban areas, and the 2010 to 2015 annual rate of urbanization was estimated at 1.0 percent. The capital and largest city is Paris (with a 2009 population estimated at 10.4 million). The July 2012 population growth rate was 0.5 percent, the birth rate 12.8 births per 1,000 population, the net migration rate 1.1 migrants per 1,000, and the total fertility rate 2.1 children per woman.

France acquired many colonies in the 19th and 20th centuries, but most have since become independent; as of 2012, France includes five Overseas Departments: Guadeloupe, Martinique, French Guiana, Réunion, and Mayotte. France ranked tied for 25th among 183 countries on the *Corruption Perceptions Index 2011,* with a score of 7.0 (on a scale where 0 indicates highly corrupt and 10 very clean). In 2011, France was classified as a country with very high human development (the highest of four categories) on the United Nations Development Programme's (UNDP's) Human Development Index (HDI), with a score of 0.884 (on a scale where 1 denotes high development and 0 low development). Life expectancy at birth in 2012 was estimated at 81.46 years, among the highest in the world, and per capita gross domestic product (GDP) in 2011 was estimated at $35,000. In 2008, the Gini Index (a measure of dispersion, in which perfect equality is denoted by 0 and maximum inequality is denoted by 100) for family income was 32.7. According to the World Economic Forum's *Global Gender Gap Index 2011*, France ranked 48th out of 135 countries on gender equality with a score of 0.702 (on a scale with a theoretical range of 1 for equality to 0 for inequality and an actual range in 2011 from 0.8530 to 0.4873).

Emergency Health Services

France's laws governing the emergency health system date from the 1990s; by law, free access to hospitals for emergency care is provided for all persons, including the uninsured. Funding for the emergency system is from multiple sources for outpatient care, and firefighters regularly substitute for ambulance services; in-hospital care is funded entirely from public sources. France has only one national telephone number (the number 15)for medical emergencies (not the European Union, or EU, standard of 112); the country has 103 dispatch centers that are interconnected.

Doctors Without Borders (Médecins Sans Frontières, or MSF) began working in France in 1987 and had 14 staff members in the country at the close of 2010. MSF established a psychological services center for asylum seekers in Paris; most are refugees from armed conflict. MSF also provided medical consultations for migrants during an outbreak of scabies in mid-2009, providing more than 1,900 consultations. MSF established a health center on Mayotte, a French island off the east coast of Africa, providing basic health care for more than 7,500 patients, many without clear legal status, between May 2009 and September 2010; the clinic closed in September 2010 when it became clear that care was available from other sources.

Insurance

In 2000, a study by the World Health Organization (WHO) ranked France first in health care among the 191 countries that are WHO members, based on factors including population health, system responsiveness, and fairness; this was the first time WHO produced such a ranking, and it has not been repeated due to the amount of time required to produce the report. France has a statutory health insurance system (SHI), in which all insurers are part of a single national union. Hospital care, ambulatory care, and prescription drugs are covered by health insurance, along with minimal coverage for outpatient dental and eye care, and some preventive services. The insurance system is paid for out of general tax revenues and an earmarked income and payroll tax collected from employers and employees. Health coverage is universal, and the state pays for services for illegal residents and other residents not eligible for the general public insurance program. The French SHI includes several types of cost sharing, including coinsurance, copayments, and extra billing. For instance, hospital care includes a 20 percent coinsurance and a daily copayment of 16 to 20 euros and physician visits a 30 percent coinsurance. There are some exemptions from cost sharing, including low-income patients and patients with chronic conditions. In 2004, a voluntary gatekeeping system began for persons age 16 or older, with financial incentives for both physicians and patients.

About 20 percent of those covered under the French SHI purchase private insurance that provides cost sharing and some amenities, and 10 percent choose private coverage (opting out of the SHI system). There is no cap on out-of-pocket expenses, although certain categories (including children, the disabled, low-income people, and the chronically ill) are exempt from some cost-sharing provisions. Primary care is paid for on a fee-for-service basis, while hospital payments are handled through a combination of global budgets and case-based payments; hospital payments include physician costs.

A 2004 study by WHO found that, in 2000, a marginal proportion of the French population had substitutive voluntary health insurance (covering services that would other be available from the state), and 94 percent had complementary voluntary health insurance (covering services not covered or not fully covered by the state). Much of the growth in the voluntary insurance market is attributed to increased cost sharing as a state strategy to control health care expenditures; reducing the out-of-pocket burden of copayments is a primary reason complementary insurance coverage has increased steadily over the last half-century, from about 33 percent in 1960 to 50 percent in 1970, 70 percent in 1980, 85 percent in 1998, and 94 percent in 2004. Coverage by voluntary insurance is associated with higher income and occupational status and negatively associated with foreign origins. According to Ke Xu and colleagues, in 2003, less than 0.1 percent of households in France experienced catastrophic health expenditures annually; "catastrophic" was defined as exceeding 40 percent of household income remaining after basic needs were met.

Selected Health Indicators: France Compared With the Organisation for Economic Co-operation and Development (OECD) Country Average

	France	OECD average (2010 or nearest year)
Male life expectancy at birth, 2010	78	77
Female life expectancy at birth, 2010	84.7	82.5
Infant mortality (deaths per 1,000 live births), 2010	3.6	4.3
Total expenditure on health (percent of GDP), 2010	11.6	9.5
Total expenditure on health (per capita, USD purchasing power parity), 2010	3,974	3,265
Average length of hospital stay for a normal delivery (days), 2010	4.3	3.1
Cesarean sections (per 1,000 live births), 2010	203	261
Alcohol consumption (liters per capita [age 15+]), 2010	12	9.4
Tobacco consumption (percent of population 15+ who are daily smokers), 2010	23.3	21.1

Source: OECD Health Data 2012 (Organisation for Economic Co-operation and Development, 2012).
*Estimated.

Costs of Hospitalization

According to Donald West and colleagues, about 62 percent of hospital beds in France are located in public hospitals; about 18 percent are in hospitals managed by private nonprofits, and 20 percent are in hospitals managed by for-profit companies. France's 2012 Hospital Plan committed 10 billion euros to improve hospital care; specific areas of focus include increasing collaboration, improving computer systems to reduce duplication of services, and improving security systems.

Traditionally, hospitals have been funded through an endowment system from insurance funds, but France is shifting toward a diagnosis-related group (DRG) system for all hospitals. The Ministry of Health is responsible for central planning, including the number and size of hospitals, the supply of specialty awards, and the provision of major technologies such as magnetic resonance imaging (MRI) and computer tomography (CT) machines. According to Organisation for Economic Co-operation and Development (OECD) data, in 2009, hospital spending per capita in France was $1,366 (adjusted for differences in the cost of living), and hospital spending per

discharge came to $5,204 in 2011. The average length of stay in acute care was 5.2 days in 2008, and there were 263 hospital discharges per 1,000 population.

Access to Health Care

In 2009, according to OECD data, the French had an average of 6.9 physician visits. According to WHO, in 1993 (the most recent year for which data is available), 99 percent of births were attended by skilled personnel (for example, physicians, nurses, or midwives). The 2010 immunization rates for 1-year-olds were 99 percent for diphtheria and pertussis (DPT3), 90 percent for measles (MCV), and 97 percent for Hib (Hib3). In 2010, almost two-thirds (62 percent) of the French population reported that, when sick, they were able to get a medical appointment the same day or the next day. However, a similar proportion (63 percent) reported it was very or somewhat difficult to get medical care after usual office hours. For those who needed particular types of care, more than one-quarter (28 percent) reported they waited two or more months to see a specialist (of those who needed to see a specialist in the prior two years), but only 7 percent reported waiting four or more months for elective surgery (of those who required elective surgery in the prior two years), and only 13 percent reported they had experienced an access barrier due to cost in the previous two years; an access barrier was defined as failing to fill or refill a prescription, failing to visit a physician, or failing to get recommended care. According to Donald West and colleagues, France has a cooperative plan between the public and private hospital systems that helps patients avoid long waiting times; the private system provides more than 60 percent of care for cancer and more than 50 percent of surgeries.

In 2010, about one in seven (14 percent) of French people reported experiencing a medical, medication, or lab test error in the previous two years, and 28 percent of those who needed to visit a specialist in the previous two years reported that the specialist did not have information about their medical history at the time of the appointment. More than two-thirds (71 percent) reported experiencing a gap in hospital discharge planning in the previous two years (due to any of the following: did not receive a written plan for care, did not have arrangements made for follow-up visits, did not know whom to contact with questions, or did not receive instruction about when to seek further care).

A 2011 Commonwealth Fund Survey compared access to health care for "sicker adults" (those 18 and older in self-reported poor or fair health who had been treated for a serious illness or injury in the past year or been hospitalized in the past two years) in 11 OECD countries. This survey found that 19 percent of sicker French people surveyed reported having experienced an access problem related to cost in the previous year; the most common result was failing to fill a prescription or skipping doses of a prescribed drug. Other problems reported include having serious problems paying their medical bills (5 percent), waiting six days or longer for needed care (8 percent), having difficulty getting after-hours care except in an emergency room (55 percent), and experiencing coordination gaps in care (53 percent).

Cost of Drugs

According to Elizabeth Docteur, France uses internal reference pricing to determine the price at which a new drug will be reimbursed. The Transparency Commission (Amélioration du service medical rendu) considers the therapeutic value and advantage (in relation to drugs already on the market) of a new drug and rates its innovation on a give-point scale, from major

therapeutic progress (1) to absence of improvement (5); to be included on the positive list (drugs that will be reimbursed), those classified in category 5 must offer a lower price than drugs already on the market, while those in categories 1 through 4 may be allowed to name a higher price.

In 2009, according to OECD data, pharmaceutical spending per capita in France was $640 (adjusted for differences in the cost of living). Patients pay coinsurance for prescription drugs based on their effectiveness: There is no coinsurance for highly effective drugs, 100 percent coinsurance for drugs of limited therapeutic value, and coinsurance of 35 percent or 65 percent for drugs between those two extremes. A copayment, which cannot be reimbursed through private insurance, of 0.50 euros ($0.74) is charged for each prescription.

According to Douglas Ball, as of 2011, France charged a lower value-added tax (VAT) for medicines (2.1 percent for reimbursable drugs and 5.5 percent for nonreimbursable drugs) than for other goods (the standard VAT is 19.6 percent). The dispensing fee is 0.53 euros for reimbursable medicines. The wholesale and pharmacy markups are regulated for reimbursable medicines; for wholesale, the markup ranges from 2.0 percent to 10.3 percent of the "ex-factory price" (the manufacturer's list price before discounts), and for pharmacies, it ranges from 6.0 percent to 26.1 percent of the ex-factory price.

France is the third-largest purchaser of pharmaceuticals, after the United States and Japan, accounting for 6 percent of global pharmaceutical sales. Real annual growth in pharmaceutical expenditures in France grew 4.2 percent from 1997 to 2005, about the same as the 4.1 percent growth of total health expenditure (minus pharmaceutical expenditures) over those years. According to Elizabeth Docteur, in 2004, France ranked sixth-lowest among OECD countries in terms of the use of generics; generic drugs represented 6 percent of the market share by value and 12 percent of the market share by volume of the total pharmaceutical market.

Health Care Facilities

In 2008, France had 7.11 hospital beds per 1,000 population, among the 20 highest ratios in the world. Most (62 percent) hospital beds are in public hospitals, with 20 percent in private, for-profit hospitals, and 18 percent in private, not-for-profit hospitals. French citizens have smart cards encoded with their insurance information, which is used to access care. Physicians are required to share medical records, according to Donald West and colleagues. In 2009, France had 6.4 magnetic resonance imaging (MRI) machines per 1 million population, and 55.2 MRI exams were performed per 100,000 population. About two-thirds (68 percent) of primary care physicians used electronic medical records in 2009.

Major Health Issues

In 2008, WHO estimated that 6 percent of years of life lost in France were due to communicable diseases, 80 percent to noncommunicable diseases, and 14 percent to injuries. In 2008, the age-standardized estimate of cancer deaths was 183 per 100,000 for men and 94 per 100,000 for women; for cardiovascular disease and diabetes, 128 per 100,000 for men and 69 per 100,000 for women; and for chronic respiratory disease, 19 per 100,000 for men and seven per 100,000 for women.

In 2010, tuberculosis incidence was 9.3 per 100,000 population, tuberculosis prevalence 12.0 per 100,000, and deaths due to tuberculosis among human immunodeficiency virus (HIV)-negative people 0.71 per 100,000. As of 2009, an estimated 0.4 percent of adults age 15 to 49 were living with HIV or acquired immune deficiency syndrome (AIDS). France ranked 10th among more developed countries in the 2011 Mothers' Index, produced by the international nongovernmental organization (NGO) Save the Children, based on a number of health and social factors relating to women, children, and maternal and child care. The maternal mortality rate (death from any cause related to or aggravated by pregnancy) in France in 2008 was eight maternal deaths per 100,000 live births, among the lowest in the world. The infant mortality rate, defined as the number of deaths of infants younger than 1 year, was 3.37 per 1,000 live births as of 2012, the 10th-lowest in the world.

Health Care Personnel

France has 45 medical schools. The basic degree course requires 8 or 8.5 years to complete. The degree awarded is the Diplôme d'État de Docteur en Médicine (doctor of medicine, state diploma) for those who hold the French Baccalauréat and Diplôme d'Université de Docteur en Médicine (doctor of medicine, university diploma) for those who do not.

France, as a member of the European Union (EU), cooperates with other countries in recognizing physicians qualified to practice in other EU countries,

as specified by Directive 2005/36/EC of the European Parliament. This allows qualified professionals to practice their profession in other EU states on a temporary basis and requires that the host country automatically recognize qualifications for certain professions, including physicians, nurses, dentists, midwives, and pharmacists, if certain conditions have been met (for instance, facility in the language of the host country may be required). In 2008, France had 4.54 physicians per 1,000 population and in 2009, had 1.23 pharmaceutical personnel per 1,000, 0.68 dentistry personnel per 1,000, and 8.94 nurses and midwives per 1,000. In 2000 only 2.2 percent of practicing physicians in France were trained abroad, primarily in other European countries or in north Africa.

Government Role in Health Care

According to WHO, in 2010, France spent $304 billion on health care, an amount that comes to $4,691 per capita. All health care funding was provided from domestic sources. More than three-quarters (78 percent) of health care spending was provided by government expenditures, with 7 percent coming from spending by households and 15 percent from other sources. In 2010, France allocated 16 percent of its total government expenditures to health, and government expenditures on health came to 9 percent of GDP; both figures place France in the low range when compared to other high-income European countries. The French government establishes reference prices for professional services, although physicians and dentists may charge above this rate based on their levels of professional experience; the extra billing charges are paid by the patient or by private insurance policies.

Public Health Programs

France has two national institutes concerned with public health: the French Institute for Public Health Surveillance (InVS, Institut de Veille Sanitaire) and the National Institute of Health and Medical Research (INSERM, Institut National de la Sante et de la Recherche Medicale). The InVS focuses on injuries, infectious and chronic disease, international health, tropical diseases, and environmental and occupational health. Activities of the InVS include collecting and analyzing population health data, working with other members of the national health network, collecting and analyzing information about health risks, managing emergency health situations, and notifying the Minister of Health about any threats to population health. Priorities established in 2004 include environmental health, cancer, violence, rare diseases, health risk behaviors, addiction, and the quality of life for chronic disease patients. More recent national priorities include national plans for Alzheimer's disease, HIV/AIDS and sexually transmitted diseases (STDs), occupational health, and antibiotics. Reducing health inequalities is also a priority, as is increasing the vaccination rate in the population. In 2010, regional agencies were created to monitor health and reduce inequalities across the country.

INSERM was created in 1964 and is the successor of the National Institute of Hygiene, founded in 1941. INSERM has 13,000 employees working in the fields of medicine, public health, and biology and acts as an independent scientific expert for other government departments in the field of public health. INSERM also collects and analyzes expert scientific information to guide in the decision-making process for medical screening, treatment, and prevention activities and helps identify public health needs for medical research.

In 2010, access to improved sanitary facilities and improved sources of drinking water was essentially universal in France. According to the World Higher Education Database (WHED), six universities in France offer programs in epidemiology or public health: the School of Advanced Studies in Public Health in Rennes, the University of Versailles Saint-Quentin-en-Yvelines, the University of Paris 7 (Universite Denis Diderot), the University of Lille II, the University of Paris-South 11, and the University of Bordeaux II.

GABON

Gabon is a country in west central Africa, sharing borders with Cameroon, Republic of the Congo, and Equatorial Guinea and having a coastline on the south Atlantic Ocean. The area of 103,347 square miles (267,667 square kilometers) is similar to Colorado, and the July 2012 population was estimated at 1.6 million. In 2010, 86 percent of the population lived in urban areas, and the 2010 to 2015 annual rate of urbanization was estimated at 2.1 percent. The capital and largest city is Libreville (with a 2009 population estimated at 619,000). The July 2012 population growth rate was 2.0 percent; a high birth rate

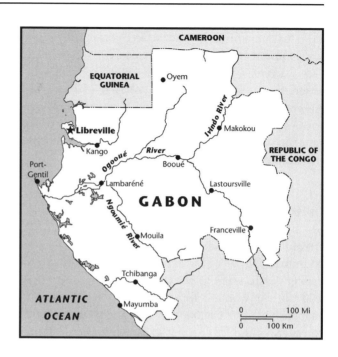

(35 births per 1,000 population, the 27th-highest in the world) and high total fertility rate (4.6 children per woman, the 29th-highest in the world) are balanced by a negative net migration rate (negative 2.2 migrants per 1,000 population). The United Nations High Commissioner for Refugees (UNHCR) estimates that, in 2010, there were 9,015 refugees and persons in refugee-like situations in Gabon.

A former French colony, Gabon became independent in 1960. For much of its history, it was ruled by Omar Bongo Ondimba from 1967 to 2009; he was succeeded after his death in 2009 by his son Ali Ben Bongo. According to the Ibrahim Index, in 2011, Gabon ranked 26th among 53 African countries in terms of governance performance, with a score of 51 (out of 100). Gabon ranked tied for 100th among 183 countries in on the *Corruption Perceptions Index 2011*, with a score of 3.0 (on a scale where 0 indicates highly corrupt and 10 very clean). In 2011, Gabon was classified as a country with medium human development (the second from the lowest of four categories) on the United Nations Development Programme's (UNDP's) Human Development Index (HDI), with a score of 0.674 (on a scale where 1 denotes high development and 0 low development). Life expectancy at birth in 2012 was estimated at 52.29 years, among the 20 lowest in the world; per capita gross domestic product (GDP) in 2011 was estimated at $16,100, and unemployment in 2006 was estimated at 21.0 percent.

Emergency Health Services

According to the U.S. State Department, the cities of Libreville, Port Gentil, and Franceville have emergency numbers comparable to 911 in the United States.

Insurance

Gabon has a social insurance and social assistance system providing maternity and medical benefits only. The social insurance system covers the employed and their dependents, and the social assistance system covers residents and citizens of Gabon older than 15 who earn less than the minimum wage. The system is paid for through payroll contributions from employers; the Family Benefits system is also paid for through employer payroll contributions. There are no cash sickness benefits, but employers are required to provide paid sick leave for up to six months. The maternity befit is 50 percent of monthly earnings for up to six weeks before and eight weeks after birth. The social insurance system provides care through National Social Security Fund hospitals and dispensaries, including hospitalization, outpatient treatment, medicine, and transportation. Maternity care and medicine are free, but other services require cost sharing. The social assistance system provides a broader range of services through clinics, hospitals, and other facilities affiliated with the National Health Insurance and Social Assistance Fund, including hospitalization, physician care, vaccinations, generic medicines, lab work and X-rays, and appliances. Copayments or coinsurance are required for most services.

The Family Benefits system covers employed people and pensioners, with special programs from the self-employed, military personnel, civil servants, and state contract workers. The system provides a prenatal allowance (CFA 13,500; the mother is required to undergo medical exams), a birth grant (CFA 8,000 plus CFA 45,000 for a layette; the mother is required to undergo medical exams), school allowances (CFA 20,000 annually for dependents attending school), and family allowances (for children younger than 16, younger than 17 if an apprentice, or younger than 20 if disabled or attending school). Some health services are also provided for mothers and children. As of 2010, almost one-third (32.6 percent) of the population of Gabon was covered by public health insurance and 10 percent by private health insurance. Insured patients pay a 10 percent coinsurance for treatment for chronic conditions and 20 percent coinsurance for acute conditions; the uninsured pay flat fees.

Costs of Hospitalization

No data available.

Access to Health Care

According to the World Health Organization (WHO), in 2000 (the most recent year for which data is available), 87 percent of births were attended by skilled personnel (for example, physicians, nurses, or midwives). In 2000, 63 percent of pregnant women received at least four prenatal care visits. The 2010 immunization rates for 1-year-olds were 45 percent for diphtheria and pertussis (DPT3), 55 percent for measles (MCV), and 45 percent for Hib (Hib3). In 2010, an estimated 53 percent of persons with advanced human immunodeficiency virus (HIV) infection were receiving antiretroviral therapy in accordance with the 2010 WHO guidelines. According to WHO, in 2010, Gabon had 1.38 magnetic resonance imaging (MRI) machines per 1 million population, 4.14 computer tomography (CT) machines per 1 million, 0.69 telecolbalt units per 1 million, and 0.69 radiotherapy machines per 1 million.

Cost of Drugs

Total pharmaceutical expenditures in Gabon in 2008 were 31.8 million Central African (CFA) francs ($68.2 million), and per capita expenditure was 15,587.8 CFA francs ($39.90). Pharmaceutical expenditures came to 15.9 percent of total health expenditures, and 0.5 percent of GDP; almost one-quarter (23 percent) of pharmaceutical expenses were paid for with public funds. Medications are provided free in public health facilities to pregnant women, children under age 5, elderly persons, and the poor. Private insurance provides drugs for individuals in these populations at a discounted rate (80 percent of the cost is covered by insurance). The public health system supplies drugs on the Essential Medications List (EML) for free as well as drugs to treat malaria, tuberculosis, and human immunodeficiency virus and acquired immune deficiency syndrome (HIV/AIDS); vaccines on WHO's Expanded Programme for Immunization (EPI) list are also provided free. Medicines for leprosy and trypanosomiasis are provided for free through WHO programs.

Health Care Facilities

As of 2010, according to WHO, Gabon had 32.68 health posts per 100,000 population, 2.46 health centers per 100,000, 2.72 district or rural hospitals per 100,000, 0.80 provincial hospitals per 100,000, and

0.40 specialized hospitals per 100,000. In 2008, Gabon had 1.25 hospital beds per 1,000 population.

Major Health Issues

In 2008, WHO estimated that 69 percent of years of life lost in Gabon were due to communicable diseases, 21 percent to noncommunicable diseases, and 9 percent to injuries. In 2008, the age-standardized estimate of cancer deaths was 79 per 100,000 for men and 72 per 100,000 for women; for cardiovascular disease and diabetes, 396 per 100,000 for men and 343 per 100,000 for women; for chronic respiratory disease, 109 per 100,000 for men and 48 per 100,000 for women.

In 2008, the age-standardized death rate from malaria was 23.2 per 100,000 population. In 2010, tuberculosis incidence was 553.0 per 100,000 population, tuberculosis prevalence 676.0 per 100,000, and deaths due to tuberculosis among HIV-negative people 70.00 per 100,000. As of 2009, an estimated 5.2 percent of adults age 15 to 49 were living with HIV or AIDS. Gabon's maternal mortality rate (death from any cause related to or aggravated by pregnancy) was estimated in 2008 as 260 maternal deaths per 100,000 live births. The infant mortality rate, defined as the number of deaths of infants younger than 1 year, was estimated at 49.00 per 1,000 live births as of 2012.

Health Care Personnel

Gabon has one medical school, the Centre Universitaire des Sciences de la Santé in Libreville, which began offering instruction in 1973. The basic medical degree course requires seven years to complete, and the degree awarded is the Docteur d'État en Médecine (doctor of medicine). In 2004, Gabon had 0.29 physicians per 1,000 population, 0.05 pharmaceutical personnel per 1,000, 0.20 laboratory health workers per 1.000, 0.11 health management and support workers per 1,000, 0.05 dentistry personnel per 1,000, and 5.02 nurses and midwives per 1,000. The global "brain drain" (international migration of skilled personnel) plays a small role in the relative undersupply of medical personnel in Gabon: Michael Clemens and Bunilla Petterson estimate that 15 percent of Gabon-born physicians and 6 percent of Gabon-born nurses are working in one of nine developed countries, primarily in France.

Government Role in Health Care

The right to health, including access to essential medicines and medical technologies, is recognized at the national level. Gabon's national pharmaceutical plan includes selection of essential medicines; financing, pricing, purchase, distribution, and regulation of drugs; pharmacovigilance; rational usage of medicines; human resource development; research; and traditional medicine. Promotion and advertising of prescription drugs is regulated, and direct advertising to the public is forbidden.

According to WHO, in 2010, Gabon spent $455 million on health care, an amount that comes to $302 per capita. Most (98 percent) health care funding was provided from domestic sources, with 2 percent provided by sources from abroad. Health care funding was almost evenly divided between government expenditures (53 percent) and household spending (47 percent). In 2010, Gabon allocated 7 percent of its total government expenditures to health, and government expenditures on health came to 2 percent of GDP; both figures place Gabon in the low range when compared to other upper-middle-income African countries. In 2009, according to WHO, official development assistance (ODA) for health in Gabon came to $11.10 per capita.

Public Health Programs

According to WHO, in 2004, Gabon had 0.11 environmental and public health workers per 1,000 population. In 2010, 33 percent of the population had access to improved sanitation facilities (30 percent in rural areas and 33 percent in urban), and 87 percent had access to improved sources of drinking water (41 percent in rural areas and 95 percent in urban).

According to the World Higher Education Database (WHED), no university in Gabon offers programs in epidemiology or public health.

GAMBIA, THE

The Gambia is a west African country, sharing borders with Senegal and having a north Atlantic coastline; the country consists primarily of the flood plains of the Gambia River. The area of 4,361 square miles (11,295 square kilometers) is about twice that of Delaware, and the July 2012 population was estimated at 1.8 million. In 2010, 58 percent of the population lived in urban areas, and the 2010 to 2015 annual rate of urbanization was estimated at 3.7 percent. The capital and largest city is Banjul (with a 2009 population estimated at

436,000). The population growth rate in 2012 was 2.3 percent despite a negative net migration rate of negative 2.5 migrants per 1,000 population; the total fertility rate was 4.1 children per woman (the 36th-highest in the world), and the birth rate was 33.4 births per 1,000 population (the 31st-highest in the world). The United Nations High Commissioner for Refugees (UNHCR) estimated that, in 2010, there were 8,330 refugees and persons in refugee-like situations in The Gambia.

A former British colony, The Gambia became independent in 1965 and formed a federation with Senegal from 1982 to 1989. According to the Ibrahim Index, in 2011, The Gambia ranked 24th among 53 African countries in terms of governance performance, with a score of 52 (out of 100). The Gambia ranked tied for 77th among 183 countries on the *Corruption Perceptions Index 2011* with a score of 3.5 (on a scale where 0 indicates highly corrupt and 10 very clean). In 2011, The Gambia was classified as a country with low human development (the lowest of four categories) on the United Nations Development Programme's (UNDP's) Human Development Index (HDI), with a score of 0.420 (on a scale where 1 denotes high development and 0 low development). In 2012, the World Food Programme estimated that 206,000 people in The Gambia were food insecure, primarily in 19 rural districts suffering from drought. Life expectancy at birth in 2012 was estimated at 63.82 years, and estimated gross domestic product (GDP) per capita in

2011 was $2,100. Income distribution in The Gambia is relatively unequal: In 1998, the Gini Index (a measure of dispersion, in which perfect equality is denoted by 0 and maximum inequality is denoted by 100) for family income was 50.2. According to the World Economic Forum's *Global Gender Gap Index 2011*, The Gambia ranked 77th out of 135 countries on gender equality with a score of 0.676 (on a scale with a theoretical range of 1 for equality to 0 for inequality and an actual range in 2011 from 0.8530 to 0.4873).

Emergency Health Services

According to the World Health Organization (WHO), as of 2007, The Gambia had a formal and publicly available emergency care (prehospital care) system accessible through a national universal access telephone number.

Insurance

Most (80 percent) of the population of The Gambia was covered by the public health system as of 2007. No information is available about the proportion holding private health insurance.

Costs of Hospitalization

No data available.

Access to Health Care

According to WHO, in 2006, 57 percent of births in The Gambia were attended by skilled personnel (for example, physicians, nurses, or midwives). The 2010 immunization rates for 1-year-olds were 98 percent for diphtheria and pertussis (DPT3), 97 percent for measles (MCV), and 98 percent for Hib (Hib3). In 2010, an estimated 35 percent of persons with advanced human immunodeficiency virus (HIV) infection were receiving antiretroviral therapy in accordance with the 2010 WHO guidelines. According to WHO, in 2010, The Gambia had 0.60 magnetic resonance imaging (MRI) machines per 1 million population and 1.20 computer tomography (CT) machines per 1 million population.

Cost of Drugs

The Gambia has a National Medicines Policy (NMP), created by the Federal Ministry of Health in 2005, and an Essential Medicines List (EML), created by the Ministry of Health in 2009; the EML contains 358 medicines, including formulations specifically for children. The NMP includes the selection of

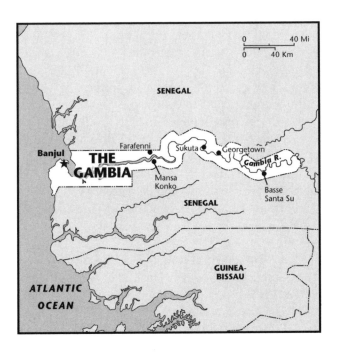

essential medicines, financing and pricing of medicines, and procurement, distribution, and regulation of medicines. Access to essential medicines and medical technologies is recognized as part of the right to health, as specified in national legislation. As of 2007, medicines have been provided without charge to the poor, children under age 5, and pregnant women. The public health system provides medicines on the EML for free, and medicines to treat malaria, tuberculosis, and human immunodeficiency virus and acquired immune deficiency syndrome (HIV/AIDS) are provided for free, as are the vaccines on WHO's Expanded Programme on Immunization (EPI) list. Private health insurance programs are required to provide coverage for medicines listed on the EML.

The Gambia is a member of WHO and is using the Trade-Related Aspects of Intellectual Property (TRIPS) flexibilities to promote access to medications permitted in the transitional period to 2016; specifically, The Gambia's law recognizes the right to compulsory licensing (allowing others than the patent owner to produce a patented product) for reasons of public health. Advertising and promotion of prescription drugs is regulated by the Medicines Board, and direct marketing of prescription medications to the public is forbidden. Private health insurance programs are required to provide coverage for medicines listed on the EML.

Health Care Facilities

As of 2010, according to WHO, The Gambia had 28.47 health posts per 100,000 population, 1.79 health centers per 100,000, 0.41 district or rural hospitals per 100,000, 0.23 provincial hospitals per 100,000, and 0.12 specialized hospitals per 100,000. In 2009, The Gambia had 1.13 hospital beds per 1,000 population.

Major Health Issues

In 2008, WHO estimated that 73 percent of years of life lost in The Gambia were due to communicable diseases, 20 percent to noncommunicable diseases, and 7 percent to injuries. In 2008, the age-standardized estimate of cancer deaths was 112 per 100,000 for men and 87 per 100,000 for women; for cardiovascular disease and diabetes, 401 per 100,000 for men and 433 per 100,000 for women; and for chronic respiratory disease, 110 per 100,000 for men and 66 per 100,000 for women.

In 2010, tuberculosis incidence was 273.0 per 100,000 population, tuberculosis prevalence 460.0 per 100,000, and deaths due to tuberculosis among HIV-negative people 49.00 per 100,000. As of 2009, an estimated 2.0 percent of adults age 15 to 49 were living with HIV or AIDS. In 2010, 116,353 cases of malaria were reported.

The Gambia's maternal mortality rate (death from any cause related to or aggravated by pregnancy) is high by global standards, estimated at 400 maternal deaths per 100,000 live births as of 2008. A 2005 to 2006 survey estimated the prevalence of female genital mutilation at 78.3 percent. The infant mortality rate, defined as the number of deaths of infants younger than 1 year, is also high, at 69.58 per 1,000 live births as of 2012 data. In 2006, 16.8 percent of children under age 5 were underweight (defined as 2 kilograms [kg] below standard weight-for-age at age 1, 3 kg below for ages 2 to 3, and 4 kg below for ages 4 to 5). In 2008, the age-standardized death rate from malaria was 53.7 per 100,000 population.

Health Care Personnel

In 2006, WHO identified The Gambia as one of 57 countries with a critical deficit in the supply of skilled health workers. The Gambia has one medical school, the School of Medicine and Allied Health Sciences of the University of The Gambia. The medical school was established with the assistance of Cuba, which provided the initial faculty, and began operation in October 1999. The medical course lasts six years: one year of premedical studies and five years of medical studies. The School of Medicine and Allied Health Sciences also offers degrees in nursing, midwifery, and public health. In 2008, The Gambia had 0.04 physicians per 1,000 population, 0.03 pharmaceutical personnel per 1,000, 0.06 laboratory health workers per 1,000, 0.85 health management and support workers per 1,000, 0.07 community and traditional health workers per 1,000, and 0.57 nurses and midwives per 1,000. The global "brain drain" (international migration of skilled personnel) plays a small role in the relative undersupply of medical personnel in The Gambia: Michael Clemens and Bunilla Petterson estimate that 53 percent of The Gambia-born physicians and 66 percent of The Gambia-born nurses are working in one of nine developed countries, primarily in the United States.

Government Role in Health Care

The Gambia has a National Health Policy (NHP), created in 2011, and a plan to implement it. The Gambia also has a National Medicines Policy (NMP), created in 2007. National legislation in The Gambia recognizes the right to health. According to WHO, in 2010, The Gambia spent $45 million on health care, an amount that comes to $26 per capita. Over half (59 percent) of health care funding was provided from domestic sources, with the remaining 41 percent provided by sources from abroad. Just over half (51 percent) of health care funding was paid for through government expenditures, with the remainder split almost evenly between household spending (24 percent) and other sources (25 percent). In 2010, The Gambia allocated 1 percent of its total government expenditures to health, and government expenditures on health came to 3 percent of GDP; both figures place The Gambia in the median range when compared to other low-income African countries. In 2009, according to WHO, official development assistance (ODA) for health in The Gambia came to $9.88 per capita.

Public Health Programs

According to WHO, in 2008, The Gambia had 0.05 environmental and public health workers per 1,000 population. In 2010, 68 percent of the population of The Gambia had access to improved sanitation facilities (65 percent in rural areas and 70 percent in urban), and 89 percent had access to improved sources of drinking water (85 percent in rural areas and 92 percent in urban). According to the World Higher Education Database (WHED), no university in The Gambia offers programs in epidemiology or public health.

GEORGIA

Georgia is a country in southwestern Asia, sharing borders with Russia, Turkey, Armenia, and Azerbaijan and having a coastline on the Black Sea. The area of 69,700 square miles (180,522 square kilometers) is similar to South Carolina, and the July 2012 population was estimated at 4.6 million. In 2010, 53 percent of the population lived in urban areas, and the 2010 to 2015 annual rate of urbanization was estimated at negative 0.4 percent. The capital is Tbilisi. The July 2012 population growth rate was among the 20 lowest in the world, at negative 0.33 percent; the net migration rate is negative 4.0 migrants per 1,000 population, the birth rate 10.8 per 1,000, and the total fertility rate 1.5 children per woman. The United Nations High Commissioner for Refugees (UNHCR)

estimated that, in 2010, there were 639 refugees and persons in refugee-like situations in Georgia.

Georgia became independent from the Soviet Union in 1991; Russia has fueled unrest in the country by supporting separatist movements in Abkhazia and South Ossetia. Georgia ranked tied for 64th among 183 countries on the *Corruption Perceptions Index 2011*, with a score of 4.1 (on a scale where 0 indicates highly corrupt and 10 very clean). In 2011, Georgia was classified as a country with high human development (the second-highest category) on the United Nations Development Programme's (UNDP's) Human Development Index (HDI), with a score of 0.733 (on a scale where 1 denotes high development and 0 low development). Life expectancy at birth in 2012 was estimated at 77.32 years, and the estimated gross domestic product (GDP) per capita in 2011 was $5,400. In 2009, the Gini Index (a measure of dispersion, in which perfect equality is denoted by 0 and maximum inequality is denoted by 100) for family income was 40.8. According to the World Economic Forum's *Global Gender Gap Index 2011*, Georgia ranked 86th out of 135 countries on gender equality, with a score of 0.662 (on a scale with a theoretical range of 1 for equality to 0 for inequality and an actual range in 2011 from 0.8530 to 0.4873).

Emergency Health Services

According to the World Health Organization (WHO), as of 2007, Georgia had a formal and publicly available emergency care (prehospital care) system accessible through a national universal access telephone number. Doctors Without Borders (Médecins Sans Frontières, or MSF) began working in Georgia in 1993 and had 133 staff members in the country at the close of 2010. MSF began a program to manage drug-resistant tuberculosis in Zugdidi (western Georgia) in 2006; this program was transferred to the Ministry of Health in September 2010. MSF also runs a program to increase health care access in Abkhazia (northwestern Georgia), but this program has been considerably reduced due to improved services provided by the national authorities.

Insurance

Georgia has a social insurance system covering some benefits to the employed (sickness) and to employed and self-employed women (maternity) and a social assistance system providing medical benefits to the poor and disabled. The social insurance system is paid for by a contribution of 25 percent of taxable

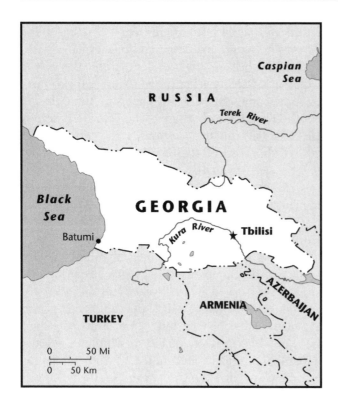

75 percent of pregnant women received at least four prenatal care visits. The 2010 immunization rates for 1-year-olds were 91 percent for diphtheria and pertussis (DPT3), 94 percent for measles (MCV), and 67 percent for Hib (Hib3). In 2010, an estimated 65 percent of persons with advanced human immunodeficiency virus (HIV) infection were receiving antiretroviral therapy in accordance with the 2010 WHO guidelines.

Cost of Drugs
No data available.

Health Care Facilities
Georgia had an extensive, well-funded health system during its time as a Soviet republic, and many officials from other parts of the Soviet Union travelled to Georgia to take a "cure" in one of the country's health spas. However, decreased funding after independence led to some deterioration of the infrastructure. As of 2010, according to WHO, Georgia had 13.76 health posts per 100,000 population and 2.21 specialized hospitals per 100,000. In 2007, Georgia had 3.32 hospital beds per 1,000 population.

Major Health Issues
In 2008, WHO estimated that 15 percent of years of life lost in Georgia were due to communicable diseases, 75 percent to noncommunicable diseases, and 10 percent to injuries. In 2008, the age-standardized estimate of cancer deaths was 116 per 100,000 for men and 78 per 100,000 for women; for cardiovascular disease and diabetes, 650 per 100,000 for men and 376 per 100,000 for women; and for chronic respiratory disease, 15 per 100,000 for men and eight per 100,000 for women.

Georgia's maternal mortality rate (death from any cause related to or aggravated by pregnancy) was estimated in 2008 as 48 maternal deaths per 100,000 live births. The infant mortality rate, defined as the number of deaths of infants younger than 1 year, was 14.68 per 1,000 live births as of 2012. In 2010, tuberculosis incidence was 107.0 per 100,000 population, tuberculosis prevalence 118.0 per 100,000, and deaths due to tuberculosis among HIV-negative people 4.60 per 100,000. As of 2009, an estimated 0.1 percent of adults age 15 to 49 were living with HIV or acquired immune deficiency syndrome (AIDS).

Health Care Personnel
Georgia has two medical schools: the AIETI Medical School in Tbilisi, founded in 1991, and Tbilisi

income from the employed and self-employed; the government provides subsidies as needed for the social insurance system and covers the total cost of the social assistance system. Medical benefits are provided to the poor and disabled at government clinics, hospitals, and other institutions; recipients of benefits must pass a means test. The cash sickness benefit is 100 percent of daily wages; the maternity benefit is 100 percent of daily wages, with the employer paying some of the benefit for high-wage workers (over GEL 600). The Social Services Agency administers the program, with general supervision and coordination from the Ministry of Labor, Health, and Social Affairs.

Costs of Hospitalization
Georgia introduced a new method of hospital payments in 1995 based on a case-mix system and 30 disease categories, which includes estimated indirect costs as well as direct costs for treatment for an average length of stay; the categories are revised annually.

Access to Health Care
According to WHO, in 2005, 98 percent of births in Georgia were attended by skilled personnel (for example, physicians, nurses, or midwives). In 2005,

State Medical University, founded in 1921. The basic medical degree course lasts six or seven years. In 2007, Georgia had 4.54 physicians per 1,000 population, 0.06 pharmaceutical personnel per 1,000, 0.28 health management and support workers per 1,000, and 3.89 nurses and midwives per 1,000.

Government Role in Health Care

According to WHO, in 2010, Georgia spent $1.2 billion on health care, an amount that comes to $272 per capita. Almost all (97 percent) of health care funding was provided from domestic sources, with the remaining 3 percent provided by sources from abroad. More than two-thirds (68 percent) of health care funding was paid for through household spending, with the remainder provided through government expenditures (24 percent) and other sources (8 percent).

In 2010, Georgia allocated 7 percent of its total government expenditures to health, placing Georgia in the low range compared to other lower-middle-income Asian countries; government expenditures on health came to 2 percent of GDP, placing Georgia in the median range compared to other lower-middle-income Asian countries. In 2009, according to WHO, official development assistance (ODA) for health in Georgia came to $5.46 per capita.

Public Health Programs

In 2010, 95 percent of the population of Georgia had access to improved sanitation facilities (93 percent in rural areas and 96 percent in urban) and 98 percent had access to improved sources of drinking water (96 percent in rural areas and 100 percent in urban). According to the World Higher Education Database (WHED), eight universities in Georgia offer programs in epidemiology or public health: the Georgian Institute of Economics and Law, Shota Rustaveli State University, Sukhishvili University, Tbilisi State Medical University, Tbilisi University, the University of Georgia, AIETI Medical School, and Interpharm Plus University.

GERMANY

Germany is a western European country, sharing borders with nine countries and having coastlines on the North Sea and Baltic Sea. Germany's area of 137,847 square miles (357,022 square kilometers) makes it similar in size to Montana, and the July 2012 population was estimated at 81.3 million (the second-largest in Europe and 16th-largest in the world). In 2010, 74 percent of the population lived in urban areas, and the 2010 to 2015 annual rate of urbanization was estimated at 0.0 percent. Berlin is the capital and largest city (with a 2009 population estimated at 3.4 million). The July 2012 population growth rate was negative 0.2 percent despite a positive net migration rate (0.7 migrants per 1,000 population); the birth rate is 8.3 births per 1,000 population, and the total fertility rate is 1.4 children per woman.

Germany was divided into two countries in 1949: The German Democratic Republic (East Germany), which had a communist government, and the Federal Republic of Germany (West Germany), which was democratic and a leader in Western economic and strategic organizations; the two countries were reunited in 1990. The German government has a reputation for honesty and transparency, ranking tied for 14th among 183 countries on the *Corruption Perceptions Index 2011*, with a score of 8.0 (on a scale where 0 indicates highly corrupt and 10 very clean).

Germany has the largest economy in Europe and was notably unaffected by the sovereign debt crisis affecting some European countries from 2011 to 2012. Germany ranked sixth (tied with Liechtenstein) in 2011 on the United Nations Development Programme's (UNDP's) Human Development Index (HDI), with a score of 0.905 (on a scale where 1 denotes high development and 0 low development). Life expectancy at birth in 2012 was estimated at 80.19 years, among the highest in the world, and per capita gross domestic product (GDP) in 2011 was estimated at $37,900. Income distribution is among the most equal in the world: In 2006, the Gini Index (a measure of dispersion, in which perfect equality is denoted by 0 and maximum inequality is denoted by 100) for family income was 27.0. Germany has achieved a high level of gender equality: According to the World Economic Forum's *Global Gender Gap Index 2011*, Germany ranked 11th out of 135 countries on gender equality, with a score of 0.759 (on a scale with a theoretical range of 1 for equality to 0 for inequality and an actual range in 2011 from 0.8530 to 0.4873).

Emergency Health Services

Germany's laws governing the emergency health system date from the 2000s, and emergency medicine has been recognized as a medical specialty since the 1990s;

by law, free access to hospitals for emergency care is provided for all persons, including the uninsured. Funding for the emergency system comes from multiple sources. Germany has two national telephone numbers for medical emergencies, 112 (the European Union, or EU, standard) and 19222; the country's dispatch centers are interconnected.

Insurance

Germany has a statutory health insurance system (SHI) with 292 competing "sickness funds" (insurers) as of 2004; those with high income can also choose private coverage and opt out of the SHI system. The SHI system is paid for through general tax revenues and an earmarked payroll tax paid by employers and employees. About 85 percent of the population is covered through the SHI scheme, with about 10 percent through private insurance and the remainder through programs for special categories of individuals, such as police and soldiers. The SHI benefit covers most services, including physician services, hospital care, prescription drugs, dental care, mental health care, preventive services, rehabilitation, and sick leave compensation; long-term care is covered under a separate and mandatory insurance program.

Since 2004, the SHI scheme has included copayments for medical services such as physician and dentist office visits for adults (age 18 and older), prescriptions, inpatient hospital care, and prescribed medical

aids. About 20 percent of those covered by one of the German health care programs purchase private insurance that provides amenities and cost sharing, and about 10 percent opt out of the SHI system and purchase private insurance instead. Out-of-pocket expenses are capped at 2 percent of income and at 1 percent for persons with low income or chronic illness; children are exempt from out-of-pocket expenses. Primary care is paid for on a fee-for-service basis, while hospital payments are handled through a combination of global budgets and case-based payments; hospital payments do not include physician costs. Patients are not required to register with a general practice physician, but since 2004, sickness funds have been required to offer a family physician care model to their members; some of these plans offer bonuses for complying with gatekeeping rules.

A 2004 study by the World Health Organization (WHO) found that 9 percent of the German population had substitutive voluntary health insurance (covering services that would otherwise be available from the state) and 9 percent either complementary voluntary health insurance (covering services not covered or not fully covered by the state) or supplementary health insurance (providing increased choice or faster access to services). A recent survey found that substitutive policyholders are most likely to be young and affluent working adults; only 1 percent of unemployed people had substitutive insurance. Substitutive insurance is also more common among people who grew up in the former West Germany (10.1 percent) as opposed to those who grew up in the former East Germany (3.6 percent). According to Ke Xu and colleagues, in 2003, fewer than 0.1 percent of households in Germany experienced catastrophic health expenditures annually; "catastrophic" was defined as exceeding 40 percent of household income remaining after basic needs were met.

Costs of Hospitalization

Most German hospitals are nonprofit, with about half of all hospital beds in public facilities and about one-third in private, nonprofit facilities. According to Organisation for Economic Co-operation and Development (OECD) data, in 2009, hospital spending per capita in Germany was $1,200 (adjusted for differences in the cost of living), and hospital spending per discharge came to $15,072 in 2011. The average length of stay in acute care was 7.5 days in 2008, and there were 237 hospital discharges per 1,000 population. In 2008, according to the OECD, hospital spending in Germany represented 29.4 percent of total spending on health; hospitals were paid based on global budgets and payment per case or diagnosis-related group (DRG).

Access to Health Care

According to WHO, in 2006, 100 percent of births were attended by skilled personnel (for example, physicians, nurses, or midwives). The 2010 immunization rates for 1-year-olds were 93 percent for diphtheria and pertussis (DPT3), 96 percent for measles (MCV), and 94 percent for Hib (Hib3). In 2009, according to OECD data, Germans had an average of 8.2 physician visits. In 2010, almost two-thirds (66 percent) reported that, when sick, they were able to get a medical appointment the same day or the next day. A somewhat lower proportion (57 percent) reported it was very or somewhat difficult to get medical care after usual office hours. For those who needed particular types of care, only 7 percent reported they waited two or more months to see a specialist (of those who needed to see a specialist in the prior two years), none reported waiting four or more months for elective surgery (of those who required elective surgery in the prior two years), but 25 percent reported they had experienced an access barrier due to cost in the previous two years; an access barrier was defined as failing to fill or refill a prescription, failing to visit a physician, or failing to get recommended care.

In 2010, one in 10 (10 percent) of German people reported experiencing a medical, medication, or lab test error in the previous two years, and 32 percent of those who needed to visit a specialist in the previous two years reported that the specialist did not have information about their medical history at the time of the appointment. More than three-fifths (61 percent) reported experiencing a gap in hospital discharge planning in the previous two years (due to any of the following: did not receive a written plan for care, did not have arrangements made for follow-up visits, did not know whom to contact with questions or did not receive instruction about when to seek further care).

A 2011 Commonwealth Fund Survey compared access to health care for "sicker adults" (those 18 and older in self-reported poor or fair health who had been treated for a serious illness or injury in the past year or been hospitalized in the past two years) in 11 OECD countries. This survey found that 22 percent of sicker Germans surveyed reported having experienced an access problem related to cost in the previous year; the most common result was failing to fill a prescription or skipping doses of a prescribed drug. Other problems reported include having serious problems paying their medical bills (6 percent), waiting six days or longer for needed care (23 percent, the highest proportion among the surveyed countries), having difficulty getting after-hours care except in an emergency room (40 percent), and experiencing coordination gaps in care (56 percent, the highest in the 11 countries surveyed).

Cost of Drugs

In 2009, according to OECD data, pharmaceutical spending per capita in Germany was $628 (adjusted for differences in the cost of living). While prescription drugs are covered under the SHI, since 2004, a copayment of 5 to 10 euros ($7 to $17) for prescriptions has been required, except for drugs whose price is 30 percent or more below the reference price (a category including more than 12,000 drugs as of 2010). The reference price is the maximum reimbursable amount for drugs determined to be of equivalent effectiveness to the drug in question.

According to Douglas Ball, Germany charged a 19 percent value-added tax (VAT) on medicines as of January 2007 and allowed a dispensing fee of 8.10 euros for prescription-only medicines. The wholesale markup for prescription-only medicines ranges from 6 to 15 percent of the ex-factory price (the manufacturer's list price before discounts), with a cap of 72 euros; for reimbursable over-the-counter medicines, the markup ranges from 3 to 21 percent of the ex-factory price, with a cap of 61.63 euros. The pharmacy markup for prescription-only medicines is 3 percent of the wholesale price; for reimbursable over-the counter medicines, it ranges from 8.26 to 68.00 percent of the wholesale price, with a cap of 118.24 euros.

Germany is the world's fourth-largest purchaser of pharmaceuticals, after the United States, Japan, and France; Germany accounts for 5 percent of global pharmaceutical sales. Real annual growth in pharmaceutical expenditures in Germany grew 3.7 percent from 1997 to 2005, much faster than the 1.9 percent growth of total health expenditure (minus pharmaceutical expenditure) over those years. According to Elizabeth Docteur, in 2004, generic drugs represented 23 percent of the market share by value and 41 percent of the market share by volume of the total pharmaceutical market.

Health Care Facilities

In 2008, Germany had 8.17 hospital beds per 1,000 population, the seventh-highest ratio in the world. In 2009, Germany had 9.5 magnetic resonance imaging (MRI) units per million population and 17.2 computer tomography (CT) scanners per million and conducted 17.3 MRI exams per 1,000 population; all are below OCED averages. In 2009, about three-quarters (72 percent) of primary care physicians in Germany used electronic medical records.

Major Health Issues

In 2008, WHO estimated that 5 percent of years of life lost in Germany were due to communicable diseases, 87 percent to noncommunicable diseases, and 8 percent to injuries. In 2008, the age-standardized estimate of cancer deaths was 156 per 100,000 for men and 99 per 100,000 for women; for cardiovascular disease and diabetes, 207 per 100,000 for men and 134 per 100,000 for women; and for chronic respiratory disease, 24 per 100,000 for men and 11 per 100,000 for women.

The maternal mortality rate (death from any cause related to or aggravated by pregnancy) in Germany in 2008 was seven maternal deaths per 100,000 live births, among the lowest in the world. The infant mortality rate, defined as the number of deaths of infants younger than 1 year, was 3.51 per 1,000 live births as of 2012, among the lowest in the world. In 2010, tuberculosis incidence was 4.8 per 100,000 population, tuberculosis prevalence 5.9 per 100,000, and deaths due to tuberculosis among human immunodeficiency virus (HIV)-negative people 0.25 per 100,000. As of 2009, an estimated 0.1 percent of adults age 15 to 49 were living with HIV or acquired immune deficiency syndrome (AIDS).

Health Care Personnel

Germany has 39 medical schools, several of which have been offering instruction since the 14th or 15th century. The duration of the basic degree course is 6 or 6.5 years, and another 1.5 years of practical training is also required. The degree awarded is the Staatsexamen und Arzt im Praktikum (state examination and completion of compulsory practical training). Physicians must register with the General Medical Council of the province in which they will practice. Foreigners from outside the European Union (EU) may be granted only a temporary license.

Selected Health Indicators: Germany Compared With the Organisation for Economic Co-operation and Development (OECD) Country Average

	Germany	OECD average (2010 or nearest year)
Male life expectancy at birth, 2010	78	77
Female life expectancy at birth, 2010	83	82.5
Total expenditure on health (percent of GDP), 2010	11.6	9.5
Total expenditure on health (per capita, USD purchasing power parity), 2010	4,338.4	3,265
Public expenditure on health (per capita, USD purchasing power parity), 2010	3,331	2,377.8
Public expenditure on health (percent total expenditure on health), 2010	76.8	72.2
Pharmaceutical expenditure (percent total expenditure on health), 2010	14.8	16.6
Pharmaceutical expenditure (per capita, USD purchasing power parity), 2010	640	495.4

Source: OECD Health Data 2012 (Organisation for Economic Co-operation and Development, 2012).

Germany, as a member of the EU, cooperates with other countries in recognizing physicians qualified to practice in other EU countries, as specified by Directive 2005/36/EC of the European Parliament. This allows qualified professionals to practice their profession in other EU states on a temporary basis and requires that the host country automatically recognize qualifications for certain professions, including physicians, nurses, dentists, midwives, and pharmacists, if certain conditions have been met (for instance, facility in the language of the host country may be required).

In 2008, Germany had 3.53 physicians per 1,000 population, 0.60 pharmaceutical personnel per 1,000, 0.77 dentistry personnel per 1,000, and 10.82 nurses and midwives per 1,000. In 2000, 3.5 percent of physicians practicing in Germany were trained abroad, primarily in other European countries.

Government Role in Health Care

According to WHO, in 2010, Germany spent $382 billion on health care, or $4,668 per capita. Health care funding was provided exclusively from domestic sources. Over three-fourths (77 percent) of health care funding was paid for through government expenditures, with the remainder provided through household spending (13 percent) and other sources (10 percent). In 2010, Germany allocated 19 percent of its total government expenditures to health, and government expenditures on health came to 9 percent of GDP; both place Germany in the high range compared to other high-income European countries.

Public Health Programs

The Robert Koch Institut (RKI), located in Berlin and headed by Reinhard Burger, is Germany's central institution for public health and the federal authority for prevention and control of disease. RKI is also responsible for analysis of diseases that have health-related political significance or that have a high prevalence in the country. RKI includes about 1,000 staff members divided into four departments: infectious disease, epidemiology and health reporting (focusing on noncommunicable disease), infectious disease epidemiology, and biological safety (including viral and bacterial toxins and pathogens). In 2005, a national plan was created to provide coordinated response for influenza outbreaks, and in 2008, the RKI completed the German Health Interview and Examination Survey for Children and Adolescents, gathering information from almost 18,000 adolescents and children.

The German Network for Antimicrobial Resistance Surveillance (GENARS) evaluates data on pathogens with antibiotic resistance and provides information to hospitals regarding antibiotic resistance.

In 2010, access to improved methods of sanitation and improved sources of drinking water was essentially universal in Germany. According to the World Higher Education Database (WHED), 11 universities in Germany offer programs in epidemiology or public health.

GHANA

Ghana is a west African nation, sharing borders with Côte d'Ivoire, Burkina Faso, and Togo and having a coastline on the Gulf of Guinea. The total area of 92,098 square miles (238,533 square kilometers) is similar to Oregon, and the July 2012 population was estimated at 25.3 million. In 2010, 51 percent of the population lived in urban areas, and the 2010 to 2015 annual rate of urbanization was estimated at 3.4 percent. The July 2012 population growth rate was 1.8 percent despite a negative net migration rate (negative 0.6 migrants per 1,000 population); the birth rate was 270 births per 1,000 population, and the total fertility rate was 3.4 children per woman. The United Nations High Commissioner for Refugees (UNHCR) estimated that, in 2010, there were 13,828 refugees and persons in refugee-like situations in Ghana.

A former British colony, in 1957, Ghana became the first sub-Saharan colony to become independent. The country suffered many coups, followed by single-party rule, until a new constitution was approved in 1992. According to the Ibrahim Index, in 2011, Ghana ranked seventh among 53 African countries in terms of governance performance, with a score of 66 (out of 100), and ranked tied for 69th among 183 countries on the *Corruption Perceptions Index 2011,* with a score of 3.9 (on a scale where 0 indicates highly corrupt and 10 very clean). In 2011, Ghana was classified as a country with medium human development (the second from the lowest of four categories) on the United Nations Development Programme's (UNDP's) Human Development Index (HDI), with a score of 0.541 (on a scale where 1 denotes high development and 0 low development). Life expectancy at birth in 2012 was estimated at 61.45 years, and the estimated

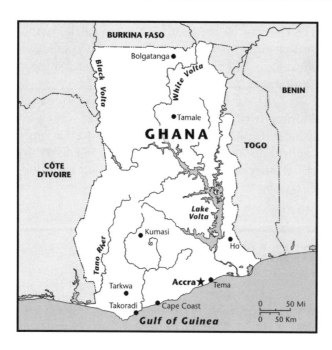

gross domestic product (GDP) per capita in 2011 was $3,100. In 2006, the Gini Index (a measure of dispersion, in which perfect equality is denoted by 0 and maximum inequality is denoted by 100) for family income was 39.4. According to the World Economic Forum's *Global Gender Gap Index 2011*, Ghana ranked 70th out of 135 countries on gender equality with a score of 0.681 (on a scale with a theoretical range of 1 for equality to 0 for inequality and an actual range in 2011 from 0.8530 to 0.4873).

Emergency Health Services

According to the World Health Organization (WHO), as of 2007, Ghana had a formal and publicly available emergency care (prehospital care) system accessible through a national universal access telephone number.

Insurance

According to the *2010 World Health Report* published by WHO, Ghana provided free medical care to its citizens following independence in 1957, with services financed through general taxation, but in the 1980s, Ghana introduced fees in the public market and allowed private insurance schemes; the result was that the use of health care services dropped, and those who required treatment often faced financial ruin becuase they had to pay high out-of-pocket costs. In 2004, Ghana introduced a National Health Insurance Scheme, and as

of 2009, over two-thirds (67.5 percent) of Ghanaian citizens were registered with it. This system resulted in lowered out-of-pocket payments and increased use of medical services (for example, outpatient visits increased from approximately 12 million to 18 million from 2005 to 2008). The national scheme is made up of separate mutual insurance schemes in each district, and so each composes a separate risk pool, a situation leading to fragmentation. Nonetheless, the system has greatly increased access to care and diminished the reliance on direct payment from those requiring care.

The system is funded by contributions from the employed (5.5 percent of earnings), the self-employed (18.5 percent of declared income), voluntary members (18.5 percent of declared income), informal sector employers (a flat-rate monthly contribution based on a means test), and employers (13 percent of payroll). The government covers the cost of benefits for children up to age 18 (if both parents contribute), the aged, and the poor. Medical benefits are provided through the National Health Insurance program. The Social Security and National Insurance Trust administers the program. According to Ke Xu and colleagues, in 2003, 1.3 percent of households in Ghana experienced catastrophic health expenditures annually; "catastrophic" was defined as exceeding 40 percent of household income remaining after basic needs were met.

Costs of Hospitalization

No data available.

Access to Health Care

A 2004 survey found that the government provided the most care in urban areas, amounting to about 60 percent of the total; the mission sector provided the most care in rural areas, amounting to the remaining 40 percent of care provided. Medicines were found to be unaffordable for a large proportion of the Ghanaian population, and medicines for chronic diseases less affordable than those for acute conditions. In the public sector, Ghana procured generic medicines at a median price ratio of 0.95 as compared to the international reference price, meaning that Ghana paid on average 5 percent below the international market price for these drugs. However, certain drugs were much more expensive: For instance, the median price ratio for albendazole was 9.27 (more than nine times the international reference price), and the median price ratio for the lowest-priced generic ciprofloxacin was 7.05. The median price ratio for the lowest-priced generic drugs was 2.43, with a range of 0.88 to 23.17. Prices for generics were much higher at private pharmacies, with the lowest-priced generic having a median price ratio of 4.12. Only three innovator brands were found in the public sector, and these were sold with median price ratios of 7.35 to 66.94. In the nongovernmental organization (NGO) sector, the median price ratio for procurement was 1.31 for the lowest-priced generic, and the median price ratio for the consumer price was 2.75.

According to WHO, in 2008, 58.7 percent of births were attended by skilled personnel (for example, physicians, nurses, or midwives). In 2008, 78 percent of pregnant women received at least four prenatal care visits. The 2010 immunization rates for 1-year-olds were 94 percent for diphtheria and pertussis (DPT3), 93 percent for measles (MCV), and 94 percent for Hib (Hib3). In 2010, an estimated 35 percent of persons with advanced human immunodeficiency virus (HIV) infection were receiving antiretroviral therapy in accordance with the 2010 WHO guidelines. According to WHO, in 2010, Ghana had 0.26 computer tomography (CT) machines per 1 million population, 0.09 telecolbalt units per 1 million, and 0.09 radiotherapy machines per 1 million.

Cost of Drugs

The Central Medical Store (CMS) of Ghana procures pharmaceuticals through competitive bidding with international firms and also through local supplies. The Regional Medical Stores (RMS) and teaching hospitals are expected to procure pharmaceuticals from the CMS and regional hospital and facilities from the RMS. However, a significant proportion of purchases are also made through the private sector. There is no effective pricing policy, and patients tend to pay more for drugs in remote areas than in the cities. Patients pay fees for most medicines, with the exception of some poor or vulnerable population groups, who are subsidized by the Ministry of Health.

According to WHO, in 2004, the median availability of selected generic drugs in the public sector in Ghana was 17.9 percent; in the private sector, the mean availability was 44.6 percent. The median price ratio (comparing the price in Ghana to the international reference price) was 2.4 in the public sphere for selected generic medicines and 3.8 in the private sphere, indicating that median prices in the public sphere were over twice as high and, in the private sphere, almost four times as high as the international reference prices.

Health Care Facilities

As of 2010, according to WHO, Ghana had 1.18 health posts per 100,000 population, 9.69 health centers per 100,000, 1.38 district or rural hospitals per 100,000, 0.03 provincial hospitals per 100,000, and 0.04 specialized hospitals per 100,000. In 2009, Ghana had 0.93 hospital beds per 1,000 population.

Major Health Issues

In 2008, WHO estimated that 66 percent of years of life lost in Ghana were due to communicable diseases, 25 percent to noncommunicable diseases, and 9 percent to injuries. In 2008, the age-standardized estimate of cancer deaths was 90 per 100,000 for men and 99 per 100,000 for women; for cardiovascular disease and diabetes, 427 per 100,000 for men and 344 per 100,000 for women; and for chronic respiratory disease, 126 per 100,000 for men and 55 per 100,000 for women.

In 2008, the age-standardized death rate from malaria was 31.8 per 100,000 population. In 2010, tuberculosis incidence was 86.0 per 100,000 population, tuberculosis prevalence 106.0 per 100,000, and deaths due to tuberculosis among HIV-negative people 8.70 per 100,000.

As of 2009, an estimated 1.8 percent of adults age 15 to 49 were living with HIV or acquired immune deficiency syndrome (AIDS). In 2010, 68 percent of pregnant women tested positive for HIV. The mother-to-child transmission rate for HIV in 2010 was estimated at 30 percent, and in 2009, 4.1 percent of deaths to children under age 5 were attributed to HIV. In 2010, almost 1.1 million cases of malaria were reported.

Ghana's maternal mortality rate (death from any cause related to or aggravated by pregnancy) is high by global standards, estimated at 350 maternal deaths per 100,000 live births as of 2008 data. A 2006 survey estimated the prevalence of female genital mutilation at 3.8 percent. The infant mortality rate, defined as the number of deaths of infants younger than 1 year, was estimated at 47.26 per 1,000 live births as of 2012 data. In 2008, 14.3 percent of children under age 5 were underweight (defined as 2 kilograms [kg] below standard weight-for-age at age 1, 3 kg below for ages 2 to 3, and 4 kg below for ages 4 to 5).

Health Care Personnel

In 2006, WHO identified Ghana as one of 57 countries with a critical deficit in the supply of skilled health workers. Ghana has two medical schools, the University of Ghana Medical School in Accra, which began offering instruction in 1963, and the School of Medical Sciences of the University of Science and Technology in Kumasi, which began offering instruction in 1975. A private university, St. Luke's School of Medicine, also operated an unaccredited medical school in Ghana for a few years beginning in 1999. The medical degree course requires six years to complete, and the degrees awarded are bachelor of medicine and bachelor of surgery. Graduates must complete a one-year internship before receiving a medical license. One year of government service is obligatory after graduation. Foreigners who graduated from foreign medical schools must complete a one-year internship in a recognized hospital. Ghana has an agreement with the United Kingdom (UK).

In 2009, Ghana had 0.09 physicians per 1,000 population, 0.07 pharmaceutical personnel per 1,000, 0.01 laboratory health workers per 1,000, 1.39 health management and support workers per 1,000, 0.01 dentistry personnel per 1,000, 0.19 community and traditional health workers per 1,000, and 10.82 nurses and midwives per 1,000. The global "brain drain" (international migration of skilled personnel) plays a role in the relative undersupply of medical personnel in Ghana: Michael Clemens and Bunilla Petterson estimate that 56 percent of Ghana-born physicians and 24 percent of Ghana-born nurses are working in one of nine developed countries, primarily in the United States and the UK.

Using Fitzhugh Mullan's methodology, Ghana has an emigration factor of 30.0, representing a high ratio of Ghanaian physicians working outside the country (in the United States, UK, Canada, or Australia) relative to those working in Ghana. Alok Bhargava and colleagues place Ghana 12th among countries most affected by the medical "brain drain" in 2004 and second among countries with populations of more than 4 million.

Government Role in Health Care

According to WHO, in 2010 Ghana spent $1.6 billion on health care, an amount that comes to $67 per capita. Health care funding was provided primarily (83 percent) from domestic sources, with the remaining 17 percent of funding provided by overseas sources. Over half (59 percent) of health care funding was paid for through government expenditures, with the remainder provided through household spending (27 percent) and other sources (14 percent). In 2010, Ghana allocated 12 percent of its total government expenditures to health, in the high range compared to other lower-middle-income African countries; government expenditures on health came to 3 percent of GDP; both place Ghana in the median range compared to other lower-middle-income African countries. In 2009, according to WHO, official development assistance (ODA) for health in Ghana came to $14.39 per capita.

Public Health Programs

The Ghana Health Service (GHS), located in Accra and headed by Dr. E. K. Sory, was created in 1996 as an executive agency responsible for implementing national strategies aimed at making the health care system more accessible, equitable, efficient, and responsive. Functions of the GHS include managing and administering health resources; promoting good health habits in the population; establishing mechanisms for the surveillance, prevention, and control of diseases; determining charges for health services; and providing continuous education.

The Noguchi Memorial Institute for Medical Research (NMIMR), located within the College of Health Sciences of the University of Ghana, was founded in 1979 and is a biomedical research institution with approximately 280 members. The focus of the NMIMR is infectious disease, and the staff is organized into nine departments: bacteriology, clinical pathology, electron microscopy, histopathology, epidemiology, immunology, nutrition, parasitology, and virology. The NMIMR conducts clinical trials and preclinical studies; provides technical assistance and training for efforts to fight diseases such as malaria, avian flu, lymphatic filiariasis, and guinea worm; and is also expanding research into noncommunicable diseases such as cancer and heart disease.

According to WHO, in 2008, Ghana had fewer than 0.01 environmental and public health workers per 1,000 population. In 2010, 14 percent of the population had access to improved sanitation facilities (8 percent in rural areas and 19 percent in urban), and 86 percent had access to improved sources of drinking water (80 percent in rural areas and 91 percent in urban). According to the World Higher Education Database (WHED), two universities in Ghana offer programs in epidemiology or public health: the Catholic University College of Ghana in Sunyani and the University of Ghana in Accra.

GREECE

Greece is a southern European country consisting of a mainland and many islands; it shares borders with Albania, Macedonia, Bulgaria, and Turkey and has an extensive (8,498-mile or 13,676-kilometer) coastline on the Mediterranean Sea. The area of 50,949 square miles (131,957 square kilometers) makes Greece slightly smaller than Alabama, and the July 2012 population was estimated at 10.8 million. In 2010, 61 percent of the population lived in urban areas, and the 2010 to 2015 annual rate of urbanization was estimated at 0.6 percent. The capital and largest city is Athens (with a 2009 population estimated at 3.3 million). The July 2012 population growth rate was less than 0.1 percent; the total birth rate was 1.39 children per woman, and the total fertility rate was 9.1 births per 1,000 population, both among the 20 lowest in the world.

Greece became independent from the Ottoman Empire in 1830. The country had a military coup in 1967 but held democratic elections and became a parliamentary republic in 1974. Greece ranked tied for 80th among 183 on the *Corruption Perceptions Index 2011*, with a score of 3.4 (on a scale where 0 indicates highly corrupt and 10 very clean). In 2011, Greece was classified as a country with very high human development (the highest of four categories) on the United Nations Development Programme's (UNDP's) Human Development Index (HDI), with a score of 0.861 (on a scale where 1 denotes high development and 0 low development). Life expectancy at birth in 2012 was estimated at 80.05 years, among the highest in the world, and per capita gross domestic product (GDP) in 2011 was estimated at $27,600. In 2005, the Gini Index (a measure of dispersion, in which perfect equality is denoted by 0 and maximum inequality is denoted by 100) for family income was 33.0.

In December 2011, the unemployment rate was 21.0 percent. However, a sovereign debt crisis from 2011 to 2012 severely increased unemployment and lowered standards of living for many Greek citizens, forcing reductions in government benefits. According to the World Economic Forum's *Global Gender Gap Index 2011*, Greece ranked 56th out of 135 countries on gender equality with a score of 0.692 (on a scale with a theoretical range of 1 for equality to 0 for inequality and an actual range in 2011 from 0.8530 to 0.4873).

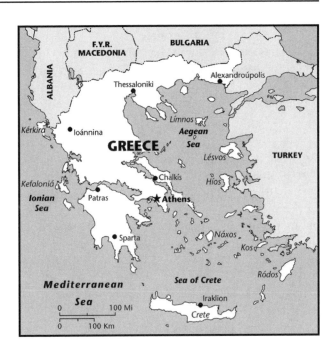

Emergency Health Services

Greek laws governing the emergency health system date from the 1980s; by law, free access to hospitals for emergency care is provided for all persons, including the uninsured. Funding for the emergency system comes entirely from the state budget for both inpatient and outpatient care.

Greece has only one national telephone number for medical emergencies, 166 (not 112, the European Union, or EU, standard); the country has 12 dispatch centers that are interconnected. Greek patients are entitled to use the emergency department of any public or privately contracted hospital, and charges for emergency department visits are low, so many use this method to access care in the hospital of their choice, even if their condition could be treated on an outpatient basis.

Doctors Without Borders (Médecins Sans Frontières, or MSF) began working in Greece in 2008 and had eight staff members in the country at the close of 2010. MSF provides psychological support to migrants and asylum seekers in detention centers; the June 2010 report *Migrants in Detention: Lives on Hold* documents the abuses MSF staff observed in these centers and the psychological effects on those held there. In December 2010, MSF began providing emergency medical care and humanitarian assistance to people held in detention centers; more than 850 patients were treated in December 2010.

Insurance

Greece has a social insurance system, as provided in the Social Security Law No. 1846 of 1951 and the National Health System Law No. 1397 of 1983; the 1983 system is called the ESY. The system covers people working in industry, commerce, and related occupations. Some urban self-employed people and some pensioners are covered for medical benefits. There are special systems for many classes of employees, including doctors and dentists, public-sector employees, agricultural workers, tradesmen, and craftsmen; persons covered by approved funds providing equivalent benefits to the national program are excluded from the national system. The system is funded by wage contributions (0.4 percent of covered monthly earnings for the cash benefit system and 2.15 percent for medical benefits), contributions from the self-employed (0.4 percent of covered monthly earnings for the cash benefit system and 2.15 percent for medical benefits), contributions from pensioners (4 percent of the monthly pension), and employer contributions (0.8 percent of covered monthly payroll for the cash benefit system and 4.30 percent for medical benefits); the government provides a guaranteed subsidy.

Medical benefits are provided directly to patients through the facilities of the Social Insurance Institute; covered benefits include hospitalization, general and specialist medical care, maternity care, medicine, dental care, appliances, and transportation. Cost sharing is required for some services, with a lower rate paid by pensioners. The maternity benefit is 50 percent of earnings plus a dependent's supplement for 56 days before and 63 days after childbirth. The sickness benefit is 50 percent of daily earnings, plus a dependent's supplement, with a maximum daily benefit. A birth grant (928.10 euros) is paid for each child, and a lump sum grant is paid for funerals (at least eight times earnings). The system is administered through the Social Insurance Institute with general supervision from the Ministry of Labor and Social Security.

A 2004 study by the World Health Organization (WHO) found none of the Greek population had substitutive voluntary health insurance (covering services that would otherwise be available from the state), and 10 percent had supplementary health insurance (providing increased choice or faster access to services). Holders of voluntary policies tend to be white-collar professionals living in urban areas and between the ages of 35 and 45. According to Ke Xu and colleagues, in 2003, 2.2 percent of households in Greece experienced catastrophic health expenditures annually; "catastrophic" was defined as exceeding 40 percent of household income remaining after basic needs were met.

Costs of Hospitalization

ESY hospitals have fixed budgets to cover capital investment and operational costs and are reimbursed for services delivered, a system that creates no incentive to improve efficiency. Physicians working in public hospitals and health centers are salaried.

Access to Health Care

Health is recognized as a social right in the Greek constitution, and citizens are entitled to health care through the ESY system, often through services provided based on occupational status and through payment of contributions to an insurance fund. Hospitals do not have a gatekeeping system, and patients may use any public or privately contracted hospital; demand is great for the best-equipped hospitals in Athens and for care at university hospitals, which sometimes results in waiting periods for university services. In rural areas, most health care is provided free of charge through a network of 201 health centers, and medical graduates are required to work for one year in a rural area after graduation. However, staffing is often inadequate in rural centers (for example, with approximately 50 percent of medical positions vacant). There is an oversupply of specialists relative to general practitioners throughout the country.

Much primary care is provided through local authorities and is free of charge; in Athens, these services are used primarily by the uninsured and by immigrants. There is also a public system of primary care paid for by out-of-pocket payments or private insurance payments; the private system includes about 400 private diagnostics centers and more than 25,000 private medical practices.

The 2010 immunization rates for 1-year-olds were 99 percent for diphtheria and pertussis (DPT3), 99 percent for measles (MCV), and 83 percent for Hib (Hib3).

Cost of Drugs

All prescription-only medicines are covered by social insurance in Greece, with patients paying a 25 percent copayment, which is lowered or waived for people with chronic conditions, low-income retirees, and the very poor. Prices for medicines (both branded and generic) are set by the government. Wholesale and pharmacy markups are both fixed by law: The wholesale markup is 8.43 percent of the ex-factory price (the manufacturer's list price before discounts), and for pharmacies, it is 35 percent of the wholesale price. There is no regulated dispensing fee.

Health Care Facilities

As of 2010, Greece had 132 public hospitals in the ESY system, including seven university hospitals and 23 specialized hospitals. In addition, 23 public hospitals operated outside the ESY system, including 14 military hospitals, and 218 private, for-profit hospitals also operated in the country. In 2008, Greece had 4.77 hospital beds per 1,000 population, among the 50 highest rates in the world. As of 2001, the average bed occupancy rate for acute care hospital beds was 75.1 percent. Average hospital length of stay declined from 10.2 days in 1980 to 5.6 days in 2005, and the hospital discharge rate was 18.8 per 100,000 population.

Major Health Issues

In 2008, WHO estimated that 5 percent of years of life lost in Greece were due to communicable diseases, 83 percent to noncommunicable diseases, and 12 percent to injuries. In 2008, the age-standardized estimate of cancer deaths was 167 per 100,000 for men and 87 per 100,000 for women; for cardiovascular disease and diabetes, 215 per 100,000 for men and 158 per 100,000 for women; and for chronic respiratory disease, 27 per 100,000 for men and 16 per 100,000 for women.

In 2010, tuberculosis incidence was 4.6 per 100,000 population, tuberculosis prevalence 5.7 per 100,000, and deaths due to tuberculosis among human immunodeficiency virus (HIV)-negative people 0.71 per 100,000. As of 2009, an estimated 0.1 percent of adults age 15 to 49 were living with HIV or acquired immune deficiency syndrome (AIDS). In 2003, an estimated 23.5 percent of adults in Greece were obese (defined as a body mass index, or BMI, of 30 or greater). The maternal mortality rate (death from any cause related to or aggravated by pregnancy) in Greece in 2008 was three maternal deaths per 100,000 live births, the lowest in the world. The infant mortality rate, defined as the number of deaths of infants younger than 1 year, was 4.92 per 1,000 live births as of 2012.

Health Care Personnel

Greece has seven medical schools, located in Athens, Alexandropoulos, Ioannina, Heraklion, Larissa, Patras, and Thessaloniki. The basic course of training requires six years, and the degree awarded is Ptychion iatrikis (diploma of medicine). One year of government service in a rural area is required after graduation. Greece, as a member of the EU, cooperates with other countries in recognizing physicians qualified to practice in other EU countries, as specified by Directive 2005/36/EC of the European Parliament. This allows qualified professionals to practice their profession in other EU states on a temporary basis and requires that the host country automatically recognize qualifications for certain professions, including physicians, nurses, dentists, midwives, and pharmacists, if certain conditions have been met (for instance, facility in the language of the host country may be required). In 2008, Greece had 6.04 physicians per 1,000 population, 0.88 pharmaceutical personnel per 1,000, 1.32 dentistry personnel per 1,000, and 3.66 nurses and midwives per 1,000.

Government Role in Health Care

According to WHO, in 2010, Greece spent $31 billion on health care, an amount that comes to $2,729 per capita. Health care funding was provided entirely from domestic sources. More than half (59 percent) of health care funding was paid for through government expenditures, with the remainder provided through household spending (38 percent) and other sources (2 percent). In 2010, Greece allocated 12 percent of its total government expenditures to health, placing Greece in the low range compared to other high-income European countries; government expenditures on health came to 6 percent of GDP, placing Greece in the median range compared to other high-income European countries.

Public Health Programs

Public health services are organized at the national level by the Directorate General for Public Health in the Ministry of Health and Social Solidarity; specific charges of the directorate include epidemiological monitoring, public health risk management, maternal and child health, control of sexually transmitted diseases (STDs), workplace health and safety, sourcing and quality control of vaccines, and school health. The Directorate for Environmental Health is responsible for water treatment and waste disposal, sanitation in health care and housing units, air pollution, radioactivity, and regulation. In 2010, access to improved sanitary facilities was close to universal in Greece (98 percent overall with 97 percent in rural areas and 99 percent in urban), and access to improved supplies of drinking water was essentially universal. According to the World Higher Education Database (WHED), two universities in Greece offer programs in epidemiology or public health: the Technological Educational Institute of Athens and the Technological Educational Institute of Larissa.

GRENADA

Grenada is an island nation in the Caribbean Sea, consisting of one large island (Grenada) and numerous smaller islands (the Grenadines). The area of 133 square miles (344 square kilometers) is about twice the size of Washington, D.C., and makes Grenada one of the smallest countries in the Western hemisphere; the July 2012 population was estimated at 109,011. In 2010, 39 percent of the population lived in urban areas, and the 2010 to 2015 annual rate of urbanization was estimated at 1.6 percent. St. George's is the capital and largest city (with a 2009 population estimated at 40,000). The July 2012 population growth rate was 0.5 percent due in part to a high emigration rate (net migration of negative 3.4 migrants per 1,000 population), a moderate birth rate (16.8 births per 1,000 population), and a total fertility rate of 2.1 children per woman.

Grenada was a French then a British colony; it was granted autonomy in 1967 and full independence in 1974. Grenada was seized by a Marxist military council in 1983, but the island was invaded by armed forces from the United States and other Caribbean countries, and free elections were reinstated. Grenada was severely damaged in 2004 by Hurricane Ivan. In 2011, Grenada was classified as a country with high human development (the second-highest category) on the United Nations Development Programme's (UNDP's) Human Development Index (HDI), with a score of 0.748 (on a scale where 1 denotes high development and 0 low development). Life expectancy at birth in 2012 was estimated at 73.50 years, and per capita gross domestic product (GDP) in 2011 was estimated at $13,300. Unemployment in 2008 was estimated at 25.0 percent.

Emergency Health Services

Emergency health services are provided mainly through public facilities, and 24-hour accident and emergency care is provided through the General Hospital in Roseau. From 2003 to 2005, 76,133 people were seen at the General Hospital's accident and emergency department, of whom 20,977 were admitted to the hospital.

Insurance

Grenada has a social insurance system covering the employed and self-employed from ages 16 to 59; only cash benefits are provided, and there are no statutory medical benefits. The system is funded through contributions from the employed (4 percent of covered earnings), the self-employed (9 percent of monthly covered earnings), and employers (5 percent of covered payroll); for all three, there is a ceiling of XCD 3,500 on monthly earnings used to calculate contributions. The maternity benefit is 65 percent of average covered earnings for six weeks before and after birth, with employers making an additional contribution (40 percent of average covered earnings) for the first two months of leave. The sickness benefit is 65 percent of average covered earnings for up to 26 weeks and for up to 52 weeks if the person has made at least 75 weeks of contributions into the system in the last three years. The system also covers funeral grants (XCD 2,320 for the insured, XCD 1,740 for the insured's spouse, and XCD for the insured's child).

Costs of Hospitalization

No data is available.

Access to Health Care

Grenada is divided into seven health districts, six of which have health centers; 30 medical stations are located throughout the country so that every person lives no more than 3 miles from a health facility. According to the World Health Organization (WHO), in 2007, 99 percent of births were attended by skilled personnel (for example, physicians, nurses, or midwives). The 2010 immunization rates for 1-year-olds were 97 percent for diphtheria and pertussis (DPT3), 95 percent for measles (MCV), and 97 percent for Hib (Hib3). According to WHO, in 2010, Grenada had 09.66 magnetic resonance imaging (MRI) machines per 1 million population and 19.32 computer tomography (CT) machines per 1 million. All high-technology medical equipment for the public sector is located at the General Hospital in Roseau, while the private sector also provides some laboratory and other technical services; CT scans are available only through the private sector.

Cost of Drugs

Health supplies, including drugs, are obtained by the Procurement Unit; about 85 percent of drugs used in the public health sector are obtained through the Regional Organization of Eastern Caribbean States Pharmaceutical Procurement Services. Grenada's national formulary is based on a regional formulary that is updated every 18 months.

Health Care Facilities

The General Hospital in St. George's is Grenada's main hospital and oversees the operations of the Princess Alice Hospital in St. Andrews, Princess Royal Hospital in Carriacou, the Mt. Gay Psychiatric Hospital, and the Richmond Home (a geriatric facility). Patients must have a referral from a physician or a district medical officer to be admitted to one of the hospitals. Grenada also has a Community Health Service providing care through six district health centers and 30 medical stations spread across the country. As of 2010, according to WHO, Grenada had 34.45 health posts per 100,000 population, 4.79 health centers per 100,000, and 0.96 district or rural hospitals per 100,000.

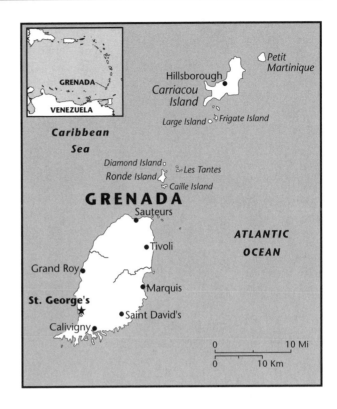

Major Health Issues

In 2008, WHO estimated that 17 percent of years of life lost in Grenada were due to communicable diseases, 70 percent to noncommunicable diseases, and 13 percent to injuries. In 2008, the age-standardized estimate of cancer deaths was 215 per 100,000 for men and 111 per 100,000 for women; for cardiovascular disease and diabetes, 346 per 100,000 for men and 253 per 100,000 for women; and for chronic respiratory disease, 29 per 100,000 for men and 9 per 100,000 for women. The infant mortality rate, defined as the number of deaths of infants younger than 1 year, was 11.12 per 1,000 live births as of 2012. No information is available from WHO on the maternal mortality rate in Grenada. In 2010, tuberculosis incidence was 4.1 per 100,000 population, tuberculosis prevalence 4.1 per 100,000, and deaths due to tuberculosis among human immunodeficiency virus (HIV)-negative people 0.33 per 100,000.

Health Care Personnel

Grenada has one medical school, St. George's University School of Medicine. The basic medical degree requires 4.5 years (11 terms) to complete, and the fifth and sixth study terms are spent at Kingstown Medical College in Saint Vincent and the Grenadines. Students

supported by government grants must complete three years of government service after graduation. Physicians must register with the Medical Registration Board of the Ministry of Health, and medical licenses are granted to graduates holding degrees from St. George's University School of Medicine or the equivalent. Grenada has agreements with British Commonwealth countries, eastern Caribbean countries, and the United States.

In 1998, Grenada had 0.98 physicians per 1,000 population, 0.84 pharmaceutical personnel per 1,000, 0.24 dentistry personnel per 1,000, 0.49 community and traditional health workers per 1,000, and 3.98 nurses and midwives per 1,000. Despite the location of a medical school on Grenada, the country has a relative undersupply of physicians because most of the students are foreigners who do not stay to practice in Grenada. Almost 70 percent are U.S. citizens, and an additional 17 percent are U.S. permanent residents. The non-U.S. citizens enrolled come primarily from Trinidad and Tobago (more than 70 percent) with about 12 percent from Grenada. Alok Bhargava and colleagues placed Grenada second among countries most affected by medical "brain drain" (international migration of skilled personnel) in 2004.

Government Role in Health Care

According to WHO, in 2010, Grenada spent $46 million on health care, an amount that comes to $439 per capita. Health care funding was provided almost entirely (94 percent) from domestic sources, with the remaining 6 percent coming from overseas sources. More than half (54 percent) of health care funding was paid for through expenditures by households, with the remainder provided through government spending (45 percent) and other sources (1 percent). In 2010, Grenada allocated 8 percent of its total government expenditures to health, and government expenditures on health came to 3 percent of GDP; both figures place Grenada in the low range as compared with other upper-middle-income countries in the Americas region.

Public Health Programs

The Environment Health Department of Grenada is responsible for vector control, food safety, disease surveillance, water quality and waste management, hazardous materials, and public education. St. George's University offers a master's of public health (MPH) program of which about 70 percent of the students are U.S. citizens and another 20 percent U.S. permanent residents. According to WHO, in 2003, Grenada had 0.19 environmental and public health workers per 1,000 population. In 2010, 97 percent of the population of Grenada had access to improved sanitation facilities (77 percent in rural areas and 96 percent in urban), and 97 percent of the urban population had access to improved sources of drinking water (no information is available on rural areas).

GUATEMALA

Guatemala is a Central American country, sharing borders with Mexico, Belize, Honduras, and El Salvador and having coastlines on the north Pacific Ocean and the Caribbean Sea. The area of 42,042 square miles (108,889 square kilometers) makes Guatemala similar in size to Tennessee, and the July 2012 population was estimated at 14.1 million. In 2010, 49 percent of the population lived in urban areas, and the 2010 to 2015 annual rate of urbanization was estimated at 3.4 percent. Guatemala City is the capital and the largest (with a 2009 population estimated at 1.1 million).

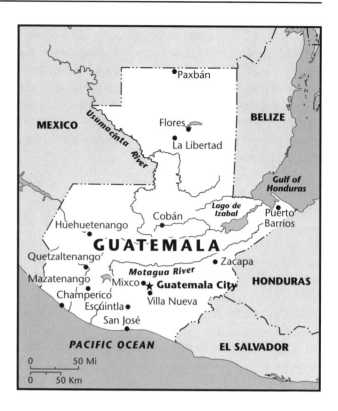

Population growth in 2012 was 1.9 percent despite a negative net migration rate (negative 2.1 migrants per 1,000 population); the birth rate was 26.5 births per 1,000 population, and the total fertility rate was 3.2 children per woman. The United Nations High Commissioner for Refugees (UNHCR) estimated that, in 2010, there were seven refugees and persons in refugee-like situations in Guatemala.

Guatemala achieved independence from Spain in 1821. In the second half of the 20th century, it suffered through a guerrilla war and a succession of military governments; the conflicts were formally concluded in 1996. Guatemala ranked tied for 120th among 183 countries in terms of perceived public-sector corruption on the *Corruption Perceptions Index 2011,* with a score of 2.7 (on a scale where 0 indicates highly corrupt and 10 very clean). In 2011, Guatemala was classified as a country with medium human development (the second from the lowest of four categories) on the United Nations Development Programme's (UNDP's) Human Development Index (HDI), with a score of 0.574 (on a scale where 1 denotes high development and 0 low development). Life expectancy at birth in 2012 was estimated at 71.17 years, and estimated gross domestic product (GDP) per capita in 2011 was $5,000. Income distribution in Guatemala is relatively unequal: In 2007, the Gini Index (a measure of dispersion, in which perfect equality is denoted by 0 and maximum inequality is denoted by 100) for family income was 55.1, among the highest in the world. According to the World Economic Forum's *Global Gender Gap Index 2011*, Guatemala ranked 112th out of 135 countries on gender equality, with a score of 0.623 (on a scale with a theoretical range of 1 for equality to 0 for inequality and an actual range in 2011 from 0.8530 to 0.4873).

Emergency Health Services

According to the World Health Organization (WHO), as of 2007, Guatemala did not have a formal and publicly available system for providing prehospital care (emergency care). Doctors Without Borders (Médecins Sans Frontières, or MSF) began working in Guatemala in 1984 and had 39 staff members in the country at the close of 2010. MSF's primary focus in Guatemala is caring for victims of sexual violence, including treatment to reduce the risk of human immunodeficiency virus (HIV) infection, psychological care, medical care, and assistance from a social worker; more than 870 new patients were treated in 2010. MSF also provided emergency care after the volcanic eruption and tropical storm in May 2010.

Insurance

Guatemala has a social insurance system covering employees of companies with at least three workers and transport enterprises with at least one worker. The self-employed and elected officials are not included. The system is funded by wage contributions (2 percent of gross earnings), employer contributions (4 percent of gross payroll), and government contributions (1 percent of gross payroll). Medical services are provided directly to patients through the facilities of the Social Security Institute; covered services include hospitalization; general, specialist, and maternity care; lab services; medicine; X-rays; rehabilitation and retraining; appliances; and transportation. Emergency medical services are provided to the uninsured for free. Coverage for dependents varies by region, but in most of the country, the wife or partner of an insured man receives the same benefits as an insured woman. The maternity benefit is 100 percent of earnings 30 days before and 54 days after the due date. The cash sickness benefit is 66.7 percent of earnings and is paid for 26 weeks, with extensions possible to 39 weeks. The program is administered through the Social Security Institute with general supervision from the Ministry of Labor and Social Welfare.

Costs of Hospitalization

No data available.

Access to Health Care

Health is recognized as a fundamental right in the constitution, and the country is moving toward a system to provide integrated health care to everyone. Beginning in 2005, free basic health services have been provided to the Guatemala's poorest citizens. However, according to Latinobarometer, an annual public opinion survey conducted in Latin America, 39 percent of citizens in Guatemala are satisfied with the level of health care available to them (the regional average is 51.9 percent). According to WHO, in 2009, 51.3 percent of births in Guatemala were attended by skilled personnel (for example, physicians, nurses, or midwives). The 2010 immunization rates for 1-year-olds were 94 percent for diphtheria and pertussis (DPT3), 93 percent for measles (MCV), and 94 percent for Hib (Hib3). In 2010, an estimated 53 percent of persons with advanced human immunodeficiency virus (HIV) infection were receiving antiretroviral therapy in accordance with the 2010 WHO guidelines.

Cost of Drugs

Pharmaceuticals in Guatemala are sold through a pharmacy network including both public and private outlets, and drugs are manufactured in 85 national and two foreign laboratories. In 1997, the Ministry of Public Health and Social Welfare, the Guatemalan Social Security Institute, and the Military Medical Center created a system to negotiate drug prices. In 1999, the Ministry of Public Health and Social Welfare spent $17.7 million on drugs, the Guatemalan Social Security Institute $24.0 million, and the private sector $129.8 million.

Health Care Facilities

In 1999, Guatemala's Ministry of Public Health and Social Welfare operated more than 1,000 public health establishments, including 43 hospitals, and the Guatemalan Social Security Institute operated an additional 24 hospitals as well as 30 consultation offices and 18 primary care posts. As of 2010, according to WHO, Guatemala had 3.81 health posts per 100,000 population, 0.54 health centers per 100,000, 0.30 district or rural hospitals per 100,000, 0.03 provincial hospitals per 100,000, and 0.03 specialized hospitals per 100,000. In 2009, Guatemala had 0.60 hospital beds per 1,000 population, one of the 30 lowest rates in the world.

Major Health Issues

In 2008, WHO estimated that 45 percent of years of life lost in Guatemala were due to communicable diseases, 31 percent to noncommunicable diseases, and 24 percent to injuries. In 2008, the age-standardized estimate of cancer deaths was 110 per 100,000 for men and 119 per 100,000 for women; for cardiovascular disease and diabetes, 189 per 100,000 for men and 190 per 100,000 for women; and for chronic respiratory disease, 23 per 100,000 for men and 18 per 100,000 for women.

In 2008, the age-standardized death rate from malaria was 0.1 per 100,000 population. In 2010, tuberculosis incidence was 62.0 per 100,000 population, tuberculosis prevalence 111.0 per 100,000, and deaths due to tuberculosis among HIV-negative people 3.90 per 100,000. As of 2009, an estimated 0.8 percent of adults age 15 to 49 were living with HIV or acquired immune deficiency syndrome (AIDS). The maternal mortality rate (death from any cause related to or aggravated by pregnancy) in Guatemala in 2008 was 110 maternal deaths per 100,000 live births. The infant mortality rate, defined as the number of deaths of infants younger than 1 year, was estimated at 25.16 per 1,000 live births as of 2012. In 2002, 17.7 percent of children under age 5 were underweight (defined as

2 kilograms [kg] below standard weight-for-age at age 1, 3 kg below for ages 2 to 3, and 4 kg below for ages 4 to 5).

Health Care Personnel

Guatemala has two medical schools, the Facultad de Ciencias Medicas of the University of San Carlos (which began offering instruction in 1676) and the Facultad de Medicins of the Universidad Francisco Marroquin (which began offering instruction in 1978). Both are located in Guatemala City. The basic degree course requires six to seven years to complete and the degree awarded is Médico y Cirujano (physician and surgeon). In 1999, Guatemala had 0.90 physicians per 1,000 population, 0.18 dentistry personnel per 1,000, and 4.05 nurses and midwives per 1,000.

Government Role in Health Care

According to WHO, in 2010, Guatemala spent $2.8 billion on health care, an amount that comes to $196 per capita. Health care funding was provided almost entirely (98 percent) from domestic sources, with the remaining 2 percent coming from overseas sources. More than half (54 percent) of health care funding was paid for through expenditures by households, with the remainder provided through government spending (36 percent) and other sources (10 percent). In 2010, Guatemala allocated 16 percent of its total government expenditures to health, placing it in the high range

Selected Health Indicators: Guatemala Compared With the Global Average (2010)

	Guatemala	Global Average
Male life expectancy at birth* (years)	66	66
Female life expectancy at birth* (years)	73	71
Under-5 mortality rate, both sexes (per 1,000 live births)	32	57
Adult mortality rate, both sexes* (probability of dying between 15 and 60 years per 1,000 population)	214	176
Maternal mortality ratio (per 100,000 live births)	120	210
HIV prevalence* (per 1,000 adults aged 15 to 49)	8	8
Tuberculosis prevalence (per 100,000 population)	111	178

Source: World Health Organization Global Health Observatory Data Repository.
*Data refers to 2009.

among lower-middle-income countries in the Americas region; government expenditures on health came to 3 percent of GDP, placing Guatemala in the low range as compared with other lower-middle-income countries in the Americas region. In 2009, according to WHO, official development assistance (ODA) for health in Guatemala came to $3.44 per capita.

Public Health Programs

In 2010, 78 percent of the population of Guatemala had access to improved sanitation facilities (70 percent in rural areas and 87 percent in urban), and 92 percent had access to improved sources of drinking water (87 percent in rural areas and 98 percent in urban areas). According to the World Higher Education Database (WHED), no university in Guatemala offers programs in epidemiology or public health.

GUINEA

Guinea is a west African country sharing borders with Guinea-Bissau, Senegal, Mali, Côte d'Ivoire, Liberia, and Sierra Leone and having a coastline on the north Atlantic. The area of 94,926 square miles (245,857 square kilometers) makes Guinea similar in size to Oregon, and the July 2012 population was estimated at 10.9 million. In 2010, 35 percent of the population lived in urban areas, and the 2010 to 2015 annual rate of urbanization was estimated at 4.3 percent. Conakry is the capital and largest city (with a 2009 population estimated at 1.6 million). The July 2012 population growth rate was 2.6 percent (the 21st-highest in the world); the birth rate was 36.6 births per 1,000 population (the 26th-highest), the net migration rate 0.0 migrants per 1,000, and the total fertility rate 5.0 children per woman (the 17th-highest in the world). The United Nations High Commissioner for Refugees (UNHCR) estimates that, in 2010, there were 14,113 refugees and persons in refugee-like situations in Guinea.

Guinea became independent from France in 1958 and has had a history of authoritarian rule since then, although free and fair elections were held in 2010. According to the Ibrahim Index, in 2011, Guinea ranked 43rd among 53 African countries in terms of governance performance, with a score of 38 (out of 100). Guinea's government is perceived as corrupt, 164th among 183 countries on the *Corruption Perceptions Index 2011*,

with a score of 2.1 (on a scale where 0 indicates highly corrupt and 10 very clean). In 2011, Guinea was classified as a country with low human development (the lowest of four categories) on the United Nations Development Programme's (UNDP's) Human Development Index (HDI), with a score of 0.344 (on a scale where 1 denotes high development and 0 low development), the 10th-lowest in the world. Life expectancy at birth in 2012 was estimated at 58.61 years, and estimated gross domestic product (GDP) per capita in 2011 was $1,100, among the 20 lowest in the world. In 2007, the Gini Index (a measure of dispersion, in which perfect equality is denoted by 0 and maximum inequality is denoted by 100) for family income was 39.4.

Emergency Health Services

Doctors Without Borders (Médecins Sans Frontières, or MSF) began working in Guinea in 1984 and had 213 staff members in the country at the close of 2010. MSF efforts are focused on providing pediatric care and treatment for human immunodeficiency virus and acquired immune deficiency syndrome (HIV/AIDS) and malaria in Conakry (the national capital) and Guéckédou (in southeastern Guinea).

Insurance

Guinea has a social insurance system covering employed persons; maternity benefits are provided under the Family Allowances system. The social insurance system is financed through wage contributions (2.5 percent of covered earnings) and employer payroll contributions (4 percent of covered payroll). Medical benefits are provided through hospitals, physicians, and pharmacists paid by the National Social Security Fund. Cost sharing is required for medicine (30 percent), but care for some diseases is covered 100 percent (tuberculosis, tetanus, cancer, cholera, and smallpox). The insured's spouse and children under age 17 are also covered (children to age 21 if disabled or a student). The maternity benefit is 100 percent of earnings for six weeks before and eight weeks after birth (10 weeks after for multiple births and 12 weeks after if there are complications). The cash sickness benefit is 100 percent for 26 weeks (52 weeks if the insured has at least one full year of employment). According to Guinea's *Pharmaceutical Sector Country Profile* (published by the World Health Organization [WHO]), in 2010, about 5 percent of the population of Guinea was covered by public health insurance and 0.4 percent by private health insurance.

Costs of Hospitalization
No data available.

Access to Health Care
According to WHO, in 2007, 46.1 percent of births were attended by skilled personnel (for example, physicians, nurses, or midwives). In 2007, 50 percent of pregnant women received at least four prenatal care visits. The 2010 immunization rates for 1-year-olds were 57 percent for diphtheria and pertussis (DPT3), 51 percent for measles (MCV), and 57 percent for Hib (Hib3). In 2010, an estimated 57 percent of persons with advanced HIV infection were receiving antiretroviral therapy in accordance with the 2010 WHO guidelines.

Cost of Drugs
In 2010, total pharmaceutical expenditures in Guinea were GNF 227.8 billion ($460.3 million) and per capita pharmaceutical expenditures GNF 20,782 ($3). Pharmaceutical expenditures totaled 19 percent of total health expenditures. Medicines are provided free of charge for certain population groups, including pregnant women, children under the age of 5, and the poor. Medicines to treat certain conditions are also provided for free, including malaria, tuberculosis, HIV/AIDS, and leprosy. Vaccines on WHO's Expanded Programme on Immunization (EPI) list are provided free, as are kits for cesarean deliveries, ivermectin (an

antiparasitic), Vitamin A, and mebendazole (an anthelmintic). Drugs are partially covered under both private and public insurance schemes; in the former, reimbursement ranges from 70 to 100 percent.

Health Care Facilities
As of 2010, according to WHO, Guinea had 7.34 health posts per 100,000 population, 4.15 health centers per 100,000, 0.31 district or rural hospitals per 100,000, 0.10 provincial hospitals per 100,000, and 0.03 specialized hospitals per 100,000. In 2005, Guinea had 0.31 hospital beds per 1,000 population, one of the 10 lowest rates in the world.

Major Health Issues
In 2008, WHO estimated that 73 percent of years of life lost in Guinea were due to communicable diseases, 19 percent to noncommunicable diseases, and 8 percent to injuries. In 2008, the age-standardized estimate of cancer deaths was 98 per 100,000 for men and 106 per 100,000 for women; for cardiovascular disease and diabetes, 544 per 100,000 for men and 495 per 100,000 for women; and for chronic respiratory disease, 154 per 100,000 for men and 79 per 100,000 for women.

In 2008, the age-standardized death rate from malaria was 90.4 per 100,000 population, the ninth-highest in the world. Rates of other vector-borne diseases, including yellow fever, also remain high, as are infectious diseases such as Lassa fever, schistosomiasis, meningococcal meningitis, cholera, and measles. In 2010, tuberculosis incidence was 334.0 per 100,000 population, tuberculosis prevalence 525.0 per 100,000, and deaths due to tuberculosis among HIV-negative people 59.0 per 100,000. As of 2009, an estimated 1.3 percent of adults age 15 to 49 were living with HIV or AIDS. As of December 2010, an estimated 66 percent of adults and 14 percent of children who needed antiretroviral therapy were receiving it. In 2008, the age-standardized death rate from childhood-cluster diseases (pertussis, polio, diphtheria, measles, and tetanus) was 20.9 per 100,000 population, the sixth-highest in the world.

Guinea's maternal mortality rate (death from any cause related to or aggravated by pregnancy) is quite high by global standards, estimated at 680 maternal deaths per 100,000 live births as of 2008. A 2005 survey estimated the prevalence of female genital mutilation at 95.6 percent. The infant mortality rate, defined as the number of deaths of infants younger than 1 year, also has been high, at 59.04 per 1,000 live births as of 2012. In 2008, 20.8 percent of children under age 5 were underweight (defined as 2 kilograms [kg] below standard weight-for-age at age 1, 3 kg below for ages 2 to 3, and 4 kg below for ages 4 to 5).

Health Care Personnel

In 2006, WHO identified Guinea as one of 57 countries with a critical deficit in the supply of skilled health workers. Guinea has one medical school, the Faculte de Medecine, Pharmacie et Odonto-Stomatologie of the University of Conakry, which began offering instruction in 1967. The basic medical training course lasts eight years, and the degree awarded is Docteur en Médecine (doctor of medicine). In 2005, Guinea had 0.10 physicians per 1,000 population, 0.02 dentistry personnel per 1,000, 0.03 laboratory health workers per 1,000, 0.05 health management and support workers per 1,000, 0.02 community and traditional health workers per 1,000, and 0.04 nurses and midwives per 1,000. The global "brain drain" (international migration of skilled personnel) is a minor factor in the supply of health care services in Guinea: Michael Clemens and Bunilla Petterson estimate that 11 percent of Guinea-born physicians and 6 percent of Guinea-born nurses are working in one of nine developed countries, primarily in France (physicians) and the United States (nurses).

Government Role in Health Care

The right to health, including access to essential medicines and medical technologies, is recognized in Guinea's 2009 constitution. Guinea has a National Health Policy (NHP), written in 1997, a plan to implement it, written in 2004, and a National Medicines Policy (NMP), written in 2007, that includes selection of essential medicines; financing, pricing, purchase, distribution, and regulation of drugs; rational usage of medicines; human resource development; research; and traditional medicine.

According to WHO, in 2010, Guinea spent $230 million on health care, an amount that comes to $23 per capita. Health care funding was provided primarily (89 percent) from domestic sources, with the remaining 11 percent coming from overseas sources. Almost all (88 percent) of health care funding was paid for through expenditures by households, with the remainder provided through government spending (11 percent) and other sources (1 percent). In 2010, Guinea allocated 2 percent of its total government expenditures to health, and government expenditures

on health came to 1 percent of GDP; both figures place Guinea in the low range as compared with other low-income African countries. In 2009, according to WHO, official development assistance (ODA) for health in Guinea came to $3.29 per capita.

Public Health Programs

The National Institute of Public Health Guinea (INSP), located in Conakry and headed by Dr. Lamine Koivogui, has 45 staff members working in the National Public Health Lab, the Community Health Department, and the Chemical and Pharmaceutical Department. The INSP concentrates on tropical infectious diseases, including malaria and cholera, and intends to begin a program of epidemiologic surveillance in the future. In 2010, the INSP completed the first phase of a program of malaria surveillance and research in conjunction with the London School of Hygiene and Tropical Medicine, and the microbiology lab within INSP was involved in the early diagnosis of cholera, shigella, and yellow fever, allowing preventive actions to prevent epidemic outbreaks.

According to WHO, in 2005, Guinea had 0.01 environmental and public health workers per 1,000 population. In 2010, 18 percent of the population had access to improved sanitation facilities (11 percent in rural areas and 32 percent in urban), and 74 percent had access to improved sources of drinking water (65 percent in rural areas and 90 percent in urban).

According to the World Higher Education Database (WHED), one university in Guinea offers programs in epidemiology or public health: Gamal Abdel Nasser University of Conakry.

GUINEA-BISSAU

Guinea-Bissau is a west African country, sharing borders with Senegal and Guinea and having a coastline on the north Atlantic Ocean; it consists of a mainland portion and many islands. The area of 13,948 square miles (36,125 square kilometers) makes Guinea-Bissau about three times the size of Connecticut; the July 2012 population was estimated at 1.6 million. In 2010, 30 percent of the population lived in urban areas, and the 2010 to 2015 annual rate of urbanization was estimated at 3.0 percent. Bissau is the capital and largest city (with an estimated 2009 population of 302,000). The July 2012 population growth rate was 2.0 percent; the birth rate was 34.7 births per 1,000 population (the 34th-highest in the world), the net migration rate 0.0 migrants per 1,000, and the total fertility rate 4.4 children per woman (the 31st-highest in the world). The United Nations High Commissioner for Refugees (UNHCR) estimated that, in 2010, there were 7,679 refugees and persons in refugee-like situations in Guinea-Bissau.

According to the Ibrahim Index, in 2011, Guinea-Bissau ranked 44th among 53 African countries in terms of governance performance, with a score of 37 (out of 100). Guinea-Bissau ranked tied for 152nd among 183 countries on the *Corruption Perceptions Index 2011,* with a score of 2.2 (on a scale where 0 indicates highly corrupt and 10 very clean). A military coup in April 2012 caused disruption in an already weak system for delivering human services. In 2011, Guinea-Bissau was classified as a country with low human development (the lowest of four categories) on the United Nations Development Programme's (UNDP's) Human Development Index (HDI), with a score of 0.353 (on a scale where 1 denotes high development and 0 low development). Life expectancy at birth in 2012 was estimated at 49.1 years, among the five lowest rates in the world, and estimated gross domestic product (GDP) per capita in 2011 was $1,100, among the 20 lowest in the world.

Emergency Health Services

According to the World Health Organization (WHO), as of 2007, Guinea-Bissau had a formal and publicly available emergency care (prehospital care) system accessible through a national universal access telephone number.

Insurance

No data available.

Costs of Hospitalization

No data available.

Access to Health Care

According to WHO, in 2006, 39 percent of births were attended by skilled personnel (for example, physicians, nurses, or midwives). The 2010 immunization rates for 1-year-olds were 76 percent for diphtheria and pertussis (DPT3), 71 percent for measles (MCV), and 76 percent for Hib (Hib3). In 2010, an estimated 48 percent of persons with advanced human immunodeficiency virus (HIV) infection were receiving

antiretroviral therapy in accordance with the 2010 WHO guidelines.

Cost of Drugs

Medications in Guinea-Bissau are provided free to pregnant women and children under the age of 5. Medicines are provided free to treat tuberculosis and human immunodeficiency virus and acquired immune deficiency syndrome (HIV/AIDS), and some antimalarial drugs are free. All vaccinations on WHO's Expanded Programme on Immunization (EPI) list are provided free.

Health Care Facilities

As of 2010, according to WHO, Guinea-Bissau had 6.34 health posts per 100,000 population, 37.09 health centers per 100,000, 28.84 district or rural hospitals per 100,000, and 34.65 specialized hospitals per 100,000. In 2009, Guinea-Bissau had 0.96 hospital beds per 1,000 population.

Major Health Issues

In 2008, WHO estimated that 79 percent of years of life lost in Guinea-Bissau were due to communicable diseases, 15 percent to noncommunicable diseases, and 6 percent to injuries. In 2008, the age-standardized estimate of cancer deaths was 90 per 100,000 for men and 98 per 100,000 for women; for cardiovascular disease and diabetes, 502 per 100,000 for men and

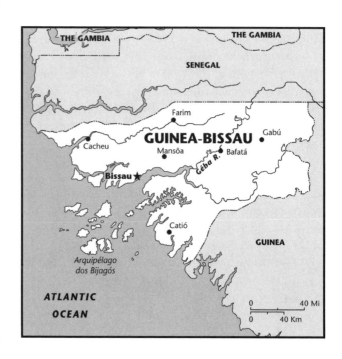

523 per 100,000 for women; and for chronic respiratory disease, 140 per 100,000 for men and 83 per 100,000 for women.

In 2008, the age-standardized death rate from malaria was 108.7 per 100,000 population, the fourth-highest in the world, and the rates of infection from other vector-borne and water-borne diseases such as yellow fever, cholera, typhoid, and meningococcal meningitis are also high. In 2010, tuberculosis incidence was 233.0 per 100,000 population, tuberculosis prevalence 303.0 per 100,000, and deaths due to tuberculosis among HIV-negative people 327.00 per 100,000. As of 2009, an estimated 2.5 percent of adults age 15 to 49 were living with HIV or AIDS. In 2008, the age-standardized death rate from childhood-cluster diseases (pertussis, polio, diphtheria, measles, and tetanus) was 20.9 per 100,000 population, the sixth-highest in the world.

Guinea-Bissau's maternal mortality rate (death from any cause related to or aggravated by pregnancy) is the fourth-highest in the world, estimated at 1,000 per 100,000 live births as of 2008. A 2006 survey estimated the prevalence of female genital mutilation at 44.5 percent. The infant mortality rate, defined as the number of deaths of infants younger than 1 year, is the sixth-highest in the world, at 94.40 per 1,000 live births as of 2012. In 2008, 17.2 percent of children under age 5 were underweight (defined as 2 kilograms [kg] below standard weight-for-age at age 1, 3 kg below for ages 2 to 3, and 4 kg below for ages 4 to 5).

Health Care Personnel

In 2006, WHO identified Guinea-Bissau as one of 57 countries with a critical deficit in the supply of skilled health workers. Guinea-Bissau has one medical school, the Escola Superior de Medicina Eduardo Mondlane in Bissau, which began offering instruction in 1986. The basic medical course requires six years to complete, and the degree awarded is Doctor en Medicina (doctor of medicine). Guinea-Bissau has agreements with several other countries, including Brazil, Cuba, and some European and North American countries, which allow students from Guinea-Bissau to receive medical training in those countries. Physicians must register with the Ministry of Public Health. Graduates of foreign medical schools must have their degrees certified, and foreigners must have a work and residence permit to practice. In 2008, Guinea-Bissau had 0.05 physicians per 1,000 population, 0.02 pharmaceutical personnel per 1,000, 0.12 laboratory health workers per 1,000, 0.79 health management and support workers per 1,000, and 0.55 nurses and midwives per 1,000. The global "brain drain" (international migration of skilled personnel) plays a role in the relative undersupply of medical personnel in Guinea-Bissau: Michael Clemens and Bunilla Petterson estimate that 71 percent of Guinea-Bissau–born physicians and 25 percent of Guinea-Bissau–born nurses are working in one of nine developed countries, primarily in Portugal.

Government Role in Health Care

The right to health, recognized in national legislation in Guinea-Bissau, includes the right to access to essential medicines and medical technologies. The country has a National Health Policy (NHP), written in 1993, a plan to implement the national health policy, written in 2008, and a National Medicines Plan (NMP), written in 2009. The NMP includes selection of essential medicines; financing, pricing, purchase, distribution, and regulation of drugs; pharmacovigilance; rational usage of medicines; and evaluation and monitoring.

According to WHO, in 2010, Guinea-Bissau spent $71 million on health care, an amount that comes to $47 per capita. Health care funding was provided primarily (77 percent) from domestic sources, with the remaining 23 percent coming from overseas sources. Almost two-thirds (66 percent) of health care funding was paid for through expenditures by households, with the remainder provided through government spending (10 percent) and other sources (24 percent). In 2010, Guinea-Bissau allocated 4 percent of its total government expenditures to health, and government expenditures on health came to 1 percent of GDP; both figures place Guinea-Bissau in the low range as compared with other low-income African countries. In 2009, according to WHO, official development assistance (ODA) for health in Guinea-Bissau came to $12.18 per capita.

Public Health Programs

The National Institute of Public Health (INASA), located in Bissau and headed by Amabelia Rodrigues, was created in 2008 to rebuild the nation's public health system after the civil war. Four organizations came together under the guidance of the Ministry of Health to create the INASA: the National Public Health Laboratory, the Ministry of Health's Center for Epidemiology and Community Health, the National School of Public Health, and the Center for Tropical Medicine. Current projects include creating malaria-control policies, creating a course on malaria control, and building financial management capacity within the INASA.

According to WHO, in 2008, Guinea-Bissau had 0.03 environmental and public health workers per 1,000 population. In 2010, 20 percent of the population had access to improved sanitation facilities (9 percent in rural areas and 44 percent in urban), and 64 percent had access to improved sources of drinking water (53 percent in rural areas and 91 percent in urban). According to the World Higher Education Database (WHED), one university in Guinea-Bissau offers programs in epidemiology or public health: the Lusophone University of Guinea, located in Bissau.

GUYANA

Guyana is a country in northern South America, sharing borders with Venezuela, Brazil, and Suriname and having a coastline on the north Atlantic Ocean. The area of 83,000 square miles (214,969 square kilometers) makes Guyana slightly smaller than Idaho, and the July 2012 population was 741,908. In 2010, 29 percent

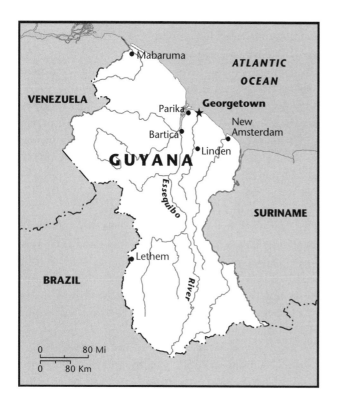

of the population lived in urban areas, and the 2010 to 2015 annual rate of urbanization was estimated at 0.5 percent. Georgetown is the capital and largest city (with a 2009 population estimated at 132,000). The population growth rate in 2012 was negative 0.3 percent due in large part to high emigration; Guyana had the seventh-lowest net migration rate in the world, negative 12.78 migrants per 1,000 population. The birth rate (16.7 births per 1,000 population) and total fertility rate (2.3 children per woman) were both in the middle range as compared to other countries.

Guyana was a Dutch colony, then a British possession, before becoming independent in 1966. Guyana ranked tied for 134th among 183 countries on the *Corruption Perceptions Index 2011,* with a score of 2.5 (on a scale where 0 indicates highly corrupt and 10 very clean). In 2011, Guyana was classified as a country with medium human development (the second from the lowest of four categories) on the United Nations Development Programme's (UNDP's) Human Development Index (HDI), with a score of 0.633 (on a scale where 1 denotes high development and 0 low development). Life expectancy at birth in 2012 was estimated at 67.39 years, and estimated gross domestic product (GDP) per capita in 2011 was $7,500. In 2007, the Gini Index (a measure of dispersion, in which perfect equality is denoted by 0 and maximum inequality is denoted by 100) for family income was 44.6. According to the World Economic Forum's *Global Gender Gap Index 2011,* Guyana ranks 38th out of 135 countries on gender equality with a score of 0.708 (on a scale with a theoretical range of 1 for equality to 0 for inequality and an actual range in 2011 from 0.8530 to 0.4873).

Emergency Health Services
According to the World Health Organization (WHO), as of 2007, Guyana had a formal and publicly available emergency care (prehospital care) system accessible through regional telephone access numbers, but not a national universal access telephone number. Public and some private hospitals provide ambulance services, as do some private security firms, but there is no national ambulance service.

Insurance
Guyana has a social insurance program providing cash benefits only; there is no national health insurance system, but medical care is provided free through a network of public facilities. The social insurance system includes employed and self-employed people

ages 16 to 59, along with casual employees, family labor, and those with very low wages (less than GYD 7.50 weekly). Persons up to age 60 may join the system voluntarily. The system is funded through wage contributions (5.2 percent of covered earnings; there is a cap on the amount of earnings covered), contributions from the self-employed (11.5 percent of covered income up to a cap), voluntary contributions (9.3 percent of average wages when in covered employment), and employer contributions (7.8 percent of covered monthly payroll).

Medical care is available in public health centers and hospitals, with cost sharing required based on income. The maternity benefit is 70 percent of average wages for 13 weeks, with an extension to 26 weeks possible if there are birth complications. The cash sickness benefit is 70 percent of average earnings for up to 26 weeks. The program is administered by the Ministry of Labour, Human Services, and Social Security and supervised by the Ministry of Finance. According to Ke Xu and colleagues, in 2003, 0.6 percent of households in Guyana experienced catastrophic health expenditures annually; "catastrophic" was defined as exceeding 40 percent of household income remaining after basic needs were met.

Costs of Hospitalization

In 2005, 36.7 percent of recurrent government health expenditures were allocated to the Georgetown Public Hospital Corporation. Health care in public facilities is provided at no charge.

Access to Health Care

According to WHO, in 2006, 83 percent of births in Guyana were attended by skilled personnel (for example, physicians, nurses, or midwives). The 2010 immunization rates for 1-year-olds were 95 percent for diphtheria and pertussis (DPT3), 95 percent for measles (MCV), and 95 percent for Hib (Hib3). In 2010, an estimated 84 percent of persons with advanced human immunodeficiency virus (HIV) infection were receiving antiretroviral therapy in accordance with the 2010 WHO guidelines. According to WHO, in 2010, Guyana had 1.31 magnetic resonance imaging (MRI) machines per 1 million population and 3.93 computer tomography (CT) machines per 1 million.

Cost of Drugs

The Materials Management Unit is responsible for procuring medicines for use in the public sector,

based on an essential drugs list (EDL) and on recommendations from WHO; the purpose of the EDL is to eliminate redundancies and prevent prescription of an expensive drug when an equally good and cheaper alternative exists. Medicines are obtained through the National Procurement and Tender Administration Board, and as of 2010, Guyana considered pooling its procurements with those of other Caribbean countries.

Health Care Facilities

Guyana's health care system is divided into five levels. The first level is health posts providing primary and preventive care in remote areas. Level 2 includes health centers and clinics providing maternal and child care, infectious disease care, outpatient services, dentistry, pharmacy services, and so on. Level 3 includes district hospitals, providing limited surgery and inpatient care. Level 4 includes regional hospitals and diagnostic centers, proving specialized care, surgery, and diagnostics. Level 5 includes national hospitals providing specialty care as well as care in private facilities and in other countries, subsidized by the Ministry of Health, for those in need of care not available in Guyana's public health system. As of 2010, according to WHO, Guyana had 27.17 health posts per 100,000 population, 15.64 health centers per 100,000, 2.12 district or rural hospitals per 100,000, 1.33 provincial hospitals per 100,000, and 0.13 specialized hospitals per 100,000. In 2007, Guyana had 1.90 hospital beds per 1,000 population.

Major Health Issues

In 2008, WHO estimated that 32 percent of years of life lost in Guyana were due to communicable diseases, 47 percent to noncommunicable diseases, and 31 percent to injuries. In 2008, the age-standardized estimate of cancer deaths was 85 per 100,000 for men and 80 per 100,000 for women; for cardiovascular disease and diabetes, 475 per 100,000 for men and 428 per 100,000 for women; and for chronic respiratory disease, 27 per 100,000 for men and 14 per 100,000 for women.

In 2008, the age-standardized death rate from malaria was 5.3 per 100,000 population. In 2010, tuberculosis incidence was 111.0 per 100,000 population, tuberculosis prevalence 115.0 per 100,000, and deaths due to tuberculosis among HIV-negative people 13.00 per 100,000. As of 2009, an estimated 1.2 percent of adults age 15 to 49 were living with HIV or acquired immune deficiency syndrome (AIDS). In 2010, 22,935 cases of malaria were reported.

Guyana's maternal mortality rate (death from any cause related to or aggravated by pregnancy) was estimated in 2008 as 270 maternal deaths per 100,000 live births. The infant mortality rate, defined as the number of deaths of infants younger than 1 year, was estimated at 35.59 per 1,000 live births as of 2012. In 2007, 10.8 percent of children under age 5 were underweight (defined as 2 kilograms [kg] below standard weight-for-age at age 1, 3 kg below for ages 2 to 3, and 4 kg below for ages 4 to 5).

Health Care Personnel
Guyana has two medical schools, the School of Medicine of the University of Guyana in Georgetown, which began offering instruction in 1985, and the American International School of Medicine, also in Georgetown, which began offering instruction in 2000. The basic medical training course is five years, and the degree awarded is doctor of medicine. In 2000, Guyana had 0.48 physicians per 1,000 population, 0.04 dentistry personnel per 1,000, and 2.29 nurses and midwives per 1,000.

Government Role in Health Care
According to WHO, in 2010, Guyana spent $120 million on health care, an amount that comes to $159 per capita. Health care funding was provided primarily (73 percent) from domestic sources, with the remaining 27 percent coming from overseas sources. Most (85 percent) of health care funding was paid for through government expenditures, with the remainder provided through household expenditures (15 percent).

In 2010, Guyana allocated 15 percent of its total government expenditures to health, and government expenditures on health came to 5 percent of GDP; the former figures place Guyana in the median range as compared with other lower-middle-income countries in the Americas region, while the latter places Guyana in the high range. In 2009, according to WHO, official development assistance (ODA) for health in Guyana came to $36.29 per capita.

Public Health Programs
In 2010, 84 percent of the population of Guyana had access to improved sanitation facilities (82 percent in rural areas and 88 percent in urban), and 94 percent had access to improved sources of drinking water (93 percent in rural areas and 98 percent in urban). According to the World Higher Education Database

(WHED), no university in Guyana offers programs in epidemiology or public health.

HAITI

Haiti is a Caribbean country occupying the western third of the island of Hispaniola and sharing a border with the Dominican Republic. The area of 10,714 square miles (27,750 square kilometers) makes Haiti similar in size to Maryland; the July 2012 population was estimated at 9.8 million. In 2010, 52 percent of the population lived in urban areas, and the 2010 to 2015 annual rate of urbanization was estimated at 3.2 percent. Port au Prince is the capital and largest city, with a 2010 estimated population of 2.1 million. The population growth rate in 2012 was 0.9 percent, with a negative net migration rate (negative 6.90 migrants per 1,000 population), a birth rate of 23.9 births per 1,000 population, and a total fertility rate of 3.0 children per woman.

Haiti was a French colony, with an economy based on slave labor, and in 1804, became the first black-majority country to achieve independence. Haiti's

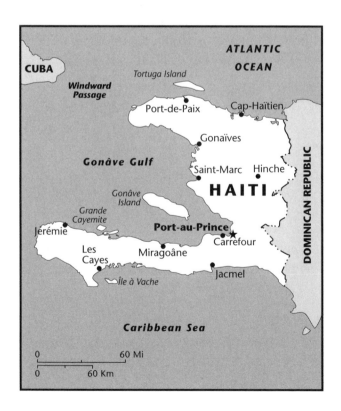

history in the 20th century was largely one of violence and political corruption, and it remains the poorest country in the Western hemisphere; however, democratic elections were held in 2006. A severe earthquake in 2010 killed more than 300,000 people and left an estimated 1 million homeless. As of May 2012, the World Food Programme estimated that 421,000 people in Haiti were still living in emergency camps, and 212,000 were food insecure. Haiti's government is perceived as corrupt, ranking tied for 175th among 183 on the *Corruption Perceptions Index 2011,* with a score of 1.8 (on a scale where 0 indicates highly corrupt and 10 very clean).

In 2011, Haiti was classified as a country with low human development (the lowest of four categories) on the United Nations Development Programme's (UNDP's) Human Development Index (HDI), with a score of 0.454 (on a scale where 1 denotes high development and 0 low development). In 2011, the International Food Policy Research Institute (IFPRI) classified Haiti as a country with an "alarming" hunger problem, with a Global Hunger Index (GHI) score of 28.2, the sixth-highest in the world. Life expectancy at birth in 2012 was estimated at 62.51 years, and the estimated gross domestic product (GDP) per capita in 2011 was $1,200, among the 20 lowest in the world. Income distribution in Haiti is relatively unequal: In 2001, the Gini Index (a measure of dispersion, in which perfect equality is denoted by 0 and maximum inequality is denoted by 100) for family income was 59.2, among the highest in the world. Unemployment in 2010 was estimated at 40.6 percent, among the highest rates in the world.

Emergency Health Services

Doctors Without Borders (Médecins Sans Frontières, or MSF) began working in Haiti in 1991 and had 2,918 staff members in the country at the close of 2010. In response to the January 2010 earthquake in Haiti, MSF mobilized the largest emergency response in its history; medical teams performed more than 16,500 surgeries and treated more than 358,000 people between January and October. More than 3,400 MSF staff provided care in hospitals and mobile clinics, distributed humanitarian supplies, and ensured provision of safe water and sanitary facilities. MSF also treated more than 91,000 people in the cholera epidemic that began in October.

More than 400 humanitarian health entities took part in the emergency response to the Haitian earthquake on January 12, 2010; the effort was coordinated by the Haitian Ministry of Public Health and Population and the World Health Organization (WHO). Haitian national health authorities, supported by WHO, also mounted a response to a cholera outbreak in October 2010, which began in the northern part of the country but quickly became national; more than 171,000 cholera cases were reported from October to December 2010, and 3,650 deaths were related to cholera. Emergency response and treatment and continuing surveillance were able to stabilize the outbreak and bring the case fatality rate down to 1.1 percent.

The International Federation of Red Cross and Red Crescent Societies (IFRC) deployed 21 emergency response units (ERU) to aid victims of the 2010 Haitian earthquake; the Haitian Red Cross also deployed approximately 1,000 staff members and volunteers. More than 100,000 people were treated by these IFRC ERUs from January to May 2010, and by May, essentially all displaced persons had received emergency shelter materials; the IFRC also raised more than CHF 250 million to assist earthquake victims. The IFRC operation in Haiti was expected to continue for three years.

Insurance

Haiti does not have a national, universal program for health care or social insurance; instead, health care is provided from four separate sectors. The public sector includes the Ministry of Public Health and Population and the Ministry of Social Affairs, which oversee and coordinate health facilities, the national bureaus and coordinating units dealing with infectious diseases, the departmental health bureaus, and the community health units. The private, for-profit sector is concentrated in Haiti's cities and includes health professionals in private practice; private facilities, which include labs, pharmacies, and clinics, do not participate in national health programs or epidemiological surveillance activities.

The mixed, nonprofit sector is made up of facilities run by religious organizations, nongovernmental organizations (NGOs), or the private sector, but staffed by employees of the Ministry of Public Health and Population. Traditional medicine includes alternative healers (for example, voodoo priests or spiritualists) as well as more medically recognized specialties, such as midwives and bonesetters. As of 2007, the public sector accounted for more than one-third (35.7 percent) of Haiti's health infrastructure, the private sector almost another third (32.5 percent),

Selected Health Indicators: Haiti Compared With the Global Average (2010)

	Haiti	Global Average
Male life expectancy at birth* (years)	60	66
Female life expectancy at birth* (years)	63	71
Under-5 mortality rate, both sexes (per 1,000 live births)	165	57
Adult mortality rate, both sexes* (probability of dying between 15 and 60 years per 1,000 population)	251	176
Maternal mortality ratio (per 100,000 live births)	350	210
HIV prevalence* (per 1,000 adults aged 15 to 49)	19	8
Tuberculosis prevalence (per 100,000 population)	314	178

Source: World Health Organization Global Health Observatory Data Repository.
*Data refers to 2009.

and the mixed private sector almost another third (31.5 percent).

Because unemployment in Haiti is high (54 percent in 2007) and many of those who do work do so in the informal sector, employment-based health insurance is not a likely model for Haiti. About 2 percent of the population is covered under a national assistance program covering illness and death, and 1 to 3 percent of those working in the formal employment sector are covered by government-sponsored social protection programs. Government employees and their dependents are covered by a separate insurance system, but the services provided are widely considered unsatisfactory, particularly outside Port au Prince. The Office of Labor, Illness, and Maternity Insurance offers some medical coverage for private employees, including indemnity for disability and access to a hospital offering basic and some specialized services; in 2007, about 43,000 people were enrolled in this system.

Costs of Hospitalization
No data available.

Access to Health Care
According to a 2007 report by the Pan American Health Organization (PAHO), in some departments (analogous to states or counties) in Haiti less than 40 percent of residents have access to basic health services; traditional healers are more commonly used in some areas. The Haitian system requires people to pay before receiving care, and many cannot afford to do so; this is particularly true given extreme inflation in the 1980s and 1990s: For instance, a medical consultation cost HTG 25 in the late 1980s but HTG 1,200 in 2007. Overall, half (50 percent) of Haitians lack access to basic drugs, and almost half (47 percent) lack access to basic medical care.

Prenatal care is an exception: A 2005 to 2006 survey found that 85 percent of pregnant women had one or more appointments with a health professional while pregnant (up from 67.7 percent in 1995), and 60 percent of births were attended by a skilled professional (up from 46 percent in 1994). However, a 2001 survey found that less than a quarter (24.7 percent) of childbirths took place in a health facility. According to WHO, in 2006, 26 percent of births were attended by skilled personnel (for example, physicians, nurses, or midwives). In 2006, 54 percent of pregnant women received at least four prenatal care visits.

The 2010 immunization rates for 1-year-olds were 59 percent for diphtheria and pertussis (DPT3) and 59 percent for measles (MCV). In 2010, an estimated 51 percent of persons with advanced human immunodeficiency virus (HIV) infection were receiving antiretroviral therapy in accordance with the 2010 WHO guidelines.

Cost of Drugs

Four labs in Haiti, run by the private sector, are authorized to produce drugs for use within the country; they provide 30 to 40 percent of the drugs used in Haiti. Quality monitoring is carried out by WHO and PAHO. A 2004 census found that 42 different agencies were authorized to import pharmaceutical products, and some NGOs also import and distribute pharmaceuticals. Haiti has a program to distribute essential drugs throughout the country; the value of drugs distributed in 2005 through the Pan American Health Organization's Essential Drug Program (PROMESS) was more than $4.3 million. This is much lower than in 2001, when PROMESS distributed more than $7.7 million worth of drugs.

Health Care Facilities

As of 2010, according to WHO, Haiti had 0.30 health centers per 100,000, 0.17 district or rural hospitals per 100,000, 0.04 provincial hospitals per 100,000, and 0.04 specialized hospitals per 100,000. In 2007, Haiti had 1.30 hospital beds per 1,000 population.

Major Health Issues

In 2008, WHO estimated that 72 percent of years of life lost in Haiti were due to communicable diseases, 22 percent to noncommunicable diseases, and 6 percent to injuries. In 2008, the age-standardized estimate of cancer deaths was 119 per 100,000 for men and 87 per 100,000 for women; for cardiovascular disease and diabetes, 428 per 100,000 for men and 394 per 100,000 for women; and for chronic respiratory disease, 45 per 100,000 for men and 22 per 100,000 for women.

In 2008, the age-standardized death rate from malaria was 5.2 per 100,000 population. In 2010, tuberculosis incidence was 230.0 per 100,000 population, tuberculosis prevalence 314.0 per 100,000, and deaths due to tuberculosis among HIV-negative people 29.00 per 100,000. As of 2009, an estimated 1.9 percent of adults age 15 to 49 were living with HIV or acquired immune deficiency syndrome (AIDS). Malaria is endemic in Haiti, and in 2010, 84,152 cases of malaria were reported. Lymphatic filariasis is found in both rural and urban areas, and in some cities the infection rate is more than 20 percent.

Haiti's maternal mortality rate (death from any cause related to or aggravated by pregnancy) was estimated in 2008 as 300 maternal deaths per 100,000 live births. The infant mortality rate, defined as the number of deaths of infants younger than 1 year, was estimated at 52.44 per 1,000 live births as of 2012. A 2005 to 2006 survey found that 24 percent of children age 5 or under had had at least one episode of diarrheal disease in the previous two weeks. In 2006, 18.9 percent of children under age 5 were underweight (defined as 2 kilograms [kg] below standard weight-for-age at age 1, 3 kg below for ages 2 to 3, and 4 kg below for ages 4 to 5).

Health Care Personnel

In 2006, WHO identified Haiti as one of 57 countries with a critical deficit in the supply of skilled health workers; not only does Haiti have an undersupply of medical personnel, but they are also distributed unequally around the country. Haiti has two medical schools, the École de Medecine et de Pharmacie of the Université d'Etat d'Haiti in Port-au-Prince (which began offering instruction in 1867) and the Faculté de Medecine et des Sciences de la Santé of the Université Notre-Dame d'Haiti, also in Port-au-Prince, which began offering instruction in 1996. The course of training requires six years followed by one year of social service, and the degree awarded is Docteur en Médecine (doctor of medicine). Physicians must register with the Ministère de la Santé publique et de la Population, and those who attended foreign medical school must have their degrees validated. Foreigners require special authorization to practice in Haiti.

In 1998, Haiti had 0.25 physicians per 1,000 population, 0.01 dentistry personnel per 1,000, and 0.11 nurses and midwives per 1,000. The global "brain drain" (international migration of skilled personnel) plays a role in the relative undersupply of medical personnel in Haiti: Using Fitzhugh Mullan's methodology, Haiti has an emigration factor of 41.4, representing a high ratio of Haitian physicians working in the United States, the United Kingdom, Canada, or Australia relative to those working in Haiti. Alok Bhargava and colleagues place Haiti 14th among countries most affected by the medical "brain drain" in 2004 and third among countries with populations of more than 4 million.

Government Role in Health Care

In 2005, the Haitian Ministry of Public Health and Population published a national strategic plan for reforming the health sector; this plan recognized health as a basic human right. In 2006, a Pharmacy, Drug, and Traditional Medicine Bureau was created within the Ministry of Public Health and Population to develop a National Medicine Policy (NMP). According to WHO, in 2010, Haiti spent $464 million on health care, an amount that comes to $46 per capita. About two-thirds (62 percent) of health care funding was provided from domestic sources, with the remaining 38 percent coming from overseas sources. The largest proportion (40 percent) of health care funding was paid for through household expenditures, with the remainder provided through government expenditures (21 percent) and other sources (38 percent). In 2010, Haiti allocated 5 percent of its total government expenditures to health, and government expenditures on health came to 1 percent of GDP; both figures place Haiti in the median range as compared with other low-income countries in the Americas region. In 2009, according to WHO, official development assistance (ODA) for health in Haiti came to $18.08 per capita.

Public Health Programs

Haiti has many unmet public health needs. According to a 2007 report, more than 40 percent of households are reported to have food insecurity, and 23 percent of children under age 5 suffer from chronic malnutrition. In 2010, just 17 percent of the population had access to improved sanitation facilities (10 percent in rural areas and 24 percent in urban), and 69 percent had access to improved sources of drinking water (51 percent in rural areas and 85 percent in urban). Ongoing public health problems are exacerbated by the country's chronic poverty, civil unrest, and vulnerability to natural disasters.

Haiti's Bureau of Epidemiology, Laboratories, and Research was created in 2006 and is charged with conducting research contributing to disease prevention and control; however, personnel shortages and financial restraints have prevented this research from being carried out. According to the World Higher Education Database (WHED), no university in Haiti offers programs in epidemiology or public health.

HONDURAS

Honduras is a Central American country, sharing borders with Nicaragua, El Salvador, and Guatemala and having coastlines on the north Pacific Ocean and the Caribbean Sea. The area of 43,278 square miles (112,090 square kilometers) makes Honduras similar in size to Tennessee; the July 2012 population was

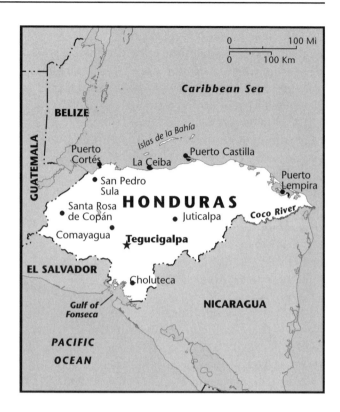

estimated at 8.3 million. In 2010, 52 percent of the population lived in urban areas, and the 2010 to 2015 annual rate of urbanization was estimated at 3.1 percent. Population growth in 2012 was 1.8 percent; the net migration rate was negative 1.2 migrants per 1,000 population, the birth rate 24.7 births per 1,000, and the total fertility rate 3.0 children per woman.

Honduras is a former Spanish colony and became independent in 1821. Honduras was ruled by a series of military governments from 1961 to 1982, when an elected civilian government took power. Honduras ranked tied for 129th among 183 countries on the *Corruption Perceptions Index 2011,* with a score of 2.6 (on a scale where 0 indicates highly corrupt and 10 very clean). Honduras was severely damaged by Hurricane Mitch in 1998. In 2011, Honduras was classified as a country with medium human development (the second from the lowest of four categories) on the United Nations Development Programme's (UNDP's) Human Development Index (HDI), with a score of 0.625 (on a scale where 1 denotes high development and 0 low development). Life expectancy at birth in 2012 was estimated at 70.71 years, and estimated gross domestic product (GDP) per capita in 2011 was $4,300. Income distribution in Honduras is relatively unequal: In 2007, the Gini Index (a measure of dispersion, in which perfect equality is denoted by 0 and maximum inequality is denoted by 100) for family income was 57.7, among the highest in the world. According to the World Economic Forum's *Global Gender Gap Index 2011*, Honduras ranked 54th out of 135 countries on gender equality with a score of 0.694 (on a scale with a theoretical range of 1 for equality to 0 for inequality and an actual range in 2011 from 0.8530 to 0.4873).

Emergency Health Services

According to the World Health Organization (WHO), as of 2007 Honduras had a formal and publicly available emergency care (prehospital care) system accessible through a national universal access telephone number. Doctors Without Borders (Médecins Sans Frontières, or MSF) began working in Honduras in 1988 and had 28 staff members in the country at the close of 2010. MSF operated a center for homeless young people (23 and younger) in Tegucigalpa (the national capital), including medical care and psychological services. In 2010, MSF began a new approach, providing outreach to vulnerable groups rather than expecting them to come to the center. MSF also provided medical care, community education, and vector control in a dengue fever outbreak in Tegucigalpa in mid-2010.

Insurance

Honduras has a social insurance system (the IHSS system) providing medical benefits, cash sickness benefits, and maternity benefits to a somewhat overlapping population group. Medical benefits are provided to most employees (including those working in the public sector and for industrial and commercial firms), pensioners, the unemployed, the self-employed, and household workers; temporary and casual workers, and people working for their families, are excluded. The cash sickness benefits plan covers most employees (including those working in the public sector and for industrial and commercial firms), pensioners, and the unemployed; the self-employed are excluded, as are temporary, agricultural, and family workers. Cash maternity benefits are provided to most employees, the self-employed, and those on disability pensions; the unemployed are excluded, as are agricultural, family, and temporary workers. The system is funded by an earnings tax (2.5 percent of covered earnings for employees and 8.5 percent for the self-employed), employer payroll contributions (5 percent of covered payroll), and

government contributions (0.5 percent of total covered earnings). The Social Security Institute provides medical services in its health facilities, including hospitalization, surgery, general and specialist care, medicine, lab services, appliances, and maternity and dental care. Children of insured people are provided with pediatric care up to the age of 5, and wives are provided with maternity care.

The maternity benefit is 66 percent of earnings for 6 weeks before and after the due date; employers must provide maternity leave to employees not included in the social insurance system. The cash sickness benefit is 66 percent of earnings for up to 26 weeks, with possible extensions for another 26 weeks; employers are required to provide sick leave to employees not in the social insurance system. The system is administered by the Social Security Institute under the general supervision of the Secretariat of Labor and Social Security.

Costs of Hospitalization

No data available.

Access to Health Care

In 2004, 83.1 percent of Hondurans were classified by the Pan American Health Organization (PAHO) as being without health insurance and 30.1 percent as being without health care; as of 2007, about 11 percent of the population (37 percent of the working population) was covered by the IHSS system. However, according to Latinobarometer, an annual public opinion survey conducted in Latin America, 55 percent of citizens in Honduras are satisfied with the level of health care available to them (the regional average is 51.9 percent). According to WHO, in 2006, 67 percent of births were attended by skilled personnel (for example, physicians, nurses, or midwives). In 2006, 81 percent of pregnant women received at least four prenatal care visits. The 2010 immunization rates for 1-year-olds were 98 percent for diphtheria and pertussis (DPT3), 99 percent for measles (MCV), and 98 percent for Hib (Hib3). In 2010, an estimated 51 percent of persons with advanced human immunodeficiency virus (HIV) infection were receiving antiretroviral therapy in accordance with the 2010 WHO guidelines.

Cost of Drugs

As of 2007, an estimated 16,000 drugs were available in Honduras, most of them imported brand-name drugs. The Ministry of Health regulates the drug supply and has the power to shut down pharmacies that do not comply with regulations.

Health Care Facilities

In 2002, Honduras' Ministry of Health operated 28 hospitals and 1,241 outpatient and maternal and child health care facilities, and nongovernmental organizations (NGOs) operated 108 hospitals and 820 outpatient facilities. As of 2010, according to WHO, Honduras had 18.74 health posts per 100,000 population, 0.78 health centers per 100,000, 0.21 district or rural hospitals per 100,000, 0.08 provincial hospitals per 100,000, and 0.09 specialized hospitals per 100,000. In 2009, Honduras had 0.80 hospital beds per 1,000 population, one of the 30 lowest rates in the world. Most medical care is available in the major cities, with services in rural areas much rarer. According to WHO, in 2010, Honduras had 1.23 magnetic resonance imaging (MRI) machines per 1 million population, 2.32 computer tomography (CT) machines per 1 million, 0.55 telecolbalt units per 1 million, and 0.55 radiotherapy machines per 1 million.

Major Health Issues

In 2008, WHO estimated that 42 percent of years of life lost in Honduras were due to communicable diseases, 43 percent to noncommunicable diseases, and 14 percent to injuries. In 2008, the age-standardized estimate of cancer deaths was 137 per 100,000 for men and 131 per 100,000 for women; for cardiovascular disease and diabetes, 410 per 100,000 for men and 342 per 100,000 for women; and for chronic respiratory disease, 47 per 100,000 for men and 30 per 100,000 for women. In 2008, the age-standardized death rate from malaria was 0.1 per 100,000 population.

Honduras' maternal mortality rate (death from any cause related to or aggravated by pregnancy) was estimated in 2008 as 110 maternal deaths per 100,000 live births. The infant mortality rate, defined as the number of deaths of infants younger than 1 year, was estimated at 19.85 per 1,000 live births as of 2012. In 2010, an estimated 51 percent of persons with advanced HIV infection were receiving antiretroviral therapy in accordance with the 2010 WHO guidelines. In 2010, tuberculosis incidence was 51.0 per 100,000 population, tuberculosis prevalence 65.0 per 100,000, and deaths due to tuberculosis among HIV-negative people 5.20 per 100,000. As of 2009, an estimated 0.8 percent of adults age 15 to 49 were living with HIV or acquired immune deficiency syndrome (AIDS).

Health Care Personnel

In 2006, WHO identified Honduras as one of 57 countries with a critical deficit in the supply of skilled health workers. Honduras has one medical school, the Facultad de Ciencias Medicas of the Universidad Nacional Autonoma de Honduras in Tegucigalpa, which began offering instruction in 1907. The basic course of study requires eight years of training, with an additional two years of practice (one year of social service and one year as an intern) before the degree Doctor en medicina y Cirugía is awarded. Physicians must register with the Colegio Médico de Honduras, and those who attended a foreign medical school must have their degrees validated. Foreigners must have a residence permit to practice. Honduras has agreements with El Salvador and Guatemala. In 2000, Honduras had 0.57 physicians per 1,000 population, 0.14 pharmaceutical personnel per 1,000, 0.21 dentistry personnel per 1,000, and 2.29 nurses and midwives per 1,000.

Government Role in Health Care

According to WHO, in 2010, Honduras spent $1.0 billion on health care, an amount that comes to $137 per capita. Almost all (94 percent) of health care funding was provided from domestic sources, with the remaining 6 percent coming from overseas sources. The largest proportion (65 percent) of health care funding was paid for through government expenditures, with the remainder provided through household expenditures (31 percent) and other sources (4 percent). In 2010, Honduras allocated 17 percent of its total government expenditures to health, and government expenditures on health came to 4 percent of GDP; both figures place Honduras in the high range as compared with other lower-middle-income countries in the Americas region. In 2009, according to WHO, official development assistance (ODA) for health in Honduras came to $7.46 per capita.

Public Health Programs

According to WHO, in 2000, Honduras had 0.03 environmental and public health workers per 1,000 population. In 2010, 77 percent of the population had access to improved sanitation facilities (69 percent in rural areas and 85 percent in urban), and 87 percent had access to improved sources of drinking water (79 percent in rural areas and 95 percent in urban).

According to the World Higher Education Database (WHED), no university in Honduras offers programs in epidemiology or public health.

HUNGARY

Hungary is a landlocked country in central Europe, sharing borders with Austria, Croatia, Romania, Serbia, Slovakia, Slovenia, and Ukraine. The area of 25,918 square miles (93,028 square kilometers) is similar to Indiana, and the 2012 population was estimated at 10.0 million. In 2010, 68 percent of the population lived in urban areas, and the 2010 to 2015 annual rate of urbanization is estimated at 0.3 percent. Budapest is the capital and largest city (with a 2009 population estimated at 1.7 million). The population growth rate in 2012 was negative 0.2 percent despite a positive net migration rate (1.4 migrants per 1,000 population); the birth rate was 9.5 births per 1,000 population, and the total fertility rate was 1.4 children per woman.

Hungary was part of the Soviet sphere of influence after World War II, and the country was invaded by the Soviet Union in 1956 after announcing its withdrawal from the Warsaw Pact. In 1990, Hungary held the first multiparty elections in its history and began to operate as a free market economy. Hungary ranked tied for 54th among 183 countries on the *Corruption Perceptions Index 2011,* with a score of 4.6 (on a scale where 0 indicates highly corrupt and 10 very clean). In 2011, Hungary was classified as a country with very high human development (the highest of four categories) on the United Nations Development Programme's (UNDP's) Human Development Index (HDI), with a score of 0.816 (on a scale where 1 denotes high development and 0 low development). Life expectancy at birth in 2012 was estimated at 75.02 years, and per capita gross domestic product (GDP) in 2011 was estimated at $19,600. Income distribution is among the most equal in the world: In 2009, the Gini Index (a measure of dispersion, in which perfect equality is denoted by 0 and maximum inequality is denoted by 100) for family income was 24.7. According to the World Economic Forum's *Global Gender Gap Index 2011,* Hungary ranked 85th out of 135 countries on gender equality with a score of 0.664 (on a scale with a theoretical range of 1 for equality to 0 for inequality and an actual range in 2011 from 0.8530 to 0.4873).

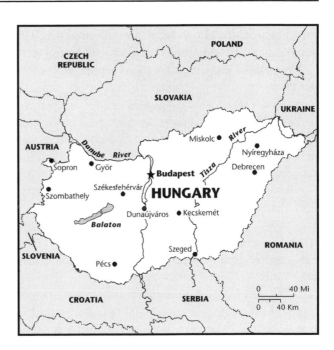

Emergency Health Services

Hungary's laws governing the emergency health system date from the 1990s; by law, free access to hospitals for emergency care is provided for all persons, including the uninsured. Emergency medicine has been recognized as a medical specialty since 1979. Funding for the emergency system is provided entirely from the state budget for both inpatient and outpatient care. Hungary has two national telephone numbers for medical emergencies: 112 (the European Union, or EU, standard) and 104; the country has 26 dispatch centers that are interconnected.

Insurance

Hungary has a social insurance system for health care, as specified by law in 1997, with amendments in 2004 and 2005. Those eligible for the cash sickness benefits system include employed and self-employed persons, members of cooperatives, apprentices, independent farmers, lawyers, performing artists, and those receiving unemployment benefits. Everyone eligible for cash sickness benefits is also in the medical benefits system, along with recipients of social assistance, pensioners, full-time students residing in Hungary and who are Hungarian citizens, and dependent family members. People otherwise exempted from the medical benefits system must still pay into it if they do not have alternative insurance. The social insurance system is covered by contributions from wages (6 percent of gross monthly earnings), contributions from the self-employed (15 percent of declared monthly earnings), and employers (2.0 percent of gross monthly income plus HUF 1,950 per employee); the government makes up any deficits. According to Ke Xu and colleagues, in 2003, 0.2 percent of households in Hungary experienced catastrophic health expenditures annually; "catastrophic" was defined as exceeding 40 percent of household income remaining after basic needs were met.

Medical benefits are provided through health facilities that contract with the National Health Insurance Institute. Services covered include general and specialist medical care, preventive care, basic dental care, hospitalization and home nursing, maternity care, medical rehabilitation, ambulance services, sanatorium care, and medical exams. Cost sharing is required for some procedures and drugs. The maternity benefit is 70 percent of average earnings for four weeks before and 20 weeks after the due date or 24 weeks after (the mother can choose). A child-care fee of 70 percent of average gross earnings (with a ceiling of twice the minimum wage) is paid for the first two years of a child's life. The sickness benefit is 60 percent of average gross earnings for up to one year, with lower rates for people with less than two years of coverage in the system and reduced time of coverage if the person has been in the system for less than one year. Contributions are collected by the Hungarian Tax Authority, the National Health Insurance Fund administers cash benefits, and the program is supervised by the Ministry of Social Affairs and Labor.

Costs of Hospitalization

In 2008, according to the Organisation for Economic Co-operation and Development (OECD), hospital spending in Hungary represented 33.1 percent of total spending on health, and per capita spending was $463; hospitals were paid based on payment per case or diagnosis-related group (DRG). As of 2002, Hungary had total expenditure caps for primary care, outpatient care, and inpatient care.

Access to Health Care

According to the World Health Organization (WHO), in 2008, 99.5 percent of births were attended by skilled personnel (for example, physicians, nurses, or midwives). The 2010 immunization rates for 1-year-olds were 99 percent for diphtheria and pertussis (DPT3), 99 percent for measles (MCV), and 99 percent for Hib (Hib3). In 2010, an estimated 38 percent of persons with advanced human immunodeficiency virus (HIV) infection were receiving antiretroviral therapy in accordance with the 2010 WHO guidelines. According to WHO, in 2010, Hungary had 1.40 magnetic resonance imaging (MRI) machines per 1 million population, 6.59 computer tomography (CT) machines per 1 million, 0.60 positron emission tomography (PET) machines per 1 million, 0.70 telecolbalt units per 1 million, and 0.70 radiotherapy machines per 1 million.

Cost of Drugs

According to Douglas Ball, Hungary charges a lower value-added tax (VAT) for medicines at rate of 15 percent for pharmaceuticals as opposed to the standard rate of 25 percent. The maximum wholesale markup ranges from 5 to 12 percent of ex-factory price (the manufacturer's list price before discounts) and the pharmacy markup from 17 to 26 percent of the ex-factory price, with a cap of HUF 850 (3.43 euros). Real annual growth in pharmaceutical expenditures in Hungary grew 9.0 percent from 1997 to 2005, faster than the 6.5 percent growth of total health expenditure (minus pharmaceutical expenditures) over those years. According to Elizabeth Docteur, in 2004, generic drugs represented 35 percent of the market share by value (the third-highest among OECD countries) and 50 percent of the market share by volume of the total pharmaceutical market. Prescription drugs are free for hospital treatment, for disabled people, for the low-income elderly, for maternity and infant care, and for life-saving care. In all other cases, drugs are subsidized by the National Health Insurance Fund according to a schedule specified by law.

Health Care Facilities

As of 2010, according to WHO, Hungary had 5.78 health posts per 100,000 population, 0.11 health centers per 100,000, 0.74 district or rural hospitals per 100,000, 0.17 provincial hospitals per 100,000, and 0.11 specialized hospitals per 100,000. In 2008, Hungary had 7.04 hospital beds per 1,000 population, among the 20 highest ratios in the world.

Major Health Issues

In 2008, WHO estimated that 3 percent of years of life lost in Hungary were due to communicable diseases, 87 percent to noncommunicable diseases, and 10 percent to injuries. In 2008, the age-standardized estimate of cancer deaths was 255 per 100,000 for men and 134 per 100,000 for women; for cardiovascular disease and diabetes, 416 per 100,000 for men and 241 per 100,000 for women; and for chronic respiratory disease, 43 per 100,000 for men and 17 per 100,000 for women.

In 2010, tuberculosis incidence was 15.0 per 100,000 population, tuberculosis prevalence 19.0 per 100,000, and deaths due to tuberculosis among HIV-negative people 1.30 per 100,000. As of 2009, an estimated 0.1 percent of adults age 15 to 49 were living with HIV or acquired immune deficiency syndrome (AIDS). The maternal mortality rate (death from any cause related to or aggravated by pregnancy) in Hungary in 2008 was 13 maternal deaths per 100,000 live births. The infant mortality rate, defined as the number of deaths of infants younger than 1 year, was 5.24 per 1,000 live births as of 2012.

Health Care Personnel

Hungary has four medical schools, located in Budapest, Debrecen, Pecs, and Szeged. The basic course of study lasts six years and the degree granted is Orvosdoktor (doctor of medicine). Hungary, as a member of the EU, cooperates with other countries in recognizing physicians qualified to practice in other EU countries, as specified by Directive 2005/36/EC of the European Parliament. This allows qualified professionals to practice their profession in other EU states on a temporary basis and requires that the host country automatically recognize qualifications for certain professions, including physicians, nurses, dentists, midwives, and pharmacists, if certain conditions have been met (for instance, facility in the language of the host country may be required). In 2008, Hungary had 3.10 physicians per 1,000 population, 0.58 pharmaceutical personnel per 1,000, 0.51 dentistry personnel per 1,000, and 6.33 nurses and midwives per 1,000.

Government Role in Health Care

According to WHO, in 2010, Hungary spent $9.4 billion on health care, an amount that comes to $942 per capita. Health care funding was provided entirely from domestic sources. The largest proportion (69 percent) of health care funding was paid for through government expenditures, with the remainder provided through household expenditures (24 percent) and other sources (7 percent). In 2010, Hungary allocated 10 percent of its total government expenditures to health, and government expenditures on health came to 5 percent of GDP; both figures place Hungary in the low range as compared with other high-income countries in the European region.

Public Health Programs

The National Center for Epidemiology (NCE), located in Budapest and headed by Marta Melles, focuses on infectious disease, particularly those preventable by vaccines, and includes surveillance and epidemiologic and microbiological research. The NCE is a European Centre for Disease Prevention and Control and, in 2008, modernized its information technology system. Hungary enjoys a high level of infrastructure development, and in 2010, access to improved sanitation facilities and access to improved sources of drinking water were both essentially universal. According to the World Higher Education Database (WHED), one university in Hungary offers programs in epidemiology or public health: the University of Pecs.

ICELAND

Iceland is an island nation in the north Atlantic, just south of the Arctic Circle. The area of 39,768 square miles (103,000 square kilometers) is similar to Kentucky, and the July 2012 population was estimated at 313,183. In 2010, 93 percent of the population lived

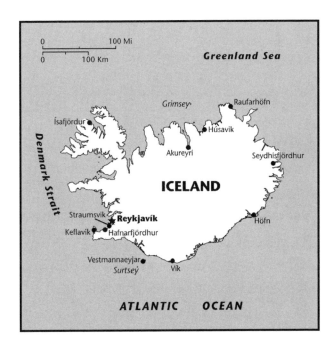

in urban areas, and the 2010 to 2015 annual rate of urbanization was estimated at 1.5 percent. Reykjavik is the capital and largest city (with a 2009 population estimated at 198,000); about two-thirds of the population lives in the southern region surrounding Reykjavik. The 2012 population growth rate was 0.7 percent, the net migration rate 0.5 migrants per 1,000 population, the birth rate 13.2 births per 1,000 population, and the total fertility rate 1.9 children per woman.

Iceland was ruled by both Norway and Denmark before being granted home rule in 1874 and complete independence is 1944. The country has achieved a high standard of living, although its economy was hurt by the global financial crisis of 2008, during which the banking system collapsed. Iceland is home to a groundbreaking study in which genetic and medical information for most of the country's population was collected; the company collecting the information, deCODE, declared bankruptcy in 2009 but continues to operate.

Iceland's government has a reputation for honesty and transparency, ranking 13th among 183 countries in terms on the *Corruption Perceptions Index 2011*, with a score of 8.3 (on a scale where 0 indicates highly corrupt and 10 very clean). In 2011, Iceland was classified as a country with very high human development (the highest of four categories) on the United Nations Development Programme's (UNDP's) Human Development Index (HDI), with a score of 0.898 (on a scale where 1 denotes high development and 0 low development). Life expectancy at birth in 2012 was estimated at 81.0 years, among the highest in the world, and per capita gross domestic product (GDP) in 2011 was estimated at $38,000. Income distribution is among the most equal in the world: In 2006, the Gini Index (a measure of dispersion, in which perfect equality is denoted by 0 and maximum inequality is denoted by 100) for family income was 28.0.

Iceland has also achieved a high level of gender equality: According to the World Economic Forum's *Global Gender Gap Index 2011*, Iceland ranked first out of 135 countries on gender with a score of 0.853 (on a scale with a theoretical range of 1 for equality to 0 for inequality and an actual range in 2011 from 0.8530 to 0.4873).

Emergency Health Services

According to the World Health Organization (WHO), as of 2007, Iceland had a formal and publicly available emergency care (prehospital care) system accessible through a national universal access telephone number.

Selected Health Indicators: Iceland Compared With the Organisation for Economic Co-operation and Development (OECD) Country Average

	Iceland	OECD average (2010 or nearest year)
Male life expectancy at birth, 2011	79.9	77
Female life expectancy at birth, 2011	83.6	82.5
Doctor consultations (number per capita), 2010	6.3	6.4
Practicing physicians (per 1,000 population), 2011	3.6	3.1
Practicing nurses (per 1,000 population), 2010	3.5	8.6
Medical graduates (per 100,000 population), 2010	13.8	10.3
Nursing graduates (per 100,000 population), 2010	78	39.8
MRI units (per 1,000,000 population), 2011	22.7	12.5
CT scanners (per 1,000,000 population), 2011	42.2	22.6

Source: OECD Health Data 2012 (Organisation for Economic Co-operation and Development, 2012).

Insurance

All residents of Iceland are covered under a medical benefits system, with employed and self-employed people also eligible for cash sickness and maternity benefits. The medical benefits and cash sickness benefits are funded by the government; the cash maternity and paternity benefits are funded by wage and payroll taxes, which also fund unemployment and work injury benefits. A minimal fee is charged for some medical benefits, including physician visits, transportation, X-rays, and some medications; hospitalization is free, as is medication for some diseases. Children under 18 receive partial reimbursement for costs, and partial reimbursement for dental care is paid to age 21.

The combined maternal and paternal benefit for the birth of a child is 3 months and must be taken before the child is 18 months old. The benefit for maternity and paternity benefits is 80 percent of the insured average wage if the insured worked full time, with minimum payments for those employed part time. Icelandic Health Insurance and the Social Insurance Administration administer the program with supervision from the Ministry of Social Affairs and Social Security.

According to Ke Xu and colleagues, in 2003, 0.3 percent of households in Iceland experienced catastrophic health expenditures annually; "catastrophic" was defined as exceeding 40 percent of household income remaining after basic needs were met.

Costs of Hospitalization

In 2008, according to the Organisation for Economic Co-operation and Development (OECD), hospital spending in Iceland represented 40.6 percent of total spending on health, and per capita spending was $1,363; hospitals were paid based on a prospective global budget.

Access to Health Care

Iceland ranked second (tied with Australia) among more developed countries in the 2011 Mothers' Index, produced by the international nongovernmental organization (NGO) Save the Children, based on a number of health and social factors relating to women, children, and maternal and child care. The maternal mortality ratio in 2008 was five deaths per 100,000 births, and the infant mortality rate was 3.18 deaths per 1,000 live births as of 2012. The 2010 immunization rates for 1-year-olds were 96 percent for diphtheria and pertussis (DPT3), 93 percent for measles (MCV), and 96 percent for Hib (Hib3). According to WHO, in 2010, Iceland had 22.19 magnetic resonance imaging (MRI) machines per 1 million population and 41.21 computer tomography (CT) machines per million.

Cost of Drugs

According to Douglas Ball, Iceland charges a lower value-added tax (VAT) for medicines (14 percent) than the standard (24.5 percent). There is no fixed dispensing fee for pharmaceuticals. The wholesale and pharmacy markups for prescription-only medications are set by law; there is no regulation of markup for over-the-counter medicines. Real annual growth in pharmaceutical expenditures grew 4.8 percent from 1997 to 2005, slower than the 6.8 percent growth of total health expenditure (minus pharmaceutical expenditures).

Health Care Facilities

As of 2010, according to WHO, Iceland had 17.80 health posts per 100,000 population, 1.87 health centers per 100,000, 2.19 district or rural hospitals per 100,000, 0.94 provincial hospitals per 100,000, and 0.62 specialized hospitals per 100,000. In 2007, Iceland had 5.79 hospital beds per 1,000 population, among the 30 highest ratios in the world.

Major Health Issues

In 2008, WHO estimated that 5 percent of years of life lost in Iceland were due to communicable diseases, 77 percent to noncommunicable diseases, and 18 percent to injuries. In 2008, the age-standardized estimate of cancer deaths was 131 per 100,000 for men and 105 per 100,000 for women; for cardiovascular disease and diabetes, 156 per 100,000 for men and 86 per 100,000 for women; and for chronic respiratory disease, 19 per 100,000 for men and 16 per 100,000 for women.

In 2010, tuberculosis incidence was 5.0 per 100,000 population, tuberculosis prevalence 5.2 per 100,000, and deaths due to tuberculosis among human immunodeficiency virus (HIV)-negative people 0.40 per 100,000. As of 2009, an estimated 0.3 percent of adults age 15 to 49 were living with HIV or acquired immune deficiency syndrome (AIDS). The maternal mortality rate (death from any cause related to or aggravated by pregnancy) in 2008 was five maternal deaths per 100,000 live births, among the lowest in the world. The infant mortality rate, defined as the number of deaths of infants younger than 1 year, was 3.18 per 1,000 live births as of 2012, the eighth-lowest in the world.

Health Care Personnel

Iceland has one medical school, the Haskoli Islands Laeknadeild in Reykjavik, which began offering instruction in 1876. The basic training course lasts six years, and the degree awarded is the Candidatus Medicinae et Chirurgiae (candidate of medicine and surgery). In 2008, Iceland had 3.10 physicians per 1,000 population, 1.18 pharmaceutical personnel per 1,000, 0.51 dentistry personnel per 1,000, and 16.48 nurses and midwives per 1,000. Alok Bhargava and colleagues placed Iceland 13th among countries most affected by the medical "brain drain" (international migration of skilled personnel) in 2004.

Government Role in Health Care

According to WHO, in 2010, Iceland spent $1.2 billion on health care, an amount that comes to $3.72 per capita. Health care funding was provided entirely from domestic sources. The largest proportion (81 percent) of health care funding was paid for through government expenditures, with the remainder provided through household expenditures (18 percent) and other sources (1 percent). In 2010, Iceland allocated 15 percent of its total government expenditures to health, and government expenditures on health came to 8 percent of GDP, placing Iceland in the median and high ranges, respectively, as compared with other high-income countries in the European region.

Public Health Programs

The Directorate of Health, located in Reykjavik, is headed by Geir Gunnlaugsson, the Medical Director of Health. It was established in 2003 to improve public knowledge of the factors—social, environmental, and lifestyle—related to health and to ensure that this knowledge would be reflected in the actions of employers, the government, and others in Iceland. The 2010 Icelandic National Health Plan and the guidelines of WHO are the guiding principles for the activities of the Directorate of Health. Current topics under research include prevention of tobacco, alcohol and drug abuse; prevention of accidents; mental health; physical activity; nutrition; and dental health. According to WHO, in 2010, Iceland had 0.18 environmental and public health workers per 1,000 population. Iceland has a modern, highly developed infrastructure, and access to improved sanitary facilities and improved sources of drinking water was essentially universal in 2010. According to the World Higher Education Database

(WHED), no university in Iceland offers programs in epidemiology or public health.

INDIA

India is a country in southwest Asia, sharing borders with Bangladesh, Bhutan, Burma, China, Nepal, and Pakistan and having a long (4,350-mile or 7,000-kilometer) coastline on the Indian Ocean. India is the second-most populous country in the world, with an estimated population, as of July 2012, of 1.2 billion people; it is also the seventh-largest country in the world by area (3,705,375 square miles or 9,596,877 square kilometers). In 2010, 30 percent of the population lived in urban areas, and the 2010 to 2015 annual rate of urbanization was estimated at 2.4 percent. New Delhi is the capital and largest city (with a 2009 population estimated at 21.7 million). Population growth in 2012 was 1.3 percent; the birth rate was 20.6 births per 1,000 population, and the total fertility rate was 2.6 children per woman. The United Nations High Commissioner for Refugees (UNHCR) estimated that, in 2010, there were 14,823 refugees and persons in refugee-like situations in India.

India is home to one of the oldest civilizations in the world. Several European countries established colonies in India, with Great Britain becoming the dominant power in the 19th century. In 1947, India became independent, and the region divided into two countries, India and Pakistan. India ranked tied for 95th among 183 countries on the *Corruption Perceptions Index 2011*, with a score of 3.1 (on a scale where 0 indicates highly corrupt and 10 very clean). In 2011, India was classified as a country with medium human development (the second from the lowest of four categories) on the United Nations Development Programme's (UNDP's) Human Development Index (HDI), with a score of 0.547 (on a scale where 1 denotes high development and 0 low development). In 2011, the International Food Policy Research Institute (IFPRI) classified India as a country with an "alarming" hunger problem, with a Global Hunger Index (GHI) score of 23.7, the highest in the world (where 0 reflects no hunger and higher scores more hunger). Life expectancy at birth in 2012 was estimated at 67.14 years, and estimated gross domestic product (GDP) per capita in 2011 was $3,700. In 2004, the Gini Index

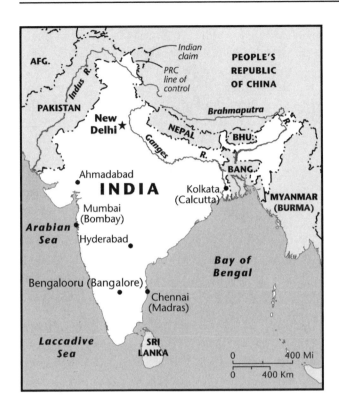

(a measure of dispersion, in which perfect equality is denoted by 0 and maximum inequality is denoted by 100) for family income was 36.8.

Emergency Health Services

According to the World Health Organization (WHO), as of 2007, India had a formal and publicly available emergency care (prehospital care) system, accessible through both a national universal access telephone number and regional access numbers.

Doctors Without Borders (Médecins Sans Frontières, or MSF) began working in India in 1989 and had 656 staff members in the country at the close of 2010. MSF provides free diagnosis and treatment for *kala azar* (visceral leishmaniasis); more than 7,000 patients were treated between July 2007 and January 2011. MSF operates health care clinics in Chhattisgarh and on the border between Andhra Pradesh and Chhattisgarh, areas beset by violence between government forces and Naxalite groups; almost 60,000 consultations were provided in 2010. MSF provides treatment for human immunodeficiency virus and acquired immune deficiency syndrome (HIV/AIDS) and tuberculosis in Mumbai, including 310 patients receiving antiretrovirals. MSF provides mental health care in Kashmir to patients suffering from the aftereffects of violence as well as basic health care in rural regions of India-administered Kashmir (more than 16,500 consultations in 2010). MSF provided emergency services to victims of the May 2010 cyclone in Andhra Pradesh, for an outbreak of malaria in Mumbai, and for an outbreak of severe diarrhea in south Chhattisgarh.

Insurance

India has a social insurance and social assistance system. The social insurance system applies to employees working in certain types of businesses with at least 10 workers (manufacturing) or 20 workers (other businesses) who make INR 15,000 or less per month. Employees may contract out of the system if they are covered by equivalent plans and work for government-run businesses. Some states in India are not currently included in the plan, which is gradually being extended. The self-employed, agricultural workers, seasonal workers, and workers in certain industries are excluded from the system. Most states are included in a national health insurance scheme covering hospitalization and transportation for the poor, and some artisans working in the informal sector are covered by separate plans. Poor women are entitled to assistance for their first two births. The system is funded by wage contributions (1.75 percent of earnings) for those making at least INR 70 per day and payroll contributions of 4.75 percent. State governments pay 12.5 percent of the costs for medical benefits as well as medical care for the recipients of unemployment benefits and the recipients' dependents. According to Donald West and colleagues, only about 11 percent of India's population had any health insurance from 2004 to 2005, and about 1 percent had private insurance.

Medical care is arranged by state governments, with different systems used in different states, including services provided by private physicians contracting with the state, state governments services, or social insurance hospitals and dispensaries; reimbursement for services is provided by the Employees' State Insurance Corporation. In model hospitals and in the National Capital Territory of Delhi, the Employees' State Insurance Corporation provides medical care directly. Benefits covered include hospitalization, surgery, physician care, obstetric care, lab services, imaging, and transportation; drugs and appliances are provided free. The Employees' State Insurance Corporation is managed by a director general and a board, and the system is supervised by the Ministry of Labor and Employment. However, a 2004 survey found that 70 percent of the population also used the private health care system.

Costs of Hospitalization

Private firms provide about 40 percent of hospital beds and 60 percent of outpatient care, according to Donald West and colleagues. While there are severe shortages of hospital beds and necessary personnel and equipment in public hospitals, at the same time India has experienced substantial growth in high-level hospitals providing specialized care to medical tourists and those covered by private insurance in fields such as cardiology, transplant surgery, orthopedic surgery, and joint replacements; many of these hospitals are partnerships with foreign entities (for example, a chain of hospitals developed to serve medical tourists has been developed through a partnership of Wockhardt Hospitals Group and Harvard Medical International).

Access to Health Care

According to Donald West and colleagues, India has a two-tier health care system; middle- and upper-class Indians and medical tourists receive high-quality, Western care, while most residents have no access to adequate medical care. Western medicine is practiced primarily in cities, where two-thirds of health centers and hospitals are located. The health care industry is growing rapidly, and expenditures are primarily (80 percent) private. The need for care far outstrips the supply: For instance, a 2007 WHO study estimated that India would need an additional 450,000 hospital beds by 2010, and Donald West and colleagues predict that an additional 1.75 million hospital beds are needed by 2025. To provide adequate basic care, India needs about 75,000 community health centers but has less than half that number, according to Donald West and colleagues; in addition, more than half of existing medical labs are underequipped or understaffed, and at least 11 states have no labs equipped for testing drugs. There is also a severe shortage of trained medical personnel, particularly in rural areas.

According to Donald West and colleagues, telemedicine is increasingly used in India, in part to offset the disparities in care between urban and rural sectors; as of 2010, the country had about 120 telemedicine centers, with at least 160 more in development. The Indian Space Research Organization (ISRO) planned to link 25 major and 650 district hospitals by 2011.

According to WHO, in 2008, 46.9 percent of births were attended by skilled personnel (for example, physicians, nurses, or midwives). In 2008, 50 percent of pregnant women received at least four prenatal care visits. The 2010 immunization rates for 1-year-olds were 72 percent for diphtheria and pertussis (DPT3) and 74 percent for measles (MCV).

Cost of Drugs

According to Ibis Sanchez-Serrano, in 2009, the pharmaceutical market in India was valued at $8.4 billion and was projected to reach $16.5 billion by 2014. The Indian government has begun tracking the drug supply. According to a 2011 report from WHO, India regulates the maximum retail price for selected medicines using implicit markups of 8 percent for retailers and 16 percent for wholesalers.

A 2004 survey in Maharashtra State found that many essential medicines (including antibacterials, antihypertensive drugs, and anticonvulsant medications) were not commonly available in the public sector: The median availability was 15.8 percent, with a range of 8.0 to 45.0 percent; the only medicines commonly available in the facilities surveyed were paracetamol (94.7 percent) and chloroquine (78.9 percent). Most of the drugs stocked were low-priced generics, with a median price ratio of less than 1 (meaning that the drugs were sold in India for less than the international reference price). Medicines were relatively affordable, with most costing less than half of one day's wages for the lowest-paid government worker. The lowest-priced generics were more available in private facilities, with a median availability of 57.3; the most common generics had a median availability of 50.0 and brand-name drugs of 2.1. Drugs to treat common conditions such as diabetes, malaria, and hypertension were available in more than three-quarters of private sector facilities. The median price ratio in private facilities was 1.9 for the lowest-priced and most-sold generics and almost four for brand-name drugs.

Health Care Facilities

According to Donald West and colleagues, an estimated 469,672 hospital beds are available in India's public sector and about 265,000 beds in the private sector. This is far beneath the number required to provide basic care to India's population. In addition to hospitals providing Western medical care, an estimated 1,110 hospitals offer care based on Indian systems of medicine and homeopathy, with an estimated 24,880 beds available in these hospitals. In 2005, India had 0.90 hospital beds per 1,000 population.

Major Health Issues

In 2008, WHO estimated that 52 percent of years of life lost in India were due to communicable diseases, 35 percent to noncommunicable diseases, and 13 percent to injuries. In 2008, the age-standardized estimate of cancer deaths was 79 per 100,000 for men and 72 per 100,000 for women; for cardiovascular disease and diabetes, 386 per 100,000 for men and 283 per 100,000 for women; and for chronic respiratory disease, 178 per 100,000 for men and 125 per 100,000 for women.

In 2008, the age-standardized death rate from malaria was 1.8 per 100,000 population. In 2008, the age-standardized death rate from childhood-cluster diseases (pertussis, polio, diphtheria, measles, and tetanus) was 16.0 per 100,000 population, the 10th-highest in the world. In 2010, tuberculosis incidence was 185.0 per 100,000 population, tuberculosis prevalence 256.0 per 100,000, and deaths due to tuberculosis among human immunodeficiency virus (HIV)-negative people 26.00 per 100,000. An estimated 2.1 percent of new tuberculosis cases and 15 percent of retreatment cases are multidrug resistant. WHO estimates that the case detection rate in 2010 was 59 percent. As of 2009, an estimated 0.3 percent of adults age 15 to 49 were living with HIV or acquired immune deficiency syndrome (AIDS). In 2010, 23 percent of pregnant women tested positive for HIV. As of 2009, an estimated 2.4 million people in India were living with HIV or AIDS, by far the largest number in the world. Polio remained a problem in India long after it was eradicated from most industrialized countries; in 1991, an estimated 6,028 cases were reported. However, extensive eradication efforts led to a sharp drop in the number of cases (741 in 2009, 42 in 2010, and 1 in 2011); as of January 13, 2012, one year had passed without a new case of polio being reported.

India's maternal mortality rate (death from any cause related to or aggravated by pregnancy) was estimated in 2008 as 230 maternal deaths per 100,000 live births. The infant mortality rate, defined as the number of deaths of infants younger than 1 year, was estimated at 46.07 per 1,000 live births as of 2012. Child malnutrition is a serious problem: In 2005, 43.5 percent of children under age 5 were underweight (defined as 2 kilograms [kg] below standard weight-for-age at age 1,

3 kg below for ages 2 to 3, and 4 kg below for ages 4 to 5), one of the highest rates in the world.

Health Care Personnel

In 2006, WHO identified India as one of 57 countries with a critical deficit in the supply of skilled health workers. In 2007, India had 150 medical schools. The basic course of training requires four to six years followed by one year of internship before awarding a degree bachelor of medicine or bachelor of surgery degree. The internship may be served in an approved hospital or in the Armed Forces Medical Service. Physicians must register with the Medical Council of India in New Delhi. Foreigners with recognized qualifications may be granted medical licenses to practice for limited periods.

In 2006, India had 0.60 physicians per 1,000 population, 0.52 pharmaceutical personnel per 1,000, 0.07 dentistry personnel per 1,000, and 1.30 nurses and midwives per 1,000. The global "brain drain" (international migration of skilled personnel) plays a role in the relative undersupply of medical personnel in India. Overall, India is the largest exporter of physicians among developing countries, and emigration of top students is a particular concern. According to research by Manas Kaushik and colleagues, from 1989 to 2000, almost 54 percent of the graduates of India's top-ranked medical school, the All India Institute of Medical Sciences (AIIMS), emigrated, with the highest percentage (85.4 percent) emigrating to the United States. Individuals receiving multiple academic awards were 35 percent more likely to emigrate than those receiving no awards. Graduates admitted under affirmative action programs (for scheduled castes and scheduled tribes) were significantly less likely to emigrate.

Government Role in Health Care

According to WHO, in 2010, India spent $1.2 billion on health care, an amount that comes to $3,722 per capita. Health care funding was provided almost entirely (99 percent) from domestic sources, with the remaining 1 percent coming from overseas sources. The largest proportion (61 percent) of health care funding was paid for through household expenditures, with the remainder provided through government expenditures (29 percent) and other sources (10 percent). In 2010, India allocated 4 percent of its total government expenditures to health, and government expenditures on health came to 4 percent of GDP, placing India in the low range as compared with other lower-middle-income countries in the southeast Asia region. In 2009, according to WHO, official development assistance (ODA) for health in India came to $0.90 per capita.

Public Health Programs

The National Center for Disease Control (NCDC), located in Delhi and headed by Dr. L. S. Chauhan, has more than 400 staff members in six departments: epidemiology and parasitic diseases, microbiology, AIDS and related diseases, entomology, zoonosis, and study of malaria and its prevention. The NCDC also has programs devoted to eliminating yaws and Guinea worm, to polio surveillance and eradication, and to control of the H1N1 and severe acute respiratory syndrome (SARS) viruses. The NCDC works with the various states in India to control infectious disease outbreaks, improve surveillance, create networks of public health labs, and build capacity. Current goals include national surveillance of diseases preventable by vaccines, study of the animal and human disease interface, furthering the Field Epidemiology and Laboratory Training Program, and developing an epidemiologic information service.

According to WHO, in 1991 (the most recent year for which data was available), India had 0.05 environmental and public health workers per 1,000 population. In 2010, 34 percent of the population of India had access to improved sanitation facilities (23 percent in rural areas and 58 percent in urban), and 92 percent had access to improved sources of drinking water (90 percent in rural areas and 97 percent in urban). According to the World Higher Education Database (WHED), nine universities in India offer programs in epidemiology or public health: the Indian Veterinary Research Institute, the International Institute for Population Sciences, Jawaharial Nehru University, Jodhpur National University, Panjab University, Punjab Agricultural University, the Shere-e-Kashmir University of Agricultural Sciences and Technology-Jammu, SRM University, and the Tamil Nadu Doctor M.G.R. Medical University.

INDONESIA

Indonesia is an island nation located between the Indian Ocean and north Pacific Ocean, sharing land borders with Papua New Guinea (on the island of New Guinea), East Timor (on the island of Timor), and Malaysia (on the island of Borneo). It is the 15th-largest country in the world by area (735,358 square miles or 1,904,569 square kilometers) and the fourth largest by population (with a July 2012 estimated population of 248.2 million); Indonesia is home to the world's largest Muslim population and is also the world's third-most populous democracy. In 2010, 44 percent of the population lived in urban areas, and the 2010 to 2015 annual rate of urbanization was estimated at 1.7 percent. Jakarta, located on the island of Java, is the capital and largest city (with a 2009 population estimated at 9.1 million). The population growth rate in 2012 was 1.0 percent, the net migration rate negative 1.1 migrants per 1,000 population, the birth rate 17.8 births per 1,000, and the fertility rate 2.2 children per woman. The United Nations High Commissioner for Refugees (UNHCR) estimated that, in 2010, there were 811 refugees and persons in refugee-like situations in Indonesia.

Indonesia achieved independence from the Netherlands in 1949. After decades of authoritarian rule, Indonesia held free elections in 1999. Indonesia ranked tied for 100th among 183 countries on the *Corruption Perceptions Index 2011,* with a score of 3.0 (on a scale where 0 indicates highly corrupt and 10 very clean). In 2011, Indonesia was classified as a

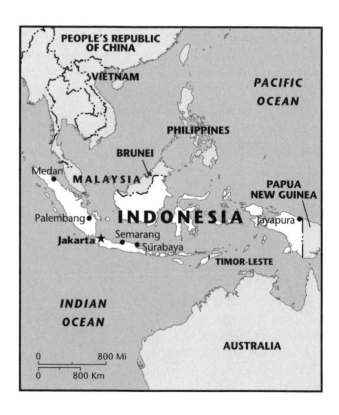

country with medium human development (the second from the lowest of four categories) on the United Nations Development Programme's (UNDP's) Human Development Index (HDI), with a score of 0.617 (on a scale where 1 denotes high development and 0 low development). In 2012, the World Food Programme estimated that 25 million people in Indonesia were vulnerable to food insecurity, primarily those engaged in agriculture in eastern Indonesia. Life expectancy at birth in 2012 was estimated at 71.62 years, and estimated gross domestic product (GDP) per capita in 2011 was $4,700. In 2009, the Gini Index (a measure of dispersion, in which perfect equality is denoted by 0 and maximum inequality is denoted by 100) for family income was 36.8. According to the World Economic Forum's *Global Gender Gap Index 2011*, Indonesia ranked 90th out of 135 countries on gender equality, with a score of 0.659 (on a scale with a theoretical range of 1 for equality to 0 for inequality and an actual range in 2011 from 0.8530 to 0.4873).

Emergency Health Services

According to the World Health Organization (WHO), as of 2007, Indonesia had a formal and publicly available emergency care (prehospital care) system accessible through a national universal access telephone number.

Insurance

Indonesia has a social insurance system, the Jamsostek system, for medical benefits only. It includes employees of companies with a monthly payroll of at least IDR 1 million or with at least 10 employees; coverage is being extended to workers in smaller companies and to informal-sector workers including fisherman, employees in rural cooperatives, and those working for their families. Employees working on labor contracts of less than three months are exempt, as are employees whose employers provide more comprehensive benefits than the Jamsostek system. Several classes of workers are in separate systems, including veterans, civil servants, and national independence pioneers. The system is funded by employer payroll contributions (3 percent of monthly payroll for single employees and 6 percent for married) and contributions by the self-employed (3 percent of monthly declared earnings if single and 6 percent if married). Individuals must register with a primary care physician under contract with Jamsostek, and a referral is required for hospital and specialist care.

Medical benefits provided include medicine; hospitalization; and primary, specialist, emergency, dental and eye care. Glasses, hearing aids, and prostheses are subsidized up to a set maximum. Maternity care is covered for three children, and up to three children plus the spouse are eligible to be covered as dependents. The Employees Social Security System (Jamsostek) collects contributions and contracts with health care providers; the Ministry of Manpower and Transmigration supervises the system and grants exemptions to employers providing benefits more comprehensive than those in the Jamsostek system. Indonesia also has a private care system, paid for primarily by out-of-pocket payments. According to Ke Xu and colleagues, in 2003, 1.3 percent of households in Indonesia experienced catastrophic health expenditures annually; "catastrophic" was defined as exceeding 40 percent of household income remaining after basic needs were met.

Costs of Hospitalization

No data available.

Access to Health Care

According to WHO, in 2007, 73 percent of births were attended by skilled personnel (for example, physicians, nurses, or midwives). In 2007, 82 percent of pregnant women received at least four prenatal care visits. The 2010 immunization rates for 1-year-olds were 83 percent for diphtheria and pertussis (DPT3) and 89 percent for measles (MCV). In 2010, an estimated 24 percent of persons with advanced human immunodeficiency virus (HIV) infection were receiving antiretroviral therapy in accordance with 2010 WHO guidelines.

Cost of Drugs

The Indonesian government regulates the price of 153 unbranded generic medicines in both the public and private sectors, while the other 216 drugs on the National Essential Medicines List (EML) are not subject to price controls; branded medications are also not subject to price controls. Medicines are procured and distributed to public primary health care centers by District Health Boards. The median price ratio for public-sector procurement of the lowest-priced generic medications was 1.74, or 74 percent higher than the international reference price; for most-sold generics, the median price ratio was 1.44. However, the median price ratio was much higher for a few drugs, including the lowest-priced generic ranitidine (8.43) and the lowest-priced generic ciprofloxacin

Health Expenditures: Indonesia Compared With the Global Average (2009)

	Indonesia	Global Average
Out-of-pocket expenditure as percent of private expenditure on health	75.2	50.2
Private prepaid plans as percent of private expenditure on health	3.1	38.9
Per capita total expenditure on health at average exchange rate (USD)	56	900
Per capita total expenditure on health (purchasing power parity, international dollars)	100	990
Per capita government expenditure on health at average exchange rate (USD)	26	549
Per capita government expenditure on health (purchasing power parity, international dollars)	46	584

Source: 2011 World Health Organization Global Health Expenditure Atlas.

(6.34). Patient prices were high in the public sector, with a median price ratio of 2.54 for the lowest-priced generics, 5.51 for the most-sold generics, and 21.8 for originator brands.

For some drugs, patient prices varied widely by outlet; for instance, the minimum median price ratio for diazepam was 0.97, and the maximum was 16.12. The median availability for lowest-priced generics was 46.7 percent, as compared to 20 percent for most-sold generics and 6.7 percent for originator brands. In the private sector, prices tended to be higher; the median price ratio was 2.78 for the lowest-priced generics, 6.74 for the most-sold generics, and 22.78 for originator brands. Medicines ranged from affordable to unaffordable, depending on the specific condition treated and whether the lowest-priced generic medication for a condition was available. The lowest-paid government worker would have to spend 0.2 to 5.7 days' wages to purchase the lowest-priced generics for common acute disease and 0.1 to 17.2 days' wages to purchase the lowest-priced generic drugs to treat common chronic diseases. If only brand-name drugs were available, it would take an average of 2.4 to 12.3 days' wages to treat common acute conditions and 4.1 to 41.0 days' wages to treat common chronic conditions.

Health Care Facilities

As of 2010, according to WHO, Indonesia had 9.66 health posts per 100,000 population, 3.56 health centers per 100,000, and 0.45 district or rural hospitals per 100,000. In 2002, Indonesia had 0.60 hospital beds per 1,000 population, one of the 20 lowest rates in the world.

Major Health Issues

In 2008, WHO estimated that 41 percent of years of life lost in Indonesia were due to communicable diseases, 45 percent to noncommunicable diseases, and 13 percent to injuries. In 2008, the age-standardized estimate of cancer deaths was 136 per 100,000 for men and 109 per 100,000 for women; for cardiovascular disease and diabetes, 400 per 100,000 for men and 300 per 100,000 for women; and for chronic respiratory disease, 102 per 100,000 for men and 52 per 100,000 for women.

In 2008, the age-standardized death rate from malaria was 3.1 per 100,000 population. In 2010, tuberculosis incidence was 189.0 per 100,000 population, tuberculosis prevalence 289.0 per 100,000, and deaths due to tuberculosis among HIV-negative people 27.00 per 100,000. WHO estimates that the case detection rate in 2010 was 66 percent. An estimated 1.8 percent of new tuberculosis cases and 17 percent of retreatment cases are multidrug resistant. As of 2009, an estimated 0.2 percent of adults age 15 to 49 were living with HIV or acquired immune deficiency syndrome (AIDS).

Indonesia's maternal mortality rate (death from any cause related to or aggravated by pregnancy) was estimated in 2008 as 240 maternal deaths per 100,000 live births. The infant mortality rate, defined as the number of deaths of infants younger than 1 year, was estimated at 26.99 per 1,000 live births as of 2012. In 2007, 19.6 percent of children under age 5 were underweight (defined as 2 kilograms [kg] below standard weight-for-age at age 1, 3 kg below for ages 2 to 3, and 4 kg below for ages 4 to 5).

Health Care Personnel

In 2006, WHO identified Indonesia as one of 57 countries with a critical deficit in the supply of skilled health workers. Indonesia has 32 medical schools. The basic course of training is six to eight years and the degree granted is Dokter (doctor). Physicians must register with the Ministry of Health in Jakarta, while the license to practice medicine is granted by provincial health authorities. In 2007, Indonesia had 0.29 physicians per 1,000 population, 0.14 pharmaceutical personnel per 1,000, and 0.06 dentistry personnel per 1,000. In 2005, Indonesia had 0.05 community and traditional health workers per 1,000 and 1.30 nurses and midwives per 1,000.

Government Role in Health Care

According to WHO, in 2010, Indonesia spent $18 billion on health care, an amount that comes to $77 per capita. Health care funding was provided almost entirely (99 percent) from domestic sources, with the remaining 1 percent coming from overseas sources. The largest proportion (49 percent) of health care funding was paid for through government expenditures, with the remainder provided through household expenditures (38 percent) and other sources (13 percent). In 2010, Indonesia allocated 8 percent of its total government expenditures to health, placing Indonesia in the high range as compared with other lower-middle-income countries in the southeast Asia region; government expenditures on health came to 1 percent of GDP, placing Indonesia in the low range as compared with other lower-middle-income countries in the southeast Asia region. In 2009, according to WHO, official development assistance (ODA) for health in Indonesia came to $1.27 per capita.

Public Health Programs

According to WHO, in 2002, Indonesia had 0.03 environmental and public health workers per 1,000 population. In 2010, 54 percent of the population had access to improved sanitation facilities (39 percent in rural areas and 73 percent in urban), and 82 percent had access to improved sources of drinking water (74 percent in rural areas and 82 percent in urban). According to the World Higher Education Database (WHED), 29 universities in Indonesia offer programs in epidemiology or public health.

IRAN

Iran is a country in the Middle East, sharing borders with Afghanistan, Armenia, Azerbaijan, Iraq, Pakistan, Turkey, and Turkmenistan. It has coastlines on the Persian Gulf and the Gulf of Oman and a shoreline on the Caspian Sea. The area of 636,372 square miles (1,648,195 square kilometers, slightly smaller than Alaska) makes Iran the 18th-largest country in the world, and Iran also ranks 18th in terms of population (with a July 2012 estimated population 78.9 million). In 2010, 71 percent of the population lived in urban areas, and the 2010 to 2015 annual rate of urbanization was estimated at 1.9 percent. The capital and largest city is Tehran (population 7.2 million). Population growth in 2012 was 1.2 percent, with net migration of negative 0.1 migrants per 1,000 population, a birth rate of 18.5 births per 1,000, and a total fertility rate of 1.9 children per woman. The United Nations High Commissioner for Refugees (UNHCR) estimated that, in 2010, there were 1,073,366 refugees and persons in refugee-like situations in Iran.

Iran became an Islamic Republic in 1979, overthrowing the monarchy of Shah Mohammad Reza Pahlavi. A war with Iraq from 1980 to 1988 resulted in severe infrastructure damage and economic losses as well as civilian and military injuries and deaths (estimations of Iranian casualties vary widely). Iran ranked tied for 120th among 183 countries on the *Corruption Perceptions Index 2011*, with a score of 2.7 (on a scale where 0 indicates highly corrupt and 10 very clean). In 2011, Iran was classified as a country with high human development (the second-highest category) on the United Nations Development Programme's (UNDP's) Human Development Index (HDI), with a score of 0.707 (on a scale where 1 denotes high development and 0 low development). Life expectancy at birth in 2012 was estimated at 70.35 years, and per capita gross domestic product (GDP) in 2011 was estimated at $12,200. In 2006, the Gini Index (a measure of dispersion, in which perfect equality is denoted by 0 and maximum inequality is denoted by 100) for family income was 44.5. According to the World Economic Forum's *Global Gender Gap Index 2011*, Iran ranked 125th out of 135 countries on gender equality with a score of 0.589 (on a scale with a theoretical range of 1 for equality to 0 for inequality and an actual range in 2011 from 0.8530 to 0.4873).

Emergency Health Services

According to the World Health Organization (WHO), as of 2007, Iran had a formal and publicly available emergency care (prehospital care) system accessible through a national universal access telephone number. Doctors Without Borders (Médecins Sans Frontières, or MSF) began working in Iran in 1996 and had 94 staff members in the country at the close of 2010. MSF provides services in Sistan-Baluchestan, a province in southeastern Iran, concentrating on providing care to underserved groups, including refugees from Afghanistan. In 2010, staff in clinics in Zahedan provided more than 6,300 consultations monthly; a fourth clinic provides maternal and pediatric care. Staff also make home visits, identifying individual needs and referring patients to appropriate care while also providing basic health education.

Insurance

Iran has a social insurance system (Social Security Organization, or SSO) covering all employed persons, with special systems covering the military (the Armed Forces Medical Service Organization) and government employees, the self-employed, and others (the Medical Service Insurance Organization, or MSIO); the MSIO is obligatory for government employees and voluntary for everyone else. Individuals may also have private insurance, and the Imam Khomeini Relief Foundation finances care for the poor. As of 1997, 23.4 million people were covered through the SSO, 29.1 million through the MSIO, 3.1 million through the Imam Komeini Foundation and other charities, and 5.4 million had no insurance.

The government system is funded by contributions from earnings and payroll and is part of the same system that finances old age, disability, and survivor benefits. Medical care is provided directly through SSO facilities. Care is also available in public and private hospitals and clinics and from contracted physicians, with cost sharing and reimbursement varying by the service provided. A dental grant is provided to cover the cost of dentures. The wife and first three children of an insured person are covered as dependents; children are covered to age 18, or age 20 if a student, with no age limit for unmarried daughters or disabled children. The maternity benefit is 66 percent of average earnings and is paid for six months (one year for triplets). The sickness benefit is 75 percent of average earnings for a worker with dependents and 66 percent for a worker with no dependents.

Costs of Hospitalization

As of 1999, persons covered under the SSO system were not charged for services in SSO facilities but faced cost sharing of 10 percent for inpatient care in non-SSO-contracted facilities and, if treated in a facility that was neither part of the SSO system or contracted by SSO, patients had to pay the difference between SSO payment levels and the charges at the facility. For people covered under the MSIO system, inpatient care required a 10 percent copayment (25 percent for rural households).

Access to Health Care

According to WHO, in 2005, 97 percent of births were attended by skilled personnel (for example, physicians, nurses, or midwives). In 2005, 94 percent of pregnant women received at least four prenatal care visits. The 2010 immunization rates for 1-year-olds were 99 percent for diphtheria and pertussis (DPT3) and 99 percent for measles (MCV). In 2010, an estimated 7 percent of persons with advanced human immunodeficiency virus (HIV) infection were receiving antiretroviral therapy in accordance with the 2010 WHO guidelines.

Cost of Drugs

The National Pharmaceutical Authority oversees the provision and utilization of medicines, and both public and private health facilities and pharmacies obtain their medicines from the same distributors. National law promotes the use of generics, and only drugs included on the Iranian Drug List (about 3,750 products) are legal. Prices, markups, and margins are established by the Commission on Pricing. Most drug costs are covered by health insurance, and the government subsidizes the costs for some medicines and vaccines. A 2007 survey found that the government procured medicine at reasonable prices, the government set prices for medicine, and those prices were the same in the public and private spheres; the

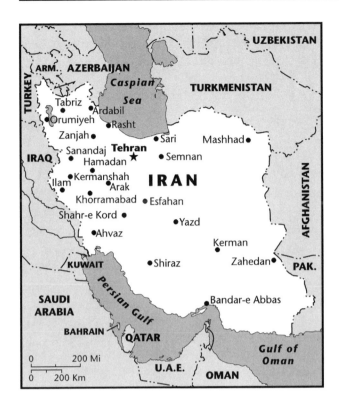

to injuries. In 2008, the age-standardized estimate of cancer deaths was 113 per 100,000 for men and 70 per 100,000 for women; for cardiovascular disease and diabetes, 421 per 100,000 for men and 348 per 100,000 for women; and for chronic respiratory disease, 42 per 100,000 for men and 29 per 100,000 for women.

Iran's maternal mortality rate (death from any cause related to or aggravated by pregnancy) in 2008 was 30 maternal deaths per 100,000 live births. The infant mortality rate, defined as the number of deaths of infants younger than 1 year, was estimated at 41.11 per 1,000 live births as of 2012. In 2010, tuberculosis incidence was 17.0 per 100,000 population, tuberculosis prevalence 23.0 per 100,000, and deaths due to tuberculosis among HIV-negative people 1.80 per 100,000. As of 2009, an estimated 0.2 percent of adults age 15 to 49 were living with HIV or acquired immune deficiency syndrome (AIDS).

Health Care Personnel

Iran has 46 medical schools. The basic medical degree requires seven years to complete, and two years of work in government service is then required before the degree doctor of medicine can be awarded. Physicians must register with the Medical Council of Iran in Teheran. In 2005, Iran had 0.89 physicians per 1,000 population, 0.20 pharmaceutical personnel per 1,000, 0.19 dentistry personnel per 1,000, and 1.60 nurses and midwives per 1,000. In 2004, Iran had 0.29 laboratory health workers per 1,000, 1.04 health management and support workers per 1,000, and 0.36 community and traditional health workers per 1,000.

Government Role in Health Care

Medical treatment and care is guaranteed as a right in the Iranian constitution. According to WHO, in 2010, Iran spent $23 billion on health care, an amount that comes to $317 per capita. Health care funding was provided entirely from domestic sources. The largest proportion (58 percent) of health care funding was paid for through household expenditures, with the remainder provided through government expenditures (40 percent) and other sources (2 percent). In 2010, Iran allocated 11 percent of its total government expenditures to health, placing Iran in the median range as compared with other upper-middle-income countries in the eastern Mediterranean region; government expenditures on health came to 2 percent of GDP, placing Iran in the low range as compared with other upper-middle-income countries in the eastern

prices paid by patients for the lowest-price generic medicines were reasonable; a minimum-wage worker could afford medicines for most illnesses and conditions. Only a few originator medicines were available, and they were priced much higher than their generic equivalents. The mean availability of generics in public facilities was 92.7 percent, as opposed to only 20 percent of originator brands. In private facilities, the mean availability of generic drugs was 92.8 percent, while for originator brands it was only 35.8 percent. A dispensing fee of IRR 5,000 (about $0.50) was charged for each prescription; cumulative markups ranged from 29 to 174 percent.

Health Care Facilities

About 10 percent of hospital beds in Iran are in private institutions and 80 percent in institutions run by the Ministry of Health and Medical Education (MOHME); occupancy in MOHME hospitals is about 56 percent. In 2006, Iran had 1.38 hospital beds per 1,000 population.

Major Health Issues

In 2008, WHO estimated that 28 percent of years of life lost in Iran were due to communicable diseases, 49 percent to noncommunicable diseases, and 23 percent

Mediterranean region. In 2009, according to WHO, official development assistance (ODA) for health in Iran came to $0.16 per capita.

Public Health Programs

The National Health Research Institute of Iran, located in Tehran and headed by Arash Rashidian, is responsible for monitoring the nation's health status and promoting the use of scientific evidence by those who set the national health policy. The institute also promotes networking and cooperation among researchers and policy makers and produces research and reports to inform national health policies. Institute departments include Population-Based Health Services; Health in Emergencies and Disasters; Social Determinants of Health; the Health Care Provision System; Quality in Health Care; Human Resources for Health; Management and Procurement of Facilities, Equipment, and Medicines; Health Care Financing and Payment; and Health Care Law and Ethics.

According to WHO, in 2004, Iran had 0.14 environmental and public health workers per 1,000 population. In 2010, essentially all the population had access to improved sanitation facilities (87 percent in rural areas and 83 percent in urban), and 96 percent had access to improved sources of drinking water (92 percent in rural areas and 97 percent in urban). According to the World Higher Education Database (WHED), 11 universities in Iran offer programs in epidemiology or public health.

IRAQ

Iraq is a country in the Middle East, sharing borders with Iran, Jordan, Kuwait, Saudi Arabia, Syria, and Turkey and having a small (36-mile or 58-kilometer) coastline on the Persian Gulf. Iraq's area is 169,235 square miles (438,317 square kilometers, about twice the size of Idaho), and the July 2012 population was estimated at 31.1 million. In 2010, 66 percent of the population lived in urban areas, and the 2010 to 2015 annual rate of urbanization was estimated at 2.6 percent. Baghdad is the capital and largest city (with a 2009 population estimated at 5.8 million). The population growth rate in 2012 was 2.3 percent (the 33rd-highest in the world); the birth rate was 28.2 births per 1,000 population, the net migration rate 0.0 migrants per 1,000, and the

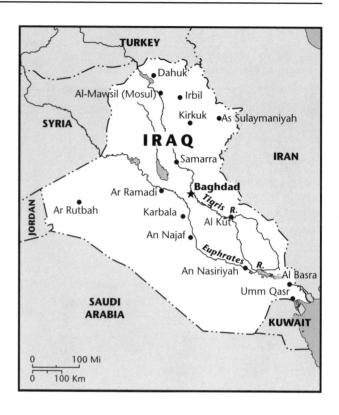

total fertility rate 3.6 children per woman. The United Nations High Commissioner for Refugees (UNHCR) estimated that, in 2010, there were 34,655 refugees and persons in refugee-like situations in Iraq and 294,770 internally displaced persons and persons in internally displaced-person-like situations.

Iraq was part of the Ottoman Empire, was occupied by Great Britain during World War II, and became independent in 1932. Iraq invaded Iran in 1980, beginning the Iran–Iraq War (from 1980 to 1988), and invaded Kuwait in 1990; the latter prompted the Gulf War, in which a coalition force led by the United States resulted in Iraq's defeat.

The current Iraqi government is perceived as corrupt, ranking tied for 172nd among 183 countries on the *Corruption Perceptions Index 2011,* with a score of 1.9 (on a scale where 0 indicates highly corrupt and 10 very clean). In 2011, Iraq was classified as a country with medium human development (the second from the lowest of four categories) on the United Nations Development Programme's (UNDP's) Human Development Index (HDI), with a score of 0.573 (on a scale where 1 denotes high development and 0 low development). Life expectancy at birth in 2012 was estimated at 70.85 years, and estimated gross domestic product (GDP) per capita in 2011 was $3,900.

Emergency Health Services

According to the World Health Organization (WHO), as of 2007, Iraq had a formal and publicly available emergency care (prehospital care) system accessible through a national universal access telephone number. Doctors Without Borders (Médecins Sans Frontières, or MSF) began working in Iraq in 2003 and had 273 staff members in the country at the close of 2010. Although MSF activities are limited by violence in parts of Iraq, the organization provides specialized care and training in surgery as well as reconstructive surgery for the severely injured; the latter is provided in Jordan. Hospital staff trained by MSF provided more than 5,000 consultations in Baghdad and Fallujah in 2010, and MSF has instituted programs to improve hospital care in Al Zahra and Basra; an Iraqi MSF surgical team in Hawijah performs approximately 300 operations monthly. MSF has also provided triage training for physicians working in hospitals in Kirkuk and Ninewa.

Insurance

Iraq has a social insurance program providing cash and medical benefits. The system covers employees of companies with at least five workers; servants, temporary employees, agricultural employees, and family labor are excluded. Medical benefits are provided through government health centers and hospitals supported by the Labor and Social Security Institute. The Ministry of Health purchases and distributes pharmaceuticals and manages ancillary and public health services. A small private-sector health care industry also exists. Maternity benefits are 100 percent of wages for at least 10 weeks and may be extended to nine months in the case of complications. Maternity is provided for the first child only and is 50 percent of wages for up to six months during the child's first four years. The cash sickness benefit is 75 percent of the average wage for up to six months; in the case of incurable or malignant disease, the benefit may be paid at 100 percent of the average wage for up to two years. The system is administered by the Labor and Social Security Institute under the general supervision of the Ministry of Labor and Social Affairs.

Costs of Hospitalization

No data available.

Access to Health Care

According to WHO, in 2007, 79.7 percent of births were attended by skilled personnel (for example,

physicians, nurses, or midwives). The 2010 immunization rates for 1-year-olds were 65 percent for diphtheria and pertussis (DPT3) and 73 percent for measles (MCV). According to WHO, in 2010, Iraq had 1.26 magnetic resonance imaging (MRI) machines per 1 million population and 1.56 computer tomography (CT) machines per 1 million.

Cost of Drugs

As of 2007, Kimadia, an arm of the Ministry of Health in Iraq, is responsible for procuring drugs for both the public and private sectors; the latter includes about 700 private pharmacies established since 1994. About 50 percent of pharmaceuticals are manufactured domestically from about 15 licensed operations. In 2005, Iraq spent about $174.2 million on importing pharmaceuticals. Drugs are not promoted or marketed in Iraq.

Health Care Facilities

Iraq had an extensive network of primary, secondary, and tertiary health care facilities prior to August 1990, and the Iraqi government estimated that 79 percent of the rural population and 97 percent of the urban population had access to health care. However, since the Gulf War and the sanctions that followed, conditions have become much worse, and the system was estimated to be functioning at about one-third of prewar levels in 1997. As of 2003, the public system in Iraq had 166 public hospitals, 90 specialized treatment centers, 17 dental health centers, 1,641 primary health centers, and 894 dispensary health laboratories. In the private sector, there were 361 public clinics, 232 health insurance clinics, 205 chronic illness pharmacies, 31 pharmacies specializing in rare drugs, 73 hospitals, 3,052 pharmacies, and 490 clinical laboratories. As of 2010, according to WHO, Iran had 7.36 health posts per 100,000 population, 0.82 provincial hospitals per 100,000, and 0.19 specialized hospitals per 100,000. In 2009, Iraq had 1.30 hospital beds per 1,000 population.

Major Health Issues

In 2008, WHO estimated that 35 percent of years of life lost in Iraq were due to communicable diseases, 25 percent to noncommunicable diseases, and 40 percent to injuries. In 2008, the age-standardized estimate of cancer deaths was 121 per 100,000 for men and 82 per 100,000 for women; for cardiovascular disease and diabetes, 471 per 100,000 for men and 376 per 100,000 for women; and for chronic respiratory disease, 51 per 100,000 for men and 33 per 100,000 for women.

Iraq's maternal mortality rate (death from any cause related to or aggravated by pregnancy) was estimated in 2008 as 75 maternal deaths per 100,000 live births. The infant mortality rate, defined as the number of deaths of infants younger than 1 year, was estimated at 40.25 per 1,000 live births as of 2012. In 2010, tuberculosis incidence was 64.0 per 100,000 population, tuberculosis prevalence 117.0 per 100,000, and deaths due to tuberculosis among human immunodeficiency virus (HIV)-negative people 12.00 per 100,000. As of 2009, an estimated 0.1 percent of adults age 15 to 49 were living with HIV or acquired immune deficiency syndrome (AIDS).

Health Care Personnel

In 2006, WHO identified Iraq as one of 57 countries with a critical deficit in the supply of skilled health workers. In 2009, Iraq had 0.69 physicians per 1,000 people, 0.17 pharmaceutical personnel per 1,000, 0.15 dentistry personnel per 1,000, and 1.38 nurses and midwives per 1,000. In 2004, Iraq had 0.47 laboratory health workers per 1,000, 1.33 health management and support workers per 1,000, and 0.08 community and traditional health workers per 1,000.

Iraq has 10 medical schools. The basic medical degree course lasts six years and a two-year internship is then required: one year of rural service and one year of national service. The degree awarded is a bachelor of medicine and bachelor of surgery or bachelor of science in medicine and general surgery. Physicians must register with the Iraqi Medical Association in Baghdad. Foreign graduates must have their degrees validated, and a foreign physician may practice in Iraq if his or her country has a reciprocal agreement with Iraq or if he or she holds a contract with a government agency.

Government Role in Health Care

The Iraqi constitution states that every citizen has the right to health. According to WHO, in 2010, Iraq spent $6.9 billion on health care, an amount that comes to $247 per capita. Health care funding was provided primarily (97 percent) from domestic sources, with the remaining 3 percent provided by funding from abroad. Most (81 percent) of health care funding was paid for through government expenditures, with the remaining 19 percent provided through household expenditures. In 2010, Iraq allocated 9 percent of its total government expenditures to health, and

government expenditures on health came to 7 percent of GDP; both figures place Iraq in the high range as compared with other lower-middle-income countries in the eastern Mediterranean region. In 2009, according to WHO, official development assistance (ODA) for health in Iraq came to $3.03 per capita.

Public Health Programs

According to WHO, in 2004, Iraq had 0.10 environmental and public health workers per 1,000 population. In 2010, 73 percent of the population of Iraq had access to improved sanitation facilities (67 percent in rural areas and 76 percent in urban), and 79 percent had access to improved sources of drinking water (56 percent in rural areas and 91 percent in urban). According to the World Higher Education Database (WHED), one university in Iraq offers programs in epidemiology or public health: Hawler Medical University, located in Erbil, Kurdistan.

IRELAND

Ireland is an island nation in the north Atlantic, sharing a land border with the United Kingdom (Northern Ireland) and having 900 miles (1,448 kilometers) of coastline. The area of 27,133 square miles (70,273 square kilometers) makes Ireland about the size of West Virginia, and the July 2012 population was estimated at 4.7 million. In 2010, 62 percent of the population lived in urban areas, and the 2010 to 2015 annual rate of urbanization was estimated at 1.8 percent. Dublin is the capital and largest city, with a 2009 population estimated at 1.1 million; about one-quarter of the population lives within 62 miles (100 kilometers) of Dublin. The population growth rate in 2012 was 1.1 percent, with a positive net migration rate of 1.7 migrants per 1,000 population, a birth rate of 15.8 births per 1,000, and a total fertility rate of 2.0 children per woman.

Ireland became independent of the United Kingdom (UK) in 1921; six counties remained part of the UK, and this area remains disputed and is sometimes the source of violent conflicts. The Irish government has a reputation for transparency and honesty, ranking tied for 19th on the *Corruption Perceptions Index 2011,* with a score of 7.5 (on a scale where 0 indicates highly corrupt and 10 very clean). Ireland ranked

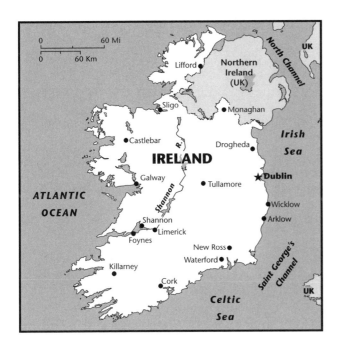

sixth (tied with Canada) in 2011 on the United Nations Development Programme's (UNDP's) Human Development Index (HDI), with a score of 0.908 (on a scale where 1 denotes high development and 0 low development). Life expectancy at birth in 2012 was estimated at 80.32 years, among the highest in the world, and per capita gross domestic product (GDP) in 2011 was estimated at $39,500. In 2010, the Gini Index (a measure of dispersion, in which perfect equality is denoted by 0 and maximum inequality is denoted by 100) for family income was 33.9. Ireland enjoyed a booming economy in the late 1990s and early 2000 but was hit hard in the global financial crisis of 2008 and went into recession; unemployment was reported at 14.3 percent in 2011. According to the World Economic Forum's *Global Gender Gap Index 2011*, Ireland ranked fifth out of 135 countries on gender equality, with a score of 0.783 (on a scale with a theoretical range of 1 for equality to 0 for inequality and an actual range in 2011 from 0.8530 to 0.4873).

Emergency Health Services

Ireland's laws governing the emergency health system date from the 1970s; by law, free access to hospitals for emergency care is provided for all persons, including the uninsured. Emergency medicine was recognized as a medical specialty in the 1990s. Funding for the outpatient emergency system comes entirely from the state budget, while funding for in-hospital emergency care

comes from multiple sources. Ireland has two national telephone numbers for medical emergencies, 112 (the European Union, or EU, standard) and 999; the country has 14 dispatch centers that are not interconnected.

Insurance

Ireland has a universal medical care system covering everyone residing in Ireland and a cash sickness and maternity benefits system covering employees age 65 and younger; self-employed persons are also eligible for cash maternity benefits. The system is funded through contributions from wages (on a sliding scale based on income), contributions from self-employed persons (also on a sliding scale), and employer contributions (also on a sliding scale). The government bears part of the cost of the system and the total cost for low-income residents.

Medical care is provided in public clinics and hospital wards and in contracted facilities; services are free for those who meet a means test and require cost sharing for those who do not. Benefits include medical care, lab services, maternity and infant care, medicines (free for those who meet a means test, otherwise with cost sharing), and optical, dental, and hearing care. The maternity benefit is 80 percent of earnings for 26 weeks, with a weekly minimum of 225.80 euros and a maximum of 270 euros The cash sickness benefit depends on income, up to 196 euros per week for up to one year (up to two years if the insured has paid into the system for at least 260 weeks). The Health Service Executive provides and contracts for services, and the Department of Social and Family Affairs administers benefits.

A 2004 study by the World Health Organization (WHO) found that none of the Irish population had substitutive voluntary health insurance (covering services that would otherwise be available from the state), and 45 percent had complementary voluntary health insurance (covering services not covered or not fully covered by the state) or supplementary health insurance (providing increased choice or faster access to services). Voluntary subscribers tend to have higher incomes and educational levels than nonsubscribers, are less likely to be in poor health, and are more likely to live in Dublin rather than in the countryside or in a small town.

Costs of Hospitalization

Persons ordinarily resident in Ireland (by the determination of the Health Service Executive, or HSE) are entitled to free treatment in HSE hospitals and voluntary hospitals; some others are also entitled to care, for example, residents of other EU countries. There are charges for some services, with holders of medical cards (primarily the poor and children in foster care) exempt from these charges. The inpatient charges in a public hospital are 75 euros per day and up to 750 euros per year; women receiving maternity services, those being treated for infectious diseases, and a few other categories are exempt. As of 1995, hospitals in Ireland were stratified according to teaching status and were funded based on the basis of historical costs (85 percent) and case mix adjustment (15 percent).

Access to Health Care

According to WHO, in 2007, 100 percent of births were attended by skilled personnel (for example, physicians, nurses, or midwives). The 2010 immunization rates for 1-year-olds were 94 percent for diphtheria and pertussis (DPT3), 90 percent for measles (MCV), and 95 percent for Hib (Hib3). According to WHO, in 2010, Ireland had 2.03 magnetic resonance imaging (MRI) machines per 1 million population, 4.73 computer tomography (CT) machines per 1 million, 0.45 positron emission tomography (PET) machines per 1 million, 0.23 telecolbalt units per 1 million, and 0.23 radiotherapy machines per 1 million.

Cost of Drugs

According to Douglas Ball, Ireland charges no value-added tax (VAT) on oral medicines and the standard VAT (21 percent) on other medicines. The pharmacy dispensing fee depends on the patient's coverage: For General Medical Services (GMS) patients, there is a fixed fee of 3.26 euros, while for those covered by the Drug Payment Scheme (DPS) and Long Term Illness (LTI) schemes, the flat fee is 2.86 euros. The wholesale markup is 15 percent of the ex-factory price (the manufacturer's list price before discounts), while the retail markup depends on the patient's insurance: The markup is 0 percent for GMS patients and 50 percent for those covered by the DPS or LTI schemes. Real annual growth in pharmaceutical expenditures in Ireland grew 10.1 percent from 1997 to 2005, faster than the 8.8 percent growth of total health expenditure (minus pharmaceutical expenditures) over those years. According to Elizabeth Docteur, in 2004, Ireland ranked third-lowest among Organisation for Economic Co-operation and Development (OECD) countries in terms of the use of generics; generic

drugs represented 5 percent of the market share by value and 13 percent of the market share by volume of the total pharmaceutical market.

Health Care Facilities

Ireland has three types of hospitals: HSE hospitals, voluntary public hospitals funded primarily by the government (although they may be owned by a religious order or other private body), and private hospitals that do not receive state funding. In 2007, Ireland had 5.17 hospital beds per 1,000 population, among the 50 highest rates in the world.

Major Health Issues

In 2008, WHO estimated that 6 percent of years of life lost in Ireland were due to communicable diseases, 78 percent to noncommunicable diseases, and 16 percent to injuries. In 2008, the age-standardized estimate of cancer deaths was 153 per 100,000 for men and 119 per 100,000 for women; for cardiovascular disease and diabetes, 179 per 100,000 for men and 104 per 100,000 for women; and for chronic respiratory disease, 34 per 100,000 for men and 21 per 100,000 for women.

In 2010, tuberculosis incidence was 8.1 per 100,000 population, tuberculosis prevalence 9.7 per 100,000, and deaths due to tuberculosis among human immunodeficiency virus (HIV)-negative people 0.49 per 100,000. As of 2009, an estimated 0.2 percent of adults age 15 to 49 were living with HIV or acquired immune deficiency syndrome (AIDS). The maternal mortality rate (death from any cause related to or aggravated by pregnancy) in Ireland in 2008 was three maternal deaths per 100,000 live births, the second-lowest in the world. The infant mortality rate, defined as the number of deaths of infants younger than 1 year, was 3.81 per 1,000 live births as of 2012.

Health Care Personnel

Ireland has five medical schools, located in Cork, Dublin, and Galway. The basic medical degree course requires five to six years to complete, and graduates must complete a one-year internship (six months in medicine and six months in surgery). Ireland has agreements with other EU countries and certain universities in Australia, New Zealand, and South Africa. Ireland, as a member of the EU, cooperates with other countries in recognizing physicians qualified to practice in other EU countries, as specified by Directive 2005/36/EC of the European Parliament. This allows qualified professionals to practice their profession in other EU states on a temporary basis and requires that the host country automatically recognize qualifications for certain professions, including physicians, nurses, dentists, midwives, and pharmacists, if certain conditions have been met (for instance, facility in the language of the host country may be required).

In 2009, Ireland had 3.19 physicians per 1,000 population, 1.02 pharmaceutical personnel per 1,000, 0.62 dentistry personnel per 1,000, and 15.67 nurses and midwives per 1,000. Global movement of the trained workforce plays a role in the supply of medical personnel in Ireland. In 2001, 13.1 percent of practicing physicians in Ireland were trained abroad, primarily in the UK and other EU countries. Using Fitzhugh Mullan's methodology, Ireland has an emigration factor of 41.4, representing a high ratio of Irish physicians working in the United States, UK, Canada, or Australia relative to those working in Ireland. Alok Bhargava and colleagues place Ireland fifth among countries most affected by medical "brain drain" (international migration of skilled personnel) in 2004.

Government Role in Health Care

According to WHO, in 2010, Ireland spent $19 billion on health care, an amount that comes to $4,242 per capita. Health care funding was provided entirely from domestic sources. More than two-thirds (69 percent) of health care funding was paid for through government expenditures, with the remainder provided through household expenditures (15 percent) and other sources (16 percent). In 2010, Ireland allocated 10 percent of its total government expenditures to health, and government expenditures on health came to 6 percent of GDP; both figures place Ireland in the low range as compared with other high-income European countries.

Public Health Programs

The Institute of Public Health (IPH) in Ireland, located in Dublin and headed by Owen Metcalfe, was created in 1998. The mission of the IPH is to build public health capacity and strengthen public health intelligence; it works with a variety of partners to promote actions that will result in improvements in health. The IRH is a key partner in two research centers: the UK Clinical Research Collaboration (UKCRC) Center for Public Health in Northern Ireland, and the national Heart Rate Variability (HRV) Centre for Health and Diet Research. In addition, the

IPH is a leader in national discussions of public health and has held more than 30 conferences and published more than 50 publications in the past 10 years.

The infrastructure of Ireland is highly developed, and in 2010, nearly all (99 percent) of the population of Ireland had access to improved sanitation facilities (98 percent in rural areas and 100 percent in urban), and access to improved sources of drinking water was essentially universal. According to the World Higher Education Database (WHED), five universities in Ireland offer programs in epidemiology or public health: University College Dublin, University College Cork, the Royal College of Surgeons in Ireland (Dublin), the Royal College of Physicians in Ireland (Dublin), and University College Galway.

ISRAEL

Israel is a country in the Middle East, sharing borders with Egypt, Jordan, Lebanon, and Syria and having a coastline on the Mediterranean Sea. The area of 8,019 square miles (20,770 square kilometers) makes Israel about the size of New Jersey, and the July 2012 population was estimated at 7.6 million. In 2010, 92 percent of the population lived in urban areas, and the 2010 to 2015 annual rate of urbanization was estimated at 1.5 percent. Jerusalem is the capital and Tel Aviv the largest city (with a 2009 population estimated at 3.2 million). The population growth rate in 2012 was 1.5 percent, the net migration rate 1.9 migrants per 1,000 population, the birth rate 19.0 births per 1,000, and the total fertility rate 2.7 children per woman. The United Nations High Commissioner for Refugees (UNHCR) estimated that, in 2010, there were 9,587 refugees and persons in refugee-like situations in Israel.

Israel was created through the partition of Palestine after World War II; it became an independent country in 1948. The borders of Israel, and for some the legitimacy of the original partition, remain in dispute. Israel withdrew from the Gaza Strip, a 139-square-mile (360-square-kilometer) area bordering the Mediterranean Sea, in 2005, but continues to control access to this area. Parts of the West Bank are controlled by the Palestinian Authority, and other parts are controlled by Israel. Some countries (more than 100 as of December 2011) recognize Palestine (consisting of the Gaza Strip plus parts of the West Bank) as a separate country, but

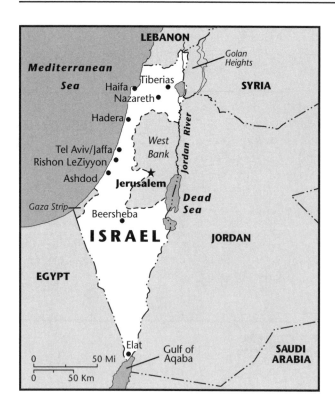

neither Israel nor the United Nations does; however, some health and welfare statistics are reported separately for these areas because living conditions are substantially different than they are for Israel.

In 2011, Israel was classified as a country with very high human development (the highest of four categories) on the United Nations Development Programme's (UNDP's) Human Development Index (HDI), with a score of 0.888 (on a scale where 1 denotes high development and 0 low development). Life expectancy at birth in 2012 was estimated at 81.07 years, among the highest in the world, and per capita gross domestic product (GDP) in Israel in 2011 was estimated at $31,000. In 2008, the Gini Index (a measure of dispersion, in which perfect equality is denoted by 0 and maximum inequality is denoted by 100) for family income in Israel was 39.2.

In 2011, the Occupied Palestinian Territory was classified as a region with medium human development (the second from the lowest of four categories) on the UNDP's HDI, with a score of 0.641. In the West Bank, per capita GDP in 2008 was estimated at $2,900. In the Gaza Strip, unemployment in 2010 was estimated at 40.0 percent, among the highest rates in the world; in the West Bank, unemployment in 2011 was estimated at 23.5 percent; in contrast, unemployment

in Israel was estimated at 5.6 percent in 2011. In 2011, the World Food Programme estimated that 44 percent of households in the Gaza Strip were food insecure, as were 17 percent of households in the West Bank.

Emergency Health Services

As of 2005, all general hospitals in Israel are required to provide emergency medical care. The Israeli Association for Emergency Medicine was created in 1992 to improve the quality of emergency medical care and create training programs for emergency medicine physicians, and in 1993, six institutions were designated as Level I Trauma Centers offering around-the-clock care from trained trauma surgeons.

Doctors Without Borders (Médecins Sans Frontières, or MSF) began working in the Occupied Palestinian Territory in 1989 and had 169 staff members in the area at the close of 2010. MSF has been present in the Gaza Strip and currently concentrates on training the Palestinian staff, providing specialized surgery, and providing rehabilitation and medical and psychosocial assistance to victims of trauma. MSF provided more than 33,000 physiotherapy sessions, more than 180 surgeries, and more than 3,400 mental health consultations in the Gaza Strip in 2010. In Nablus and Qalqilya, MSF provided more than 2,700 psychological consultations in 2010 and more than 1,000 individual and 350 group counseling sessions in Hebron and East Jerusalem; more than 300 medical consultations were also provided in Hebron and East Jerusalem. MSF planned to offer medical services and humanitarian aid to nomadic Bedouins in Negev and to migrants crossing from Egypt.

As of January 2012, the United Nations Relief and Works Agency for Palestine Refugees (UNRWA) operated 19 camps in the West Bank, with 874,627 registered persons, including 727,471 registered refugees, and eight camps in the Gaza Strip, with 1.22 million registered persons, including 1.17 million registered refugees.

Insurance

Israel has a social insurance system providing medical benefits to all residents of Israel, sickness benefits to employees, and maternity benefits to the employed, unemployed, and people in vocational training who are 18 or older. According to Donald West and colleagues, Israel's 1995 National Health Insurance Law (NHI) requires all residents to register with a sick fund; the funds provide a legally defined basket of medical services. The system is funded through wage contributions, contributions from self-employed persons, and employer contributions, all calculated on a sliding scale according to income. Medical benefits are provided by physicians and hospitals operated by or contracting with the sick fund. Patients pay a share of the costs of drugs and appliances. Covered benefits include hospitalization, general and specialist care, medicine, lab services, and rehabilitation.

The maternity allowance is 100 percent of average net income for 14 weeks, and a maternity grant is paid for each birth (ILS 1,615 for the first child, ILS 727 for the second, and ILS 484 for each subsequent child). The cash sickness benefit is at least 75 percent of earnings for 90 days. Four funds administer sickness insurance and medical care under rules defined by the Ministry of Health: the Leumit Sick Fund, the Clalit Sick Fund (covering just over half the Israeli population), Maccabi Health Care Services, and the Meuhedet Sick Fund; the National Insurance Institute collects contributions, pays benefits, and administers the program.

According to Ke Xu and colleagues, in 2003, 0.4 percent of households in Israel experienced catastrophic health expenditures annually; "catastrophic" was defined as exceeding 40 percent of household income remaining after basic needs were met.

Costs of Hospitalization

Hospitals receive capped budgets from the sickness funds based on expected use and determined by a system, including per-diem payments, fee-for-service payments, and payments based on diagnosis-related groups (DRGs); once costs exceed the cap, the sickness funds pay 50 percent of the standard rate, creating an incentive to channel patients to hospitals that have exceeded their caps. Reimbursement rates are set by the Ministry of Health, and this system has been effective in controlling cost inflation. Health professionals, including physicians and nurses, belong to national professional associations who negotiate salaries on their behalf; many physicians in public hospitals also have after-hours practices and perform procedures in public hospitals.

Access to Health Care

Access to health care is universal, provided through four regulated sick funds (registration with a sick fund is mandatory) providing a basic package of benefits; individuals can also elect to pay for supplementary insurance, either through the sick fund or through private health insurance. A public committee, established in 1998, determines which services will be provided by the plans; Israelis can theoretically choose which hospital to be treated in; in reality, referrals usually specify a provider. Despite universal coverage, studies have found that members of minorities (for example, Israeli Arabs) are less likely to use medical services than the majority population.

The 2010 immunization rates for 1-year-olds were 96 percent for diphtheria and pertussis (DPT3), 98 percent for measles (MCV), and 93 percent for Hib (Hib3).

All hospitals and sick funds use electronic patient records (EPRs), but they are not standardized, and sometimes more than one type of EPR is used within a single hospital. According to WHO, in 2010, Israel had 1.42 magnetic resonance imaging (MRI) machines per 1 million population, 8.23 computer tomography (CT) machines per 1 million, 0.85 positron emission tomography (PET) machines per 1 million, 0.14 telecolbalt units per 1 million, and 0.14 radiotherapy machines per 1 million.

Cost of Drugs

Patients are required to make copayments for most prescription drugs, but the total amount a family must pay annually is capped, and there are many exemptions from these copayments.

Health Care Facilities

As of 2010, according to the World Health Organization (WHO), Israel had 0.01 health centers per 100,000, 0.50 provincial hospitals per 100,000, and 0.08 specialized hospitals per 100,000. In 2007, Israel had 5.83 hospital beds per 1,000 population, among the 30 highest ratios in the world.

Major Health Issues

In 2008, WHO estimated that 10 percent of years of life lost in Israel were due to communicable diseases, 78 percent to noncommunicable diseases, and 12 percent to injuries. In 2008, the age-standardized estimate of cancer deaths was 132 per 100,000 for men and 101 per 100,000 for women; for cardiovascular disease and diabetes, 139 per 100,000 for men and 94 per 100,000 for women; and for chronic respiratory disease, 25 per 100,000 for men and 15 per 100,000 for women. In 2001, an estimated 22.9 percent of adults in Israel were obese (defined as a body mass index, or BMI, of 30 or greater).

In 2010, tuberculosis incidence was 4.9 per 100,000 population, tuberculosis prevalence 5.6 per 100,000, and deaths due to tuberculosis among human immunodeficiency virus (HIV)-negative people 0.23 per 100,000. As of 2009, an estimated 0.2 percent of adults age 15 to 49 in Israel were living with HIV or acquired immune deficiency syndrome (AIDS). Compared to other countries at a similar level of development, Israel ranked second among 80 less-developed countries on the 2011 Mothers' Index, produced by the international nongovernmental organization (NGO) Save the Children, based on a number of health and social factors relating to women, children, and maternal and child care. The maternal mortality rate (death from any cause related to or aggravated by pregnancy) in Israel in 2008 was seven maternal deaths per 100,000 live births, among the lowest in the world. The infant mortality rate, defined as the number of deaths of infants younger than 1 year, was 4.07 per 1,000 live births as of 2012. However, conditions were much worse in the Gaza Strip and West Bank. The infant mortality rate, defined as the number of deaths of infants younger than 1 year, in the Gaza Strip was estimated at 16.55 per 1,000 live births as of 2012 and, in the West Bank, as 14.47 per 1,000 live births as of 2012.

Health Care Personnel

Israel has four medical schools, located in Beer Sheva, Haifa, Jerusalem, and Tel Aviv. The course of training is six to seven years, and the degree awarded is doctor of medicine. According to Eric Gould and Omer Moav, Israel suffers from a "brain drain" (international migration of skilled personnel). Between 1995 and 2002, 4.8 percent of physicians emigrated, the second-highest level among professions (only university professors had a higher emigration rate); physician emigration was higher among physicians born in Israel (almost 7 percent) as opposed to immigrants to Israel. In 2007, Israel had 3.63 physicians per 1,000 population, 0.76 pharmaceutical personnel per 1,000, 1.12 dentistry personnel per 1,000, and 6.15 nurses and midwives per 1,000.

Government Role in Health Care

According to WHO, in 2010, Israel spent $17 billion on health care, an amount that comes to $2,183 per capita. Health care funding was provided entirely from domestic sources. The majority (60 percent) of health care funding was paid for through government expenditures, with the remainder provided through household expenditures (29 percent) and other sources (11 percent). In 2010, Israel allocated 10 percent of its total government expenditures to health, and government expenditures on health came to 5 percent of GDP; both figures place Israel in the low range as compared with high-income European countries.

Public Health Programs

The Israel Center for Disease Control (ICDC) was created in 1994 and is headed by Tamy Shohat. The ICDC is part of the Israeli Ministry of Health (MOH) and its objectives include establishing health-related databases, determining areas in which the current data are weak, providing support for database users, undertaking applied research and national health surveys, reporting on the health status of the population, advising the MOH on policy alternatives, and monitoring unusual patterns of disease. The ICDC conducted a national survey for rehabilitation and outcomes for patients with hip fracture and played a key role in monitoring and responding to the 2009 to 2010 influenza pandemic. The ICDC's focus is on integrating information from sources such as health maintenance organizations (HMOs) into existing databases in order to upgrade the ICDC's status as a public health research institute and to ensure quality in rehabilitation services within Israel. Israel has a highly developed infrastructure, and in 2010, access to improved sanitary facilities and improved sources of drinking water was essentially universal in Israel. According to the World Higher Education Database (WHED), three universities in Israel offer programs in epidemiology or public health: the Hebrew University of Jerusalem, Ben-Gurion University of the Negev, and Tel Aviv University.

ITALY

Italy is a southern European country consisting of a peninsula, two large islands, and numerous smaller islands; Italy shares borders with Austria, France, Vatican City (the Holy See), San Marino, Switzerland, and Slovenia and has an extensive coastline (4,722 miles or 7,600 kilometers) on the Mediterranean Sea. The area of 116,348 square miles (301,340 square kilometers) makes Italy slightly larger than Arizona, and the July

2012 population was estimated at 61.3 million (the 23rd-largest in the world). In 2010, 68 percent of the population lived in urban areas, and the 2010 to 2015 annual rate of urbanization was estimated at 0.5 percent. Rome is the capital and largest city (with a 2009 population estimated at 3.4 million). The population growth rate in 2012 was 0.4 percent, the birth rate was 9.1 births per 1,000 population, the net migration rate 4.7 migrants per 1,000 (the 22nd-highest in the world), and the total fertility rate 1.27 children per woman, one of the 20 lowest in the world.

Italy became a unified nation-state in 1861. Benito Mussolini established a fascist dictatorship in the 1920s, and Italy sided with Germany in World War II; however, a democratic republic was reestablished in 1946. Italy ranked tied for 69th among 183 countries on the *Corruption Perceptions Index 2011*, with a score of 3.9 (on a scale where 0 indicates highly corrupt and 10 very clean). In 2011, Italy was classified as a country with very high human development (the highest of four categories) on the United Nations Development Programme's (UNDP's) Human Development Index (HDI), with a score of 0.874 (on a scale where 1 denotes high development and 0 low development). Life expectancy at birth in 2012 was estimated at 81.86 years, among the highest in the world, and per capita gross domestic product (GDP) in 2011 was estimated at $30,100. In 2006, the Gini Index (a measure of dispersion, in which perfect equality is denoted by 0 and maximum inequality is denoted by 100) for family income was 32.0. According to the World Economic Forum's *Global Gender Gap Index 2011*, Italy ranked 74th out of 135 countries on gender equality with a score of 0.680 (on a scale with a theoretical range of 1 for equality to 0 for inequality and an actual range in 2011 from 0.8530 to 0.4873).

Emergency Health Services

Italy's laws governing the emergency health system date from the 1990s, as does recognition of emergency medicine as a medical specialty; by law, free access to hospitals for emergency care is provided for all persons, including the uninsured. Funding for the emergency system is provided entirely from the state budget for both inpatient and outpatient services. Italy has only one national telephone number for medical emergencies, 118 (not 112, the European Union, or EU, standard); the country has 113 dispatch centers that are interconnected. Since 2007, Italy has applied a copayment of 24 euros ($37) for the use of emergency medical services judged to be noncritical and not urgent.

Insurance

Italy has a national health service (Servizio Sanitario Nazionale, or SSN) financed through regional tax revenues, a value-added tax (VAT), and an earmarked business tax. The SSN covers medical expenses such as hospital care, physician services, and some prescription drugs but does not cover most dental care or eye care. The SSN is modeled on the British National Health Service and provides uniform comprehensive care. Primary care is free at point of use, but copayments are required for some specialist services and prescription drugs. Illegal immigrants have been granted access to basic services since 1998. Citizens are allowed to purchase supplemental private insurance, and about 15 percent do. Out-of-pocket expenses are partially subsidized once a maximum is reached (129 euros, or $179). Some individuals are exempt from cost sharing, including children, pregnant women, the elderly, those with low incomes, and persons with some disabilities or chronic conditions. Primary care is paid for through a mix of fee for service and capitation, while hospital payments are handled through a combination of global budgets and case-based payments; hospital payments include physician costs. Patients are not required to register with a general practice physician.

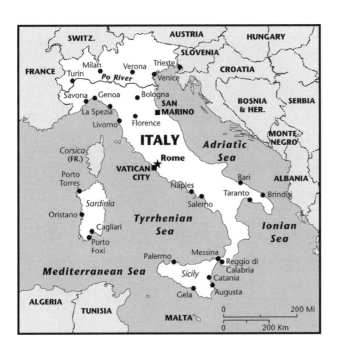

A 2004 study by the World Health Organization (WHO) found that none of the Italian population had substitutive voluntary health insurance (covering services that would otherwise be available from the state), and 15.6 percent had complementary voluntary health insurance (covering services not covered or not fully covered by the state) or supplementary health insurance (providing increased choice or faster access to services). Persons who hold voluntary policies are likely to have high educational levels and incomes, to live in urban areas, and to live in northeastern Italy.

Costs of Hospitalization

As of 2002, hospitals in Italy were funded on a capitation basis by local health units; in 1995, tariffs based on diagnosis-related groups (DRGs) began to be used to fund cross-boundary activity at hospitals outside local health units.

Access to Health Care

According to WHO, in 2003, 99 percent of births were attended by skilled personnel (for example, physicians, nurses, or midwives), and 68 percent of pregnant women received at least four prenatal care visits.

The 2010 immunization rates for 1-year-olds were 96 percent for diphtheria and pertussis (DPT3), 90 percent for measles (MCV), and 95 percent for Hib (Hib3). According to WHO, in 2010, Italy had 18.40 magnetic resonance imaging (MRI) machines per 1 million population, 29.95 computer tomography (CT) machines per 1 million, and 1.76 positron emission tomography (PET) machines per 1 million.

Cost of Drugs

The SSN issues an annual list of services covered, including a ranking of prescription drugs into three tiers, based on effectiveness and, in some cases, cost-effectiveness. Drugs in the first tier are covered by the SSN, drugs in the second tier are covered only in hospitals, and drugs in the third tier are not covered at all. According to Elizabeth Docteur, in 2004, Italy ranked lowest among Organisation for Economic Co-operation and Development (OECD) countries in terms of the use of generics; generic drugs represented 2 percent of the market share by value and 4 percent of the market share by volume of the total pharmaceutical market. In 2009, according to OECD data, pharmaceutical spending per capita in Italy was $572 (adjusted for

Selected Health Indicators: Italy Compared With the Organisation for Economic Co-operation and Development (OECD) Country Average

	Italy	OECD average (2010 or nearest year)
Male life expectancy at birth, 2009	79.4	77
Female life expectancy at birth, 2009	84.6	82.5
Total expenditure on health (percent of GDP), 2011	9.1	9.5
Total expenditure on health (per capita, USD purchasing power parity), 2010	2,963.7	3,265
Public expenditure on health (per capita, USD purchasing power parity), 2010	2,358.9	2,377.8
Public expenditure on health (percent total expenditure on health), 2011	79	72.2
Out-of-pocket expenditure on health (percent total expenditure on health), 2011	18.3	19.5
Out-of-pocket expenditure on health (per capita, USD purchasing power parity), 2010	527.9	558.4

Source: OECD Health Data 2012 (Organisation for Economic Co-operation and Development, 2012).

differences in the cost of living). Real annual growth in pharmaceutical expenditures in Italy grew 2.6 percent from 1997 to 2005, slower than the 3.4 percent growth of total health expenditure (minus pharmaceutical expenditures) over those years.

According to Douglas Ball, Italy charges a lower VAT for medicines (10 percent) than for other goods (the standard VAT is 20 percent). There is no fixed pharmaceutical dispensing fee. The wholesale fixed margin for reimbursable medicines is 6.65 percent of the retail price, and the margin for nonreimbursable medicines is about 8 percent of the retail price. The pharmacy markup is 26.7 percent of the retail price for reimbursable medicines; the pharmacy margin for nonreimbursable drugs is not regulated.

Health Care Facilities
As of 2010, according to WHO, Italy had 0.11 district or rural hospitals per 100,000, 1.84 provincial hospitals per 100,000, and 0.14 specialized hospitals per 100,000. In 2008, Italy had 3.70 hospital beds per 1,000 population. Most (94 percent) of primary care physicians used electronic medical records (EMRs) in 2009. According to OECD data, in Italy, the average length of stay in acute care was 7.7 days (in 2008), and there were 130 hospital discharges per 1,000 population (in 2009).

Major Health Issues
In 2008, WHO estimated that 5 percent of years of life lost in Italy were due to communicable diseases, 86 percent to noncommunicable diseases, and 9 percent to injuries. In 2008, the age-standardized estimate of cancer deaths was 158 per 100,000 for men and 91 per 100,000 for women; for cardiovascular disease and diabetes, 156 per 100,000 for men and 102 per 100,000 for women; and for chronic respiratory disease, 25 per 100,000 for men and 9 per 100,000 for women.

In 2010, tuberculosis incidence was 4.9 per 100,000 population, tuberculosis prevalence 6.0 per 100,000, and deaths due to tuberculosis among human immunodeficiency virus (HIV)-negative people 0.44 per 100,000. As of 2009, an estimated 0.3 percent of adults age 15 to 49 were living with HIV or acquired immune deficiency syndrome (AIDS). The maternal mortality rate (death from any cause related to or aggravated by pregnancy) in Italy in 2008 was five maternal deaths per 100,000 live births, among the lowest in the world. The infant mortality rate, defined as the number of deaths of infants younger than 1 year, was 3.36 per 1,000 live births as of 2012, the ninth-lowest in the world.

Health Care Personnel
Italy has 34 medical schools. The basic medical degree requires six to seven years to complete, and the degree awarded is Laurea in Medicine e Cirurgia (diploma in medicine and surgery). Italy, as a member of the EU, cooperates with other countries in recognizing physicians qualified to practice in other EU countries, as specified by Directive 2005/36/EC of the European Parliament. This allows qualified professionals to practice their profession in other EU states on a temporary basis and requires that the host country automatically recognize qualifications for certain professions, including physicians, nurses, dentists, midwives, and pharmacists, if certain conditions have been met (for instance, facility in the language of the host country may be required). In 2008, Italy had 4.24 physicians per 1,000 population, 1.02 pharmaceutical personnel per 1,000, 0.49 dentistry personnel per 1,000, and 6.52 nurses and midwives per 1,000.

Government Role in Health Care
According to WHO, in 2010, Italy spent $196 billion on health care, an amount that comes to $3,248 per capita. Health care funding was provided entirely from domestic sources. More than three-quarters (78 percent) of health care funding was paid for through government expenditures, with the remainder provided through household expenditures (20 percent) and other sources (3 percent). In 2010, Italy allocated 15 percent of its total government expenditures to health, and government expenditures on health came to 7 percent of GDP; both figures place Italy in the median range as compared with other high-income European countries.

Each year, the SSN produces a list of essential levels of care (*livelli essenziali di assistenza*, or LEAs) for ambulatory and hospital care and prescription drugs. The LEAs include a positive list of services that are covered by the SSN and a negative list of services that are not covered (for example, cosmetic surgery), are covered only in some cases, or are considered inappropriate cause for a hospital admission (for example, cataract surgery).

Public Health Programs
Italy's National Institute of Health (Institute Superiore di Sanita, or ISS) is located in Rome and headed

by Enrico Garaci. The ISS is part of the National Health Service and its responsibilities include conducting research, certifying the quality of medicines and medical devices, monitoring trends in disease and mortality, and providing technical support for public health problems, including health-related environmental surveys and epidemic investigations. The ISS also provides training activities to meet the needs of the National Health Services and promotes international cooperation, including scientific partnerships in industrialized countries, scientific and development projects in countries where the economy is in transition, and development partnerships in developing and war-torn countries in need of humanitarian and technical assistance. Italy has a highly developed infrastructure, and in 2010, access to improved sources of drinking water was essentially universal.

According to the World Higher Education Database (WHED), three universities in Italy offer programs in epidemiology or public health: the University of Aquila, the University of Florence, and the University of Milan.

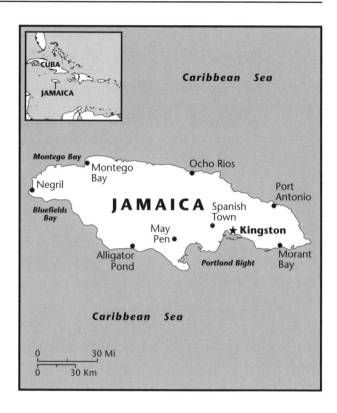

JAMAICA

Jamaica is a mountainous island nation in the Caribbean Sea. Jamaica's area of 4,244 square miles (10,991 square kilometers) makes Jamaica about the size of Connecticut, and the July 2012 population was estimated at 2.9 million. In 2010, 52 percent of the population lived in urban areas, and the 2010 to 2015 annual rate of urbanization was estimated at 0.6 percent. Kingston is the capital and largest city (with a 2009 population estimated at 580,000). The 2012 population growth rate was 0.7 percent, the net migration rate negative 5.2 migrants per 1,000 population (one of the 30 highest emigration rates in the world), the birth rate 18.9 births per 1,000, and the total fertility rate 2.1 children per woman. The United Nations High Commissioner for Refugees (UNHCR) estimated that, in 2010, there were 20 refugees and persons in refugee-like situations in Jamaica. Jamaica was colonized in the 17th century by England, which used the island as a plantation; after slavery was abolished in 1834, many former slaves became small farmers. In 1958, Jamaica joined the Federation of the West Indies and gained full independence from Great Britain in 1962.

Jamaica ranked tied for 86th among 183 countries on the *Corruption Perceptions Index 2011*, with a score of 3.3 (on a scale where 0 indicates highly corrupt and 10 very clean). In 2011, Jamaica was classified as a country with high human development (the second-highest category) on the United Nations Development Programme's (UNDP's) Human Development Index (HDI), with a score of 0.727 (on a scale where 1 denotes high development and 0 low development). Life expectancy at birth in 2012 was estimated at 73.43 years, and per capita gross domestic product (GDP) in 2011 was estimated at $9,000.

In 2004, the Gini Index (a measure of dispersion, in which perfect equality is denoted by 0 and maximum inequality is denoted by 100) for family income was 45.5. According to the World Economic Forum's *Global Gender Gap Index 2011*, Jamaica ranked 47th out of 135 countries on gender equality, with a score of 0.703 (on a scale with a theoretical range of 1 for equality to 0 for inequality and an actual range in 2011 from 0.8530 to 0.4873).

Emergency Health Services

The first emergency department in Jamaica was established in 1988 at the University Hospital of the West Indies (UWHI); this unit was divided into an

Accident and Emergency unit to care for trauma and emergency cases and an ambulatory care unit for nonurgent cases; the Accident and Emergency unit was administered through the department of surgery. Emergency medicine is now an accepted specialty in Jamaica; in 1995, a training course in emergency medicine was established for nurses. Most emergency care in Jamaica is provided through the country's 23 public hospitals. Two major adult hospitals (Kingston Regional Hospital and the UWHI) provide 24-hour adult emergency services for Kingston, and Bustamante Children's Hospital does the same for pediatric emergencies.

Jamaica is prone to natural disasters, including hurricanes and earthquakes; the National Disaster Committee manages disaster response, and the Office of Disaster Preparedness and Emergency Management creates response plans and informs the public of disaster threats.

Insurance

Jamaica has a social insurance system providing medical benefits to all residents of Jamaica and cash maternity benefits to employed women age 18 or older. Medical benefits are funded primarily through general tax revenues, with cash benefits funded through contributions from wages (2.5 percent of covered earnings, up to a maximum, for most employed persons—JMD 25 per week for members of the armed forces; JMD 50 per week for those voluntarily joining the system; JMD 50 per week and 5 percent of covered earnings, up to a maximum, for the self-employed) and employer payroll contributions (2.5 percent of covered payroll or JMD 25 per week for the military); these contributions also support the pension system.

Medical benefits are provided at nominal cost or free through public hospitals and dispensaries, and the National Health Fund covers prescription drugs for some illnesses. Social insurance pensioners receive additional coverage through the National Insurance Gold program, funded by earmarked alcohol and tobacco taxes. The maternity benefit is equal to the national minimum wage and is paid for eight weeks. The program is administered by the Ministry of Labor and Social Security. According to Ke Xu and colleagues, in 2003, 1.9 percent of households in Jamaica experienced catastrophic health expenditures annually; "catastrophic" was defined as exceeding 40 percent of household income remaining after basic needs were met.

Costs of Hospitalization

No data available.

Access to Health Care

According to the World Health Organization (WHO), in 2008, 98 percent of births were attended by skilled personnel (for example, physicians, nurses, or midwives). In 2008, 87 percent of pregnant women received at least four prenatal care visits. The 2010 immunization rates for 1-year-olds were 98 percent for diphtheria and pertussis (DPT3), 88 percent for measles (MCV), and 98 percent for Hib (Hib3). In 2010, an estimated 57 percent of persons with advanced human immunodeficiency virus (HIV) infection were receiving antiretroviral therapy in accordance with the 2010 WHO guidelines.

According to WHO, in 2010, Jamaica had 1.48 magnetic resonance imaging (MRI) machines per 1 million population, 1.48 computer tomography (CT) machines per 1 million, 1.11 telecolbalt units per 1 million, and 1.11 radiotherapy machines per 1 million.

Cost of Drugs

Drugs are procured for the public sector by Health Corporation Limited, an agency of the Ministry of Health. Most (over 90 percent) of vaccines for the national immunization program are obtained through the Pan American Health Organization's (PAHO's) Revolving Fund for Vaccine Procurement. In the public sector, prescriptions are guided by the Vital Essential and Necessary (VEN) list, while the National Drug Formulary guides prescribing in the private sector. About 20 percent of government health expenditures from 2004 to 2005 were for pharmaceuticals. The National Health Fund, established in 2002 and funded by taxes, provides assistance for those needing drugs to treat specific chronic diseases. The Jamaican Drugs for the Elderly also provides assistance specifically to older persons suffering from chronic diseases.

Health Care Facilities

The University Hospital of the West Indies (UWHI) and Kingston Regional Hospital, both in Jamaica, are the primary referral hospitals for Jamaica; the UWHI is a teaching hospital and has all the major disciplines and referral tools.

As of 2010, according to WHO, Jamaica had 0.40 district or rural hospitals per 100,000, 0.29 provincial hospitals per 100,000, and 0.07 specialized hospitals per 100,000. In 2009, Jamaica had 1.70 hospital beds per 1,000 population.

Major Health Issues

In 2008, WHO estimated that 37 percent of years of life lost in Jamaica were due to communicable diseases, 42 percent to noncommunicable diseases, and 41 percent to injuries. In 2008, the age-standardized estimate of cancer deaths was 126 per 100,000 for men and 120 per 100,000 for women; for cardiovascular disease and diabetes, 246 per 100,000 for men and 249 per 100,000 for women; and for chronic respiratory disease, 51 per 100,000 for men and 42 per 100,000 for women.

Jamaica's maternal mortality rate (death from any cause related to or aggravated by pregnancy) was estimated in 2008 as 89 maternal deaths per 100,000 live births. The infant mortality rate, defined as the number of deaths of infants younger than 1 year, was 14.30 per 1,000 live births as of 2012. In 2010, tuberculosis incidence was 6.6 per 100,000 population, tuberculosis prevalence 7.6 per 100,000, and deaths due to tuberculosis among HIV-negative people 0.59 per 100,000. As of 2009, an estimated 1.7 percent of adults age 15 to 49 were living with HIV or acquired immune deficiency syndrome (AIDS).

Health Care Personnel

Jamaica has one medical school, the Faculty of Medical Sciences of the UWHI in Kingston, which began offering instruction in 1948. UWHI is supported by and serves students from countries of the Commonwealth Caribbean. The basic medical course requires five years to complete, and the degrees awarded are bachelor of medicine and bachelor of surgery.

In 2007, Jamaica had a shortage of health personnel in many categories, particularly nurses, due to high emigration. In 2003, Jamaica had 0.85 physicians per 1,000 population, 0.08 dentistry personnel per 1,000, and 1.65 nurses and midwives per 1,000. Using Fitzhugh Mullan's methodology, Jamaica has an emigration factor of 41.4, representing a high ratio of Jamaican physicians working outside Jamaica (in the United States, United Kingdom, Canada, or Australia) relative to those working in Jamaica. Alok Bhargava and colleagues place Jamaica eighth among countries most affected by the medical "brain drain" (international migration of skilled personnel) in 2004.

Government Role in Health Care

According to WHO, in 2010, Jamaica spent $678 million on health care, an amount that comes to $247 per capita. Health care funding was provided primarily (88 percent) from domestic sources, with the remaining 2 percent of funding coming from overseas sources. Just over half (54 percent) of health care funding was paid for through government expenditures, with the remainder provided through household expenditures (33 percent) and other sources (14 percent). In 2010, Jamaica allocated 6 percent of its total government expenditures to health, and government expenditures on health came to 3 percent of GDP; both figures place Jamaica in the low range as compared with other upper-middle-income countries in the Americas region. In 2009, according to WHO, official development assistance (ODA) for health in Jamaica came to $3.44 per capita.

Public Health Programs

The 2004 National Policy for the Promotion of Healthy Lifestyles focuses on chronic diseases, high-risk sexual behavior, violence, physical activity, nutrition, and smoking prevention and cessation. In 2010, 80 percent of the population of Jamaica had access to improved sanitation facilities (82 percent in rural areas and 78 percent in urban), and 93 percent had access to improved sources of drinking water (88 percent in rural areas and 99 percent in urban). According to the World Higher Education Database (WHED), no university in Jamaica offers programs in epidemiology or public health.

JAPAN

Japan is an island nation in the north Pacific, consisting of four large islands and numerous smaller ones. The area of 145,914 square miles (377,915 square kilometers) makes Japan similar in size to California, and the July 2012 population was estimated at 127.4 million (the 10th-largest in the world; Japan's coastline of 18,486 miles (29,751 kilometers) is also one of the longest in the world. In 2010, 67 percent of the population lived in urban areas, and the 2010 to 2015 annual rate of urbanization was estimated at 0.2 percent. Tokyo is the capital and largest city (with a 2009 population estimated at 36.5 million, making it the largest city in

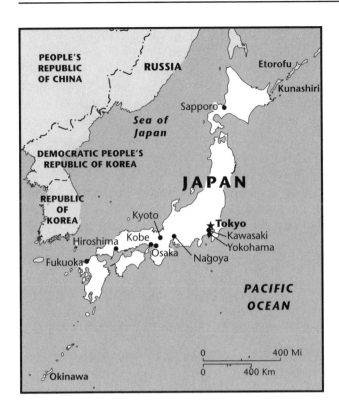

at $34,300. In 2008, the Gini Index (a measure of dispersion, in which perfect equality is denoted by 0 and maximum inequality is denoted by 100) for family income was 37.6. According to the World Economic Forum's *Global Gender Gap Index 2011*, Japan ranked 98th out of 135 countries on gender equality, with a score of 0.651 (on a scale with a theoretical range of 1 for equality to 0 for inequality and an actual range in 2011 from 0.8530 to 0.4873).

Emergency Health Services

According to the World Health Organization (WHO), as of 2007, Japan had a formal and publicly available emergency care (prehospital care) system accessible through a national universal access telephone number.

Insurance

Japan has a statutory health insurance system (SHI) with more than 3,500 noncompeting insurers (public, quasi-public, and employer-based). The system is financed through general tax revenue and insurance premiums. Most citizens buy private insurance that covers care in private facilities and some cost sharing. Out-of-pocket expenses for coinsurance are reduced after a monthly cap of 80,100 yen ($1,050) is reached. The out-of-pocket cap is lower for those with low incomes, and copayments are lower for the elderly and children. Primary care is paid for on a fee-for-service basis, while hospital payments are handled through a combination of global budgets (about 50 percent) and case-based payments (about 50 percent); hospital payments include physician costs. Patients are not required to register with a general practice physician.

Costs of Hospitalization

According to Organisation for Economic Co-operation and Development (OECD) data, in 2009, hospital spending per capita in Japan was $1,355 (adjusted for differences in the cost of living), and hospital spending per discharge came to $12,650 in 2011.

Access to Health Care

In 2009, according to OECD data, the Japanese had an average of 13.2 physician visits. According to WHO, in 2006, 100 percent of births were attended by skilled personnel (for example, physicians, nurses, or midwives). The 2010 immunization rates for 1-year-olds were 98 percent for diphtheria and pertussis (DPT3) and 94 percent for measles (MCV). According to

the world). Population growth in 2012 was slightly negative (negative 0.1 percent), the total fertility rate was 1.4 children per woman, the net migration rate 0.0 migrants per 1,000 population, and the birth rate 8.4 births per 1,000, one of the lowest in the world. The United Nations High Commissioner for Refugees (UNHCR) estimated that, in 2010, there were 727 refugees and persons in refugee-like situations in Japan.

Japan became a regional power in the 20th century and occupied large areas of Asia during World War II. After defeat in the war, Japan quickly rebuilt and became an industrial and economic power. Japan's government has a reputation for transparency, ranking tied for 14th among 183 countries on the *Corruption Perceptions Index 2011,* with a score of 8.0 (on a scale where 0 indicates highly corrupt and 10 very clean).

In 2011, Japan was classified as a country with very high human development (the highest of four categories) on the United Nations Development Programme's (UNDP's) Human Development Index (HDI), with a score of 0.901 (on a scale where 1 denotes high development and 0 low development). Life expectancy at birth in 2012 was estimated at 83.91 years, the third-highest in the world, and the per capita gross domestic product (GDP) in 2011 was estimated

WHO, in 2010, Japan had 45.89 magnetic resonance imaging (MRI) machines per 1 million population, 101.07 computer tomography (CT) machines per 1 million, and 4.34 positron emission tomography (PET) machines per 1 million.

Cost of Drugs

In 2009, according to OECD data, pharmaceutical spending per capita in Japan was $558 (adjusted for differences in the cost of living). Real annual growth in pharmaceutical expenditures in Japan grew 1.7 percent from 1997 to 2005, slower than the 3.1 percent growth of total health expenditure (minus pharmaceutical expenditures) over those years. According to Douglas Ball, Japan charges the standard value-added tax (VAT) of 5 percent of medicines. The wholesale and pharmacy markups are unregulated, while the pharmacy dispensing and prescription fees vary with the class of drug and other factors. Japan is the second-largest purchaser of pharmaceuticals, after the United States, accounting for 9 percent of global pharmaceutical sales.

According to Elizabeth Docteur, in Japan, the reimbursement price for drugs is determined by the Ministry of Health, Labour, and Welfare, based on innovativeness and usefulness; drugs judged innovative or that offer therapeutic improvement when compared to existing drugs may charge a premium based on the degree of innovation or improvement. To be considered innovative, drugs must meet two of the following three requirements: offer a clinically useful and novel action mechanism, demonstrate higher safety or efficacy, or offer improved treatment for injury or illness. Premiums are also available for drugs produced using a new manufacturing technique that offers higher clinical usefulness, and for orphan drugs and pediatric drugs as well. The amount of premium ranges from 120 percent (the most innovative drugs) to 5 percent (the lowest premium for pediatric drugs) over the price of existing drugs to treat a condition based on the degree of innovation or improvement.

Health Care Facilities

In 2008, Japan had 13.75 hospital beds per 1,000 population, the highest ratio in the world.

Major Health Issues

In 2008, WHO estimated that 9 percent of years of life lost in Japan were due to communicable diseases, 77 percent to noncommunicable diseases, and 15 percent to injuries. In 2008, the age-standardized estimate of cancer deaths was 150 per 100,000 for men and 77 per 100,000 for women; for cardiovascular disease and diabetes, 118 per 100,000 for men and 65 per 100,000 for women; and for chronic respiratory disease, 23 per 100,000 for men and eight per 100,000 for women.

The maternal mortality rate (death from any cause related to or aggravated by pregnancy) in Japan in 2008 was six maternal deaths per 100,000 live births, among the lowest in the world. The infant mortality rate was 2.21 per 1,000 live births as of 2012, the second-lowest in the world. In 2010, tuberculosis incidence was 21.0 per 100,000 population, tuberculosis prevalence 27.0 per 100,000, and deaths due to tuberculosis among human immunodeficiency virus (HIV)-negative people 1.50 per 100,000. As of 2009, an estimated 0.1 percent of adults age 15 to 49 were living with HIV or acquired immune deficiency syndrome (AIDS).

Health Care Personnel

Japan has 80 medical schools. The basic degree course lasts six years, and the degree awarded is Igakushi (bachelor of medicine). The license to practice medicine is granted to graduates of recognized schools who complete the national medical exam. Graduates of foreign medical schools must have their degrees validated. In 2006, Japan had 2.06 physicians per 1,000 population, 1.26 pharmaceutical personnel per 1,000, 0.74 dentistry personnel per 1,000, and 4.14 nurses and midwives per 1,000.

Government Role in Health Care

According to WHO, in 2010, Japan spent $518 billion on health care, an amount that comes to $4,065 per capita. Health care funding was provided entirely from domestic sources. More than four-fifths (83 percent) of health care funding was paid for through government expenditures, with the remainder provided through household expenditures (14 percent) and other sources (3 percent). In 2010, Japan allocated 18 percent of its total government expenditures to health, and government expenditures on health came to 8 percent of GDP; both figures place Japan in the high range as compared with other high-income western Pacific region countries.

Public Health Programs

The National Institute of Public Health in Japan is located in Wako (in Saitama Prefecture, part of the

Greater Tokyo region) and, in 2012, was headed by Yukio Matsutani. The National Institute was created in 1938 for the purpose of conducting research in public health and training public health personnel; it took its current form in 2002 with the mergers of the Institute of Public Health and the National Institute of Health Services Management. Japan has a highly developed infrastructure, and in 2010, access to improved sanitary facilities and improved sources of drinking water was essentially universal. According to the World Higher Education Database (WHED), 26 universities in Japan offer programs in epidemiology or public health.

JORDAN

Jordan is a Middle Eastern country, sharing borders with Iraq, Israel, Saudi Arabia, Syria, and the West Bank and having a short coastline (16 miles or 26 kilometers) on the Gulf of Aqaba. The area of 34,109 square miles (88,342 square kilometers) makes Jordan similar in size to Indiana, and the July 2012 population was estimated at 6.5 million. In 2010, 79 percent of the population lived in urban areas, and the 2010 to 2015 annual rate of urbanization is estimated at 1.6 percent. Amman is the capital and largest city (with a 2009 population estimated at 1.1 million). In 2012, the population growth rate was negative 1.0 percent, among the lowest in the world, due in part to Jordan having the second-lowest net migration rate in the world, negative 33.42 migrants per 1,000 population, as of 2012 (meaning that substantially more people are leaving the country than are entering). The 2012 birth rate was 26.5 births per 1,000, and the total fertility rate was 3.4 children per woman. The United Nations High Commissioner for Refugees (UNHCR) estimated that, in 2010, there were 31,013 refugees and persons in refugee-like situations in Jordan.

Jordan was created as the region of Transjordan after World War I and became an independent country in 1946. King Abdullah ruled the country from 1953 to 1999, although parliamentary elections were reinstated in 1989 and political parties legalized in 1992. Jordan ranked 56th among 183 countries on the *Corruption Perceptions Index 2011,* with a score of 4.5 (on a scale where 0 indicates highly corrupt and 10 very clean). In 2011, Jordan was classified as a country with medium human development (the second from the lowest of four categories) on the United Nations Development Programme's (UNDP's) Human Development Index (HDI), with a score of 0.698 (on a scale where 1 denotes high development and 0 low development). Life expectancy at birth in 2012 was estimated at 80.18 years, among the highest in the world, and estimated gross domestic product (GDP) per capita in 2011 was $5,900.

In 2007, the Gini Index (a measure of dispersion, in which perfect equality is denoted by 0 and maximum inequality is denoted by 100) for family income was 39.7. According to the World Economic Forum's *Global Gender Gap Index 2011,* Jordan ranked 117th out of 135 countries on gender equality, with a score of 0.612 (on a scale with a theoretical range of 1 for equality to 0 for inequality and an actual range in 2011 from 0.8530 to 0.4873).

Emergency Health Services

According to the World Health Organization (WHO), as of 2007, Jordan had a formal and publicly available emergency care (prehospital care) system accessible through a national universal access telephone number. As of January 2012, the United Nations Relief and Works Agency for Palestine

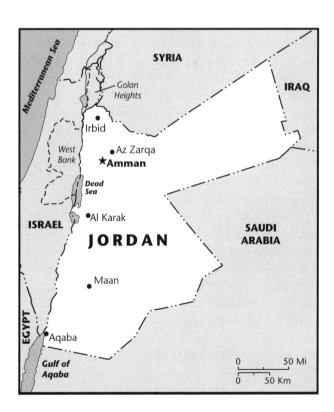

Refugees (UNRWA) operated 10 camps in Jordan with 2.05 million registered persons, including 1.98 million registered refugees.

Insurance

As of 2004, about one-third (32 percent) of the population of Jordan was uninsured. Many people had more than one type of insurance, so 21 percent of the population was covered under the Government Ministry of Health plan (including civil servants and their dependents, the poor and disabled, and blood donors); one-third (33 percent) were covered by the Royal Medical Services (including military personnel and their dependents and some public firm workers); others were covered by private insurance (8 percent), the UNRWA and similar organizations (18 percent, mainly Palestinian refugees); and 1 percent were covered by the Jordan University Hospital (employees of the hospital). As of 2011, Jordan's social insurance provided maternity benefits of 100 percent of monthly earnings for up to 10 weeks for women working in private companies with at least five employees.

Costs of Hospitalization

No data available.

Access to Health Care

Free medical care is provided to the poor in Jordan, as is comprehensive medical care for children younger than age 5. More than 200 health care centers spread throughout the country provide medical and preventive services. According to WHO, in 2007, 99 percent of births were attended by skilled personnel (for example, physicians, nurses, or midwives). In 2007, 94 percent of pregnant women received at least four prenatal care visits. The 2010 immunization rates for 1-year-olds were 98 percent for diphtheria and pertussis (DPT3), 98 percent for measles (MCV), and 98 percent for Hib (Hib3).

Access to pharmaceuticals does not appear to be a major problem in Jordan. According to Jordan's 2011 Pharmaceutical Country Profiles, a household survey indicated that more than three-quarters of Jordanians with acute illnesses took all the medicines prescribed them, and less than 1 percent indicated that cost prevented them from taking all prescribed medicines. Even in poor households, less than 1 percent of adult patients reported failing to take prescribed medication for acute conditions due to cost. According to WHO, in 2010, Jordan had 2.44 magnetic resonance imaging (MRI) machines per 1 million population, 6.52 computer tomography (CT) machines per 1 million, 0.33 positron emission tomography (PET) machines per 1 million, 0.33 telecolbalt units per 1 million, and 0.33 radiotherapy machines per 1 million.

Cost of Drugs

The sale of medicines is regulated by the Jordan Food and Drug Administration; pharmaceutical products must be registered, and this includes setting the price. In 2008, total pharmaceutical expenditures in Jordan came to JOD 496.4 ($701 million), which comes to JOD 84.9 ($120) per capita. Pharmaceutical expenditures represented more than one-third (35.9 percent) of total health expenditures, and 3.1 percent of GDP. More than one-third (38.4 percent) of pharmaceutical expenditures were paid for through public funds, for a per capita public expenditure on pharmaceuticals of JOD 32.6 ($46). A 2004 survey found that drugs were procured near the international reference price and that markups were low or nonexistent in the public sector. However, availability was low (averaging 28 percent) in the public sector, so many people were forced to purchase drugs through the private sector, where they were more available (the mean availability of generics was 80 percent and 60 percent for originator brand drugs), but prices were substantially higher (generics were priced about 10 times as high in private as opposed to public pharmacies, and originator brands were priced about twice as high).

Certain population groups are entitled to medicines free of charge, including the elderly, children less than 5 years of age, pregnant women, and the poor. Drugs for several conditions are also provided for free, including malaria, tuberculosis, sexually transmitted diseases (STDs), and human immunodeficiency virus and acquired immune deficiency syndrome (HIV/AIDS); vaccinations on the Expanded Programme on Immunization (EPI) list, created by WHO, are also provided free of charge. Public health insurance provides coverage for medicines on the Essential Medicines List (EML); private insurance provides varying levels of coverage for medications. Most (97.8 percent) of medicines prescribed in public clinics are on the EML. A 2004 survey determined brand-name drugs were sold for higher than the international reference price (almost six times higher in the public sector and 17 times higher in the private sector), while generic drugs were sold at slightly less than the international reference price in the public sector (85 percent of the

Selected Health Indicators: Jordan Compared With the Global Average (2010)

	Jordan	Global Average
Male life expectancy at birth* (years)	69	66
Female life expectancy at birth* (years)	74	71
Under-5 mortality rate, both sexes (per 1,000 live births)	22	57
Adult mortality rate, both sexes* (probability of dying between 15 and 60 years per 1,000 population)	155	176
Maternal mortality ratio (per 100,000 live births)	63	210
Tuberculosis prevalence (per 100,000 population)	8	178

Source: World Health Organization Global Health Observatory Data Repository.
*Data refers to 2009.

reference price) but more than 10 times the reference price in the private sector.

As a member of the World Trade Organization (WTO), Jordan observes patent law, but national law also includes some elements of the Trade-Related Aspects of Intellectual Property Rights (TRIPS), which provide exceptions to patent law. In Jordan, these exceptions include compulsory licensing for reasons of public health, the Bolar exception that allows manufacturers to perform research and testing to create generic drugs before a patent has expired, and parallel importing provisions (allowing import of drugs created for sale in a different country). Drugs sold in Jordan must go through an assessment process and be authorized (registered) before they may be marketed to the public; as of 2010, 7,700 pharmaceutical products were registered.

Health Care Facilities

As of 2010, according to WHO, Jordan had 22.63 health posts per 100,000 population, 1.66 district or rural hospitals per 100,000, 0.48 provincial hospitals per 100,000, and 0.13 specialized hospitals per 100,000. In 2009, Jordan had 1.80 hospital beds per 1,000 population.

Major Health Issues

In 2008, WHO estimated that 26 percent of years of life lost in Jordan were due to communicable diseases, 55 percent to noncommunicable diseases, and 19 percent to injuries. In 2008, the age-standardized estimate of cancer deaths was 110 per 100,000 for men and 89 per 100,000 for women; for cardiovascular disease and diabetes, 550 per 100,000 for men and 380 per 100,000 for women; and for chronic respiratory disease, 46 per 100,000 for men and 17 per 100,000 for women.

Jordan's maternal mortality rate (death from any cause related to or aggravated by pregnancy) was estimated in 2008 as 59 maternal deaths per 100,000 live births. The infant mortality rate, defined as the number of deaths of infants younger than 1 year, was estimated at 15.82 per 1,000 live births as of 2012. In 2010, tuberculosis incidence was 5.4 per 100,000 population, tuberculosis prevalence 8.0 per 100,000, and deaths due to tuberculosis among HIV-negative people 0.70 per 100,000. As of 2009, an estimated 0.1 percent of adults age 15 to 49 were living with HIV or AIDS.

Health Care Personnel

Jordan has three medical schools: the Faculty of Medicine of the University of Jordan in Amman, the Faculty of Medicine of Jordan University of Science and Technology in Irbid, and the Faculty of Medicine of Mu'tah University in Karak. The course of training for the basic medical degree is six years followed by an 11-month internship in a teaching hospital. The degree awarded is bachelor of medicine and surgery. Physicians must register with the Jordan Medical Association in Amman, and the medical license is granted by the Ministry of Health. Graduates of foreign medical schools must have their degrees validated, and foreigners need residence permits to practice in Jordan. Jordan has an agreement with the Arab Board of Medical Specialties that provides mutual recognition of degrees in medicine and surgery. In 2009, Jordan had 2.45 physicians per 1,000 population, 1.41 pharmaceutical personnel per 1,000, 1.00 laboratory health workers per 1,000, 3.15 health management and support workers per 1,000, 0.73 dentistry personnel per 1,000, 0.18 community and traditional health workers per 1,000, and 4.03 nurses and midwives per 1,000.

Government Role in Health Care

The right to health, including access to essential medicines and medical technology, is recognized in national legislation in Jordan, and the country has a National Health Policy (NHP), updated in 2009, although it does not have an implementation plan for the NHP. Jordan also has a National Medicines Policy (NMP), updated in 2002, including selection of essential medicines; financing, pricing, purchase, distribution, and regulation of drugs; pharmacovigilance; rational usage of medicines; human resource development; research; and evaluation and monitoring.

However, Jordan does not have an implementation plan for the NMP, nor does it regularly monitor or assess the implementation of pharmaceutical policy. According to WHO, in 2010, Jordan spent $2.2 billion on health care, an amount that comes to $347 per capita. Health care funding was provided almost entirely (96 percent) from domestic sources, with the remainder coming from sources from abroad. More than two-thirds (68 percent) of health care funding was paid for through government expenditures, with the remainder provided through household expenditures (25 percent) and other sources (7 percent). In 2010, Jordan allocated 19 percent of its total government expenditures to health, and government expenditures on health came to 5 percent of GDP; both figures place Jordan in the high range as compared with other upper middle-income eastern Mediterranean region countries. In 2009, according to WHO, official development assistance (ODA) for health in Jordan came to $6.44 per capita.

Public Health Programs

Jordan's Ministry of Health is located in Amman and is headed by Adel Belbeisi. Its duties include providing health insurance, supervising the provision of health services, and creating and managing educational and training institutes for health workers. The ministry is also involved with public health activities, including encouraging healthy behaviors in the public, monitoring the quality of the food supply, providing services for women and children, promoting breast-feeding, conducting premarital medical testing, supervising the health conditions for institutions caring for senior citizens, monitoring the environmental conditions of industrial workers, and implementing programs to fight chronic diseases such as diabetes, cancer, and cardiovascular disease.

According to WHO, in 2004, Jordan had 0.25 environmental and public health workers per 1,000 population. The infrastructure of the country is highly developed, and in 2010, 98 percent of the population of Jordan had access to improved sanitation facilities (98 percent in both rural and urban areas), and 97 percent had access to improved sources of drinking water (92 percent in rural areas and 98 percent in urban). According to the World Higher Education Database (WHED), one university in Jordan offers programs in epidemiology or public health: Mu'tah University in the Karak Governorate.

KAZAKHSTAN

Kazakhstan is a landlocked country in Central Asia, sharing borders with China, Kyrgyzstan, Russia, Turkmenistan, and Uzbekistan. The area of 1,052,090 square miles (2,724,900 square kilometers) makes Kazakhstan the ninth-largest country in the world, and the July 2012 population was estimated at 17.5 million. In 2010, 59 percent of the population lived in urban areas, and the 2010 to 2015 annual rate of urbanization was estimated at 1.1 percent. Almaty is the capital and the largest city (with a 2009 population estimated at 1.4 million). The 2012 population growth rate was 1.2 percent, the net migration rate 0.4 migrants per 1,000 population, the birth rate 20.4 births per 1,000, and the total fertility rate 2.4 children per woman. The United Nations High Commissioner for Refugees (UNHCR) estimated that, in 2010, there were 655 refugees and persons in refugee-like situations in Kazakhstan.

Kazakhstan was conquered by Russia in the 18th century, became a Soviet republic in 1936, and became

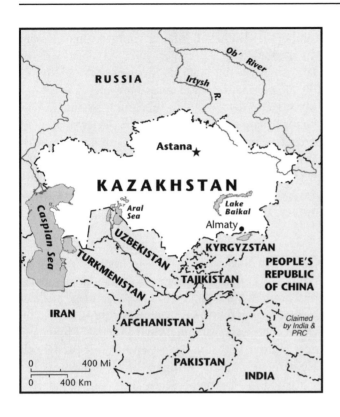

available emergency care (prehospital care) system accessible through a national universal access telephone number.

Insurance

Kazakhstan has a universal medical care system covering all permanent residents of Kazakhstan, along with a social insurance system providing maternity benefits and an employer liability system providing cash sickness benefits. The medical benefits system is funded out of general tax revenues, as is the maternity benefit system; the cash sickness benefit system is funded by employers. Medical benefits are provided through government or private health care providers; coverage includes maternity care, dental care, hospitalization, medical care, transportation, and lab services. The maternity benefit is based on the mother's average earnings, up to a maximum, and is paid for one year. The sickness benefit depends on average earnings and is calculated according to a schedule that is regularly updated to reflect changes in the consumer price index. The Ministry of Health and local health departments administer health care facilities, and the Ministry of Labor and Social Protection provides general coordination and supervision.

Costs of Hospitalization

As of 2002, a case-based system was being introduced to replace the former bed-day system of payments. In the 1990s, Kazakhstan saw a sharp drop in the number of beds and hospitals in many regions; for example, in Dzhezkazgan, the number of beds dropped from 6,225 in 1994 to 2,919 in 1997, and the number of hospitals dropped from 55 to 22 in the same time period.

Access to Health Care

According to WHO, in 2006, 100 percent of births in Kazakhstan were attended by skilled personnel (for example, physicians, nurses, or midwives). The 2010 immunization rates for 1-year-olds were 99 percent for diphtheria and pertussis (DPT3), 99 percent for measles (MCV), and 96 percent for Hib (Hib3). In 2010, an estimated 30 percent of persons with advanced human immunodeficiency virus (HIV) infection were receiving antiretroviral therapy in accordance with the 2010 WHO guidelines.

Cost of Drugs

A 2005 survey found that drugs were generally expensive in Kazakhstan and unaffordable for the average

independent in 1991. Kazakhstan ranked tied for 120th among 183 countries on the *Corruption Perceptions Index 2011,* with a score of 2.7 (on a scale where 0 indicates highly corrupt and 10 very clean). In 2011, Kazakhstan was classified as a country with high human development (the second-highest category) on the United Nations Development Programme's (UNDP's) Human Development Index (HDI), with a score of 0.745 (on a scale where 1 denotes high development and 0 low development). Life expectancy at birth in 2012 was estimated at 69.63 years, and per capita gross domestic product (GDP) in 2011 was estimated at $13,000. Income distribution is among the most equal in the world: In 2009, the Gini Index (a measure of dispersion, in which perfect equality is denoted by 0 and maximum inequality is denoted by 100) for family income was 26.7. According to the World Economic Forum's *Global Gender Gap Index 2011,* Kazakhstan ranked 49th out of 135 countries on gender equality, with a score of 0.701 (on a scale with a theoretical range of 1 for equality to 0 for inequality and an actual range in 2011 from 0.8530 to 0.4873).

Emergency Health Services

According to the World Health Organization (WHO), as of 2007, Kazakhstan had a formal and publicly worker. In the public sector, the median price ratio for the lowest-cost generic drugs was 3.02, meaning that the drugs sold on average for more than three times the international reference price. For the most-sold generic drugs, the median price ratio was 3.85, and for innovator brand drugs, it was 7.23. The median price ratio for some drugs was extremely high, for example, 55.65 for the lowest-priced generic for fluconazole and 99.62 for the innovator brand of the same drug. In the private sector, the median price ratio averaged 8.58 for innovator brand drugs, 4.65 for the most-sold generics, and 3.73 for the lowest-priced generics; however, availability was better in the private sector than in the public. The lowest-paid government worker would have required half a day's wages to pay for the lowest-priced generic drug (atenolol) for one month, 0.6 day's wages to purchase the most-sold generic, and 0.9 day's wages to purchase the innovator brand. To treat hypertension for one month, the same worker would have to work 1.0 day to purchase the lowest-cost generic, 1.5 days to purchase the most common generic, and 2.7 days to purchase the innovator brand. If a family had multiple medical needs, the necessary pharmaceuticals would quickly become unaffordable.

Health Care Facilities
As of 2010, according to WHO, Kazakhstan had 22.99 health posts per 100,000 population, 2.04 district or rural hospitals per 100,000, 1.40 provincial hospitals per 100,000, and 0.17 specialized hospitals per 100,000. In 2009, Kazakhstan had 7.60 hospital beds per 1,000 population, among the 20 highest ratios in the world and a reflection of its status as a former Soviet republic.

Major Health Issues
In 2008, WHO estimated that 16 percent of years of life lost in Kazakhstan were due to communicable diseases, 59 percent to noncommunicable diseases, and 24 percent to injuries. In 2008, the age-standardized estimate of cancer deaths was 199 per 100,000 for men and 123 per 100,000 for women; for cardiovascular disease and diabetes, 859 per 100,000 for men and 546 per 100,000 for women; and for chronic respiratory disease, 68 per 100,000 for men and 22 per 100,000 for women.

Kazakhstan's maternal mortality rate (death from any cause related to or aggravated by pregnancy) was estimated in 2008 as 45 maternal deaths per 100,000 live births. The infant mortality rate, defined as the number of deaths of infants younger than 1 year, was estimated at 23.06 per 1,000 live births as of 2012. In 2010, tuberculosis incidence was 151.0 per 100,000 population, tuberculosis prevalence 198.0 per 100,000, and deaths due to tuberculosis among HIV-negative people 23.00 per 100,000. An estimated 14 percent of new tuberculosis cases and 45 percent of retreatment cases are multidrug resistant. As of 2009, an estimated 0.1 percent of adults age 15 to 49 were living with HIV or acquired immune deficiency syndrome (AIDS).

Health Care Personnel
Kazakhstan has six medical schools, located in Akmola, Aktjubinsk, Almaty, Karaganda, Sempalatinsk, and Shymkent. The basic course for a medical degree requires five to seven years of study followed by two to three years of supervised practice. Physicians must register with the Oblast and Municipal Health Department, and the Ministry of Health grants the license to practice medicine. In 2007, Kazakhstan had 3.88 physicians per 1,000 population, 0.86 pharmaceutical personnel per 1,000, 0.39 dentistry personnel per 1,000, and 7.83 nurses and midwives per 1,000.

Government Role in Health Care
According to WHO, in 2010, Kazakhstan spent $6.3 billion on health care, an amount that comes to $393 per capita. Health care funding was provided almost entirely from domestic sources (99 percent). The largest share (59 percent) of health care funding was paid for through government expenditures, with the remainder provided through household expenditures (40 percent) and other sources (1 percent). In 2010, Kazakhstan allocated 11 percent of its total government expenditures to health, in the median range for upper-middle-income Asian countries; government expenditures on health came to 3 percent of GDP, in the low range as compared with other upper-middle-income Asian countries. In 2009, according to WHO, official development assistance (ODA) for health in Kazakhstan came to $2.24 per capita.

Public Health Programs
In 2010, 97 percent of the population of Kazakhstan had access to improved sanitation facilities (98 percent in rural areas and 97 percent in urban), and 95 percent had access to improved sources of drinking water (90 percent in rural areas and 99 percent in urban). According to the World Higher Education Database

(WHED), six universities in Kazakhstan offer programs in epidemiology or public health: Semey State Medical University, South Kazakhstan State Medical Academy, Karaganda State Medical University, S. D. Asfendiyarov Kazakh National Medical University, Astana Medical University, and Marat Ospanov Western Kazakhstan State Medical Academy.

KENYA

Kenya is an east African country, sharing borders Uganda, Ethiopia, Somalia, Sudan, and Tanzania and having a coastline on the Indian Ocean. The area of 224,081 square miles (580,367 square kilometers) makes Kenya about twice the size of Nevada, and the July 2012 population was estimated at 43.0 million (the 31st-largest in the world). In 2010, 22 percent of the population lived in urban areas, and the 2010 to 2015 annual rate of urbanization was estimated at 4.2 percent. Nairobi is the capital and largest city (with an estimated population of 3.4 million). The 2012 net migration was slightly negative (negative 0.2 migrants per 1,000 population), but the population growth rate was 2.4 percent due to a birth rate of 31.9 births per 1,000 population (the 37th-highest in the world) and a fertility rate of 4.0 children per woman. The United Nations High Commissioner for Refugees (UNHCR) estimated that, in 2010, there were 203,905 refugees and persons in refugee-like situations in Kenya.

A former British colony, Kenya achieved independence in 1963. Kenya was ruled by a single party from 1969 to 1982, and elections in the 1990s were marred by violence and fraud, as were elections in 2005 and 2007. Kenya ranked tied for 152nd among 183 countries on the *Corruption Perceptions Index 2011*, with a score of 2.2 (on a scale where 0 indicates highly corrupt and 10 very clean), and ranked 23rd among 53 African countries on the 2011 Ibrahim Index in terms of governance performance, with a score of 53 (out of 100). In 2011, Kenya was classified as a country with low human development (the lowest of four categories) on the United Nations Development Programme's (UNDP's) Human Development Index (HDI), with a score of 0.509 (on a scale where 1 denotes high development and 0 low development). Life expectancy at birth in 2012 was estimated at 63.07 years, and estimated gross domestic product (GDP) per capita in 2011 was $1,700. In 2008, the Gini Index (a measure of dispersion, in which perfect equality is denoted by 0 and maximum inequality is denoted by 100) for family income was 42.5. Unemployment in 2008 was estimated at 40.0 percent, among the highest rates in the world. In 2012, the World Food Programme estimated that 2.2 million people in Kenya were food insecure, a considerable improvement from 3.7 million in July 2011 (the latter emergency caused by poor rainfall).

According to the World Economic Forum's *Global Gender Gap Index 2011*, Kenya ranked 99th out of 135 countries on gender equality, with a score of 0.649 (on a scale with a theoretical range of 1 for equality to 0 for inequality and an actual range in 2011 from 0.8530 to 0.4873).

Emergency Health Services

According to the World Health Organization (WHO), as of 2007, Kenya did not have a formal and publicly available system for providing prehospital care (emergency care). Doctors Without Borders (Médecins Sans Frontières, or MSF) began working in Kenya in 1987 and had 691 staff members in the country at the close of 2010. Prevention and treatment of human immunodeficiency virus and acquired immune deficiency syndrome (HIV/AIDS) are a major focus of MSF's work in Kenya, as is providing care to the approximately 300,000 Somali refugees living in camps near Dadaab (eastern Kenya). In Nairobi, the national capital, MSF provides treatment for tuberculosis and HIV/AIDS, and operates clinics that aid the victims of gender-based violence. MSF also runs training programs for Ministry of Health staff to treat *kala azar* (visceral leishmaniasis), a disease spread by sand flies, and lobbies the Ministry of Health to make testing more available and provide treatment for free.

Insurance

Kenya has a social insurance system providing medical benefits; it covers employed and self-employed people earning at least KES 1,000 monthly along with their dependents; those earning less can join the system voluntarily. The system is entirely funded through contributions from the insured: KES 160 per month for voluntary contributors and from KES 30 to KES 320 per month for employed and self-employed persons. Insured persons and their dependents are reimbursed for medical and hospital treatment, up to KES 396,000 annually; the amount of reimbursement is determined by law. Those contributing to

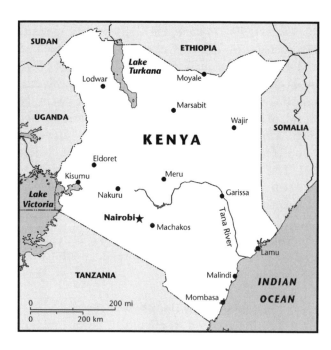

the National Social Security Fund but not covered by the medical benefits system can receive free care in government hospitals. Private hospitals may charge copayments, which are in some cases unlimited and in other cases limited to KES 15,000 (for certain faith-based and other private hospitals) for surgery. Subsidized care for government workers is provided by government hospitals, and free care in government hospitals is provided to all patients for some diseases, including AIDS, tuberculosis, and sexually transmitted diseases (STDs). According to Kenya's 2011 Pharmaceutical Country Profile, less than one-quarter of the population has health insurance, as 22 percent are covered by the national health system or another public insurance plan and 0.9 percent by private plans.

Costs of Hospitalization
No data available.

Access to Health Care
According to WHO, in 2009, 43.8 percent of births were attended by skilled personnel (for example, physicians, nurses, or midwives). In 2009, 47 percent of pregnant women received at least four prenatal care visits. The 2010 immunization rates for 1-year-olds were 83 percent for diphtheria and pertussis (DPT3), 86 percent for measles (MCV), and 83 percent for Hib (Hib3). In 2010, an estimated 61 percent of persons with advanced HIV infection were

receiving antiretroviral therapy in accordance with the 2010 WHO guidelines. According to WHO, in 2010, Kenya had 0.18 magnetic resonance imaging (MRI) machines per 1 million population, 0.28 computer tomography (CT) machines per 1 million, 0.03 telecolbalt units per 1 million, and 0.03 radiotherapy machines per 1 million.

Cost of Drugs
In 2006, total pharmaceutical expenditures in Kenya came to KES 26,796 million ($372 million), or KES 714 ($9.90) per capita. Pharmaceutical expenditures made up more than one-third (36.6 percent) of total health expenditures and 1.6 percent of GDP. Most pharmaceuticals were paid for privately, with government expenditures representing 9.0 percent of the total. Drugs are provided free to certain population groups, including the poor, children under the age of 5, pregnant women, and elderly people. Drugs are also free to treat certain conditions, including malaria, tuberculosis, STDs, and HIV/AIDS; vaccines on the Expanded Programme on Immunization (EPI) list, created by WHO, are also provided for free. The National Health Insurance Fund does not cover medications, but some private insurance plans do.

As a member of the World Trade Organization (WTO), Kenya observes patent law, but national law also includes some elements of the Trade-Related Aspects of Intellectual Property Rights (TRIPS), which provide exceptions to patent law. In Kenya, these exceptions include compulsory licensing for reasons of public health, the Bolar exception that allows manufacturers to perform research and testing to create generic drugs before a patent has expired, and parallel importing provisions (allowing import of drugs created for sale in a different country).

Drugs sold in Kenya must be registered and go through an approval process. As of 2010, about 13,000 pharmaceutical products were registered in Kenya. The government regulates promotion and advertising of medicines, and direct advertising to the general public is banned. A 2004 survey found that medications were more available in the private than in the public sector. Availability of brand-name medicines was 66 percent in the public sector and 81 percent in the private sector; for generics, availability was 36.6 percent in the public sector and 72.4 percent in the private sector. Prices for drugs were generally high, with a median price ratio (relative to the international reference price for a basket of pharmaceuticals) of 2.0

(for example, the median price in Kenya was twice the international reference price) for generic drugs in the public sector and 3.6 for brand-name drugs; in the private sector, the median price ratio was 3.3 for generics and 18.1 for brand-name drugs. However, drugs were judged relatively affordable, as it would have taken 0.2 day of wages (for the lowest-paid government worker) to purchase generic medicine (cotrimoxazole) in the public sector to treat a child's respiratory infection.

Health Care Facilities

As of 2010, according to WHO, Kenya had 8.27 health posts per 100,000 population, 6.55 health centers per 100,000, 1.55 district or rural hospitals per 100,000, 0.04 provincial hospitals per 100,000, and 0.02 specialized hospitals per 100,000. In 2006, Kenya had 1.40 hospital beds per 1,000 population.

Major Health Issues

In 2008, WHO estimated that 76 percent of years of life lost in Kenya were due to communicable diseases, 14 percent to noncommunicable diseases, and 10 percent to injuries. In 2008, the age-standardized estimate of cancer deaths was 119 per 100,000 for men and 113 per 100,000 for women; for cardiovascular disease and diabetes, 410 per 100,000 for men and 326 per 100,000 for women; and for chronic respiratory disease, 109 per 100,000 for men and 45 per 100,000 for women.

In 2008, the age-standardized death rate from malaria was 8.2 per 100,000 population. In 2010, tuberculosis incidence was 298.0 per 100,000 population, tuberculosis prevalence 283.0 per 100,000, and deaths due to tuberculosis among HIV-negative people 17.00 per 100,000. WHO estimates that the case detection rate in 2010 was 82 percent. As of 2009, an estimated 6.3 percent of adults age 15 to 49 were living with HIV or AIDS. As of 2009, an estimated 1.5 million people in Kenya were living with HIV or AIDS, the fourth-highest number in the world. In 2010, 83 percent of pregnant women tested positive for HIV. As of December 2010, an estimated 74 percent of adults and 21 percent of children who needed antiretroviral therapy were receiving it. The mother-to-child transmission rate for HIV in 2010 was estimated at 21 percent, and in 2009, 8.9 percent of deaths to children under age 5 were attributed to HIV.

Kenya's maternal mortality rate (death from any cause related to or aggravated by pregnancy) is quite high by global standards, estimated at 5,300 maternal deaths per 100,000 live births as of 2008. A 2008 through 2009 survey estimated the prevalence of female genital mutilation at 27.1 percent. The infant mortality rate, defined as the number of deaths of infants younger than 1 year, was estimated at 43.61 per 1,000 live births as of 2012. In 2003, 16.5 percent of children under age 5 were underweight (defined as 2 kilograms [kg] below standard weight-for-age at age 1, 3 kg below for ages 2 to 3, and 4 kg below for ages 4 to 5).

Health Care Personnel

In 2006, WHO identified Kenya as one of 57 countries with a critical deficit in the supply of skilled health workers. Kenya has two medical schools: the Faculty of Health Sciences of Moi University in Eldoret and the College of Health Sciences of the University of Nairobi. The basic medical degree course requires six years to complete, and the degrees awarded are bachelor of medicine and bachelor of surgery. In 2002, Kenya had 0.14 physicians per 1,000 population, 0.10 pharmaceutical personnel per 1,000, 0.22 laboratory health workers per 1,000, 0.06 health management and support workers per 1,000, 0.04 dentistry personnel per 1,000, and 1.18 nurses and midwives per 1,000. The supply of medical personnel in Kenya is affected by the global "brain drain" (international migration of skilled personnel): Michael Clemens and Bunilla Petterson estimate that 51 percent of Kenya-born physicians and 8 percent of Kenya-born nurses are working in one of nine developed countries, primarily in the United Kingdom and the United States.

Government Role in Health Care

The Kenyan constitution recognizes the right to health, including access to essential medicines and medical technology. Kenya has a National Health Policy (NHP), the Kenya Health Policy Framework, created in 1994, and a National Medicines Policy (NMP), the Kenya National Pharmaceutical Policy, updated in 2010. The Kenya National Pharmaceutical Policy covers many areas of drug policy, including selection of essential medicines; financing, pricing, purchase, distribution, and regulation of drugs; pharmacovigilance; rational usage of medicines; human resource development; research; evaluation and monitoring; and traditional medicine.

According to WHO, in 2010, Kenya spent $1.5 billion on health care, an amount that comes to $4,242 per capita. About two-thirds (64 percent) of health care funding was provided from domestic sources, with the remainder (36 percent) coming from abroad. Health care funding was paid for almost equally by household spending (43 percent) and government expenditures (44 percent), with the remaining 13 percent coming from other sources. In 2010, Kenya allocated 7 percent of its total government expenditures to health, in the low range for low-income African countries; government expenditures on health came to 2 percent of GDP, in the median range as compared with other low-income African countries. In 2009, according to WHO, official development assistance (ODA) for health in Kenya came to $16.75 per capita.

Public Health Programs

The Kenya Medical Research Institute (KEMRI), established in 1979, is located in Nairobi and headed by Solomon Mpoke. KEMRI was created after the breakup of the East African Medical Community in 1977 and was created as part of the Kenyan Science and Technology Act. Areas of research within KEMRI include infectious diseases, parasitic diseases, noncommunicable diseases, biotechnology, and epidemiology, health systems, and public health.

According to WHO, in 2004, Kenya had 0.20 environmental and public health workers per 1,000 population. In 2010, 32 percent of the population had access to improved sanitation facilities (32 percent in rural areas and 32 percent in urban), and 59 percent had access to improved sources of drinking water (52 percent in rural areas and 82 percent in urban). According to the World Higher Education Database (WHED), three universities in Kenya offer programs in epidemiology or public health: Kenyatta University in Nairobi, Maseno University, and Moi University in Eldoret.

KIRIBATI

Kiribati, formerly called the Gilbert Islands, is an island nation (33 coral atolls) in the south Pacific Ocean. The area of 313 square miles (811 square kilometers) makes Kiribati about four times the size of Washington, D.C., and the July 2012 population was estimated at 101,998. In 2010, 44 percent of the population lived in urban areas, and the 2010 to 2015 annual rate of

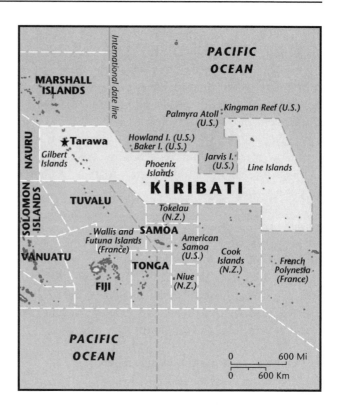

urbanization was estimated at 1.9 percent. Tarawa is the capital and largest city (with a 2009 population estimated at 43,000). The population growth rate in 2012 was 1.3 percent, the net migration rate negative 2.8 migrants per 1,000 population, the birth rate 22.4 births per 1,000, and the total fertility rate 2.7 children per woman.

Kiribati was a British protectorate and then a British colony; it achieved self-rule in 1971 and independence in 1979. Kiribati ranked tied for 95th among 183 countries on the *Corruption Perceptions Index 2011*, with a score of 3.1 (on a scale where 0 indicates highly corrupt and 10 very clean). In 2011, Kiribati was classified as a country with medium human development (the second from the lowest of four categories) on the United Nations Development Programme's (UNDP's) Human Development Index (HDI), with a score of 0.624 (on a scale where 1 denotes high development and 0 low development). Life expectancy at birth in 2012 was estimated at 64.76 years, and estimated gross domestic product (GDP) per capita in 2011 was $6,200.

Emergency Health Services

According to the World Health Organization (WHO), as of 2007, Kiribati had a formal and publicly available emergency care (prehospital care) system.

Insurance

Kiribati has a publicly funded health system administered by the Ministry of Health and Medical Services, providing primary and secondary care; patients may be referred overseas for tertiary care if they meet specified criteria.

Costs of Hospitalization

No data available.

Access to Health Care

In 2007, primary health care services were well established in the Outer Islands of Kiribati, and South Tarawa and Kiritimati Island had referral hospitals as well; however, tertiary and palliative services were limited. According to WHO, in 2005, 65 percent of births were attended by skilled personnel (for example, physicians, nurses, or midwives). The 2010 immunization rates for 1-year-olds were 91 percent for diphtheria and pertussis (DPT3), 89 percent for measles (MCV), and 91 percent for Hib (Hib3). According to WHO, in 2010, Kiribati had fewer than 0.01 magnetic resonance imaging (MRI) machines per 1 million population and fewer than 0.01 computer tomography (CT) machines per 1 million.

Cost of Drugs

No data available.

Health Care Facilities

Kiribati has a national referral hospital located in South Tawara that provides secondary care, a basic hospital on Kiribati Island, and a small hospital providing basic services in South Tawara; tertiary care is not available within the country, but patients meeting specified clinical criteria are referred for overseas care. Primary care is provided through a network of 92 health centers and dispensaries. Kiribati also has a parallel system of traditional healers and cures, and many residents use both systems. As of 2010, according to WHO, Kiribati had 85.39 health posts per 100,000 population and 144.66 health centers per 100,000. In 2008, Kiribati had 1.80 hospital beds per 1,000 population.

Major Health Issues

In 2008, WHO estimated that 36 percent of years of life lost in Kiribati were due to communicable diseases, 60 percent to noncommunicable diseases, and 4 percent to injuries. In 2008, the age-standardized estimate of cancer deaths was 39 per 100,000 for men and 64 per 100,000 for women; for cardiovascular disease and diabetes, 426 per 100,000 for men and 224 per 100,000 for women; and for chronic respiratory disease, 62 per 100,000 for men and 19 per 100,000 for women. Kiribati has one of the highest adult obesity rates in the world, estimated at 50.6 percent in 2006; obesity is defined as a body mass index (BMI) of 30 or above.

In 2008, the age-standardized death rate from malaria was 2.2 per 100,000 population. In 2010, tuberculosis incidence was 370.0 per 100,000 population, tuberculosis prevalence 550.0 per 100,000, and deaths due to tuberculosis among human immunodeficiency virus (HIV)-negative people 47.00 per 100,000. The maternal mortality rate (death from any cause related to or aggravated by pregnancy) in Kiribati in 2008 was nine maternal deaths per 100,000 live births. The infant mortality rate, defined as the number of deaths of infants younger than 1 year, was estimated at 37.68 per 1,000 live births as of 2012.

Health Care Personnel

In 2006, Kiribati had 0.30 physicians per 1,000 population, 0.01 pharmaceutical personnel per 1,000, 0.03 dentistry personnel per 1,000, and 3.02 nurses and midwives per 1,000. Kiribati does not have a school of medicine, but locally recruited students have been trained in Cuba and at the Fiji School of Medicine. There is a three-year nursing training course in Kiribati, with advanced training also available in midwifery and public health. There is a shortage of support staff and medical personnel, and many engaged in lab and radiography services lack basic training in these fields.

Government Role in Health Care

According to WHO, in 2010, Kiribati spent $16 million on health care, an amount that comes to $160 per capita. Health care funding was provided primarily (83 percent) from domestic sources, with the remainder (17 percent) coming from abroad. Most (82 percent) of health care funding was paid for through government expenditures, with the remainder provided by other sources (18 percent). In 2010, Kiribati allocated 12 percent of its total government expenditures to health, in the high range for low-middle-income western Pacific region countries; government expenditures on health came to 9 percent of GDP, in the high range as compared with other low-middle-income western Pacific region countries.

Public Health Programs

According to WHO, in 2008, Kiribati had 0.12 environmental and public health workers per 1,000 population. In 2010, 34 percent of the population had access to improved sanitation facilities (22 percent in rural areas and 49 percent in urban), and 63 percent had access to improved sources of drinking water (53 percent in rural areas and 77 percent in urban). According to the World Higher Education Database (WHED), no university in Kiribati offers programs in epidemiology or public health.

KUWAIT

Kuwait is a Middle Eastern country, sharing borders with Iraq and Saudi Arabia and having a coastline on the Persian Gulf. The area of 6,880 square miles (17,818 square kilometers) makes Kuwait similar in size to New Jersey, and the July 2012 population was estimated at 2.6 million. In 2010, 98 percent of the population lived in urban areas, and the 2010 to 2015 annual rate of urbanization was estimated at 2.1 percent. Kuwait is the capital and largest city (with a 2009

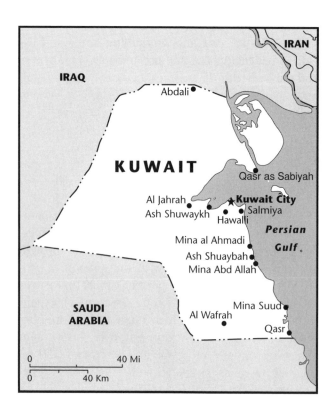

population estimated at 2.2 million). The population growth rate in 2012 was 1.9 percent, the birth rate 21.0 births per 1,000 population, the net migration rate 0.0 migrants per 1,000, and the total fertility rate 2.6 children per woman.

Kuwait's ties to Great Britain date back to the late 19th century, and after World War I, the country became a British protectorate; Kuwait became independent in 1961. Petroleum accounts for about half of Kuwait's gross domestic product (GDP), and the country has about 7 percent of the world's petroleum reserves. In 1990, Kuwait was invaded by Iraq, and the nation's infrastructure and ecology were damaged in the process; however, the country has since returned to full functioning. Kuwait ranked tied for 54th among 183 countries on the *Corruption Perceptions Index 2011*, with a score of 4.6 (on a scale where 0 indicates highly corrupt and 10 very clean). In 2011, Kuwait was classified as a country with high human development (the second-highest category) on the United Nations Development Programme's (UNDP's) Human Development Index (HDI), with a score of 0.760 (on a scale where 1 denotes high development and 0 low development). Life expectancy at birth in 2012 was estimated at 77.28 years, and per capita GDP in 2011 was estimated at $40,700. According to the World Economic Forum's *Global Gender Gap Index 2011*, Kuwait ranked 105th out of 135 countries on gender equality with a score of 0.632 (on a scale with a theoretical range of 1 for equality to 0 for inequality and an actual range in 2011 from 0.8530 to 0.4873).

Emergency Health Services

According to the World Health Organization (WHO), as of 2007, Kuwait had a formal and publicly available emergency care (prehospital care) system.

Insurance

As of 2004, health care in Kuwait was provided for free to citizens in the public sector, including all medicines required.

Costs of Hospitalization

Care is provided free of charge in public hospitals and clinics.

Access to Health Care

More than 80 percent of health care services in Kuwait are provided through the public sector, overseen by the Ministry of Health. According to WHO, in 2007, 100

Selected Health Indicators: Kuwait Compared With the Global Average (2010)

	Kuwait	Global Average
Male life expectancy at birth* (years)	78	66
Female life expectancy at birth* (years)	79	71
Under-5 mortality rate, both sexes (per 1,000 live births)	11	57
Adult mortality rate, both sexes* (probability of dying between 15 and 60 years per 1,000 population)	60	176
Maternal mortality ratio (per 100,000 live births)	14	210
Tuberculosis prevalence (per 100,000 population)	51	178

Source: World Health Organization Global Health Observatory Data Repository.
*Data refers to 2009.

percent of births were attended by skilled personnel (for example, physicians, nurses, or midwives). The 2010 immunization rates for 1-year-olds were 98 percent for diphtheria and pertussis (DPT3), 98 percent for measles (MCV), and 98 percent for Hib (Hib3).

Cost of Drugs

All government facilities in Kuwait are supplied with medicines by the Central Medical Stores, while private pharmacies are supplied by private wholesalers; the government regulates pharmaceutical prices at both the wholesale and retail levels. For generic drugs, the procurement price was 1.39 times the international reference price (that is, 39 percent higher), while for originator brands it was 2.69 times the international reference price. Some drugs are purchased through the Gulf Cooperation Council, and some drugs are thus procured below the international reference price.

Almost all drugs used in Kuwait are imported, and total annual pharmaceutical expenditure in 2001 was about $200 million. A 2004 survey found severe problems with availability in the private sector: Median availability was 12 percent for both the lowest-priced generics and for originator brands. However, availability of some generic drugs was greater than 80 percent; these included amoxicillin, atenolol, diclofenac, insulin, and paracetamol. In the private sector, the median price ratio for the lowest-priced generics was 15.72, and for originator brands, it was 17.45. Median availability in the private sector was better for originator

brands (84 percent) than for the lowest-priced generics (0 percent). The lowest-paid Kuwaiti government worker would need more than three days of wages to purchase a month's supply of ranitidine, 0.8 day's wages to purchase a month's supply of omeprazole, and 2.9 days' wages to purchase a month's supply of fluoxetine. Those medications are all provided free to Kuwaitis in government health care facilities, however, if they are available.

Health Care Facilities

Kuwait has 72 health care centers providing primary care spread throughout the country, six hospitals providing secondary care, and 10 specialized hospitals and care centers providing services such as neurosurgery, cancer diagnosis and treatment, and organ transplants. Kuwait also has five private hospitals and a number of private health care clinics; most of the private facilities are concentrated in the capital region and commercial areas, including Farwania and Hawalli.

Major Health Issues

In 2008, WHO estimated that 14 percent of years of life lost in Kuwait were due to communicable diseases, 64 percent to noncommunicable diseases, and 22 percent to injuries. In 2008, the age-standardized estimate of cancer deaths was 62 per 100,000 for men and 70 per 100,000 for women; for cardiovascular disease and diabetes, 282 per 100,000 for men and 263 per 100,000 for women; and for chronic respiratory disease, eight per 100,000 for men and 12 per 100,000 for women.

Kuwait's maternal mortality rate (death from any cause related to or aggravated by pregnancy) was estimated in 2008 as nine maternal deaths per 100,000 live births. The infant mortality rate, defined as the number of deaths of infants younger than 1 year, was 7.87 per 1,000 live births as of 2012. In 2010, tuberculosis incidence was 41.0 per 100,000 population, tuberculosis prevalence 51.0 per 100,000, and deaths due to tuberculosis among human immunodeficiency virus (HIV)-negative people 1.20 per 100,000. As of 2009, an estimated 0.1 percent of adults age 15 to 49 were living with HIV or acquired immune deficiency syndrome (AIDS).

Health Care Personnel

Kuwait has one medical school, the Faculty of Medicine of Kuwait University in Kuwait City, which began offering instruction in 1973. The basic course of study lasts seven years, and the degrees awarded are bachelor of medical science and bachelor of medicine and bachelor of surgery. In 2009, Kuwait had 1.79 physicians per 1,000 population, 0.30 pharmaceutical personnel per 1,000, 1.00 laboratory health workers per 1,000, 4.13 health management and support workers per 1,000, 0.35 dentistry personnel per 1,000, 0.18 community and traditional health workers per 1,000, and 4.55 nurses and midwives per 1,000.

Government Role in Health Care

According to WHO, in 2010, Kuwait spent $16 million on health care, an amount that comes to $160 per capita. Health care funding was provided primarily (83 percent) from domestic sources, with the remainder (17 percent) coming from abroad. More than three-quarters (82 percent) of health care funding was paid for through government expenditures, with the remainder provided from other sources (18 percent). In 2010, general government expenditures on health came to 5.6 percent of total government expenditures and 3.3 percent of GDP.

Public Health Programs

In 2010, access to improved sanitation facilities in Kuwait was essentially universal, and access to improved sources of drinking water also close to universal (99 percent). According to the World Higher Education Database (WHED), no university in Kuwait offers programs in epidemiology or public health.

KYRGYZSTAN

Kyrgyzstan is a landlocked central Asian country, sharing borders with China, Kazakhstan, Tajikistan, and Uzbekistan. The area of 77,202 square miles (199,951 square kilometers) makes Kyrgyzstan similar in size to South Dakota, and the July 2012 population was estimated at 5.5 million. In 2010, 35 percent of the population lived in urban areas, and the 2010 to 2015 annual rate of urbanization was estimated at 1.3 percent. Bishkek is the capital and largest city (with a 2009 population estimated at 854,000). The population growth rate in 2012 was 0.9 percent, the net migration rate negative 8.1 migrants per 1,000 population (one of the 20 highest emigration rates in the world), the birth rate 23.9 births per 1,000, and the total fertility rate 2.7 children per woman. The United Nations High Commissioner for Refugees (UNHCR) estimated that, in 2010, there were 958 refugees and persons in refugee-like situations in Kyrgyzstan and 200,000 internally displaced persons and persons in internally displaced-person-like situations.

Kyrgyzstan was annexed by Russia and became a Soviet republic in 1936; it achieved independence in

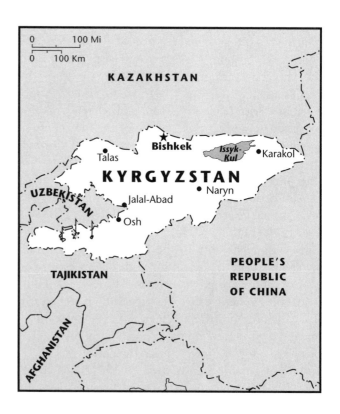

1991. President Askar Akaev ruled the country from independence to 2005, when he was ousted following nationwide demonstrations; his successor, Kurmanbek Bakiyev, resigned in 2010, also amid nationwide protests, and Kyrgyzstan also experienced widespread ethnic violence in 2010. The government is perceived as corrupt, ranking 164th among 183 countries on the *Corruption Perceptions Index 2011,* with a score of 2.1 (on a scale where 0 indicates highly corrupt and 10 very clean).

In 2011, Kyrgyzstan was classified as a country with medium human development (the second from the lowest of four categories) on the United Nations Development Programme's (UNDP's) Human Development Index (HDI), with a score of 0.615 (on a scale where 1 denotes high development and 0 low development). A March 2012 assessment by the World Food Programme estimated that 18 percent of households in Kyrgyzstan were food insecure. Life expectancy at birth in 2012 was estimated at 69.45 years, and the estimated gross domestic product (GDP) per capita in 2011 was $2,400. In 2007, the Gini Index (a measure of dispersion, in which perfect equality is denoted by 0 and maximum inequality is denoted by 100) for family income was 33.4. According to the World Economic Forum's *Global Gender Gap Index 2011,* Kyrgyzstan ranked 44th out of 135 countries on gender equality, with a score of 0.704 (on a scale with a theoretical range of 1 for equality to 0 for inequality and an actual range in 2011 from 0.8530 to 0.4873).

Emergency Health Services

According to the World Health Organization (WHO), as of 2007, Kyrgyzstan had a formal and publicly available emergency care (prehospital care) system. Doctors Without Borders (Médecins Sans Frontières, or MSF) began working in Kyrgyzstan in 2005 and had 93 staff members in the country at the close of 2010. MSF has provided care to prisoners infected with tuberculosis since 2005, provides referrals for those with drug-resistant tuberculosis, and provides care and social services after release for prisoners with tuberculosis. When violence broke out between the Kyrgyz and Uzbek communities in June 2010, MSF provided mental care, medical supplies and drugs, and health care in public health facilities.

Insurance

Kyrgyzstan has a universal medical benefits program covering all residents of the country and a social insurance system for cash sickness and maternity benefits covering employed persons, students, and members of cooperatives. The medical benefits system is entirely funded through general tax revenues, while the cash benefits system is funded through a combination of contributions from earnings (from workers and the self-employed) and payroll contributions (from employers); the same system pays for pensions. Medical benefits are provided through direct services from government- or system-administered health providers; benefits include hospitalization, medical care, dental care, maternity care, and transportation.

The maternity benefit is seven times the minimum wage, paid for a total of 126 days; it may be increased to 140 days if there are birth complications. The cash sickness benefit is 75 percent of seven times the minimum wage, raised to 100 percent for those with three or more dependent children, disabled veterans, and those disabled due to the Chernobyl disaster. Benefits are adjusted regularly to reflect changes in the cost of living. The Ministry of Health sets policy and provides supervision, coordination, and administration, along with local health departments, for health care delivery. According to Ke Xu and colleagues, in 2003, 0.6 percent of households in Kyrgyzstan experienced catastrophic health expenditures annually; "catastrophic" was defined as exceeding 40 percent of household income remaining after basic needs were met.

Costs of Hospitalization

As of 2002, Kyrgyzstan had instituted a payment system for hospitals based on a case mix with 154 categories; the health insurance fund pays only for staff, drugs, supplies, and food, amounting to less than one-third of the total costs of care.

Access to Health Care

According to WHO, in 2006, 98 percent of births were attended by skilled personnel (for example, physicians, nurses, or midwives). The 2010 immunization rates for 1-year-olds were 96 percent for diphtheria and pertussis (DPT3), 99 percent for measles (MCV), and 96 percent for Hib (Hib3). In 2010, an estimated 12 percent of persons with advanced human immunodeficiency virus (HIV) infection were receiving antiretroviral therapy in accordance with the 2010 WHO guidelines. According to WHO, in 2010, Kyrgyzstan had 0.92 magnetic resonance imaging (MRI) machines per 1 million population and 0.92 computer tomography (CT) machines per 1 million.

Cost of Drugs

As of 2005, about 10 percent of the health care budget in Kyrgyzstan was used to purchase medicines; the per capita drug expenditure was around $5, and almost all medicines were imported. The national Mandatory Health Insurance Fund includes a subsidy of 30 to 70 percent for drugs used in outpatient care. Generic substitution by pharmacists is allowed. A 2005 survey found that the median price ratio (comparing the price to the international reference price) in hospitals for the lowest-priced generic drugs procured through the public process was in the range of 1.03 to 2.04 (from just over the international reference price to twice the international reference price), with the median at 1.29 (29 percent above the national reference price). Originator brands were far more expensive, with a median price ratio of 59.47.

In the private sector (retail pharmacies), the median price ratio for the lowest-priced generics was 2.56 and, for originator brands, 5.42. There was some variation among regions; the median price ratio for the lowest-priced generics ranged from 1.8 in Bishkek (the national capital) to 2.9 in Osh and Jalalabad. For drugs that existed in both a generic and originator versions, the originator brands cost on average 3.6 times as much as the generics. Availability was generally high for the lowest-priced generics but relatively low for originator brands. Affordability was a problem: The lowest-paid government worker would have required from 1.5 to 11.5 days' wages to buy the lowest-priced generic drugs to treat common conditions such as hypertension, asthma, and a peptic ulcer.

Health Care Facilities

As of 2010, according to WHO, Kyrgyzstan had 17.77 health posts per 100,000 population, 1.86 district or rural hospitals per 100,000, 0.15 provincial hospitals per 100,000, and 0.73 specialized hospitals per 100,000. In 2007, Kyrgyzstan had 5.06 hospital beds per 1,000 population, among the 50 highest rates in the world.

Major Health Issues

In 2008, WHO estimated that 30 percent of years of life lost in Kyrgyzstan were due to communicable diseases, 55 percent to noncommunicable diseases, and 15 percent to injuries. In 2008, the age-standardized estimate of cancer deaths was 129 per 100,000 for men and 104 per 100,000 for women; for cardiovascular disease and diabetes, 697 per 100,000 for men and 516 per 100,000 for women; and for chronic respiratory disease, 101 per 100,000 for men and 49 per 100,000 for women.

Kyrgyzstan's maternal mortality rate (death from any cause related to or aggravated by pregnancy) was estimated in 2008 as 81 maternal deaths per 100,000 live births. The infant mortality rate, defined as the number of deaths of infants younger than 1 year, was estimated at 30.78 per 1,000 live births as of 2012. In 2010, tuberculosis incidence was 159.0 per 100,000 population, tuberculosis prevalence 243.0 per 100,000, and deaths due to tuberculosis among human immunodeficiency virus (HIV)-negative people 26.00 per 100,000. An estimated 14 percent of new tuberculosis cases and 39 percent of retreatment cases are multidrug resistant. As of 2009, an estimated 0.3 percent of adults age 15 to 49 were living with HIV or acquired immune deficiency syndrome (AIDS).

Health Care Personnel

Kyrgyzstan has four medical schools, located in Bishkek and Osh. The basic course of study requires five to six years, and the degree awarded is doctor of medicine. The Ministry of Health grants the license to practice medicine. Kyrgyzstan has reciprocal agreements with other Commonwealth of Independent States countries (those which were formerly part of the Soviet Union). In 2007, Kyrgyzstan had 2.30 physicians per 1,000, 0.02 pharmaceutical personnel per 1,000, 0.19 dentistry personnel per 1,000, and 5.66 nurses and midwives per 1,000.

Government Role in Health Care

According to WHO, in 2010, Kyrgyzstan spent $285 million on health care, an amount that comes to $53 per capita. Health care funding was provided primarily (87 percent) from domestic sources, with the remainder (13 percent) coming from abroad. More than half (56 percent) of health care funding was paid for through government expenditures, with the remainder provided through household expenditures (38 percent) and other sources (6 percent). In 2010, Kyrgyzstan allocated 11 percent of its total government expenditures to health, and government expenditures on health came to 3 percent of GDP; both figures place Kyrgyzstan in the high range as compared with other low-income Asian countries. In 2009, according to WHO, official development assistance (ODA) for health in Kyrgyzstan came to $4.81 per capita.

Public Health Programs

In 2010, 93 percent of the population of Kyrgyzstan had access to improved sanitation facilities (93 percent in rural areas and 94 percent in urban), and 90 percent had access to improved sources of drinking water (85 percent in rural areas and 99 percent in urban). According to the World Higher Education Database (WHED), one university in Kyrgyzstan offers programs in epidemiology or public health: Kyrgyz State Medical Academy in Bishkek.

LAOS

Laos is a landlocked country in southeastern Asia, sharing borders with Burma, Cambodia, Thailand, China, and Vietnam. The area of 91,429 square miles (236,800 square kilometers) is comparable to that of Utah, and the 2012 population was estimated at 6.6 million. In 2010, 33 percent of the population lived in urban areas, and the 2010 to 2015 annual rate of urbanization was estimated at 4.9 percent. Vientiane is the capital and largest city (with a 2009 population estimated at 799,000). The population growth rate in 2012 was 1.7 percent, the net migration rate negative 1.1 migrants per 1,000 population, the birth rate 25.7 births per 1,000, and the total fertility rate 3.1 children per woman.

A former French colony, Laos became independent in 1953; a civil war ended in 1975 with the Communist Pathet Lao movement taking power. Laos was heavily bombed during the Vietnam War, causing extensive property damage and loss of life. Laos ranked tied for 152nd among 183 countries on the *Corruption Perceptions Index 2011,* with a score of 2.2 (on a scale where 0 indicates highly corrupt and 10 very clean). In 2011, Laos was classified as a country with medium human development (the second from the lowest of four categories) on the United Nations Development Programme's (UNDP's) Human Development Index (HDI), with a score of 0.524 (on a scale where 1 denotes high development and 0 low development). In 2011, the International Food Policy Research Institute (IFPRI) classified Laos as a country with an "alarming" hunger problem, with a Global Hunger Index (GHI) score of 20.2 (where 0 reflects no hunger and higher scores more hunger). Life expectancy at birth in 2012 was estimated at

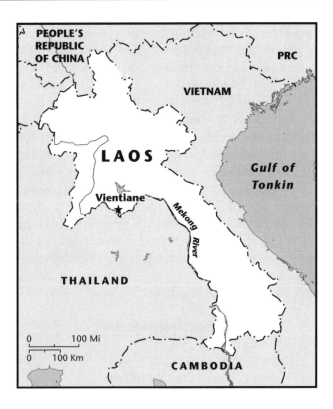

62.77 years, and estimated gross domestic product (GDP) per capita in 2011 was $2,700. In 2008, the Gini Index (a measure of dispersion, in which perfect equality is denoted by 0 and maximum inequality is denoted by 100) for family income was 36.7.

Emergency Health Services

According to the World Health Organization (WHO), as of 2007, Laos did not have a formal and publicly available system for providing prehospital care (emergency care).

Insurance

Laos has a social insurance system covering state-owned and private-sector enterprises with at least 10 employees; however, only some regions of the country currently offer coverage. Workers from international organizations and embassies and the self-employed are excluded, while workers in smaller enterprises can join voluntarily. The military, police, and civil service have a separate system. The system is funded through a combination of wage and payroll contributions and is part of the same system that funds pensions. Each insured person must register with a hospital and be treated by that hospital, except in case of emergency; the hospital may be changed once per year. Medical benefits include maternity care and preventive, curative, and rehabilitative services; however, treatment for injuries in motor vehicle accidents is excluded. The spouse and children up to age 18 of an insured person are also insured; if the child is disabled, there is no age limit for coverage, and if a full-time student, coverage continues to age 25. The maternity benefit is 100 percent of earnings for three months; a birth grant of 60 percent of the monthly minimum wage is paid as a lump sum. The cash sickness benefit is 60 percent of average covered earnings for up to 12 months, with a possible extension for another six months. Contracts are approved by the Ministry of Public Health, which supervises the program; the State Security Organization contracts with hospitals, collects contributions, and administers the cash benefit programs.

Costs of Hospitalization

No data available.

Access to Health Care

According to the World Health Organization (WHO), in 2006, 20 percent of births were attended by skilled personnel (for example, physicians, nurses, or midwives). The 2010 immunization rates for 1-year-olds were 74 percent for diphtheria and pertussis (DPT3), 64 percent for measles (MCV), and 74 percent for Hib (Hib3). In 2010, an estimated 51 percent of persons with advanced human immunodeficiency virus (HIV) infection were receiving antiretroviral therapy in accordance with the 2010 WHO guidelines. According to WHO, in 2010, Laos had fewer than 0.01 magnetic resonance imaging (MRI) machines per 1 million population and 0.81 computer tomography (CT) machines per 1 million.

Cost of Drugs

No data available.

Health Care Facilities

As of 2010, according to WHO, Laos had 10.77 health centers per 100,000 population, 2.03 district or rural hospitals per 100,000, 0.26 provincial hospitals per 100,000, and 0.11 specialized hospitals per 100,000. In 2005, Laos had 1.20 hospital beds per 1,000 population.

Major Health Issues

In 2008, WHO estimated that 58 percent of years of life lost in Laos were due to communicable diseases, 28 percent to noncommunicable diseases, and 13 percent to injuries. In 2008, the age-standardized estimate of cancer deaths was 145 per 100,000 for men and 111 per 100,000 for women; for cardiovascular disease and diabetes, 468 per 100,000 for men and 393 per 100,000 for women; and for chronic respiratory disease, 123 per 100,000 for men and 103 per 100,000 for women.

In 2008, the age-standardized death rate from malaria was 2.7 per 100,000 population. In 2010, tuberculosis incidence was 90.0 per 100,000 population, tuberculosis prevalence 130.0 per 100,000, and deaths due to tuberculosis among HIV negative people 11.00 per 100,000. As of 2009, an estimated 0.2 percent of adults age 15 to 49 were living with HIV or acquired immune deficiency syndrome (AIDS).

Compared to other countries at a similar level of development, Laos ranked eighth among 43 least-developed countries on the 2011 Mothers' Index, produced by the international nongovernmental organization (NGO) Save the Children, based on a number of health and social factors relating to women, children, and maternal and child care. The maternal mortality rate (death from any cause related to or aggravated by pregnancy) in Laos is quite high by global standards, estimated at 580 maternal deaths per 100,000 live births as of 2008. The infant mortality rate, defined as the number of deaths of infants younger than 1 year, also has been high, at 57.77 per 1,000 live births as of 2012. Child malnutrition is a serious problem: In 2006, 31.6 percent of children under age 5 were underweight (defined as 2 kilograms [kg] below standard weight-for-age at age 1, 3 kg below for ages 2 to 3, and 4 kg below for ages 4 to 5), one of the 20 highest rates in the world.

Health Care Personnel

In 2006, WHO identified Laos as one of 57 countries with a critical deficit in the supply of skilled health workers. Laos has one medical school, the Faculte des Sciences Medicales in Vientiane, which began offering instruction in 1968. The basic course of study requires six years to complete, and the degree awarded is doctor of medicine. Government service is obligatory after graduation. Physicians must register with the Ministry of Public Health, and a medical license is granted to graduates of recognized medical schools, but foreigners may only practice if they have graduated from the Faculte des Sciences Medicales in Vientiane. In 2005, Laos had 0.27 physicians per 1,000 population and 0.97 nurses and midwives per 1,000.

Government Role in Health Care

According to WHO, in 2010, Laos spent $286 million on health care, an amount that comes to $46 per capita. Health care funding was provided primarily (86 percent) from domestic sources, with the remainder (15 percent) coming from overseas. Just over half (51 percent) of health care funding was paid for through household expenditures, with the remainder provided through government expenditures (33 percent) and other sources (16 percent).

In 2010, Laos allocated 6 percent of its total government expenditures to health, and government expenditures on health came to 1 percent of GDP; both figures place Laos in the low range as compared with other low-income western Pacific region countries. In 2009, according to WHO, official development assistance (ODA) for health in Laos came to $7.42 per capita.

Public Health Programs

In 2010, 63 percent of the population of Laos had access to improved sanitation facilities (50 percent in rural areas and 89 percent in urban), and 67 percent had access to improved sources of drinking water (62 percent in rural areas and 77 percent in urban). According to the World Higher Education Database (WHED), no university in Laos offers programs in epidemiology or public health.

LATVIA

Latvia is a northern European country, sharing borders with Lithuania, Russia, Estonia, and Belarus and having a coastline on the Baltic Sea. The area of 24,938 square miles (64,589 square kilometers) makes Latvia similar in size to West Virginia, and the July 2012 population was estimated at 2.2 million. In 2010, 68 percent of the population lived in urban areas, and the 2010 to 2015 annual rate of urbanization was estimated at negative 0.4 percent.

Riga is the capital and largest city (with a 2009 population estimated at 711,000). Population growth in 2012 was negative 0.6 percent, one of the 10 lowest in the world; the net migration rate was negative 2.3 migrants per 1,000 population, the birth rate 10.0 births per 1,000, and the total fertility rate 1.33 children per woman (among the 20 lowest total fertility rates in the world).

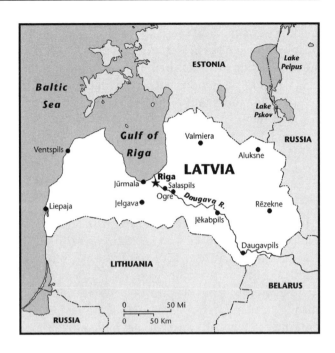

Latvia was annexed by the Soviet Union in 1940, although this act was not recognized by many countries; Latvia became independent again in 1991. The status of the substantial Russian minority (28 percent of the population) within Latvia remains a concern. Latvia ranked tied for 61st among 183 countries on the *Corruption Perceptions Index 2011,* with a score of 4.2 (on a scale where 0 indicates highly corrupt and 10 very clean). In 2011, Latvia was classified as a country with very high human development (the highest of four categories) on the United Nations Development Programme's (UNDP's) Human Development Index (HDI), with a score of 0.805 (on a scale where 1 denotes high development and 0 low development). Life expectancy at birth in 2012 was estimated at 72.93 years, and per capita gross domestic product (GDP) in 2011 was estimated at $15,400. In 2010, the Gini Index (a measure of dispersion, in which perfect equality is denoted by 0 and maximum inequality is denoted by 100) for family income was 35.2. According to the World Economic Forum's *Global Gender Gap Index 2011*, Latvia ranked 19th out of 135 countries on gender equality, with a score of 0.740 (on a scale with a theoretical range of 1 for equality to 0 for inequality and an actual range in 2011 from 0.8530 to 0.4873).

Emergency Health Services

Latvia's laws governing its emergency health system date from the 1990s, as does recognition of emergency medicine as a medical specialty; by law, free access to hospitals for emergency care is provided for all persons, including the uninsured. Funding for the emergency system is provided entirely by the state budget for both inpatient and outpatient treatment. Latvia has two national telephone numbers for medical emergencies, 112 (the European Union, or EU, standard) and 03; the country has 26 dispatch centers that are interconnected.

Insurance

Latvia has a social insurance system that provides medical benefits to all Latvian citizens residing in Latvia and noncitizens with residence permits and cash benefits to the employed and self-employed. State-guaranteed health care benefits are provided through general tax revenues, while other benefits are paid for through wage and payroll contributions (the same system that finances pensions). Medical care is provided in state-owned hospitals and in private hospitals under contract to the Health Compulsory Insurance State Agency. Benefits include hospitalization, medicine, medical care, and maternal care; dental benefits and cochlear implants are provided for children, and dental care is provided for people affected by the Chernobyl disaster. Copayments are required for some services, with exceptions for emergency care and for many population classes, including disabled persons, pregnant women and new mothers, the poor, children up to age 18, and people with certain illnesses.

The maternity benefit is 100 percent of earnings for 56 days before and after the due date, with an additional 14 days for multiple births. The paternity benefit is 80 percent of average earnings and is paid for 10 days. The cash sickness benefit is 80 percent of average earnings and is paid for up to 26 weeks with a possible extension to 52 weeks. A sick child benefit of 80 percent of average earnings is paid to an insured person caring for a child younger than 14 or if the child is receiving treatment in a hospital. The Health Payment Center administers medical benefits, the State Social Insurance Agency administers cash benefits, and the Ministry of Welfare supervises the system.

According to Ke Xu and colleagues, in 2003, 2.8 percent of households in Latvia experienced catastrophic health expenditures annually; "catastrophic" was defined as exceeding 40 percent of household income remaining after basic needs were met.

Costs of Hospitalization

As of 2002, specialized and tertiary care services are financed through a special government fund independent of the eight regional sickness funds. Government hospitals are paid on the basis of inputs (for example, personnel and beds), leading to excess capacity, and the sickness funds pay for care on the basis of bed-days, although some experiments with diagnosis-related groups (DRGs) are underway.

Access to Health Care

According to the World Health Organization (WHO), in 2006, 100 percent of births were attended by skilled personnel (for example, physicians, nurses, or midwives). The 2010 immunization rates for 1-year-olds were 89 percent for diphtheria and pertussis (DPT3), 93 percent for measles (MCV), and 88 percent for Hib (Hib3). In 2010, an estimated 18 percent of persons with advanced human immunodeficiency virus (HIV) infection were receiving antiretroviral therapy in accordance with the 2010 WHO guidelines.

Cost of Drugs

No data available.

Health Care Facilities

As of 2010, according to WHO, Latvia had 1.38 health centers per 100,000, 0.44 district or rural hospitals per 100,000, 0.31 provincial hospitals per 100,000, and 0.67 specialized hospitals per 100,000. In 2009, Latvia had 6.42 hospital beds per 1,000 population, among the 30 highest ratios in the world, reflecting its status as a former Soviet republic (and the hospital-centered model of health care typical of the Soviet Union). According to WHO, in 2010, Latvia had 6.64 magnetic resonance imaging (MRI) machines per 1 million population and 27.01 computer tomography (CT) machines per 1 million.

Major Health Issues

In 2008, WHO estimated that 5 percent of years of life lost in Latvia were due to communicable diseases, 77 percent to noncommunicable diseases, and 17 percent to injuries. In 2008, the age-standardized estimate of cancer deaths was 234 per 100,000 for men and 108 per 100,000 for women; for cardiovascular disease and diabetes, 567 per 100,000 for men and 295 per 100,000 for women; and for chronic respiratory disease, 21 per 100,000 for men and four per 100,000 for women.

The maternal mortality rate (death from any cause related to or aggravated by pregnancy) in Latvia in 2008 was 20 maternal deaths per 100,000 live births. The infant mortality rate, defined as the number of deaths of infants younger than 1 year, was 8.24 per 1,000 live births as of 2012. In 2010, tuberculosis incidence was 39.0 per 100,000 population, tuberculosis prevalence 43.0 per 100,000, and deaths due to tuberculosis among HIV-negative people 3.30 per 100,000. An estimated 10 percent of new tuberculosis cases and 24 percent of retreatment cases are multidrug resistant. As of 2009, an estimated 0.7 percent of adults age 15 to 49 were living with HIV or acquired immune deficiency syndrome (AIDS).

Health Care Personnel

Latvia has two medical schools: Latvijas Medicinas Akademija and Latvijas Universitate Medicinas Fakultate, both in Riga. The basic course of instruction requires five to six years to complete. Latvia, as a member of the EU, cooperates with other countries in recognizing physicians qualified to practice in other EU countries, as specified by Directive 2005/36/EC of the European Parliament. This allows qualified professionals to practice their profession in other EU states on a temporary basis and requires that the host country automatically recognize qualifications for certain professions, including physicians, nurses, dentists, midwives, and pharmacists, if certain conditions have been met (for instance, facility in the language of the host country may be required). In 2009, Latvia had 2.99 physicians per 1,000 population, 0.67 dentistry personnel per 1,000, and 4.84 nurses and midwives per 1,000, and in 2008, Latvia had 0.59 pharmaceutical personnel per 1,000.

Government Role in Health Care

According to WHO, in 2010 Latvia spent $1.6 billion on health care, an amount that comes to $718 per capita. Health care funding was provided entirely from domestic sources. More than three-fifths (61 percent) of health care funding was paid for through government expenditures, with the remainder provided through household expenditures (38 percent) and other sources (1 percent). In 2010, Latvia allocated 9 percent of its total government expenditures to health, in the median range as compared to other upper-middle-income European countries; government expenditures on health came to 4 percent of GDP, placing Latvia in the median range as compared with other upper-middle-income European countries.

Public Health Programs

In 2005, 78 percent of the population of Latvia had access to improved sanitation facilities (71 percent in rural areas and 82 percent in urban), and 99 percent had access to improved sources of drinking water (96 percent in rural areas and 100 percent in urban). According to the World Higher Education Database (WHED), one university in Latvia offers programs in epidemiology or public health: Riga Stradina University.

LEBANON

Lebanon is a Middle Eastern country, sharing borders with Israel and Syria and having a coastline on the Mediterranean Sea. The area of 4,015 square miles (10,400 square kilometers) makes Lebanon about 70 percent of the size of Connecticut, and the July 2012 population was estimated at 4.1 million. In 2010, 87 percent of the population lived in urban areas, and the 2010 to 2015 annual rate of urbanization was estimated at 0.9 percent. Beirut is the capital and largest city (with a 2009 population estimated at 1.9 million). The population growth rate in 2012 was negative 0.4 percent, the birth

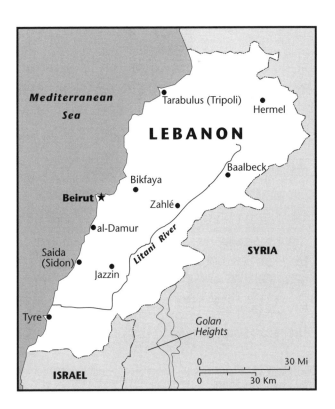

rate 14.9 births per 1,000 population, the net migration rate negative 12.1 migrants per 1,000 (among the 10 highest emigration rates in the world), and the total fertility rate 1.8 children per woman. The United Nations High Commissioner for Refugees (UNHCR) estimated that, in 2010, there were 8,063 refugees and persons in refugee-like situations in Lebanon.

The area that is now Lebanon was part of the Ottoman Empire, and France was given a mandate over it after World War I; Lebanon became an independent country in 1943. A civil war from 1975 to 1990 caused extreme infrastructure damage and human cost. Lebanon ranked tied for 134th among 183 countries on the *Corruption Perceptions Index 2011,* with a score of 2.5 (on a scale where 0 indicates highly corrupt and 10 very clean). In 2011, Lebanon was classified as a country with high human development (the second-highest category) on the United Nations Development Programme's (UNDP's) Human Development Index (HDI), with a score of 0.739 (on a scale where 1 denotes high development and 0 low development). Life expectancy at birth in 2012 was estimated at 75.23 years, and per capita gross domestic product (GDP) in 2011 was estimated at $15,600.

Gender status is unequal in Lebanon: According to the World Economic Forum's *Global Gender Gap Index 2011,* Lebanon ranked 118th out of 135 countries on gender equality, with a score of 0.608 (on a scale with a theoretical range of 1 for equality to 0 for inequality and an actual range in 2011 from 0.8530 to 0.4873).

Emergency Health Services

According to the World Health Organization (WHO), as of 2007, Lebanon did not have a formal and publicly available system for providing prehospital care (emergency care). Doctors Without Borders (Médecins Sans Frontières, or MSF) began working in Lebanon in 1975 and had 23 staff members in the country at the close of 2010. MSF opened a mental health center in Burj el-Barajneh, in the suburbs of Beirut, near a Palestinian refugee camp. MSF treated 780 new patients at this center in 2010 and also provided services within a hospital run by the Palestinian Red Crescent Society and a clinic run by the United Nations Relief and Works Agency (UNRWA), both located in the same Palestinian refugee camp. As of January 2012, the UNRWA for Palestine refugees operated 12 camps in Lebanon, with 465,798 registered persons, including 436,154 registered refugees.

Insurance

Lebanon has a social insurance program providing cash and medical benefits to many classes of employees, including teachers, those working in industry and commerce, and some agricultural workers; temporary agricultural workers and citizens of countries without reciprocal agreements are excluded from the

Selected Health Indicators: Lebanon Compared With the Global Average (2010)

	Lebanon	Global Average
Male life expectancy at birth[*] (years)	71	66
Female life expectancy at birth[*] (years)	77	71
Under-5 mortality rate, both sexes (per 1,000 live births)	22	57
Adult mortality rate, both sexes[*] (probability of dying between 15 and 60 years per 1,000 population)	124	176
Maternal mortality ratio (per 100,000 live births)	25	210
HIV prevalence[*] (per 1,000 adults aged 15 to 49)	1	8
Tuberculosis prevalence (per 100,000 population)	24	178

Source: World Health Organization Global Health Observatory Data Repository.
[*]Data refers to 2009.

program. University students, public-sector employees, dock workers, and newspaper sellers are covered only for medical benefits. The self-employed may voluntarily join the system. The government covers about 25 percent of the cost of the system through general tax funds; the remainder is paid by wage and earnings contributions (2 percent for employees and 9 percent for the self-employed) and employer contributions (7 percent of payroll). Some benefits are provided in hospitals under contract with the National Social Security Fund; if a patient is treated by a private doctor, this treatment is reimbursed at 80 percent (100 percent for maternity care). Other benefits include hospitalization, medicine, lab services, and general and specialist care. The National Social Security Fund administers the program, and the Ministry of Labor provides general supervision. According to Ke Xu and colleagues, in 2003, 5.2 percent of households in Lebanon experienced catastrophic health expenditures annually; "catastrophic" was defined as exceeding 40 percent of household income remaining after basic needs were met.

Costs of Hospitalization

No data available.

Access to Health Care

According to WHO, in 2004, 98 percent of births were attended by skilled personnel (for example, physicians, nurses, or midwives). In 2004, 71 percent of pregnant women received at least four prenatal care visits. The 2010 immunization rates for 1-year-olds were 74 percent for diphtheria and pertussis (DPT3), 53 percent for measles (MCV), and 74 percent for Hib (Hib3). In 2010, an estimated 37 percent of persons with advanced human immunodeficiency virus (HIV) infection were receiving antiretroviral therapy in accordance with the 2010 WHO guidelines. According to WHO, in 2010, Lebanon had 9.54 magnetic resonance imaging (MRI) machines per 1 million population, 28.85 computer tomography (CT) machines per 1 million, 1.43 positron emission tomography (PET) machines per 1 million, 0.72 telecolbalt units per 1 million, and 0.72 radiotherapy machines per 1 million.

Cost of Drugs

In 2005, spending on medicines accounted for more than 25 percent of government spending on health and 15.2 percent of household spending on health; if the share of hospital and ambulatory care allotted to drug purchases is included in the household total, spending on medicines comes to 21.5 percent of household expenditures. Drug prices are set by the Ministry of Health, based on the ex-factory price (the manufacturer's list price before discounts) plus specified markups for shipping and clearance fees and profit margins for wholesalers and pharmacists. There is no national policy promoting the use of generics, and pharmacists are not allowed to substitute a generic medicine for an originator brand. The National Social Security Fund, covering private employees, reimburses 80 percent of drug costs, and the Cooperative of Civil Servants, covering public sector employees, reimburses 75 percent of drug costs. Some drugs are provided for free, including those to treat cancer, multiple sclerosis, and mental illness; the United Nations Children's Fund (UNICEF) and the Young Men's Christian Association (YMCA) also provide and dispense some drugs.

A 2005 survey found that the price for drugs distributed by UNICEF were generally lower than those supplied by the government; for generic drugs, the range of median reference prices (comparing the UNICEF price to the national reference price) was between 0.59 and 1.16, while for government drugs, it was between 0.89 and 14.44. In private pharmacies, prices were substantially higher: For the lowest-priced generics, the median price ratio was 6.53, while for the most-sold generics it was 8.23 and, for innovator brands, 13.57. Availability is a problem in the public sector, forcing many patients to purchase drugs through the private sector, where the prices are high. Affordability depends on whether public- or private-sector drugs must be used and whether generics are available: For instance, a month's treatment for diabetes would cost 0.1 day's wages for the lower-paid government sector worker using the lowest-cost generic from the public sector but 0.3 day's wages for the lowest-priced generic purchased in the private sector and 1.3 days' wages for an innovator brand purchased in the private sector.

Health Care Facilities

As of 2010, according to WHO, Lebanon had 2.79 health posts per 100,000 population, 0.07 health centers per 100,000, 0.88 district or rural hospitals per 100,000, 1.89 provincial hospitals per 100,000, and 0.76 specialized hospitals per 100,000. In 2009, Lebanon had 3.50 hospital beds per 1,000 population.

Major Health Issues

In 2008, WHO estimated that 13 percent of years of life lost in Lebanon were due to communicable diseases,

70 percent to noncommunicable diseases, and 17 percent to injuries. In 2008, the age-standardized estimate of cancer deaths was 151 per 100,000 for men and 113 per 100,000 for women; for cardiovascular disease and diabetes, 404 per 100,000 for men and 263 per 100,000 for women; and for chronic respiratory disease, 44 per 100,000 for men and 23 per 100,000 for women.

Lebanon's maternal mortality rate (death from any cause related to or aggravated by pregnancy) in 2008 was 26 maternal deaths per 100,000 live births. The infant mortality rate, defined as the number of deaths of infants younger than 1 year, was 15.32 per 1,000 live births as of 2012. In 2010, tuberculosis incidence was 17.0 per 100,000 population, tuberculosis prevalence 24.0 per 100,000, and deaths due to tuberculosis among HIV-negative people 2.00 per 100,000. As of 2009, an estimated 0.1 percent of adults age 15 to 49 were living with HIV or acquired immune deficiency syndrome (AIDS).

Health Care Personnel

Lebanon has five medical schools, all located in Beirut: the Faculty of Medicine of the American University in Beirut, the Faculty of Medicine of Beirut Arab University, the Faculty of Medical Sciences of the Lebanese University, the Faculte de Medecine of the University of Saint Joseph, and the Faculty of Medicine and Medical Sciences of the University of Balamand. The basic course of study lasts four to seven years and the degree awarded is doctor of medicine. In 2009, Lebanon had 3.54 physicians per 1,000 population, 1.23 pharmaceutical personnel per 1,000, 1.33 dentistry personnel per 1,000 and 4.84 nurses and midwives per 1,000. Using Fitzhugh Mullan's methodology, Lebanon has an emigration factor of 19.3, representing a high ratio of Lebanese physicians working outside the country (in the United States, United Kingdom, Canada, or Australia) relative to those working in Lebanon.

Government Role in Health Care

According to WHO, in 2010, Lebanon spent $2.8 billion on health care, an amount that comes to $651 per capita. Health care funding was provided primarily (95 percent) from domestic sources, with the remaining 5 percent provided by overseas sources. The majority (46 percent) of health care funding was paid for through household spending, with the remainder provided through government expenditures (39 percent) and other sources (16 percent). In 2010, Lebanon allocated 10 percent of its total government expenditures to health, in the low range for upper-middle-income eastern Mediterranean region countries; government expenditures on health came to 3 percent of GDP, in the median range for upper-middle-income eastern Mediterranean region countries. In 2009, according to WHO, official development assistance (ODA) for health in Lebanon came to $2.43 per capita.

Public Health Programs

In 2010, access to improved sanitary facilities and improved sources of drinking water was essentially universal in Lebanon. According to the World Higher Education Database (WHED), seven universities in Lebanon offer programs in epidemiology or public health: Antonine University, Lebanese University, the American University of Beirut, the University of Balamand, Jinan University, Al-Manar University of Tripoli, and Saint Joseph University.

LESOTHO

Lesotho is a landlocked southern African country, completely surrounded by South Africa. The area of 11,720 square miles (30,355 square kilometers) makes Lesotho similar in size to Maryland, and the July 2012 population was estimated at 2.6 million. In 2010, 27 percent of the population lived in urban areas, and the 2010 to 2015 annual rate of urbanization is estimated at 3.4 percent. Maseru is the capital and largest city (with a 2009 population estimated at 220,000). The population growth rate in 2012 was 0.3 percent, the net migration rate negative 8.2 migrants per 1,000 population (among the 20 highest emigration rates in the world), the birth rate 26.6 births per 1,000, and the total fertility rate 2.6 children per woman.

Once known as Basutoland, Lesotho became independent from the United Kingdom in 1966. The country experienced seven years of military rule in the late 20th century, and a military mutiny in 1998 was put down by the Southern African Development Community, led by military forces from Botswana and South Africa. In 2011, Lesotho ranked eighth among 53 African countries on the Ibrahim Index (governance performance) with a score of 63 (out of 100), and tied for 77th among 183 countries on the *Corruption*

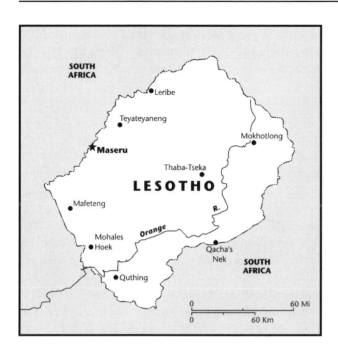

available system for providing prehospital care (emergency care). Some emergency care for remote areas is provided through the Flying Doctor Service, and Maseru Private Hospital in Thetsane has a 24-hour emergency and casualty unit.

Doctors Without Borders (Médecins Sans Frontières, or MSF) began working in Lesotho in 2006; staff working there are integrated with staff working in South Africa. MSF's major areas of focus in Lesotho are treatment for human immunodeficiency virus and acquired immune deficiency syndrome (HIV/AIDS) and tuberculosis and maternal health. In 2010, MSF completed a pilot project to integrate the treatment of HIV and tuberculosis, carried out in rural clinics and one hospital; in June, the project was handed over to the national health authority. In 2011, MSF began a program to improve health and survival among women and children by integrating HIV/AIDS and tuberculosis care with maternal care and other reproductive services.

Insurance

Lesotho has a public health system providing care through a network of health centers, clinics, and hospitals. There are also private providers of health care, particularly in Maseru, and private health insurance is available for those who can afford it.

Costs of Hospitalization

No data available.

Access to Health Care

Health care in Lesotho is organized into four tiers: small health posts, health centers, filter clinics, and network hospitals. There are also specialized facilities, including a leprosy hospital, a psychiatric hospital, and a specialized AIDS clinic. The Flying Doctor Service provides emergency services to remote mountainous areas of the country, brings in essential supplies, and has initiated rural health care programs. According to WHO, in 2009, 61 percent of births in Lesotho were attended by skilled personnel (for example, physicians, nurses, or midwives). In 2009, 70 percent of pregnant women received at least four prenatal care visits. The 2010 immunization rates for 1-year-olds were 83 percent for diphtheria and pertussis (DPT3), 85 percent for measles (MCV), and 83 percent for Hib (Hib3). In 2010, an estimated 57 percent of persons with advanced HIV infection were receiving antiretroviral therapy in accordance with the 2010 WHO guidelines.

Perceptions Index 2011, with a score of 3.5 (on a scale where 0 indicates highly corrupt and 10 very clean).

In 2011, Lesotho was classified as a country with low human development (the lowest of four categories) on the United Nations Development Programme's (UNDP's) Human Development Index (HDI), with a score of 0.450 (on a scale where 1 denotes high development and 0 low development). In 2012, the World Food Programme estimated that 514,000 people in Lesotho were facing food deficits due to low rainfall, hailstorms, and early frost that lowered agricultural output. Life expectancy at birth in 2012 was estimated at 51.86 years, among the 10 lowest in the world, and estimated gross domestic product (GDP) per capita in 2011 was $1,400, among the 30 lowest in the world. Income distribution in Lesotho is relatively unequal: In 2007, the Gini Index (a measure of dispersion, in which perfect equality is denoted by 0 and maximum inequality is denoted by 100) for family income was 61.0, among the highest in the world. According to the World Economic Forum's *Global Gender Gap Index 2011,* Lesotho ranked ninth out of 135 countries on gender equality with a score of 0.767 (on a scale with a theoretical range of 1 for equality to 0 for inequality and an actual range in 2011 from 0.8530 to 0.4873).

Emergency Health Services

According to the World Health Organization (WHO), as of 2007, Lesotho did not have a formal and publicly

Cost of Drugs

The National Drug Services Organization procures drugs for Lesotho's health system, while the Department of Pharmaceutical Services provides drugs to Lesotho's health centers and hospitals.

Health Care Facilities

Health care delivery in Lesotho is organized through Health Services Areas (HSAs), which were determined in 1979; there are 18 HSAs based on the catchment areas of 18 hospitals (nine government hospitals and nine run by the Christian Health Association of Lesotho). In 2006, Lesotho had 1.33 hospital beds per 1,000 population.

Major Health Issues

In 2008, WHO estimated that 77 percent of years of life lost in Lesotho were due to communicable diseases, 15 percent to noncommunicable diseases, and 9 percent to injuries. In 2008, the age-standardized estimate of cancer deaths was 79 per 100,000 for men and 59 per 100,000 for women; for cardiovascular disease and diabetes, 513 per 100,000 for men and 393 per 100,000 for women; and for chronic respiratory disease, 144 per 100,000 for men and 58 per 100,000 for women.

Compared to other countries at a similar level of development, Lesotho ranked third among 43 least-developed countries on the 2011 Mothers' Index, produced by the international nongovernmental organization (NGO) Save the Children, based on a number of health and social factors relating to women, children, and maternal and child care. Lesotho's maternal mortality rate (death from any cause related to or aggravated by pregnancy) is quite high by global standards, estimated at 530 maternal deaths per 100,000 live births as of 2008. The infant mortality rate, defined as the number of deaths of infants younger than 1 year, was estimated at 53.44 per 1,000 live births as of 2012. In 2005, 16.6 percent of children under age 5 were underweight (defined as 2 kilograms [kg] below standard weight-for-age at age 1, 3 kg below for ages 2 to 3, and 4 kg below for ages 4 to 5).

In 2010, tuberculosis incidence was 633.0 per 100,000 population, tuberculosis prevalence 402.0 per 100,000, and deaths due to tuberculosis among HIV-negative people 13.00 per 100,000. As of 2009, Lesotho had the third-highest HIV/AIDS rate in the world; in that year, an estimated 23.6 percent of adults age 15 to 49 were living with HIV or AIDS. In 2010, 57 percent of pregnant women tested positive for HIV. The mother-to-child transmission rate for HIV in 2010 was estimated at 26 percent, and in 2009, 30.7 percent of deaths to children under age 5 were attributed to HIV.

Health Care Personnel

In 2006, WHO identified Lesotho as one of 57 countries with a critical deficit in the supply of skilled health workers. In 2003, Lesotho had 0.05 physicians per 1,000 population, 0.03 pharmaceutical personnel per 1,000, 0.08 laboratory health workers per 1,000, 0.01 dentistry personnel per 1,000, and 0.62 nurses and midwives per 1,000. Health care professionals are unequally distributed throughout the country: For instance, in 2004, the central region had 2.04 health care personnel per 1,000 population, as compared to 1.33 per 1,000 in the northern region and 1.13 per 1,000 in the southern region. Michael Clemens and Bunilla Petterson estimate that 33 percent of Lesotho-born physicians and 3 percent of Lesotho-born nurses are working in one of nine developed countries, primarily in South Africa. Lesotho has a 20-year plan to develop human resources in health from 2005 to 2025, which is focused on increasing the supply of trained personnel.

Government Role in Health Care

According to WHO, in 2010, Lesotho spent $236 million on health care, an amount that comes to $109 per capita. Health care funding was provided primarily (81 percent) from domestic sources, with the remainder (19 percent) coming from abroad. More than three-quarters (76 percent) of health care funding was paid for through government expenditures, with the remainder provided through household expenditures (16 percent) and other sources (7 percent). In 2010, Lesotho allocated 13 percent of its total government expenditures to health, and government expenditures on health came to 8 percent of GDP; both figures place Lesotho in the high range as compared with other low-middle-income African countries. In 2009, according to WHO, official development assistance (ODA) for health in Lesotho came to $45.97 per capita.

Public Health Programs

Lesotho has 12 national public health programs organized into five sections, all within the Department of Primary Health Care of the national government. The Family Health Division includes programs for reproductive health, sexual health and family planning, immunization, control and treatment of diarrheal diseases, control and treatment of acute respiratory infections, child nutrition and household food security, and the community health work program. The Disease Control and Environmental Health Division includes programs focused on leprosy, tuberculosis, sexually transmitted diseases (STDs), acquired immune deficiency syndrome (AIDS), and environmental health. The Health Education Division promotes improved population health through health education and communication.

According to WHO, in 2003, Lesotho had 0.03 environmental and public health workers per 1,000 population. In 2010, 26 percent of the population had access to improved sanitation facilities (24 percent in rural areas and 32 percent in urban), and 78 percent had access to improved sources of drinking water (73 percent in rural areas and 91 percent in urban). According to the World Higher Education Database (WHED), no university in Lesotho offers programs in epidemiology or public health.

LIBERIA

Liberia is a west African country, sharing borders with Guinea, Sierra Leone, and Côte d'Ivoire and having a coastline on the north Atlantic Ocean. The area of 43,000 square miles (111,369 square kilometers) makes Liberia similar in size to Tennessee, and the July 2012 population was estimated at 3.9 million. In 2010, 48 percent of the population lived in urban areas, and the 2010 to 2015 annual rate of urbanization was estimated at 3.4 percent. Monrovia is the capital and largest city (with a 2009 population estimated at 882,000). The population growth rate in 2012 was 2.6 percent (the 23rd-highest in the world), the net migration rate 0.0 migrants per 1,000 population, the birth rate 36.4 births per 1,000 (the 22nd-highest in the world), and the total fertility rate 5.0 children per woman (the 18th-highest in the world). The United Nations High Commissioner for Refugees (UNHCR) estimated that, in 2010, there were 24,743 refugees and persons in refugee-like situations in Liberia.

Freed slaves from the United States began to settle in what is now Liberia in 1822 and, in 1847, formed a republic there. In 1980, Samuel Doe took power through a military coup, and in 1989, a rebellion led by Charles Taylor led to a prolonged civil war (Taylor was convicted of war crimes by a UN-backed special court in 2012). Democratic elections were held in 2005, and the UN retains a strong presence in Liberia as it rebuilds its economic and social structure. According to the Ibrahim Index, in 2011, Liberia ranked 36th among 53 African countries in terms of governance performance, with a score of 45 (out of 100). Liberia ranked tied for 91st among 183 countries on the *Corruption Perceptions Index 2011,* with a score of 3.2 (on a scale where 0 indicates highly corrupt and 10 very clean).

In 2011, Liberia was classified as a country with low human development (the lowest of four categories) on the United Nations Development Programme's (UNDP's) Human Development Index (HDI), with a score of 0.329 (on a scale where 1 denotes high development and 0 low development). In 2011, the International Food Policy Research Institute (IFPRI) classified Liberia as a country with an "alarming" hunger problem, with a Global Hunger Index (GHI) score of 21.5 (where 0 reflects no hunger and higher scores more hunger). In 2012, the World Food Programme estimated that 110,000 people in Liberia were food insecure. Life expectancy at birth in 2012 was estimated at 57.41 years, among the 30 lowest in the world, and estimated gross domestic

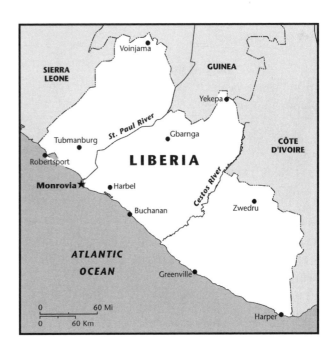

product (GDP) per capita in 2011 was $400, among the 10 lowest in the world. In 2007, the Gini Index (a measure of dispersion, in which perfect equality is denoted by 0 and maximum inequality is denoted by 100) for family income was 38.2. Unemployment in 2003 was estimated at 85.0 percent, among the highest rates in the world.

Emergency Health Services

According to the World Health Organization (WHO), as of 2007, Liberia did not have a formal and publicly available system for providing prehospital care (emergency care). Doctors Without Borders (Médecins Sans Frontières, or MSF) began working in Liberia in 1990 and had 147 staff members in the country at the close of 2010. MSF began a project in Monrovia (the national capital) to provide health, legal, and psychological care to victims of sexual violence; the center treated more than 720 patients in 2010, most (89 percent) younger than 18. Also in 2010, MSF finished the process of transferring responsibility for services it had provided during the Liberian civil war, which ended in 2003, to the Liberian Ministry of Health.

Insurance

Liberia's health system, as of 2008, was operating in partnership with various nongovernmental organizations (NGOs), churches, missions, and so on. The basis of the postconflict national health system is the provision of a Basic Package of Health Services (BPHS); by 2008, this was implemented in 40 percent of functioning facilities. Services are provided free of charge.

Costs of Hospitalization

In 2009, Liberia had 0.70 hospital beds per 1,000 population, one of the 30 lowest rates in the world.

Access to Health Care

According to WHO, in 2007, 46 percent of births in Liberia were attended by skilled personnel (for example, physicians, nurses, or midwives). In 2007, 66 percent of pregnant women received at least four prenatal care visits. The 2010 immunization rates for 1-year-olds were 64 percent for diphtheria and pertussis (DPT3), 64 percent for measles (MCV), and 64 percent for Hib (Hib3). In 2010, an estimated 27 percent of persons with advanced human immunodeficiency virus (HIV) infection were receiving antiretroviral therapy in accordance with the 2010 WHO guidelines.

Cost of Drugs

Total pharmaceutical expenditures in Liberia in 2010 came to LRD 75.8 million ($1.2 million), and per capita expenditure was LRD 19.0 ($0.30). Pharmaceutical expenditures represented 1.2 percent of national health expenditures and 0.1 percent of GDP. Pharmaceutical products must be registered in Liberia before they can be sold in the country; about 2,000 pharmaceutical products were registered as of 2010. Certain population classes are eligible for free medications, including the poor, elderly persons, children younger than age 5, and pregnant women. Due to the situation of unrest in the country, as of 2011, the government of Liberia has a policy of providing some drugs for free to everyone, including medicines on the Essential Medicines List (EML) and medications to treat malaria, tuberculosis, sexually transmitted diseases (STDs), and human immunodeficiency virus and acquired immune deficiency syndrome (HIV/AIDS); vaccines on the Expanded Programme on Immunization (EPI) list, as specified by WHO, are also provided for free.

Health Care Facilities

Liberia is rebuilding its health care system after an extended civil war. A plan to provide primary services throughout the country is being implemented, and secondary care services are available in some areas, thanks to hospital reconstruction funds provided by the Irish, Chinese, and Swiss governments. As of 2008, Liberia had only one national referral hospital, JFK Hospital in Monrovia; several other hospitals offer tertiary care. As of 2010, according to WHO, Liberia had 10.01 health posts per 100,000 population, 1.13 health centers per 100,000, 0.38 district or rural hospitals per 100,000, and 0.03 specialized hospitals per 100,000.

Major Health Issues

In 2008, WHO estimated that 82 percent of years of life lost in Liberia were due to communicable diseases, 14 percent to noncommunicable diseases, and 4 percent to injuries. In 2008, the age-standardized estimate of cancer deaths was 92 per 100,000 for men and 95 per 100,000 for women; for cardiovascular disease and diabetes, 420 per 100,000 for men and 454 per 100,000 for women; and for chronic respiratory disease, 114 per 100,000 for men and 66 per 100,000 for women.

In 2008, the age-standardized death rate from malaria was 54.1 per 100,000 population. In 2010, tuberculosis incidence was 293.0 per 100,000 population, tuberculosis prevalence 476.0 per 100,000, and deaths due to tuberculosis among HIV-negative people 48.00 per 100,000. As of 2009, an estimated 1.5 percent of adults age 15 to 49 were living with HIV or AIDS. In 2008, the age-standardized death rate from childhood-cluster diseases (pertussis, polio, diphtheria, measles, and tetanus) was 16.4 per 100,000 population, the eighth-highest in the world. Liberia's maternal mortality rate (death from any cause related to or aggravated by pregnancy) is the fifth-highest in the world, estimated at 990 per 100,000 live births as of 2008. A 2007 survey estimated the prevalence of female genital mutilation at 58.2 percent. The infant mortality rate, defined as the number of deaths of infants younger than 1 year, is also high, estimated at 72.71 per 1,000 live births as of 2012. In 2007, 20.4 percent of children under age 5 were underweight (defined as 2 kilograms [kg] below standard weight-for-age at age 1, 3 kg below for ages 2 to 3, and 4 kg below for ages 4 to 5).

Health Care Personnel

In 2006, WHO identified Liberia as one of 57 countries with a critical deficit in the supply of skilled health workers. Liberia has one medical school, the A. M. Dogliotti College of Medicine of the University of Liberia in Monrovia. (The Saint Luke School of Medicine operated in Liberia in 1999 but was shut down by the Liberian government in 2005 on charges that it was fraudulent.) The course of study for a basic medical degree lasts five years, and one year of internship and one year of service in a rural area are required after graduation before the physician can be licensed. The license to practice medicine is granted by the Liberian Medical Board.

In 2008, Liberia had 0.01 physicians per 1,000 population, 0.08 pharmaceutical personnel per 1,000, 0.03 laboratory health workers per 1,000, 0.46 health management and support workers per 1,000, 0.04 community and traditional health workers per 1,000, and 0.27 nurses and midwives per 1,000. Michael Clemens and Bunilla Petterson estimate that 63 percent of Liberia-born physicians and 81 percent of Liberia-born nurses are working in one of nine developed countries, primarily the United States. Alok Bhargava and colleagues place Liberia seventh among countries most affected by the medical "brain drain" (international migration of skilled personnel) in 2004.

Government Role in Health Care

The right to health, including the right to access to essential medicines and medical technologies, is recognized in national legislation. Liberia has a National Health Policy (NHP) covering the years 2011 to 2021, and an implementation plan for it, both written in 2011; it also has a National Medicines Policy (NMP), also written in 2011, which covers selection of essential medicines; financing, pricing, purchase, distribution, and regulation of drugs; pharmacovigilance; rational usage of medicines; human resource development; research; evaluation and monitoring; and traditional medicine.

According to WHO, in 2010, Liberia spent $116 million on health care, an amount that comes to $29 per capita. Health care funding was provided about equally from domestic (45 percent) and overseas (55 percent) sources. Health care purchasing was split fairly evenly among spending by households (35 percent), expenditures by government (33 percent), and other sources (32 percent). In 2010, Liberia allocated 11 percent of its total government expenditures to health, in the median range for low-income African countries; government expenditures on health came to 4 percent of GDP, in the high range as compared with other low-income African countries. In 2009, according to WHO, official development assistance (ODA) for health in Liberia came to $23.00 per capita.

Public Health Programs

According to WHO, in 2008, Liberia had 0.01 environmental and public health workers per 1,000 population. In 2010, 18 percent of the population had access to improved sanitation facilities (7 percent in rural areas and 29 percent in urban), and 73 percent had access to improved sources of drinking water (60 percent in rural areas and 88 percent in urban). According to the World Higher Education Database (WHED), one university in Liberia offers programs in epidemiology or public health: the University of Liberia, located in Monrovia.

LIBYA

Libya is a country in north Africa, sharing borders with Algeria, Chad, Egypt, Niger, Sudan, and Tunisia and having a coastline on the Mediterranean Sea. The area of 679,362 square miles (1,759,540 square kilometers) makes Libya similar in size to Alaska, and the July 2012 population was estimated at 27.3 million.

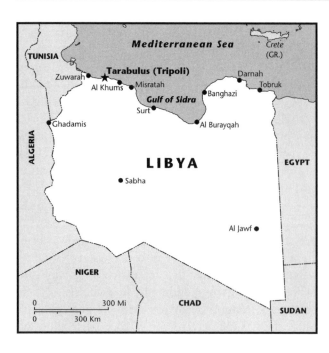

In 2010, 78 percent of the population lived in urban areas, and the 2010 to 2015 annual rate of urbanization was estimated at 2.1 percent. Tripoli is the capital and largest city (with a 2009 population estimated at 1.1 million). The population growth rate in 2012 was 2.0 percent, the net migration rate 0.0 migrants per 1,000 population, the birth rate 23.5 births per 1,000, and the total fertility rate 2.9 children per woman. The United Nations High Commissioner for Refugees (UNHCR) estimates that, in 2010, there were 1,913 refugees and persons in refugee-like situations in Libya.

The area around Tripoli was colonized by the Ottoman Empire then, in 1911, by Italy; Libya was administered by the United Nations (UN) after World War II and became independent in 1951. In 1969, Colonel Muammar al-Quadhafi took power following a military coup. Libya was isolated politically in the 1990s due to a UN sanction that was lifted in 1999; in 2008, the United States resumed normal diplomatic relations with Libya, following resolution of the Lockerbie bombing case. According to the Ibrahim Index, in 2011, Libya ranked 28th among 53 African countries in terms of governance performance, with a score of 50 (out of 100). The Libyan government is perceived as corrupt, 168th among 183 countries on the *Corruption Perceptions Index 2011,* with a score of 2.0 (on a scale where 0 indicates highly corrupt and 10 very clean). In 2011, Libya was classified as a country with high

human development (the second-highest category) on the United Nations Development Programme's (UNDP's) Human Development Index (HDI), with a score of 0.760 (on a scale where 1 denotes high development and 0 low development). Life expectancy at birth in 2012 was estimated at 77.83 years, per capita gross domestic product (GDP) in 2011 was estimated at $14,100, and unemployment in 2004 was estimated at 30.0 percent, among the highest rates in the world.

Emergency Health Services
According to the World Health Organization (WHO), as of 2007, Libya had a formal and publicly available emergency care (prehospital care) system accessible through regional access numbers, but not a national universal access telephone number. WHO has been actively involved in coordinating medical responses for refugees in neighboring countries (for example, Egypt and Tunisia) fleeing the conflict in Libya.

Insurance
Libya has an employer liability system providing cash benefits, and a social insurance system providing medical benefits for the employed and self-employed and cash benefits for the self-employed. The medical benefits system is covered by contributions from wage earners, the self-employed, employers, and the government. The social insurance system is funded by a combination of wage, income, and payroll contributions from the same system that supports pensions; government contributions cover the costs of income-tested benefits, and part of the cost of sickness benefits, pregnancy benefits, work injury benefits, and birth grants. Medical services are provided in facilities run by the Ministry for Social Security, and cost sharing may be required. Benefits available include hospitalization, maternity care, medical care, medical supplies, and rehabilitation. The maternity benefit is 100 percent of earnings for up to three months; a pregnancy benefit is paid from the fourth month until the birth, and a lump sum birth grant is also paid. The sickness benefit is 60 percent of earnings for up to one year. The Social Security Fund administers the program.

Costs of Hospitalization
No informational available.

Access to Health Care
According to WHO, in 2008, 99.8 percent of births in Libya were attended by skilled personnel (for example,

physicians, nurses, or midwives). The 2010 immunization rates for 1-year-olds were 98 percent for diphtheria and pertussis (DPT3), 98 percent for measles (MCV), and 98 percent for Hib (Hib3). In 2010, an estimated 27 percent of persons with advanced human immunodeficiency virus (HIV) infection were receiving antiretroviral therapy in accordance with the 2010 WHO guidelines.

According to WHO, in 2010, Libya had 5.08 magnetic resonance imaging (MRI) machines per 1 million population, 9.53 computer tomography (CT) machines per 1 million, 0.16 positron emission tomography (PET) machines per 1 million, 0.79 telecolbalt units per 1 million, and 0.79 radiotherapy machines per 1 million.

Cost of Drugs
No data available.

Health Care Facilities
As of 2010, according to WHO, Libya had 28.54 health posts per 100,000 population, 1.64 health centers per 100,000 1.56 district or rural hospitals per 100,000, 0.54 provincial hospitals per 100,000, and 0.49 specialized hospitals per 100,000. In 2009, Libya had 3.70 hospital beds per 1,000 population.

Major Health Issues
In 2008, WHO estimated that 21 percent of years of life lost in Libya were due to communicable diseases, 65 percent to noncommunicable diseases, and 18 percent to injuries. In 2008, the age-standardized estimate of cancer deaths was 114 per 100,000 for men and 80 per 100,000 for women; for cardiovascular disease and diabetes, 459 per 100,000 for men and 330 per 100,000 for women; and for chronic respiratory disease, 41 per 100,000 for men and 26 per 100,000 for women.

Libya's maternal mortality rate (death from any cause related to or aggravated by pregnancy) was estimated in 2008 as 64 maternal deaths per 100,000 live births. The infant mortality rate, defined as the number of deaths of infants younger than 1 year, was 19.34 per 1,000 live births as of 2012. In 2010, tuberculosis incidence was 40.0 per 100,000 population, tuberculosis prevalence 53.0 per 100,000, and deaths due to tuberculosis among HIV-negative people 4.00 per 100,000. As of 2009, an estimated 0.3 percent of adults age 15 to 49 were living with HIV or acquired immune deficiency syndrome (AIDS).

Health Care Personnel
Libya has five medical schools, located in Benghazi, Sebha, Sirte, and Tripoli. The basic course of study lasts six years and an additional year of supervised clinical practice is required. Work in government service after graduation is obligatory. The degrees awarded are bachelor of medicine and bachelor of surgery. Physicians must register with the General Medical Syndicate, and the license to practice is granted by the General Directorate for Health Affairs. Foreign medical graduates require special authorization to practice medicine. Libya has agreements with numerous universities in Europe and with other Arabic countries.

In 2009, Libya had 1.90 physicians per 1,000 population, 0.36 pharmaceutical personnel per 1,000, 0.60 dentistry personnel per 1,000, and 6.80 nurses and midwives per 1,000. Michael Clemens and Bunilla Petterson estimate that 8 percent of Libya-born physicians and 2 percent of Libya-born nurses are working in one of nine developed countries, primarily in the United Kingdom and the United States.

Government Role in Health Care
According to WHO, in 2010, Libya spent $3.1 billion on health care, an amount that comes to $484 per capita. Health care funding was provided almost entirely (9 percent) from domestic sources, with the remainder coming from abroad. More than two-thirds (69 percent) of health care funding was paid for through government expenditures, with the remainder provided through household expenditures (31 percent).

In 2010, Libya allocated 5 percent of its total government expenditures to health, and government expenditures on health came to 3 percent of gross domestic product (GDP); both figures place Libya in the low range as compared with other upper-middle-income eastern Mediterranean region countries. In 2009, according to WHO, official development assistance (ODA) for health in Libya came to $3.13 per capita.

Public Health Programs
In 2010, 97 percent of the population of Libya had access to improved sanitation facilities (96 percent in rural areas and 97 percent in urban). In 2000 (the most recent year for which data was available), 54 percent of the population had access to improved sources of drinking water (55 percent in rural areas and 54 percent in urban). According to the World Higher

Education Database (WHED), no university in Libya offers programs in epidemiology or public health.

LIECHTENSTEIN

Liechtenstein is a mountainous central European country, sharing borders with Austria and Switzerland. It is one of only two doubly landlocked countries in the world (the other is Uzbekistan). The area of 62 square miles (160 square kilometers) makes Liechtenstein slightly smaller than Washington, D.C. (in Europe, only Monaco and San Marino are smaller), and the July 2012 population was estimated at 36,713 (the third-smallest in Europe). In 2010, 14 percent of the population lived in urban areas, and the 2010 to 2015 annual rate of urbanization was estimated at 0.9 percent. Vaduz is the capital and largest city (with a 2009 population estimated at 5,000). The population growth rate in 2012 was 0.8 percent, the net migration rate 4.0 migrants per 1,000 population (the 24th highest in the world), the birth rate 10.8 births per 1,000, and the total fertility rate 1.7 children per woman.

Liechtenstein was established as part of the Holy Roman Empire in 1719, became a sovereign state in 1806, and became fully independent in 1866. It had

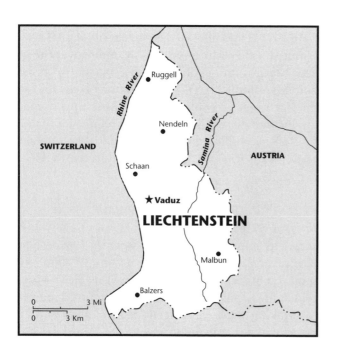

close ties to Austria until World War I and subsequently entered into a customs and monetary union with Switzerland. The country has a modern infrastructure and high standard of living. Liechtenstein ranked eighth (tied with Germany) in 2011 on the United Nations Development Programme's (UNDP's) Human Development Index (HDI). Life expectancy at birth in 2012 was estimated at 81.50 years, among the highest in the world, and per capita gross domestic product (GDP) in 2008 in Liechtenstein was estimated at $141,100, the highest in the world.

Emergency Health Services

Liechtenstein has only one hospital, located in Vaduz; patients may be admitted there for emergency treatment with a physician's referral, and everyone is entitled to treatment until the condition is stabilized, regardless of insurance status. Outside of Vaduz, physicians participate in a duty roster for after-hours care.

Insurance

Liechtenstein has a universal medical benefit that covers everyone residing, employed, or self-employed in Liechtenstein and a social insurance system that provides cash sickness and maternal benefits to employed persons from the age of 14; self-employed people may join the cash benefits system voluntarily. The system is financed through income and payroll contributions and government funding through general tax revenues. Employers must contribute at least half of the insured person's contribution, and the government pays 90 percent of the cost of medical care for children age 16 and younger, and up to 50 percent of medical benefit costs for other insured people, and subsidizes contributions for those with low incomes.

Medical care is provided by doctors and other health care professionals, hospitals, and clinics under contract to insurance funds; cost sharing is included for most services. Benefits available include hospitalization, medicines, medical treatment, maternity care, convalescence, and ambulance services. There is no family benefit because all people, including children, are insured in their own right. The maternity benefit is at least 80 percent of earnings, paid for 20 weeks. The cash sickness benefit is at least 80 percent of covered earnings for up to 720 days. Contributions and benefits are administered by Health Insurance Funds, recognized by the government and the Federation of Health Insurance Funds, and the Office for Health supervises and regulates the Health Insurance Funds.

Costs of Hospitalization

In 2010, the greatest proportion of health care expenditures went to hospital care (CHF 48.2 million), followed by physician services (CHF 48.2 million), pharmaceutical costs (CHF 23.9 million), and other professional services (CHF 24.2 million). The median length of stay in the Vaduz hospital in 2010 was approximately four days.

Access to Health Care

By law all citizens are entitled to equal access to health care. The compulsory insurance plan includes physician and specialist treatment, hospital care, prescriptions drugs, and rehabilitation services. A system of private practice physicians and private insurance exists alongside the state system.

Cost of Drugs

Prescription drugs are generally available in Liechtenstein if they have been authorized by Switzerland and must be purchased from a registered chemist, physician's practice, or hospital pharmacy. The cost of prescribed drugs is subsidized by insurance, and generics are little used (9.9 percent).

Health Care Facilities

The National Hospital, located in Vaduz, is the only hospital in Liechtenstein; however, Liechtenstein has contracts with many hospitals in Austria and Switzerland (27 in 2010), and it is not unusual for citizens of Liechtenstein to be treated in one of those countries. A number of health centers in Liechtenstein, staffed by physicians and nurses, provide general medical and dental care, maternity care, diagnostic services, and emergency medical aid.

Major Health Issues

The infant mortality rate, defined as the number of deaths of infants younger than 1 year, was 4.39 per 1,000 live births as of 2012.

Health Care Personnel

Liechtenstein has three universities, one of which, the Private University of the Principality of Liechtenstein, includes a medical school. However, many Liechtenstein students study abroad, primarily in Switzerland.

Government Role in Health Care

Liechtenstein has compulsory health insurance (OKP) and mandatory sickness insurance (OKG) supported by employer and employee contributions and covering all citizens and registered residents; however, foreign students are required to maintain their own policies. Persons exempt from contributing to the system include the unemployed, retired persons, and those on maternity leave or suffering from certain chronic conditions. The usual point of entry into the system is consultation with a general practice (GP) physician who is registered with the state insurance plan; patients may choose any physician who is so registered. The GP physician may refer patients to a specialist or to hospital admission. Cost increases are capped at 4 percent annually.

Public Health Programs

According to the World Higher Education Database (WHED), no university in Liechtenstein offers programs in epidemiology or public health.

LITHUANIA

Lithuania is a northern European country, sharing borders with Latvia, Belarus, Poland, and Russia (Kaliningrad) and having a coastline on the Baltic Sea. The area of 25,212 square miles (65,300 square kilometers) makes Lithuania similar in size to West Virginia, and the July 2012 population was estimated at 3.5 million. In 2010, 67 percent of the population lived in urban areas, and the 2010 to 2015 annual rate of urbanization was estimated at negative 0.5 percent. Vilnius is the capital and largest city (with a 2009 population estimated at 546,000). The population growth rate in 2012 was negative 0.3 percent, the net migration rate negative 0.7 migrants per 1,000 population, the birth rate 9.3 births per 1,000, and the total fertility rate 1.3 children per woman, one of the 10 lowest in the world.

In the 14th century, Lithuania was the largest state in Europe, including much of present-day Ukraine and Belarus, and in the 16th century Lithuania and Poland formed a single state. In 1795, Lithuania's territory was partitioned by surrounding countries, but after World War I, Lithuania became an independent country again. In 1940, the Soviet Union annexed Lithuania (an action not recognized by many countries), and the country became independent again in 1991, when the Soviet Union collapsed. Lithuania ranked tied for 50th among 183 countries on the *Corruption Perceptions Index 2011,* with a score of 4.8 (on a scale where 0 indicates highly corrupt and 10 very clean). In 2011, Lithuania was classified as a country with very high human development (the highest of four categories) on the United Nations Development Programme's (UNDP's) Human Development Index (HDI), with a score of 0.810 (on a scale where 1 denotes high development and 0 low development). Life expectancy at birth in 2012 was estimated at 75.55 years, and per capita gross domestic product (GDP) in 2011 was estimated at $18,700. In 2009, the Gini Index (a measure of dispersion, in which perfect equality is denoted by 0 and maximum inequality is denoted by 100) for family income was 35.5. According to the World Economic Forum's *Global Gender Gap Index 2011,* Lithuania ranked 37th out of 135 countries on gender equality, with a score of 0.703 (on a scale with a theoretical range of 1 for equality to 0 for inequality and an actual range in 2011 from 0.8530 to 0.4873).

Emergency Health Services

Lithuania's laws governing its emergency health system date from the 1990s, as does recognition of emergency medicine as a medical specialty; by law, free access to hospitals for emergency care is provided for all persons, including the uninsured. Funding for inpatient care in the emergency system is provided entirely by public sources, while funding

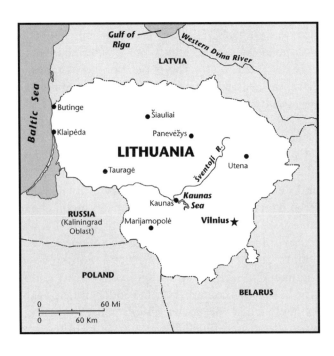

for emergency outpatient care is funded by multiple sources. Lithuania has two national telephone numbers for medical emergencies, 112 (the European Union, or EU, standard) and 03; the country has 56 dispatch centers that are interconnected.

Insurance

Lithuania has social insurance providing medical and cash benefits and covering employees in the private sector and some public-sector employees; other public-sector employees are covered by a separate program. Self-employed people may join the system voluntarily. The system is funded by contributions from wages (6 percent for medical benefits), earnings of self-employed persons (2.2 percent for cash benefits and 9 percent for medical), and employer contributions (3.4 percent of payroll for cash benefits and 3 percent for medical); the government makes up any deficit. Medical benefits include health care services and medicine. The maternity benefit is 100 percent of income for 126 days, and the child care benefit is 100 percent of income (for a child younger than 6 months) or 85 percent of income (for a child aged 6 to 12 months). The cash sickness benefit is 85 percent of average earnings, as is the occupational rehabilitation benefit. The system is administered by the State Social Insurance Board under the supervision of the Ministry of Social Security and Labor. According to Ke Xu and colleagues, in 2003, 1.3 percent of households in Lithuania experienced catastrophic health expenditures annually; "catastrophic" was defined as exceeding 40 percent of household income remaining after basic needs were met.

Costs of Hospitalization

As of 2002, Lithuanian hospitals are paid on a casemix basis, based on historical costs by specialty; for stays of less than four days, payment is by the bedday. Capital costs are reimbursed by the Ministry of Finance or municipal budgets.

Access to Health Care

According to the World Health Organization (WHO), in 2006, 100 percent of births in Lithuania were attended by skilled personnel (for example, physicians, nurses, or midwives). The 2010 immunization rates for 1-year-olds were 95 percent for diphtheria and pertussis (DPT3), 96 percent for measles (MCV), and 95 percent for Hib (Hib3). In 2010, an estimated 27 percent of persons with advanced human

Selected Health Indicators: Lithuania Compared With the Global Average (2010)

	Lithuania	Global Average
Male life expectancy at birth* (years)	68	66
Female life expectancy at birth* (years)	79	71
Under-5 mortality rate, both sexes (per 1,000 live births)	7	57
Adult mortality rate, both sexes* (probability of dying between 15 and 60 years per 1,000 population)	185	176
Maternal mortality ratio (per 100,000 live births)	8	210
HIV prevalence* (per 1,000 adults aged 15 to 49)	1	8
Tuberculosis prevalence (per 100,000 population)	94	178

Source: World Health Organization Global Health Observatory Data Repository.
*Data refers to 2009.

immunodeficiency virus (HIV) infection were receiving antiretroviral therapy in accordance with the 2010 WHO guidelines. According to WHO, in 2010, Lithuania had 5.42 magnetic resonance imaging (MRI) machines per 1 million population, 17.77 computer tomography (CT) machines per 1 million, 1.20 telecolbalt units per 1 million, and 1.20 radiotherapy machines per 1 million.

Cost of Drugs
No data available.

Health Care Facilities
As of 2010, according to WHO, Lithuania had 26.36 health posts per 100,000 population, 5.24 health centers per 100,000, 0.27 district or rural hospitals per 100,000, 1.17 provincial hospitals per 100,000, and 1.32 specialized hospitals per 100,000. In 2008, Lithuania had 6.84 hospital beds per 1,000 population, among the 20 highest ratios in the world, reflective of the hospital-centered model of health care typical in former Soviet republics.

Major Health Issues
In 2008, WHO estimated that 6 percent of years of life lost in Lithuania were due to communicable diseases, 71 percent to noncommunicable diseases, and 23 percent to injuries. In 2008, the age-standardized estimate of cancer deaths was 220 per 100,000 for men and 110 per 100,000 for women; for cardiovascular disease and diabetes, 503 per 100,000 for men and 264 per 100,000 for women; and for chronic respiratory disease, 32 per 100,000 for men and 6 per 100,000 for women.

The maternal mortality rate (death from any cause related to or aggravated by pregnancy) in Lithuania in 2008 was 13 maternal deaths per 100,000 live births. The infant mortality rate, defined as the number of deaths of infants younger than 1 year, was 6.18 per 1,000 live births as of 2012. In 2010, tuberculosis incidence was 69.0 per 100,000 population, tuberculosis prevalence 94.0 per 100,000, and deaths due to tuberculosis among HIV-negative people 1.00 per 100,000. An estimated 11 percent of new tuberculosis cases and 52 percent of retreatment cases are multidrug resistant. As of 2009, an estimated 0.1 percent of adults age 15 to 49 were living with HIV or acquired immune deficiency syndrome (AIDS).

Health Care Personnel
Lithuania has two medical schools, the Kauno Medicinos Universiteto and the Medicinos Fakultetas Vilniaus Universiteto. The course of training lasts six years. Lithuania, as a member of the European Union (EU), cooperates with other countries in recognizing physicians qualified to practice in other EU countries, as specified by Directive 2005/36/EC of the European Parliament. This allows qualified professionals

to practice their profession in other EU states on a temporary basis and requires that the host country automatically recognize qualifications for certain professions, including physicians, nurses, dentists, midwives, and pharmacists, if certain conditions have been met (for instance, facility in the language of the host country may be required). In 2008, Lithuania had 3.66 physicians per 1,000 population, 0.77 pharmaceutical personnel per 1,000, 0.65 dentistry personnel per 1,000, and 7.32 nurses and midwives per 1,000.

Government Role in Health Care

According to WHO, in 2010, Lithuania spent $2.6 billion on health care, an amount that comes to $781 per capita. Health care funding was provided almost entirely (99 percent) from domestic sources, with the remainder coming from abroad. Almost three-quarters (73 percent) of health care funding was paid for through government expenditures, with the remainder provided through household expenditures (26 percent) and other sources (1 percent). In 2010, Lithuania allocated 13 percent of its total government expenditures to health, in the median range for upper-middle-income European countries; government expenditures on health came to 5 percent of GDP; in the high range as compared with other upper-middle-income European countries.

Public Health Programs

In 2010, 86 percent of the population of Lithuania had access to improved sanitation facilities (69 percent in rural areas and 95 percent in urban), and 92 percent had access to improved sources of drinking water (81 percent in rural areas and 98 percent in urban). According to the World Higher Education Database (WHED), two universities in Lithuania offer programs in epidemiology or public health: Kaunas University of Medicine and Vilnius University.

LUXEMBOURG

Luxembourg is a landlocked western European country sharing borders with Germany, France, and Belgium. The area of 998 square miles (2,586 square kilometers) makes Luxembourg similar in size to Rhode Island, and the July 2012 population was estimated at 509,074. In 2010, 85 percent of the population lived

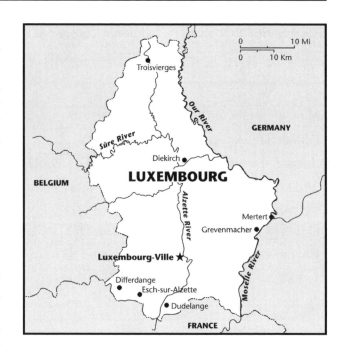

in urban areas, and the 2010 to 2015 annual rate of urbanization was estimated at 1.4 percent. Luxembourg is the capital and largest city (with a 2009 population estimated at 90,000). The population growth rate in 2012 was 1.1 percent, the net migration rate 8.2 migrants per 1,000 population (the 14th-highest in the world), the birth rate 11.7 births per 1,000, and the total fertility rate 1.8 children per woman.

Luxembourg became independent in 1867. Neutral in both World War I and World War II, it ended its neutral status in 1949 when it joined the Benelux Customs Union in 1948 (with Belgium and the Netherlands); it was also one of the founding countries in the European Economic Community (later known as the European Union, or EU). The government has a reputation for transparency and honesty, ranking 11th among 183 countries in terms of perceived public-sector corruption with a score of 8.5 (on a scale where 0 indicates highly corrupt and 10 very clean).

In 2011, Luxembourg was classified as a country with very high human development (the highest of four categories) on the United Nations Development Programme's (UNDP's) Human Development Index (HDI), with a score of 0.867 (on a scale where 1 denotes high development and 0 low development). Life expectancy at birth in 2012 was estimated at 79.75 years, and per capita gross domestic product (GDP) in 2011 in Luxembourg was estimated at $84,700, the third-highest in the world. Income distribution is among the most equal in the world: In 2005, the Gini Index (a measure of dispersion, in which perfect equality is denoted by 0 and maximum inequality is denoted by 100) for family income was 26.0. According to the World Economic Forum's *Global Gender Gap Index 2011*, Luxembourg ranked 30th out of 135 countries on gender equality, with a score of 0.722 (on a scale with a theoretical range of 1 for equality to 0 for inequality and an actual range in 2011 from 0.8530 to 0.4873).

Emergency Health Services

Luxembourg's laws governing its emergency health system date from the 1990s; by law, free access to hospitals for emergency care is provided for all persons, including the uninsured. Funding for both inpatient and outpatient care in the emergency system is provided entirely by the state budget. Luxembourg has only one national telephone number for medical emergencies, 112 (the EU standard); the country has one dispatch center.

Insurance

Luxembourg has social insurance that provides medical benefits, cash maternity and sickness benefits, and attendance (assistance with daily living) benefits. Employees and social security beneficiaries are covered in the full system, while artists, farmers, and the self-employed are covered for medical and attendance benefits. The system is financed through wage, income, and payroll contributions, with government general revenues covering maternity benefits and subsidizing other benefits (29.5 percent for cash benefits, 37 percent for health care, and 45 percent for long-term care).

Medical services are provided by hospitals and doctors under collective agreements; the insured person may choose the provider. Medical benefits include hospitalization, medical care, lab services, maternity care, dental care, medicine, appliances, transportation, and rehabilitation. Copayments are required for some services, for example, 20 percent for a physician visit, 20 percent or 60 percent for medicine, and 12.64 euros a day for hospitalization. The maternity benefit is 100 percent of earnings for eight weeks before and after the due date; those with no loss of income due to maternity receive a lump sum of 3,104.32 euros. Adoption leave is provided at 100 percent of earnings for eight weeks (12 weeks for multiple adoptions). The cash sickness benefit is 100 percent of average earnings for up to 52 weeks. The National Health Fund and the insurance funds administer benefits with supervision from the Ministry of Social Security.

A 2004 study by the World Health Organization (WHO) found that none of the population in Luxembourg had substitutive voluntary health insurance (covering services that would otherwise be available from the state), and 70 percent had complementary voluntary health insurance (covering services not covered or not fully covered by the state) or supplementary health insurance (providing increased choice or faster access to services). Most of those who do not have voluntary insurance are foreign workers residing in Luxembourg.

Costs of Hospitalization

In 2005, according to the Organisation for Economic Co-operation and Development (OECD), hospital spending in Luxembourg represented 33.4 percent of total spending on health, and per capita spending was $1,322; hospitals were paid based on a prospective global budget.

Access to Health Care

According to WHO, in 2003, 100 percent of births in Luxembourg were attended by skilled personnel (for example, physicians, nurses, or midwives). The 2010 immunization rates for 1-year-olds were 99 percent for diphtheria and pertussis (DPT3), 96 percent for measles (MCV), and 98 percent for Hib (Hib3). According to WHO, in 2010, Luxembourg had 14.57 magnetic resonance imaging (MRI) machines per 1 million population, 20.81 computer tomography (CT) machines per 1 million, 2.08 positron emission tomography (PET) machines per 1 million, and 2.08 positron emission tomography (PET) machines per 1 million.

Cost of Drugs

According to Douglas Ball, as of 2011, Luxembourg charged a lower value-added tax (VAT) for medicines (3 percent) than for other goods (the standard VAT is 15 percent). There is no fixed pharmacy dispensing. The wholesale markup is 15.21 percent for products from Belgium or Luxembourg, and the pharmacy markup is 46.7 percent for products from Belgium or Luxembourg and 50.2 percent otherwise. Real annual growth in pharmaceutical expenditures in Luxembourg grew 5.4 percent from 1997 to 2005, much slower than the 11.6 percent growth of total health expenditure (minus pharmaceutical expenditures) over those years.

Health Care Facilities

As of 2010, according to WHO, Luxembourg had 0.20 district or rural hospitals per 100,000, 0.20 provincial hospitals per 100,000, and 0.79 specialized hospitals per 100,000. In 2008, Luxembourg had 5.57 hospital beds per 1,000 population, among the 50 highest rates in the world.

Major Health Issues

In 2008, WHO estimated that 5 percent of years of life lost in Luxembourg were due to communicable diseases, 79 percent to noncommunicable diseases, and 15 percent to injuries. In 2008, the age-standardized estimate of cancer deaths was 156 per 100,000 for men and 93 per 100,000 for women; for cardiovascular disease and diabetes, 184 per 100,000 for men and 116 per 100,000 for women; and for chronic respiratory disease, 27 per 100,000 for men and 13 per 100,000 for women.

The maternal mortality rate (death from any cause related to or aggravated by pregnancy) in Luxembourg in 2008 was 17 maternal deaths per 100,000 live births. The infant mortality rate, defined as the number of deaths of infants younger than 1 year, was 4.39 per 1,000 live births as of 2012. In 2010, tuberculosis incidence was 8.8 per 100,000 population, tuberculosis prevalence 10.0 per 100,000, and deaths due to tuberculosis among human immunodeficiency virus (HIV)-negative people 0.34 per 100,000. As of 2009, an estimated 0.3 percent of adults age 15 to 49 were living with HIV or acquired immune deficiency syndrome (AIDS).

Health Care Personnel

Luxembourg, as a member of the EU, cooperates with other countries in recognizing physicians qualified to practice in other EU countries, as specified by Directive 2005/36/EC of the European Parliament. This allows qualified professionals to practice their profession in other EU states on a temporary basis and requires that the host country automatically recognize qualifications for certain professions, including physicians, nurses, dentists, midwives, and pharmacists, if certain conditions have been met (for instance, facility in the language of the host country may be required). In 2007, Luxembourg had 2.86 physicians per 1,000 population, 0.85 pharmaceutical personnel per 1,000, 0.80 dentistry personnel per 1,000, and in 2006, had 11.32 nurses and midwives per 1,000.

Government Role in Health Care

According to WHO, in 2010, Luxembourg spent $4.1 billion on health care, an amount that comes to $8,181 per capita. Health care funding was provided entirely from domestic sources. More than four-fifths (84 percent) of health care funding was paid for through government expenditures, with the remainder provided through household expenditures (11 percent) and other sources (4 percent). In 2010, Luxembourg allocated 15 percent of its total government expenditures to health, and government expenditures on health came to 7 percent of GDP; both figures place Luxembourg in the median range as compared with other high-income European countries.

Public Health Programs

In 2010, access to improved sanitary facilities and improved sources of drinking water was essentially universal in Luxembourg. According to the World Higher Education Database (WHED), one university in Luxembourg offers programs in epidemiology or public health: the International University Institute of Luxembourg, located in Munsbach.

MACEDONIA

Macedonia is a southern European country sharing borders with Albania, Bulgaria, Greece, Kosovo, and Serbia. The area of 9,928 square miles (25,713 square kilometers) makes Macedonia similar in size to Vermont, and the July 2012 population was estimated at 2.1 million. In 2010, 59 percent of the population lived in urban areas, and the 2010 to 2015 annual rate of urbanization was estimated at 0.3 percent. Skopje is the capital and largest city (with a 2009 population estimated at 480,000). The population growth rate in 2012 was 0.2 percent, the net migration rate negative 0.5 migrants per 1,000 population, the birth rate 11.8 births per 1,000, and the total fertility rate 1.6 children per woman. The United Nations High Commissioner for Refugees (UNHCR) estimated that, in 2010, there were 1,398 refugees and persons in refugee-like situations in Macedonia.

Macedonia became independent from Yugoslavia in 1991, but Greece's objection to the name led to its designation as "the Former Yugoslav Republic of Macedonia." Ethnic tensions have led to some violence (a 2002 census determined that the population was 64.2 percent Macedonian and 25.2 percent Albanian with smaller numbers of Turks, Roma, Serbs, and other minorities). Macedonia ranked tied for 69th among 183 countries on the *Corruption Perceptions Index 2011*, with a score of 3.9 (on a scale where 0 indicates highly corrupt and 10 very clean).

In 2011, Macedonia was classified as a country with high human development (the second-highest category) on the United Nations Development Programme's (UNDP's) Human Development Index (HDI), with a score of 0.728 (on a scale where 1 denotes high development and 0 low development). Life expectancy at birth in 2012 was estimated at 75.36 years, and per capita gross domestic product (GDP) in 2011 was estimated at $10,400. Unemployment in 2011 was estimated at 29.1 percent. In 2008, the Gini Index (a measure of dispersion, in which perfect equality is denoted by 0 and maximum inequality is denoted by 100) for family income was 44.2. According to the World Economic Forum's *Global Gender Gap Index 2011*, Macedonia ranked 53rd out of 135 countries on gender equality with a score of 0.697 (on a scale with a theoretical range of 1 for equality to 0 for inequality and an actual range in 2011 from 0.8530 to 0.4873).

Emergency Health Services
According to the World Health Organization (WHO), as of 2007, Macedonia had a formal and publicly

available emergency care (prehospital care) system accessible through a national access number.

Insurance
Macedonia has a social insurance system covering many population classes, including the employed, self-employed, and unemployed; relatives of covered individuals; civil servants; pensioners; recipients of social assistance; children younger than 18 (younger than 26 if a full-time student); the uninsured over age 65; and people with a contagious or severe illness. As of 2007, an estimated 90 percent of the population was covered by the national health insurance fund. The system is financed through taxes on earnings and wages and employer payroll contributions; the government covers the cost for social assistance recipients.

Medical benefits include inpatient and outpatient care, diagnostic procedures, medical exams, emergency medical care, medicines, rehabilitation, and some appliances. Most benefits require copayment, but maternity care and treatment for serious illness do not require copayment; blood donors are also exempt from copayments. The maternity benefit is 100 percent of earnings for nine months. The cash sickness benefit is 80 percent of earnings and may be also paid to an individual providing care for a family member. The Health Insurance Fund administers the program with general supervision from the Ministry of Health.

Costs of Hospitalization
No data available.

Access to Health Care
According to WHO, in 2005, 98 percent of births in Macedonia were attended by skilled personnel (for example, physicians, nurses, or midwives). The 2010 immunization rates for 1-year-olds were 95 percent for diphtheria and pertussis (DPT3), 98 percent for measles (MCV), and 89 percent for Hib (Hib3).

Cost of Drugs
Pharmaceutical products sold in Macedonia must be given marketing approval by the Drug Bureau, and those on the positive medicines list are obtained through international tender. Four local companies produce drugs, primarily generics. There is no regulation of wholesale margins, and pharmacy markups depend on whether the product in question

is reimbursed by the national health system or not. Reimbursed drugs are listed on a positive medicines list that is updated every six months and is based on the WHO essential drugs list. A tiered system of copayments for drugs has a ceiling of 20 percent, with drugs on the positive list exempt.

Health Care Facilities

In 2008, Macedonia had 4.63 hospital beds per 1,000 population, among the 50 highest rates in the world.

Major Health Issues

In 2008, WHO estimated that 6 percent of years of life lost in Macedonia were due to communicable diseases, 88 percent to noncommunicable diseases, and 6 percent to injuries. In 2008, the age-standardized estimate of cancer deaths was 165 per 100,000 for men and 96 per 100,000 for women; for cardiovascular disease and diabetes, 501 per 100,000 for men and 429 per 100,000 for women; and for chronic respiratory disease, 31 per 100,000 for men and 21 per 100,000 for women.

Compared to other countries at a similar level of development, Macedonia ranked next to last (42nd out of 43 countries) on the 2011 Mothers' Index, produced by the international nongovernmental organization (NGO) Save the Children, based on a number of health and social factors relating to women, children, and maternal and child care. The maternal mortality rate (death from any cause related to or aggravated by pregnancy) in Macedonia in 2008 was nine maternal deaths per 100,000 live births. The infant mortality rate, defined as the number of deaths of infants younger than 1 year, was 8.32 per 1,000 live births as of 2012.

In 2010, tuberculosis incidence was 21.0 per 100,000 population, tuberculosis prevalence 24.0 per 100,000, and deaths due to tuberculosis among human immunodeficiency virus (HIV)-negative people 2.00 per 100,000. As of 2009, an estimated 0.1 percent of adults age 15 to 49 were living with HIV or acquired immune deficiency syndrome (AIDS).

Health Care Personnel

Macedonia has one medical school, the Medicinski Fakultet of the Univerzitet "Sv Kiril I Metodij" Skopje. The basic medical course lasts six years, and a further period of practical training is required before award of the doctor of medicine degree. Graduates must pass a specialist exam to receive the license to practice medicine, while those with foreign degrees must have them validated and take an additional exam. Residence and work permits are also required for foreigners who want to practice in Macedonia. In 2006, Macedonia had 2.55 physicians per 1,000 population, 0.45 pharmaceutical personnel per 1,000, 0.58 dentistry personnel per 1,000, and 4.34 nurses and midwives per 1,000.

Government Role in Health Care

According to WHO, in 2010, Macedonia spent $653 million on health care, an amount that comes to $317 per capita. Health care funding was provided almost entirely (99 percent) from domestic sources, with the remaining 1 percent coming from abroad. Almost two-thirds (64 percent) of health care funding was paid for through government expenditures, with the remainder provided through household expenditures (36 percent).

In 2010, Macedonia allocated 13 percent of its total government expenditures to health, in the high range for upper-middle-income European countries; government expenditures on health came to 6 percent of GDP, in the median range for upper-middle-income European countries. In 2009, according to WHO, official development assistance (ODA) for health in Macedonia came to $2.13 per capita.

Public Health Programs

The Institute of Public Health of the Republic of Macedonia, founded in 1924, is located in Skopje and headed by Dr. Shaban Ballistic. Its mission is to improve public health within Macedonia, including conducting surveillance, research, and health promotion activities and defining priority issues at the local, regional, and national levels. The institute has more than 200 employees, organized into departments dedicated to monitoring communicable diseases, immunization, food safety, water safety and sanitation, physiology and nutrition, occupational medicine, general health, and sanitary inspection.

In 2010, 88 percent of the population of Macedonia had access to improved sanitation facilities (82 percent in rural areas and 92 percent in urban), and 100 percent had access to improved sources of drinking water (99 percent in rural areas and 100 percent in urban). According to the World Higher Education Database (WHED), one university in Macedonia offers programs in epidemiology or public health: Saints Cyril and Methodius University in Skopje.

MADAGASCAR

Madagascar is an island nation in the Indian Ocean; Mozambique is the closest country on the mainland of Africa. The area of 226,658 square miles (587,041 square kilometers) makes Madagascar about twice the size of Arizona, and the July 2012 population was estimated at 22.6 million. In 2010, 30 percent of the population lived in urban areas, and the 2010 to 2015 annual rate of urbanization was estimated at 3.9 percent. Antananarivo is the capital and largest city (with a 2009 population estimated at 1.8 million). The population growth rate in 2012 was 3.0 percent (the 18th-highest in the world), the net migration rate 0.0 migrants per 1,000 population, the birth rate 37.1 births per 1,000 (the 18th-highest in the world), and the total fertility rate 5.0 children per woman (the 19th-highest in the world).

Madagascar became a French colony in 1896 and regained its independence in 1960. According to the Ibrahim Index, in 2011, Madagascar ranked 31st among 53 African countries in terms of governance performance, with a score of 47 (out of 100). Madagascar ranked tied for 100th among 183 countries on the *Corruption Perceptions Index 2011,* with a score of 3.0 (on a scale where 0 indicates highly corrupt and 10 very clean).

In 2011, Madagascar was classified as a country with low human development (the lowest of four categories) on the United Nations Development Programme's (UNDP's) Human Development Index (HDI), with a score of 0.480 (on a scale where 1 denotes high development and 0 low development). In 2011 the International Food Policy Research Institute (IFPRI) classified Madagascar as a country with an "alarming" hunger problem, with a Global Hunger Index (GHI) score of 22.5 (where 0 reflects no hunger and higher scores more hunger), and the World Food Programme estimated that about 547,000 people in Madagascar were food insecure in 2012. Life expectancy at birth in 2012 was estimated at 64.00 years, and estimated gross domestic product (GDP) per capita in 2011 was $900, among the 10 lowest in the world. Income distribution in Madagascar is relatively unequal: In 2001, the Gini Index (a measure of dispersion, in which perfect equality is denoted by 0 and maximum inequality is denoted by 100) for family income was 57.5. According to the World Economic Forum's *Global Gender Gap Index 2011*, Madagascar ranked 71st out of 135 countries on gender equality, with a score of 0.680 (on a scale with a theoretical range of 1 for equality to 0 for inequality and an actual range in 2011 from 0.8530 to 0.4873).

Emergency Health Services

According to the World Health Organization (WHO), as of 2007, Madagascar did not have a formal and publicly available system for providing prehospital care (emergency care).

Insurance

Madagascar has a social insurance system covering maternity benefits only. Some medical services are provided by employers to the dependents of their employees, as required by law. Employed women, including salaried agricultural workers and household workers, are included in the social insurance system. The system is financed through employer contributions (2.25 percent of covered payroll, or MGA 692 per month for household workers). The maternity benefit is 50 percent of wages for six weeks before and eight weeks after the due date. Medical care during pregnancy and birth is covered also, up to MGA 5,000. Some maternity and child health services and benefits are provided through the Family Allowances System; these include a birth grant (MGA 24,000 if the mother undergoes required medical examinations and MGA 12,000 if she does not), a family allowance of MGA

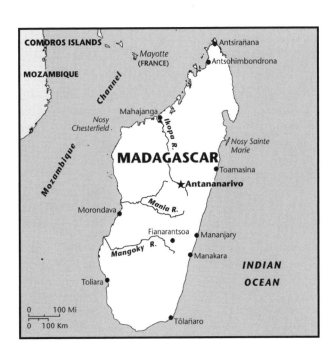

2,000 per month per child, and a prenatal allowance of MGA 18,000 if the woman undergoes required medical examinations. The system is administered by the National Social Insurance Fund with general supervision from the Ministry of Civil Service, Labor, and Social Legislation.

Costs of Hospitalization
No data available.

Access to Health Care
According to WHO, in 2009, 43.9 percent of births in Madagascar were attended by skilled personnel (for example, physicians, nurses, or midwives). In 2009, 49 percent of pregnant women received at least four prenatal care visits. The 2010 immunization rates for 1-year-olds were 74 percent for diphtheria and pertussis (DPT3), 67 percent for measles (MCV), and 74 percent for Hib (Hib3). In 2010, an estimated 1 percent of persons with advanced human immunodeficiency virus (HIV) infection were receiving antiretroviral therapy in accordance with the 2010 WHO guidelines.

Cost of Drugs
In 2010, total expenditures on pharmaceuticals in Madagascar came to MGA 115.1 billion ($62.1 million), or MGA 5,406.0 ($2.90) per capita. Pharmaceutical expenditures represented 15.9 percent of total spending on health, and 0.2 percent of GDP. As of 2009, certain populations were eligible for some free care and medications, including children under the age of 5, pregnant women, the elderly, and the poor; services provided for free vary somewhat by region. Delivery and cesarean section kits are provided for free. Some medications to treat some conditions are also free of charge, including tuberculosis, human immunodeficiency virus and acquired immune deficiency syndrome (HIV/AIDS), cancer, and malaria; vaccines on the Expanded Programme on Immunization (EPI) list, specified by WHO, are also provided free.

Health Care Facilities
As of 2010, according to WHO, Madagascar had 14.35 health posts per 100,000 population, 0.30 health centers per 100,000, 0.37 district or rural hospitals per 100,000, 0.12 provincial hospitals per 100,000, and 0.03 specialized hospitals per 100,000. In 2005, Madagascar had 0.30 hospital beds per 1,000 population, one of the 10 lowest rates in the world.

Major Health Issues
In 2008, WHO estimated that 69 percent of years of life lost in Madagascar were due to communicable diseases, 24 percent to noncommunicable diseases, and 6 percent to injuries. In 2008, the age-standardized estimate of cancer deaths was 142 per 100,000 for men and 96 per 100,000 for women; for cardiovascular disease and diabetes, 367 per 100,000 for men and 384 per 100,000 for women; and for chronic respiratory disease, 99 per 100,000 for men and 56 per 100,000 for women.

In 2008, the age-standardized death rate from malaria was 5.3 per 100,000 population. In 2010, tuberculosis incidence was 266.0 per 100,000 population, tuberculosis prevalence 489.0 per 100,000, and deaths due to tuberculosis among HIV-negative people 53.00 per 100,000. As of 2009, an estimated 0.2 percent of adults age 15 to 49 were living with HIV or AIDS. Madagascar's maternal mortality rate (death from any cause related to or aggravated by pregnancy) is high by global standards, estimated at 440 maternal deaths per 100,000 live births as of 2008 data. The infant mortality rate, defined as the number of deaths of infants younger than 1 year, was estimated at 50.09 per 1,000 live births as of 2012. Child malnutrition is a serious problem: In 2004, 36.8 percent of children under age 5 were underweight (defined as 2 kilograms [kg] below standard weight-for-age at age 1, 3 kg below for ages 2 to 3, and 4 kg below for ages 4 to 5), one of the highest rates in the world.

Health Care Personnel
In 2006, WHO identified Madagascar as one of 57 countries with a critical deficit in the supply of skilled health workers. Madagascar has two medical schools, located in Antananarivo and Mahajanga. The course of study for a basic medical degree lasts seven or eight years, and a two-year internship is also required. The degree awarded is Docteur en Médecine (Diplôme d'État), or doctor of medicine (state diploma). Physicians must register with the Ministère de la Santé et de la Population, and the license to practice is granted by the Ordre des Médecins. Foreigners wanting to practice medicine in Madagascar require authorization by the Ministry of Health. In 2007, Madagascar had 0.16 physicians per 1,000 population and 0.36 health management and support workers per 1,000, and in 2004, had 0.02 community and traditional health workers per 1,000 and 0.32 nurses and midwives per 1,000. Michael Clemens and Bunilla Petterson estimate that

39 percent of Madagascar-born physicians and 28 percent of Madagascar-born nurses are working in one of nine developed countries, primarily in France.

Government Role in Health Care

Access to essential drugs and medical technology is recognized in national legislation as part of the right to health. Madagascar has a National Health Plan (NHP), written in 2005, a plan to implement it, also written in 2005, and a National Medicines Policy (NMP), written in 2004. The NMP covers selection of essential medicines; financing, pricing, purchase, distribution, and regulation of drugs; pharmacovigilance; rational usage of medicines; human resource development; research; evaluation and monitoring; and traditional medicine.

According to WHO, in 2010, Madagascar spent $329 million on health care, an amount that comes to $16 per capita. Health care funding was provided primarily (91 percent) from domestic sources, with the remaining 9 percent coming from overseas. More than half (60 percent) of health care funding was paid for through government expenditures, with the remainder provided through household expenditures (27 percent) and other sources (13 percent). In 2010, Madagascar allocated 15 percent of its total government expenditures to health, in the high range as compared to other low-income African countries; government expenditures on health came to 2 percent of GDP, in the median range for low-income African countries. In 2009, according to WHO, official development assistance (ODA) for health in Madagascar came to $4.34 per capita.

As a member of the World Trade Organization (WTO), Madagascar observes patent law, but national law also includes some elements of the Trade-Related Aspects of Intellectual Property Rights (TRIPS), which provide exceptions to patent law. In Madagascar, these exceptions include the Bolar exception, which allows manufacturers to perform research and testing to create generic drugs before a patent has expired, and parallel importing provisions (allowing import of drugs created for sale in a different country).

Public Health Programs

According to WHO, in 2004, Madagascar had 0.01 environmental and public health workers per 1,000 population. In 2010, 15 percent of the population had access to improved sanitation facilities (12 percent in rural areas and 21 percent in urban), and 46 percent had access to improved sources of drinking water (34 percent in rural areas and 74 percent in urban). According to the World Higher Education Database (WHED), one university in Madagascar offers programs in epidemiology or public health: the University of Mahajanga.

MALAWI

Malawi is a landlocked country in southeastern Africa, sharing borders with Mozambique, Tanzania, and Zambia; it also has a long shoreline on Lake Malawi (Lake Nyasa), the eighth-largest lake in the world. The area of 45,747 square miles (118,484 square kilometers) makes Malawi similar in size to Pennsylvania, and the July 2012 population was estimated at 16.3 million. In 2010, 20 percent of the population lived in urban areas, and the 2010 to 2015 annual rate of urbanization is estimated at 5.3 percent. Lilongwe is the capital and Blantyre the largest city (with a 2009 population estimated at 856,000). The population growth rate in 2012 was 2.8 percent (the 17th-highest in the world), the net migration rate 0.0 migrants per 1,000 population, the birth rate 40.4 births per 1,000 (the ninth-highest in the world), and the total fertility rate 5.4 children per

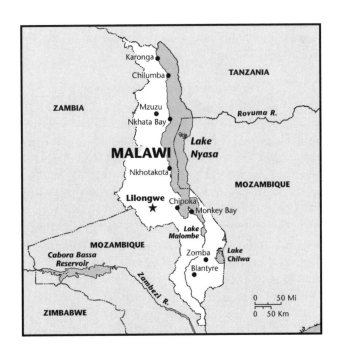

woman (the 14th-highest in the world). The United Nations High Commissioner for Refugees (UNHCR) estimates that, in 2010, there were 5,700 refugees and persons in refugee-like situations in Malawi.

Malawi was a British protectorate (known as Nyasaland) from 1891 until independence in 1964. The country was ruled by a single party until 1994, when multiparty elections were held; a new constitution came into effect in 1995.

According to the Ibrahim Index, in 2011 Malawi ranked 15th among 53 African countries in terms of governance performance, with a score of 57 (out of 100). Malawi ranked tied for 100th among 183 countries on the *Corruption Perceptions Index 2011,* with a score of 3.0 (on a scale where 0 indicates highly corrupt and 10 very clean). In 2011, Malawi was classified as a country with low human development (the lowest of four categories) on the United Nations Development Programme's (UNDP's) Human Development Index (HDI), with a score of 0.400 (on a scale where 1 denotes high development and 0 low development). Life expectancy at birth in 2012 was estimated at 52.31 years, among the 20 lowest in the world, and estimated gross domestic product (GDP) per capita in 2011 was $900, among the 10 lowest in the world. In 2004, the Gini Index (a measure of dispersion, in which perfect equality is denoted by 0 and maximum inequality is denoted by 100) for family income was 39.0.

According to the World Economic Forum's *Global Gender Gap Index 2011*, Malawi ranked 65th out of 135 countries on gender equality, with a score of 0.685 (on a scale with a theoretical range of 1 for equality to 0 for inequality and an actual range in 2011 from 0.8530 to 0.4873).

Emergency Health Services

According to the World Health Organization (WHO), as of 2007, Malawi did not have a formal and publicly available system for providing prehospital care (emergency care). Doctors Without Borders (Médecins Sans Frontières, or MSF) began working in Malawi in 1986 and had 827 staff members in the country at the close of 2010. During the measles outbreak of April and August 2010, almost 1,800 MSF staff worked on an emergency response to the outbreak, including a vaccination campaign and treatment for almost 23,000 people. MSF has been closely involved with human immunodeficiency virus and acquired immune deficiency syndrome (HIV/AIDS) care in Malawi since 2003 and currently provides antiretroviral treatment to tens of thousands

of patients in the country. MSF also provides training and scholarships to increase the supply of health care workers in rural Malawi.

Insurance

Some medical care is provided free in government health centers and hospitals. There is no statutory cash benefits program. Health services are provided through a network of government and private facilities; about 60 percent of health services are provided the government, about 35 percent by the Christian Hospital Association of Malawi, and the remainder by other private organizations.

Costs of Hospitalization

No data available.

Access to Health Care

According to WHO, in 2006, 54 percent of births in Malawi were attended by skilled personnel (for example, physicians, nurses, or midwives). In 2004, 57 percent of pregnant women received at least four prenatal care visits. The 2010 immunization rates for 1-year-olds were 93 percent for diphtheria and pertussis (DPT3), 93 percent for measles (MCV), and 93 percent for Hib (Hib3).

Cost of Drugs

Some classes of people in Malawi are entitled to receive medications for free, including children under the age of 5, pregnant women, elderly people, and the poor. Some medicines are provided free under the public health system, including medicines on the Essential Medications List (EML), antimalarials, and medicines to treat tuberculosis, sexually transmitted disease (STD), and HIV/AIDS; vaccines on the Expanded Programme on Immunization (EPI) list, created by WHO, are also provided free of charge.

Health Care Facilities

As of 2010, according to WHO, Malawi had 0.49 health posts per 100,000 population, 2.53 health centers per 100,000, 0.25 district or rural hospitals per 100,000, 0.15 provincial hospitals per 100,000, and 0.03 specialized hospitals per 100,000. In 2007, Malawi had 1.10 hospital beds per 1,000 population.

Major Health Issues

In 2008, WHO estimated that 73 percent of years of life lost in Malawi were due to communicable

Selected Health Indicators: Malawi Compared With the Global Average (2010)

	Malawi	Global Average
Male life expectancy at birth[*] (years)	44	66
Female life expectancy at birth[*] (years)	51	71
Under-5 mortality rate, both sexes (per 1,000 live births)	92	57
Adult mortality rate, both sexes[*] (probability of dying between 15 and 60 years per 1,000 population)	599	176
Maternal mortality ratio (per 100,000 live births)	460	210
HIV prevalence[*] (per 1,000 adults aged 15 to 49)	110	8
Tuberculosis prevalence (per 100,000 population)	174	178

Source: World Health Organization Global Health Observatory Data Repository.
[*]Data refers to 2009.

diseases, 17 percent to noncommunicable diseases, and 10 percent to injuries. In 2008, the age-standardized estimate of cancer deaths was 83 per 100,000 for men and 105 per 100,000 for women; for cardiovascular disease and diabetes, 674 per 100,000 for men and 500 per 100,000 for women; and for chronic respiratory disease, 145 per 100,000 for men and 58 per 100,000 for women.

In 2008, the age-standardized death rate from malaria was 48.8 per 100,000 population. In 2010, tuberculosis incidence was 219.0 per 100,000 population, tuberculosis prevalence 174.0 per 100,000, and deaths due to tuberculosis among HIV-negative people 11.00 per 100,000. Malawi has one of the highest HIV/AIDS rates in the world; as of 2009, an estimated 11.0 percent of adults age 15 to 49 were living with HIV or AIDS. In 2010, 66 percent of pregnant women tested positive for HIV. In 2009, 13.3 percent of deaths to children under 5 were attributed to HIV.

Compared to other countries at a similar level of development, Malawi ranked fourth among 43 least-developed countries on the 2011 Mothers' Index, produced by the international nongovernmental organization (NGO) Save the Children, based on a number of health and social factors relating to women, children, and maternal and child care. Malawi's maternal mortality rate (death from any cause related to or aggravated by pregnancy) is quite high by global standards, estimated at 510 maternal deaths per 100,000 live births as of 2008. The infant mortality rate, defined as the number of deaths of infants younger than 1 year, is 10th-highest in the world, at 79.02 per 1,000 live births as of 2012. In 2006, 15.5 percent of children under age 5 were underweight (defined as 2 kilograms [kg] below standard weight-for-age at age 1, 3 kg below for ages 2 to 3, and 4 kg below for ages 4 to 5).

Health Care Personnel

In 2006, WHO identified Malawi as one of 57 countries with a critical deficit in the supply of skilled health workers. Malawi has one medical school, the College of Medicine of the University of Malawi in Blantyre, which began offering instruction in 1991. The basic medical degree course lasts five years, and the degrees awarded are bachelor of medicine and bachelor of surgery. In 2008, Malawi had 0.02 physicians per 1,000 population, 0.02 pharmaceutical personnel per 1,000, 0.03 laboratory health workers per 1,000, 1.27 health management and support workers per 1,000, 0.02 dentistry personnel per 1,000, 0.73 community and traditional health workers per 1,000, and 0.28 nurses and midwives per 1,000. Michael Clemens and Bunilla Petterson estimate that 59 percent of Malawi-born physicians and 17 percent of Malawi-born nurses are working in one of nine developed countries, primarily in the United Kingdom (UK) (physicians) and the UK and the United States (nurses).

Government Role in Health Care

Malawi has a National Health Policy (NHP), written in 2007, and an implementation plan for it, written in the same year; it also has a National Medicines Policy (NMP), written in 2009. Malawi's NMP covers selection of essential medicines; financing, pricing, purchase, distribution, and regulation of drugs; pharmacovigilance; rational usage of medicines; human resource development; research; evaluation and monitoring; and traditional medicine. Promotion and advertising of prescription medications is regulated, and direct marketing to the public is prohibited.

According to WHO, in 2010, Malawi spent $382 million on health care, an amount that comes to $26 per capita. About one-third (36 percent) of health care funding was provided from domestic sources, with 64 percent coming from abroad. More than half (60 percent) of health care funding was paid for through government expenditures, with the remainder provided through household expenditures (11 percent) and other sources (29 percent). In 2010, Malawi allocated 14 percent of its total government expenditures to health, and government expenditures on health came to 4 percent of GDP; both figures place Malawi in the high range as compared with other low-income African countries. In 2009, according to WHO, official development assistance (ODA) for health in Malawi came to $19.19 per capita.

Public Health Programs

The Ministry of Health, Community Health Sciences Unit, for Malawi is located in Lilongwe and is headed by Storn Kabaluzi. Services are organized at the community health center, district hospital, and central hospital levels. At the community level, services are delivered by community health workers and health surveillance assistance, which engage in activities including health education, provision of immunizations, and distribution of mosquito nets. Health centers provide treatment for minor illnesses, while more complicated cases are referred to district and central hospitals. Public health, including disease control and prevention, is a priority for the future for the government of Malawi.

According to WHO, in 2008, Malawi had 0.02 environmental and public health workers per 1,000 population. In 2010, 51 percent of the population had access to improved sanitation facilities (51 percent in rural areas and 49 percent in urban), and 83 percent had access to improved sources of drinking water (80 percent in rural areas and 95 percent in urban). According to the

World Higher Education Database (WHED), one university in Malawi offers programs in epidemiology or public health: the University of Malawi in Blantyre.

MALAYSIA

Malaysia is a southeast Asian country, sharing borders with Brunei, Indonesia, and Thailand and having a coastline on the South China Sea; the country includes a mainland portion and a portion on the island of Borneo. The area of 127,354 square miles (329,847 square kilometers) makes Malaysia similar in size to New Mexico, and the July 2012 population was estimated at 29.2 million. In 2010, 72 percent of the population lived in urban areas, and the 2010 to 2015 annual rate of urbanization is estimated at 2.4 percent.

Kuala Lumpur is the capital and largest city (with a 2009 population estimated at 1.5 million). The population growth rate in 2012 was 1.5 percent, the net migration rate negative 0.4 migrants per 1,000 population, the birth rate 20.7 births per 1,000, and the total fertility rate 2.6 children per woman. The United Nations High Commissioner for Refugees (UNHCR)

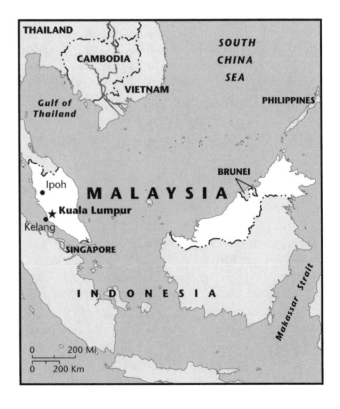

estimated that, in 2010, there were 81,516 refugees and persons in refugee-like situations in Malaysia.

Great Britain established colonies in the region that is now Malaysia in the 18th and 19th centuries. In 1948, these former British colonies (except for Singapore) became the Federation of Malaya and, in 1957, became an independent country. The areas of Sabah and Sarawak (on Borneo) became part of Malaysia in 1963, and Singapore joined Malaysia in 1963, then left in 1965. Malaysia ranked 60th among 183 countries on the *Corruption Perceptions Index 2011*, with a score of 4.3 (on a scale where 0 indicates highly corrupt and 10 very clean). In 2011, Malaysia was classified as a country with high human development (the second-highest category) on the United Nations Development Programme's (UNDP's) Human Development Index (HDI), with a score of 0.761 (on a scale where 1 denotes high development and 0 low development). Life expectancy at birth in 2012 was estimated at 74.04 years, and per capita gross domestic product (GDP) in 2011 was estimated at $15,600. Income distribution in Malaysia is relatively unequal: In 2009, the Gini Index (a measure of dispersion, in which perfect equality is denoted by 0 and maximum inequality is denoted by 100) for family income was 46.2. According to the World Economic Forum's *Global Gender Gap Index 2011*, Malaysia ranked 97th out of 135 countries on gender equality, with a score of 0.653 (on a scale with a theoretical range of 1 for equality to 0 for inequality and an actual range in 2011 from 0.8530 to 0.4873).

Emergency Health Services

According to the World Health Organization (WHO), as of 2007, Malaysia had a formal and publicly available emergency care (prehospital care) system accessible through a national universal access telephone number.

Insurance

Malaysia has a provident fund system providing medical benefits only. The system covers private-sector employees, and public-sector employees are not eligible for pensions; voluntary coverage is possible for pensionable public-sector employees, foreign workers, household workers, and the self-employed. Public-sector employees belong to a separate system. The system is funded by contributions from wages, self-employed earnings, and employer payroll and is part of the same system that funds pensions. Those covered by the fund have two accounts: Both cover old-age, disability, and survivor benefits, but one account

also covers approved investments, while the other covers home purchases, education costs, and treatment for specified illnesses (36 eligible illnesses are listed by the Employees Provident Fund Board). Fund members can withdraw savings from the latter to pay for treatment for eligible illnesses for themselves and their dependents (including children, spouses, siblings, parents, and parents-in-law) if the employer does not provide coverage. The Employees Provident Fund manages the system under the general supervision of the Ministry of Finance.

Costs of Hospitalization

No data available.

Access to Health Care

In 2000, WHO declared that the Malaysian health care system was among the best in world in terms of providing access to primary care to all sectors of society, including disadvantaged groups. According to WHO, in 2006, 100 percent of births in Malaysia were attended by skilled personnel (for example, physicians, nurses, or midwives). The 2010 immunization rates for 1-year-olds were 94 percent for diphtheria and pertussis (DPT3), 96 percent for measles (MCV), and 94 percent for Hib (Hib3). In 2010, an estimated 36 percent of persons with advanced human immunodeficiency virus (HIV) infection were receiving antiretroviral therapy in accordance with the 2010 WHO guidelines. According to WHO, in 2010, Malaysia had 3.04 magnetic resonance imaging (MRI) machines per 1 million population, 6.66 computer tomography (CT) machines per 1 million, 0.33 positron emission tomography (PET) machines per 1 million, 0.22 telecolbalt units per 1 million, and 0.22 radiotherapy machines per 1 million.

Cost of Drugs

In 1994, Malaysia privatized the drug distribution system (previously run by the government); this resulted in drug prices more than tripling by 1997, and various studies since then have shown a continuing trend toward increasing costs. Out-of-pocket expenditures on medicines are high; a 2003 survey found that 42 percent of patients obtained drugs from retail pharmacies, 37 percent from private clinics or hospitals, 13 percent from government hospitals, and 8 percent elsewhere. Branded medicines are also used widely, as opposed to generics; a 2003 survey found that more than half (56 percent) of Malaysians felt medicines were expensive, 18 percent felt they were cheap, and 26 percent felt they were priced fairly.

A 2005 survey found that, in the public sector, the median price ratio (ratio of the price to the international reference price) was 1.09 for the lowest-priced generics (meaning that the Malaysian price was 9 percent higher than the international reference price), 1.56 for the most-sold generics, and 2.41 for innovator brands. The price of some commonly used drugs, such as zidovudine and diazepam, were priced at more than twice the international reference price. In private pharmacies, the median price ratio was 6.57 for the lowest-priced generics, 6.89 for the most-sold generics, and 16.50 for innovator brands. Drugs were more expensive when obtained from dispensing physicians; for instance, the median price ratio was 7.93 for the lowest-priced generics obtained from a physician, the median price ratio for the most-sold generics 7.59, and for innovator brands, 16.09. Prices in private hospitals were also high: The median price ratio was 7.0 for the lowest-priced generics and 12.0 for innovator brands. The median availability of drugs was low in public facilities: Only 20 percent of the generics and 5 percent of innovator brands were available in all 20 public facilities surveyed. In private pharmacies, availability was higher: The median availability was 43 percent for the lowest-priced generics, 39 percent for innovator brands, and 18 percent for the most-prescribed generics. In physicians' dispensing clinics, the availability of lowest-priced generics was 45 percent, of most sold generics, 15 percent, and for innovator brands, 10 percent. In private hospitals, innovator brands were more available (60 percent) than the lowest priced generics (40 percent) and most subscribed generics (20 percent).

Health Care Facilities

As of 2010, according to WHO, Malaysia had 0.33 district or rural hospitals per 100,000, 0.07 provincial hospitals per 100,000, and 0.08 specialized hospitals per 100,000. In 2009, Malaysia had 1.82 hospital beds per 1,000 population.

Major Health Issues

In 2008, WHO estimated that 26 percent of years of life lost in Malaysia were due to communicable diseases, 58 percent to noncommunicable diseases, and 16 percent to injuries. In 2008, the age-standardized estimate of cancer deaths was 119 per 100,000 for men and 90 per 100,000 for women; for cardiovascular disease and diabetes, 319 per 100,000 for men and 236 per 100,000 for women; and for chronic respiratory disease, 75 per 100,000 for men and 42 per 100,000 for women.

In 2008, the age-standardized death rate from malaria was 0.1 per 100,000 population. In 2010, tuberculosis incidence was 82.0 per 100,000 population, tuberculosis prevalence 107.0 per 100,000, and deaths due to tuberculosis among HIV-negative people 8.50 per 100,000. As of 2009, an estimated 0.5 percent of adults age 15 to 49 were living with HIV or acquired immune deficiency syndrome (AIDS). Malaysia's maternal mortality rate (death from any cause related to or aggravated by pregnancy) in 2008 was 38 maternal deaths per 100,000 live births. The infant mortality rate, defined as the number of deaths of infants younger than 1 year, was 14.57 per 1,000 live births as of 2012.

Health Care Personnel

Malaysia has nine medical schools, located in Kuala Lumpur, Khota Bharu, Khota Samarahan, Penang, Selangor, and Bukit Baru. The course of study for the basic medical degree lasts five to six years, and an internship of one year is also required. The degree awarded is Doktor Perubatan (doctor of medicine). Physicians must register with the Malaysian Medical Council. Foreigners may receive a license to practice for a limited period, and graduates of foreign medical schools must provide evidence of sufficient experience. In 2008, Malaysia had 0.94 physicians per 1,000 population, 0.14 dentistry personnel per 1,000, and 2.73 nurses and midwives per 1,000.

Government Role in Health Care

According to WHO, in 2010, Malaysia spent $10 billion on health care, an amount that comes to $4,368 per capita. Health care funding was provided entirely from domestic sources. More than half (56 percent) of health care funding was paid for through government expenditures, with the remainder provided through household expenditures (34 percent) and other sources (10 percent). In 2010, Malaysia allocated 9 percent of its total government expenditures to health, and government expenditures on health came to 2 percent of GDP; both figures place Malaysia in the low range as compared with other upper-middle-income western Pacific region countries. In 2009, according to WHO, official development assistance (ODA) for health in Malaysia came to $0.05 per capita.

Public Health Programs

In 2010, 96 percent of the population of Malaysia had access to improved sanitation facilities (95 percent in rural areas and 96 percent in urban), and access to improved sources of drinking water was nearly universal (99 percent in rural areas and 100 percent in urban). According to the World Higher Education Database (WHED), two universities in Malaysia offer programs in epidemiology or public health: the National University of Malaysia in Bangi, Selangor, and the Universiti Sains Malaysia in Penang.

MALDIVES

The Maldives is an island nation in the Indian Ocean. The area of 115 square miles (298 square kilometers) makes the Maldives about 1.7 times the size of Washington, D.C., and the July 2012 population was estimated at 394,451; the Maldives is the smallest nation in Asia in terms of both area and population. The Maldives consists of two chains of small coral islands (of 1,190 islands, 200 are inhabited, and another 80 are tourist resorts). In 2010, 40 percent of the population

lived in urban areas, and the 2010 to 2015 annual rate of urbanization is estimated at 4.2 percent. Malé is the capital and largest city (with a 2009 population estimated at 120,000). The population growth rate in 2012 was negative 0.1 percent, the net migration rate negative 12.6 migrants per 1,000 population (one of the highest emigration rates the in the world), the birth rate 15.1 births per 1,000, and the total fertility rate 1.8 children per woman.

The Maldives became a British protectorate in 1887, became independent in 1965, and became a republic in 1968. For 30 years, the Maldives was ruled by a single party and by President Maumoon Abdul Gayoom; after riots in 2003, the government began moving toward a multiparty system, and presidential elections were held in 2008. Due to the nature of the Maldives's geography as low-lying islands, the government of the Maldives has played a prominent role in international discussions of climate change.

The Maldives ranked tied for 134th among 183 countries on the *Corruption Perceptions Index 2011*, with a score of 2.5 (on a scale where 0 indicates highly corrupt and 10 very clean). In 2011, the Maldives was classified as a country with medium human development (the second from the lowest of four categories) on the United Nations Development Programme's (UNDP's) Human Development Index (HDI), with a score of 0.661 (on a scale where 1 denotes high development and 0 low development). Life expectancy at birth in 2012 was estimated at 74.69 years, and per capita gross domestic product (GDP) in 2011 was estimated at $8,400.

According to the World Economic Forum's *Global Gender Gap Index 2011*, Maldives ranked 101st out of 135 countries on gender equality with a score of 0.648 (on a scale with a theoretical range of 1 for equality to 0 for inequality and an actual range in 2011 from 0.8530 to 0.4873).

Emergency Health Services

According to the World Health Organization (WHO), as of 2007, Maldives did not have a formal and publicly available system for providing prehospital care (emergency care).

Insurance

Maldives has a national health plan, and since the first Country Health Plan was developed in 1989, health has been considered a basic right of all citizens of the country.

Costs of Hospitalization

No data available.

Access to Health Care

The Maldives has a national health network of public facilities, including (as of 2003), two hospitals in Malé, six regional hospitals, eight atoll hospitals, 63 health centers, and 52 atoll health posts. There were also 30 private health clinics in Malé and 17 in the atolls. According to WHO, in 2009, 94.8 percent of births in the Maldives were attended by skilled personnel (for example, physicians, nurses, or midwives). In 2009, 85 percent of pregnant women received at least four prenatal care visits. The 2010 immunization rates for 1-year-olds were 96 percent for diphtheria and pertussis (DPT3) and 97 percent for measles (MCV).

In 2010, an estimated 14 percent of persons with advanced human immunodeficiency virus (HIV) infection were receiving antiretroviral therapy in accordance with the 2010 WHO guidelines. According to WHO, in 2010, Maldives had 3.28 magnetic resonance imaging (MRI) machines per 1 million population and 6.56 computer tomography (CT) machines per 1 million.

Cost of Drugs

All drugs for the Maldives must be imported. A national drug policy, including a draft formulary, was in use as of 2007, with regular drug utilization reviews, and only drugs on the national list may be imported. Drugs are procured for government health facilities and private pharmacies by the State Trading Organization. Retail price markups are regulated by the Ministry of Trade and the Ministry of Health.

Health Care Facilities

In 2003, medical facilities in the Maldives included 16 public hospitals, 63 public health centers, 52 public health posts, and 47 private health clinics. There were also 30 private health clinics in Malé and 17 in the atolls. A public health laboratory has been in operation since 1998, and the National Thalassemia Centre has been open since 1994.

As of 2010, according to WHO, the Maldives had 12.03 health posts per 100,000 population, 39.25 health centers per 100,000, 6.65 district or rural hospitals per 100,000, and 0.63 provincial hospitals per 100,000. In 2005, the Maldives had 2.60 hospital beds per 1,000 population.

Major Health Issues

In 2008, WHO estimated that 23 percent of years of life lost in the Maldives were due to communicable diseases, 56 percent to noncommunicable diseases, and 21 percent to injuries. In 2008, the age-standardized estimate of cancer deaths was 64 per 100,000 for men and 40 per 100,000 for women; for cardiovascular disease and diabetes, 369 per 100,000 for men and 333 per 100,000 for women; and for chronic respiratory disease, 93 per 100,000 for men and 111 per 100,000 for women.

In 2008, the age-standardized death rate from malaria was 0.9 per 100,000 population. In 2010, tuberculosis incidence was 36.0 per 100,000 population, tuberculosis prevalence 13.0 per 100,000, and deaths due to tuberculosis among HIV-negative people 3.40 per 100,000. As of 2009, an estimated 0.1 percent of adults age 15 to 49 were living with HIV or acquired immune deficiency syndrome (AIDS).

Compared to other countries at a similar level of development, the Maldives ranked first among 43 least-developed countries on the 2011 Mothers' Index, produced by the international nongovernmental organization (NGO) Save the Children, based on a number of health and social factors relating to women, children, and maternal and child care. The Maldives's maternal mortality rate (death from any cause related to or aggravated by pregnancy) in 2008 was 37 maternal deaths per 100,000 live births. The infant mortality rate, defined as the number of deaths of infants younger than 1 year, was estimated at 26.46 per 1,000 live births as of 2012. In 2001, 25.7 percent of children under age 5 were underweight (defined as 2 kilograms [kg] below standard weight-for-age at age 1, 3 kg below for ages 2 to 3, and 4 kg below for ages 4 to 5).

Health Care Personnel

In 2007, the Maldives had 1.60 physicians per 1,000 population, 0.82 pharmaceutical personnel per 1,000, 0.86 laboratory health workers per 1,000, 0.01 dentistry personnel per 1,000, 2.27 community and traditional health workers per 1,000, and 4.45 nurses and midwives per 1,000.

Government Role in Health Care

According to WHO, in 2010, the Maldives spent $121 million on health care, an amount that comes to $382 per capita. Health care funding was provided primarily (99 percent) from domestic sources, with 1 percent coming from abroad. More than half (60 percent) of health care funding was paid for through government expenditures, with the remainder provided through household expenditures (28 percent) and other sources (11 percent). In 2010, the Maldives allocated 9 percent of its total government expenditures to health, in the low range as compared to other upper-middle-income southeast Asian region countries; government expenditures on health came to 4 percent of GDP, in the high range as compared to other upper-middle-income southeast Asian region countries.

Public Health Programs

According to WHO, in 1996 (the most recent year for which data was available), Maldives had 0.19 environmental and public health workers per 1,000 population. In 2010, 97 percent of the population had access to improved sanitation facilities (97 percent in rural areas and 98 percent in urban), and 98 percent had access to improved sources of drinking water (97 percent in rural areas and 100 percent in urban).

MALI

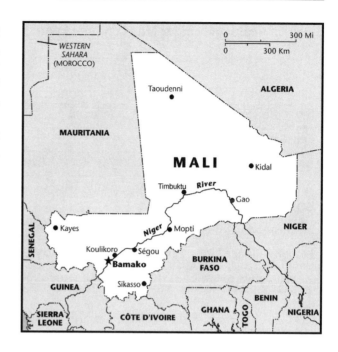

Mali is a landlocked country in west Africa, sharing borders with Algeria, Burkina Faso, Guinea, Côte d'Ivoire, Mauritania, Niger, and Senegal. The area of 478,841 square miles (1,240,192 square kilometers) makes Mali the 24th-largest country in the world (about twice the size of Texas), and the July 2012 population was estimated at 14.5 million. In 2010, 36 percent of the population lived in urban areas, and the 2010 to 2015 annual rate of urbanization is estimated at 4.4 percent. Bamako is the capital and largest city (with a 2009 population estimated at 1.6 million). The population growth rate in 2012 was 2.6 percent, the net migration rate negative 5.1 migrants per 1,000 population, the birth rate 45.2 births per 1,000 (the third-highest in the world), and the total fertility rate 6.4 children per woman (the third-highest in the world). The United Nations High Commissioner for Refugees (UNHCR) estimated that, in 2010, there were 13,558 refugees and persons in refugee-like situations in Mali.

A former French colony, Mali became independent in 1960 as the Sudanese Republic and Senegal; Senegal withdrew from the alliance after a few months, and the Sudanese Republic was named Mali. The country was ruled by a dictatorship until 1991, when a

military coup brought in a period of democratic rule. A military coup in 2012 overthrew the government, but international pressure forced the country back to democratic rule. According to the Ibrahim Index, in 2011, Mali ranked 22nd among 53 African countries in terms of governance performance, with a score of 54 (out of 100). Mali ranked tied for 118th among 183 countries on the *Corruption Perceptions Index 2011*, with a score of 2.8 (on a scale where 0 indicates highly corrupt and 10 very clean).

In 2011, Mali was classified as a country with low human development (the lowest of four categories) on the United Nations Development Programme's (UNDP's) Human Development Index (HDI), with a score of 0.359 (on a scale where 1 denotes high development and 0 low development). In 2012, the World Food Programme estimated that 3.7 million people in Mali are food insecure. Life expectancy at birth in 2012 was estimated at 53.06 years, among the 20 lowest in the world, and estimated gross domestic product (GDP) per capita in 2011 was $1,300, among the 30 lowest in the world. In 2001, the Gini Index (a measure of dispersion, in which perfect equality is denoted by 0 and maximum inequality is denoted by 100) for family income was 40.1. Unemployment in 2004 was estimated at 30 percent. According to the World Economic Forum's *Global Gender Gap Index 2011*, Mali ranked 132nd out of 135 countries on gender equality, with a score of 0.575 (on a scale with a theoretical

Selected Health Indicators: Mali Compared With the Global Average (2010)

	Mali	Global Average
Male life expectancy at birth* (years)	50	66
Female life expectancy at birth* (years)	56	71
Under-5 mortality rate, both sexes (per 1,000 live births)	178	57
Adult mortality rate, both sexes* (probability of dying between 15 and 60 years per 1,000 population)	286	176
Maternal mortality ratio (per 100,000 live births)	540	210
HIV prevalence* (per 1,000 adults aged 15 to 49)	10	8
Tuberculosis prevalence (per 100,000 population)	101	178

Source: World Health Organization Global Health Observatory Data Repository.
*Data refers to 2009.

range of 1 for equality to 0 for inequality and an actual range in 2011 from 0.8530 to 0.4873).

Emergency Health Services

According to the World Health Organization (WHO), as of 2007, Mali had a formal and publicly available emergency care (prehospital care) system accessible through a national universal access telephone number. Doctors Without Borders (Médecins Sans Frontières, or MSF) began working in Mali in 1992 and had 380 staff members in the country at the close of 2010. MSF's focus is pediatric care in the regions of Koulikoro and Sikasso; services provided include vaccination, treatment for malnutrition, rapid detection and treatment of malaria, and training of local village staff to provide basic services.

Insurance

Mali has a social insurance system providing medical and maternity benefits. Employed persons are included in the system, and the self-employed may join voluntarily; the military, magistrates, and civil servants have a separate system. The system is funded by contributions from wages (3.06 percent of gross earnings), contributions from the self-employed (6.56 percent of wage class earnings, based on a schedule of five wage classes), pensioner contributions (0.75 percent of pension), and employers (3.5 percent of gross payroll for medical benefits only). Medical care and some health

and welfare services are provided by the joint inter-employer medical services program, operated by the National Social Insurance Institute. Dependents (the children and spouse of an insured person) receive the same benefits as the insured, and insured women receive medical care for the prenatal period and birth. The cash maternity benefit is 100 percent of earnings, paid for six weeks before and eight weeks after the due date; the father receives three days of birth leave at 100 percent of salary (the father's leave may be taken any time in the first 15 days after the birth). The National Social Insurance Institute administers the program under the general supervision of the Ministry of Social Development, Solidarity, and Aged Persons.

Costs of Hospitalization

No data available.

Access to Health Care

According to WHO, in 2006, 49 percent of births in Mali were attended by skilled personnel (for example, physicians, nurses, or midwives), and 35 percent of pregnant women received at least four prenatal care visits. The 2010 immunization rates for 1-year-olds were 76 percent for diphtheria and pertussis (DPT3), 63 percent for measles (MCV), and 77 percent for Hib (Hib3). In 2010, an estimated 46 percent of persons with advanced human immunodeficiency virus (HIV) infection were receiving antiretroviral therapy in accordance with the 2010 WHO guidelines. According to WHO, in 2010, Mali had fewer than 0.01 magnetic resonance imaging (MRI) machines per 1 million population and 0.24 computer tomography (CT) machines per 1 million.

Cost of Drugs

According to Douglas Ball, Mali adopted a National Medicines Policy (NMP) in 1998 that emphasized rational prescribing and dispensing and the use of essential generic medicines. In 2006, legislation established set prices for medicines in the public sector, and a 2009 law set the maximum price for 107 essential generic medicines in the private sector; taxes on medicines were also reduced. Public medicines are sold through a central medical store to public and nonprofit facilities; the central store is also allowed to sell to for-profit retail pharmacies. Some medicines are provided free of charge to patients in public facilities. Currently, retail prices are negotiated between wholesalers and the Pharmacy and Medicines Department, and the retail price is then set; the markups of private wholesalers are estimated in the range of 13 to 30 percent for brand-name drugs and 19 to 34 percent for generic drugs. Retail markups are not directly regulated but are based on the difference between the wholesale and retail prices; the retail markup in the private retail market is estimated to be in the range of 25 percent for brand-name drugs and 28 to 45 percent for generic drugs. One study found an average price reduction of about 25 percent on a sample of essential medicines between 2006 and 2009.

Health Care Facilities

As of 2010, according to WHO, Mali had 5.68 health centers per 100,000, 0.38 district or rural hospitals per 100,000, 0.05 provincial hospitals per 100,000, and 0.03 specialized hospitals per 100,000. In 2008, Mali had 0.57 hospital beds per 1,000 population, one of the 20 lowest rates in the world.

Major Health Issues

In 2008, WHO estimated that 85 percent of years of life lost in Mali were due to communicable diseases, 11 percent to noncommunicable diseases, and 4 percent to injuries. In 2008, the age-standardized estimate of cancer deaths was 106 per 100,000 for men and 124 per 100,000 for women; for cardiovascular disease and diabetes, 419 per 100,000 for men and 393 per 100,000 for women; and for chronic respiratory disease, 117 per 100,000 for men and 55 per 100,000 for women.

In 2010, tuberculosis incidence was 68.0 per 100,000 population, tuberculosis prevalence 101.0 per 100,000, and deaths due to tuberculosis among HIV-negative people 9.70 per 100,000. As of 2009, an estimated 1.0 percent of adults age 15 to 49 were living with HIV or acquired immune deficiency syndrome (AIDS). In 2008, the age-standardized death rate from malaria was 85.2 per 100,000 population. Mali's maternal mortality rate (death from any cause related to or aggravated by pregnancy) is the 10th-highest in the world, estimated at 830 per 100,000 live births as of 2008. A 2006 survey estimated the prevalence of female genital mutilation at 12.9 percent. The infant mortality rate, defined as the number of deaths of infants younger than 1 year, was the third-highest in the world, at 109.08 per 1,000 live births in 2012. In 2006, 27.9 percent of children under age 5 were underweight (defined as 2 kilograms [kg] below standard weight-for-age at age 1, 3 kg below for ages 2 to 3, and 4 kg below for ages 4 to 5).

Health Care Personnel

In 2006, WHO identified Mali as one of 57 countries with a critical deficit in the supply of skilled health workers. Mali has one medical school, the Ecole Nationale de Medecine, de Pharmacie et d'Odontostomatologie du Mali in Bamako, which began offering instruction in 1969. The basic course of training lasts seven years. Mali has an agreement with other French-speaking African countries. In 2008, Mali had 1.60 physicians per 1,000 population, 0.02 pharmaceutical personnel per 1,000, 0.08 community and traditional health workers per 1,000, 0.14 health management and support workers per 1,000, 0.01 laboratory health workers per 1,000, and 0.30 nurses and midwives per 1,000. Michael Clemens and Bunilla Petterson estimate that 23 percent of Mali-born physicians and 15 percent of Mali-born nurses are working in one of nine developed countries, primarily in France.

Government Role in Health Care

According to WHO, in 2010, Mali spent $487 million on health care, an amount that comes to $32 per capita. The majority (73 percent) of health care funding came from domestic sources, with 27 percent coming from abroad. About half (47 percent) of health care funding was paid for through government expenditures, with the remainder provided through household expenditures (53 percent). In 2010, Mali allocated 11 percent of its total government expenditures to health, and government expenditures on health came to 2 percent of GDP; both figures are in the median range for low-income African countries. In 2009, according to WHO, official development assistance (ODA) for health in Mali came to $9.87 per capita.

Public Health Programs

According to WHO, in 2008, Mali had 0.01 environmental and public health workers per 1,000 population. In 2010, 22 percent of the population had access to improved sanitation facilities (14 percent in rural areas and 35 percent in urban), and 64 percent had access to improved sources of drinking water (51 percent in rural areas and 87 percent in urban). According to the World Higher Education Database (WHED), no university in Mali offers programs in epidemiology or public health.

MALTA

Malta is an island nation in the Mediterranean consisting of three large, inhabited islands and a number of smaller, uninhabited islands. The area of 122 square miles (316 square kilometers) makes Malta about twice the size of Washington, D.C., and the July 2012 population was estimated at 2409,836. In 2010, 95 percent of the population lived in urban areas, and the 2010 to 2015 annual rate of urbanization was estimated at 0.5 percent. Valletta is the capital and largest city (with a 2009 population estimated at 199,000). The population growth rate in 2012 was 0.4 percent, the net migration rate 2 migrants per 1,000 population (the 39th-highest in the world), the birth rate 10.3 births per 1,000, and the total fertility rate 1.5 children per woman.

Great Britain acquired Malta in 1814 with the Treaty of Paris; in 1964, Malta became independent. Malta has become an important transshipment point, financial center, and tourist destination since the 1980s. Malta ranked tied for 39th among 183 countries on the *Corruption Perceptions Index 2011,* with a score of 5.6 (on a scale where 0 indicates highly corrupt and 10 very clean).

In 2011, Malta was classified as a country with very high human development (the highest of four categories) on the United Nations Development Programme's (UNDP's) Human Development Index (HDI), with a score of 0.832 (on a scale where 1 denotes high development and 0 low development). Life expectancy at birth in 2012 was estimated at 79.85 years, and per capita gross domestic product (GDP) in 2011 was estimated at $25,700. Income distribution is among the most equal in the world: In 2007, the Gini Index (a measure of dispersion, in which perfect equality is denoted by 0 and maximum inequality is denoted by 100) for family income was 26.0. According to the World Economic Forum's *Global Gender Gap Index 2011,* Malta ranked 83rd out of 135 countries on gender equality, with a score of 0.666 (on a scale with a theoretical range of 1 for equality to 0 for inequality and an actual range in 2011 from 0.8530 to 0.4873).

Emergency Health Services

Malta's laws provide free access to hospitals, and emergency care is provided for all persons, including the uninsured. Funding for both inpatient and outpatient care in the emergency system is provided entirely by the state budget. Malta has two national telephone numbers for medical emergencies, 112 (the European Union, or EU, standard) and 196; the country has one dispatch center. Doctors Without Borders (Médecins Sans Frontières, or MSF) began working in Malta in 1981 and had nine staff members in the country at the close of 2008. In August 2008, MSF began providing medical care and psychological assistance to migrants and refugees held in detention centers in Malta; work was suspended in 2009, and poor conditions compromised the quality of medical care until MSF resumed services in June 2009. From 2008 to 2010, MSF provided health and hygiene education to almost 3,000 detainees, as well as over 4,670 medical and 724 psychological consultations. MSF also advocated for cultural mediation services to assist in providing care to the detained. By the second half of 2010, the detainee situation in Malta was no longer an emergency, and MSF shifted its attention toward creating a network to provide mental health care in the long term.

Insurance

Malta has a universal system for medical benefits (covering all resident citizens of Malta) and a social insurance system for cash sickness and maternity benefits (covering the employed and self-employed). Medical and maternity benefits are funded by general government tax revenues, while the cash benefits system is funded by contributions from wages, self-employed persons' incomes, employer payroll contributions, and general tax revenues. Medical services are provided free at public hospital services and clinics. A copayment is required for medicine and medical devices provided during outpatient care, but people with chronic diseases are exempt from the copayment for medicine. Dependents receive the same coverage as insured persons. The maternity benefit is 73.38 euros for 14 weeks. The sickness benefit is 17.88 euros per day for married people and 11.57 euros for others for up to 156 days per year; the covered period may be as long as 312 days per year for serious illness, major surgery, or severe injury. The Ministry for Health, the Elderly, and Community Care manages in-kind and medical benefits, the Ministry for the Family and Social Solidarity supervises cash benefits, and the Director General of Social Security manages the program. Malta also has a private insurance market, which developed as more private hospitals and clinics opened in the country, and tends to cover services like elective surgery and overseas treatment; as of 1999, it was unknown how many people held private insurance.

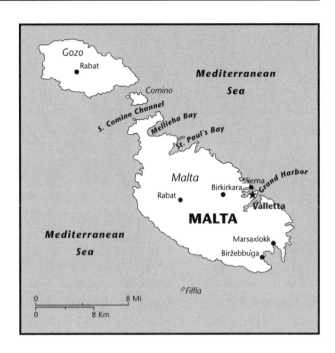

Costs of Hospitalization

As of 1999, treatment in state hospitals was provided without copayment.

Access to Health Care

According to the World Health Organization (WHO), in 2008, 99 percent of births in Malta were attended by skilled personnel (for example, physicians, nurses, or midwives). The 2010 immunization rates for 1-year-olds were 76 percent for diphtheria and pertussis (DPT3), 73 percent for measles (MCV), and 76 percent for Hib (Hib3). According to WHO, in 2010, Malta had 9.82 magnetic resonance imaging (MRI) machines per 1 million population, 9.82 computer tomography (CT) machines per 1 million, 2.45 positron emission tomography (PET) machines per 1 million, 2.45 telecolbalt units per 1 million, and 2.45 radiotherapy machines per 1 million. As of 1999, implicit rationing was a problem due to lengthy waiting lists for some types of surgery.

Cost of Drugs

As of 1999, pharmaceuticals on Malta's approved formulary were provided free to pink card holders (those with low income) and people belonging to special population groups, including some public employees, persons injured on government duty, and members of religious orders. Drugs for specific chronic conditions are also provided; the conditions covered include malignant diseases, some cardiovascular diseases, asthma and chronic respiratory failure, arthritis, lupus, schizophrenia, hemophilia, and glaucoma. Diabetics are also entitled to free treatment.

Health Care Facilities

As of 2010, according to WHO, Malta had 2.16 health posts per 100,000 population, 1.92 health centers per 100,000, 0.48 district or rural hospitals per 100,000, 0.24 provincial hospitals per 100,000, and 0.24 specialized hospitals per 100,000. In 2009, Malta had 4.88 hospital beds per 1,000 population, among the 50 highest rates in the world.

Major Health Issues

In 2008, WHO estimated that 5 percent of years of life lost in Malta were due to communicable diseases, 86 percent to noncommunicable diseases, and 9 percent to injuries. In 2008, the age-standardized estimate of cancer deaths was 137 per 100,000 for men and 92 per 100,000 for women; for cardiovascular disease and diabetes, 202 per 100,000 for men and 148 per 100,000 for women; for chronic respiratory disease, 32 per 100,000 for men and nine per 100,000 for women. In 2007, an estimated 20.7 percent of adults in Malta were obese (defined as a body mass index, or BMI, of 30 or greater).

The maternal mortality rate (death from any cause related to or aggravated by pregnancy) in Malta in 2008 was eight maternal deaths per 100,000 live births, among the lowest in the world. The infant mortality rate, defined as the number of deaths of infants younger than 1 year, was 3.65 per 1,000 live births as of 2012. In 2010, tuberculosis incidence was 12.0 per 100,000 population, tuberculosis prevalence 15.0 per 100,000, and deaths due to tuberculosis among human immunodeficiency virus (HIV)-negative people 0.70 per 100,000. As of 2009, an estimated 0.1 percent of adults age 15 to 49 were living with HIV or acquired immune deficiency syndrome (AIDS).

Health Care Personnel

Malta has one medical school, the Medical School of the University of Malta in Guardamangia. The basic degree course lasts five years, and two years of government service is obligatory after graduation. The degree awarded is Dottorat fil-Medicina u l-Kirugija (doctor of medicine and surgery). The license to practice medicine is granted by the president of Malta to graduates of a recognized medical school who have completed a two-year rotating internship in a teaching hospital. Graduates of foreign medical schools must pass a statutory examination, and foreigners can receive only temporary licenses and also need work permits to practice in Malta. Malta has agreements with Ireland and the United Kingdom.

Malta, as a member of the EU, cooperates with other countries in recognizing physicians qualified to practice in other EU countries, as specified by Directive 2005/36/EC of the European Parliament. This allows qualified professionals to practice their profession in other EU states on a temporary basis and requires that the host country automatically recognize qualifications for certain professions, including physicians, nurses, dentists, midwives, and pharmacists, if certain conditions have been met (for instance, facility in the language of the host country may be required). In 2009, Malta had 3.07 physicians per 1,000 population, 0.56 pharmaceutical personnel per 1,000, 0.44 dentistry personnel per 1,000, and 6.63 nurses and midwives per 1,000.

Government Role in Health Care

According to WHO, in 2010, Malta spent $706 million on health care, an amount that comes to $1,697 per capita. All health care funding came from domestic sources. Almost two-thirds (65 percent) of health care spending was paid for through government expenditures, with the remainder provided through household expenditures (32 percent) and other sources (2 percent). In 2010, Malta allocated 13 percent of its total government expenditures to health, and government expenditures on health came to 6 percent of GDP; both figures are in the low range for high-income European countries.

Public Health Programs

In 2010, access to improved sanitary facilities and improved sources of drinking water was essentially universal. According to the World Higher Education Database (WHED), one university in Malta offers programs in epidemiology or public health: the University of Malta, located in Msida.

MARSHALL ISLANDS

The Marshall Islands is an island nation in the north Pacific Ocean, consisting of two chains of 29 atolls plus five single islands. The area of 70 square miles (181 square kilometers) makes the Marshall Islands similar in size to Washington, D.C., and the July 2012 population was estimated at 68,480. In 2010, 72 percent of the population lived in urban areas, and the 2010 to 2015 annual rate of urbanization was estimated at 2.3 percent. Majuro is the capital and largest city (with a 2009 population estimated at 30,000). The population growth rate in 2012 was 1.9 percent, the net migration rate negative 5.1 migrants per 1,000 population, the birth rate 28.1 births per 1,000, and the total fertility rate 3.4 children per woman.

The Marshall Islands were administered by the United States after World War II until becoming independent in 1986. The country was the scene of heavy fighting during World War II and was used as a nuclear testing site by the United States from 1946 to 1958; parts of the islands remained heavily contaminated, and the United States has paid compensation to the inhabitants of some of the islands for exposure to nuclear contamination. The islands are extremely low lying (the highest point is 32.8 feet [10 meters] above sea level) and thus vulnerable to any rise in the sea level. Life expectancy at birth in 2012 was estimated at

72.03 years, estimated gross domestic product (GDP) per capita in 2011 was $2,500, and unemployment in 2008 was estimated at 36.0 percent, among the highest rates in the world.

Emergency Health Services

According to the World Health Organization (WHO), as of 2007, the Marshall Islands had a formal and publicly available emergency care (prehospital care) system accessible through a national universal access telephone number.

Insurance

The Marshall Islands have a social insurance program for medical benefits; no cash maternity or sickness benefits are paid. Medical services are delivered through a public hospital in Ebeye and a public hospital and private clinic in Majuro. Most employed and self-employed people are covered in the system, but some casual workers are excluded.

The system is funded by contributions from wages (3.5 percent), self-employed income (10 percent of 75 percent of gross income), and employers (3.5 percent of payroll or 10 percent of twice the salary of the highest-paid employee for small businesses); there is a cap on earnings used to calculate the contribution

($5,000 per quarter). The Social Security Health Fund is administered by the Ministry of Health Services, and the Social Security Administration collects contributions.

Costs of Hospitalization

No data available.

Access to Health Care

According to WHO, in 2007, 94.1 percent of births in Marshall Islands were attended by skilled personnel (for example, physicians, nurses, or midwives), and 77 percent of pregnant women received at least four prenatal care visits. The 2010 immunization rates for 1-year-olds were 94 percent for diphtheria and pertussis (DPT3), 97 percent for measles (MCV), and 92 percent for Hib (Hib3).

Cost of Drugs

No data available.

Health Care Facilities

The Marshall Islands has two hospitals in Majoru and Ebeye (both urban areas) and 60 health centers on the outer islands. As of 2010, according to WHO, the Marshall Islands had 1.85 health posts per 100,000 population, 96.23 health centers per 100,000, and 3.70 provincial hospitals per 100,000.

Major Health Issues

In 2008, WHO estimated that 27 percent of years of life lost in the Marshall Islands were due to communicable diseases, 64 percent to noncommunicable diseases, and 9 percent to injuries. In 2008, the age-standardized estimate of cancer deaths was 101 per 100,000 for men and 129 per 100,000 for women; for cardiovascular disease and diabetes, 819 per 100,000 for men and 831 per 100,000 for women; and for chronic respiratory disease, 135 per 100,000 for men and 107 per 100,000 for women.

In 2008, the age-standardized death rate from malaria was 0.9 per 100,000 population. In 2010, tuberculosis incidence was 502.0 per 100,000 population, tuberculosis prevalence 831.0 per 100,000, and deaths due to tuberculosis among human immunodeficiency virus (HIV)-negative people 81.00 per 100,000. As of 2009, an estimated 0.1 percent of adults age 15 to 49 were living with HIV or acquired immune deficiency syndrome (AIDS). The infant mortality rate, defined as the number of deaths of infants younger than 1 year, was estimated at 22.93 per 1,000 live births as of 2012.

Health Care Personnel

The Marshall Islands has no medical school. The license to practice medicine is granted by the Marshall Islands Medical Licensing Board, which requires that applicants have graduated from a recognized medical school, have a current license to practice in another country, and have no criminal record. In 2009, the Marshall Islands had 2.70 hospital beds per 1,000 population. In 2008, the Marshall Islands had 0.56 physicians per 1,000, 0.03 pharmaceutical personnel per 1,000, 0.10 dentistry personnel per 1,000, and 2.53 nurses and midwives per 1,000.

Government Role in Health Care

According to WHO, in 2010, the Marshall Islands spent $28 million on health care, an amount that comes to $520 per capita. Health care funding was evenly split between domestic (50 percent) and overseas (50 percent) sources. Most (83 percent) of health care funding was paid for through government expenditures, with the remainder provided through household expenditures (13 percent) and other sources (4 percent). In 2010, the Marshall Islands allocated 17 percent of its total government expenditures to health, and government expenditures on health came to 15 percent of GDP; both figures are in the high range for lower-middle-income western Pacific region countries.

Public Health Programs

According to WHO, in 2008, the Marshall Islands had 0.15 environmental and public health workers per 1,000 population. In 2010, 75 percent of the population had access to improved sanitation facilities (53 percent in rural areas and 83 percent in urban), and 94 percent had access to improved sources of drinking water (99 percent in rural areas and 92 percent in urban).

MAURITANIA

Mauritania is a country in north Africa, sharing borders with Algeria, Mali, Senegal, and Western Sahara and having a coastline on the north Atlantic. The area of 397,955 square miles (1,030,700 square kilometers)

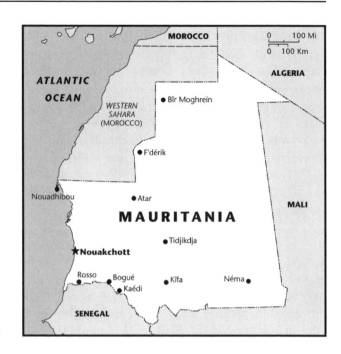

makes Mauritania the 29th-largest country in the world; the July 2012 population was estimated at 3.4 million, mostly clustered along the Senegal River and in the cities of Nouakchott and Nouadhibou. Nouakchott is the capital and largest city (with a 2009 population estimated at 709,000). In 2010, 41 percent of the population lived in urban areas, and the 2010 to 2015 annual rate of urbanization was estimated at 2.9 percent. The population growth rate in 2012 was 2.3 percent, the net migration rate negative 0.9 migrants per 1,000 population, the birth rate 32.8 births per 1,000, and the total fertility rate 4.2 children per woman. The United Nations High Commissioner for Refugees (UNHCR) estimated that, in 2010, there were 535 refugees and persons in refugee-like situations in Mauritania.

Mauritania, a former French colony, became independent in 1960. A coup in 1984 put Ould Sid Ahmed Taya in power; he was deposed in a bloodless coup in 2005, and Mauritania briefly was ruled by an elected president until another coup in 2008. The country suffers from ethnic tensions between the black African and Moorish segments of its population. According to the Ibrahim Index, in 2011, Mauritania ranked 31st among 53 African countries in terms of governance performance, with a score of 47 (out of 100). According to the Ibrahim Index, in 2011, Mauritius ranked first among 53 African countries in terms of governance performance, with a score of 82 (out of

100). Mauritania ranked tied for 143rd among 183 countries on the *Corruption Perceptions Index 2011,* with a score of 2.4 (on a scale where 0 indicates highly corrupt and 10 very clean).

In 2011, Mauritania was classified as a country with low human development (the lowest of four categories) on the United Nations Development Programme's (UNDP's) Human Development Index (HDI), with a score of 0.453 (on a scale where 1 denotes high development and 0 low development). In December 2011, the World Food Programme estimated that 700,000 people in Mauritania were food insecure due primarily to a drought. Life expectancy at birth in 2012 was estimated at 69.53 years, and estimated gross domestic product (GDP) per capita in 2011 was $2,200. In 2000, the Gini Index (a measure of dispersion, in which perfect equality is denoted by 0 and maximum inequality is denoted by 100) for family income was 39.0. Unemployment in 2008 was estimated at 30 percent, among the highest rates in the world.

According to the World Economic Forum's *Global Gender Gap Index 2011*, Mauritania ranked 114th out of 135 countries on gender equality with a score of 0.616 (on a scale with a theoretical range of 1 for equality to 0 for inequality and an actual range in 2011 from 0.8530 to 0.4873).

Emergency Health Services
According to the World Health Organization (WHO), as of 2007, Mauritania did not have a formal and publicly available system for providing prehospital care (emergency care).

Insurance
Mauritania has social insurance providing only cash maternity and medical benefits. Employed people (as defined by the labor code) and their dependents are covered under the medical system; employed women are eligible for cash maternity benefits. The system is funded by employer contributions (2 percent of covered payroll; the maximum monthly earnings used to calculate contributions is MRO 70,000). Medical services for employees and their dependents are provided through the employer's medical service program; firms with fewer than 750 workers belong to an interemployer medical service program. The cash maternity benefit is 100 percent of earnings for up to 14 weeks. The Family Allowance system, funded from employer payroll contributions, provides a prenatal allowance and birth grant if the mother and child undergo required medical examinations and a family allowance for children up to age 14 (up to age 21 if the child is disabled, a student, or an apprentice). The social insurance program and Family Benefits program are administered by the National Social Security Fund, and both are supervised by the Ministry of Civil Service and State Modernization.

Costs of Hospitalization
No data available.

Access to Health Care
According to WHO, in 2007, 61 percent of births in Mauritania were attended by skilled personnel (for example, physicians, nurses, or midwives). In 2001, 16 percent of pregnant women received at least four prenatal care visits. The 2010 immunization rates for 1-year-olds were 64 percent for diphtheria and pertussis (DPT3), 67 percent for measles (MCV), and 64 percent for Hib (Hib3). According to WHO, in 2010, Mauritania had 0.93 magnetic resonance imaging (MRI) machines per 1 million population and 1.87 computer tomography (CT) machines per 1 million.

Cost of Drugs
No data available.

Health Care Facilities
As of 2010, according to WHO, Mauritania had 13.09 health posts per 100,000 population, 4.28 health centers per 100,000, 0.78 district or rural hospitals per 100,000, 0.17 provincial hospitals per 100,000, and 0.20 specialized hospitals per 100,000. In 2006, Mauritania had 0.40 hospital beds per 1,000 population, one of the 10 lowest rates in the world.

Major Health Issues
In 2008, WHO estimated that 72 percent of years of life lost in Mauritania were due to communicable diseases, 19 percent to noncommunicable diseases, and 9 percent to injuries. In 2008, the age-standardized estimate of cancer deaths was 103 per 100,000 for men and 100 per 100,000 for women; for cardiovascular disease and diabetes, 407 per 100,000 for men and 437 per 100,000 for women; and for chronic respiratory disease, 113 per 100,000 for men and 65 per 100,000 for women.

In 2008, the age-standardized death rate from malaria was 26.0 per 100,000 population. In 2010, tuberculosis incidence was 337.0 per 100,000 population, tuberculosis prevalence 670.0 per 100,000, and deaths due to tuberculosis among human immunodeficiency virus (HIV)-negative people 79.00 per 100,000. As of 2009, an estimated 0.7 percent of adults age 15 to 49 were living with HIV or acquired immune deficiency syndrome (AIDS).

Mauritania's maternal mortality rate (death from any cause related to or aggravated by pregnancy) is quite high by global standards, estimated at 550 maternal deaths per 100,000 live births as of 2008. A 2007 survey estimated the prevalence of female genital mutilation at 72.2 percent. The infant mortality rate, defined as the number of deaths of infants younger than 1 year, also has been high, at 58.93 per 1,000 live births in 2012. In 2008, 16.7 percent of children under age 5 were underweight (defined as 2 kilograms [kg] below standard weight-for-age at age 1, 3 kg below for ages 2 to 3, and 4 kg below for ages 4 to 5).

Health Care Personnel

In 2009, Mauritania had 0.13 physicians per 1,000 population, 0.04 pharmaceutical personnel per 1,000, 0.04 laboratory health workers per 1,000, 1.30 health management and support workers per 1,000, 0.03 dentistry personnel per 1,000, 0.28 community and traditional health workers per 1,000, and 0.67 nurses and midwives per 1,000. Michael Clemens and Bunilla Petterson estimate that 11 percent of Mauritania-born physicians and 7 percent of Mauritania-born nurses are working in one of nine developed countries, primarily in France.

Government Role in Health Care

According to WHO, in 2010, Mauritania spent $148 million on health care, an amount that comes to $43 per capita. Health care funding was provided primarily (90 percent) by domestic sources, with the remainder (10 percent) coming from abroad. Just over half (53 percent) of health care funding was paid for through government expenditures, with the remainder provided through household expenditures (44 percent) and other sources (3 percent). In 2010, Mauritania allocated 7 percent of its total government expenditures to health, and government expenditures on health came to 2 percent of GDP; both figures are in the median range for lower-middle-income African countries. In 2009, according to WHO, official development assistance (ODA) for health in Mauritania came to $5.45 per capita.

Public Health Programs

According to WHO, in 2009, Mauritania had 0.06 environmental and public health workers per 1,000 population. In 2010, 26 percent of the population had access to improved sanitation facilities (9 percent in rural areas and 51 percent in urban), and 50 percent had access to improved sources of drinking water (48 percent in rural areas and 52 percent in urban). According to the World Higher Education Database (WHED), one university in Mauritania offers programs in epidemiology or public health: the University of Nouakchott.

MAURITIUS

Mauritius is an island nation in the Pacific Ocean, west of Madagascar. The area of 788 square miles (2,040 square kilometers) makes Mauritius about seven times the size of Washington, D.C., and the July 2012 population was estimated at 1.3 million. In 2010, 42 percent of the population lived in urban areas, and the 2010 to 2015 annual rate of urbanization is estimated at 0.8 percent. Port Louis is the capital and largest city (with a 2009 population estimated at 149,000). The population growth rate in 2012 was 0.7 percent, the net migration rate 0.0 migrants per 1,000 population, the birth rate 13.8 births per 1,000, and the total fertility rate 1.8 children per woman.

Mauritius was settled by the Dutch in the 17th century; France assumed control in 1715, and the United Kingdom in 1810, and the country became independent in 1968. It has enjoyed stable democratic rule since independence, attracted foreign investment, and has one of the highest per capita gross domestic products (GDPs) in Africa. Mauritius ranked tied for 46th among 183 countries on the *Corruption Perceptions Index 2011,* with a score of 5.1 (on a scale where 0 indicates highly corrupt and 10 very clean). In 2011, Mauritius was classified as a country with high human development (the second-highest category) on the United Nations Development Programme's (UNDP's) Human Development Index (HDI), with a score of 0.728 (on a scale where 1 denotes high development and 0 low development). Life expectancy at birth in 2012 was estimated at 74.71 years, and per capita GDP in 2011 was estimated at $15,000. In 2006, the Gini Index (a measure of dispersion, in which perfect equality is denoted

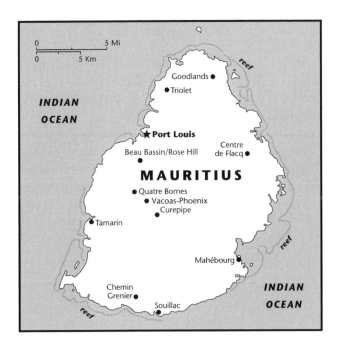

health care, but as of 2003, only about 6 percent of the population had private insurance. According to Ke Xu and colleagues, in 2003, 1.3 percent of households in Mauritius experienced catastrophic health expenditures annually; "catastrophic" was defined as exceeding 40 percent of household income remaining after basic needs were met.

Costs of Hospitalization
Care is provided at no cost to the patient in government hospitals.

Access to Health Care
According to WHO, in 2010, 99.5 percent of births in Mauritius were attended by skilled personnel (for example, physicians, nurses, or midwives). The 2010 immunization rates for 1-year-olds were 99 percent for diphtheria and pertussis (DPT3), 99 percent for measles (MCV), and 99 percent for Hib (Hib3). In 2010, an estimated 16 percent of persons with advanced human immunodeficiency virus (HIV) infection were receiving antiretroviral therapy in accordance with the 2010 WHO guidelines. According to WHO, in 2010, Mauritius had 4.69 magnetic resonance imaging (MRI) machines per 1 million population, 6.25 computer tomography (CT) machines per 1 million, 1.56 telecolbalt units per 1 million, and 1.56 radiotherapy machines per 1 million.

Cost of Drugs
Mauritius has a formal process for approving drugs, and products must be approved before being marketed in the county; as of 2008, about 3,500 products were approved. Most prescriptions are written by the generic names of the drugs, although this is not required by law; there are no incentives to promote the use of generics in pharmacies because most drugs are distributed through the private sector, which does not handle originator brands. Drugs are procured at the national level and distributed through the public sector under the auspices of the Ministry of Health. In 2007, Mauritius spent about $12 million for pharmaceuticals. The government sets the prices for drugs sold in the private sector (in the public sector, drugs are provided free to patients), but there is no national monitoring of drug prices in pharmacies.

A 2008 survey found that only generic drugs were available in the public sector in Mauritius, with a mean availability of 68.6 percent; in the private sector, generic and originator brands had approximately

by 0 and maximum inequality is denoted by 100) for family income was estimated at 39.0. According to the World Economic Forum's *Global Gender Gap Index 2011*, Mauritius ranked 95th out of 135 countries on gender equality, with a score of 0.653 (on a scale with a theoretical range of 1 for equality to 0 for inequality and an actual range in 2011 from 0.8530 to 0.4873).

Emergency Health Services
According to the World Health Organization (WHO), as of 2007, Mauritius had a formal and publicly available emergency care (prehospital care) system accessible through a national universal access telephone number.

Insurance
Mauritius does not have a public insurance plan; instead, free medical services are provided in government hospitals and clinics. The Family Benefits system, funded by general government revenues, provides a compassionate allowance (up to MUR 639 annually) for people with serious illnesses (this requires a physician's certification). Paid sick leave is provided by employers, as required in the 2008 Employment Rights Act, for 15 days annually if the employee has been on the job for at least a year. The same law requires 12 weeks of paid maternity leave or five days of paid paternity leave for employees who have been on the job for at least one year. Mauritius also has a small private sector providing

equal availability (54.9 percent for generics and 55.7 percent for originator brands). There was no general difference in availability across regions of the country, but there was a wide variability between facilities, however, and some common medicines were not available in any of the facilities. Public procurement prices were generally low, with a median price ratio of 0.66, meaning that the median price was 34 percent lower than the international reference price. In the private sector, prices were much higher: The median price ratio for the lowest-priced generics was 5.93 (meaning that the cost was almost six times above the international reference price) and 19.28 for originator brands. Besides the fact that drugs are provided in the private sector for free, the lowest-cost generics to treat common conditions such as diabetes and asthma were available in the private sector at a cost lower than the price of one day's wages for the lowest-paid government worker.

Health Care Facilities

Health care in Mauritius is based on the provision of free service in the public sector. Primary health care, including family planning, maternal and child care, and treatment of common injuries and illnesses, is provided through community health centers, area health centers, and medical clinics; dental care is also provided at area health centers. Secondary care is provided through regional and district hospitals; and tertiary care is provided through hospitals providing specialist care for mental illness, eye disease, chest disease, heart disease, and ear, nose, and throat (ENT) disease. Mauritius also has a private sector providing health care, including (as of 2008) more than 500 physicians and 13 clinics. As of 2010, according to WHO, Mauritius had 8.47 health posts per 100,000 population, 10.15 health centers per 100,000, 0.15 district or rural hospitals per 100,000, 0.38 provincial hospitals per 100,000, and 0.38 specialized hospitals per 100,000. In 2008, Mauritius had 3.33 hospital beds per 1,000 population.

Major Health Issues

In 2008, WHO estimated that 12 percent of years of life lost in Mauritius were due to communicable diseases, 76 percent to noncommunicable diseases, and 12 percent to injuries. In 2008, the age-standardized estimate of cancer deaths was 103 per 100,000 for men and 75 per 100,000 for women; for cardiovascular disease and diabetes, 545 per 100,000 for men and 345 per 100,000 for women; and for chronic respiratory disease, 54 per 100,000 for men and 26 per 100,000 for women.

Mauritius's maternal mortality rate (death from any cause related to or aggravated by pregnancy) in 2008 was 36 maternal deaths per 100,000 live births. The infant mortality rate, defined as the number of deaths of infants younger than 1 year, was 11.20 per 1,000 live births as of 2012. In 2010, tuberculosis incidence was 22.0 per 100,000 population, tuberculosis prevalence 39.0 per 100,000, and deaths due to tuberculosis among HIV-negative people 0.97 per 100,000. As of 2009, an estimated 1.0 percent of adults age 15 to 49 were living with HIV or acquired immune deficiency syndrome (AIDS).

Health Care Personnel

Mauritius has two medical schools: the Department of Medicine of the University of Mauritius in Réduit, which began offering instruction in 1998, and Sir Seewoosagar Ramgoolam Medical College (SSRMC, affiliated with the University of Mauritius), which began offering instruction in 2000. The SSRMC was established with the aid of the Indian Ocean Medical Institute Trust and serves students from the other countries on the Indian Ocean rim as well as Mauritius. One course of study lasts three years, resulting in a bachelor of science in medicine; a one-year master's program is also available. Another course lasts five years, resulting in the bachelor of medicine or bachelor of surgery degree.

In 2004, Mauritius had 1.06 physicians per 1,000 population, 1.16 pharmaceutical personnel per 1,000, 0.26 laboratory health workers per 1,000, 1.64 health management and support workers per 1,000, 0.19 dentistry personnel per 1,000, 0.19 community and traditional health workers per 1,000, and 3.73 nurses and midwives per 1,000. Michael Clemens and Bunilla Petterson estimate that 46 percent of Mauritius-born physicians and 63 percent of Mauritius-born nurses are working in one of nine developed countries, primarily in France and the United Kingdom (physicians) and the United Kingdom (nurses).

Government Role in Health Care

According to WHO, in 2010, Mauritius spent $583 million on health care, an amount that comes to $449 per capita. Health care funding was provided primarily (98 percent) through domestic sources, with 2 percent coming from abroad. Just over half (52 percent) of health care spending was paid for through household expenditures, with the remainder provided through government expenditures (42 percent) and other sources (7 percent). In 2010, Mauritius allocated 10 percent of its total government expenditures to health, in the low range for upper-middle-income African countries; government expenditures on health came to 3 percent of GDP, in the low range for upper-middle-income African countries. In 2009, according to WHO, official development assistance (ODA) for health in Mauritius came to $1.64 per capita.

Public Health Programs

According to WHO, in 2004, Mauritius had 0.19 environmental and public health workers per 1,000 population. In 2010, 89 percent of the population had access to improved sanitation facilities (88 percent in rural areas and 91 percent in urban), and 99 percent had access to improved sources of drinking water (99 percent in rural areas and 100 percent in urban). According to the World Higher Education Database (WHED), one university in Mauritius offers programs in epidemiology or public health: the University of Mauritius, located in Moka.

MEXICO

Mexico is a North American country, sharing borders with the United States, Guatemala, and Belize and having coastlines on the Gulf of Mexico and the north Pacific Ocean. The area of 758,449 square miles (1,964,375 square kilometers) makes Mexico the 14th-largest country in the world (about three times the size of Texas), and the July 2012 population was estimated at 115.0 million (the 11th-largest in the world). In 2010, 78 percent of the population lived in urban areas, and the 2010 to 2015 annual rate of urbanization is estimated at 1.2 percent. Mexico City is the capital and largest city (with a 2009 population estimated at 19.3 million, the second-largest metropolitan area in the Western Hemisphere). The population growth rate in 2012 was 1.1 percent, the net migration rate negative 3.1 migrants per 1,000 population, the birth rate 18.9 births per 1,000, and the total fertility rate 2.3 children per woman. The United Nations High Commissioner for Refugees (UNHCR) estimated that, in 2010, there were 200 refugees and persons in refugee-like situations in Mexico.

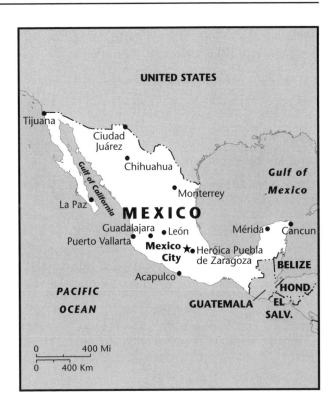

Mexico was ruled by Spain for three centuries before becoming independent in 1821. Mexico ranked tied for 100th among 183 countries on the *Corruption Perceptions Index 2011,* with a score of 3.0 (on a scale where 0 indicates highly corrupt and 10 very clean). In 2011, Mexico was classified as a country with high human development (the second-highest category) on the United Nations Development Programme's (UNDP's) Human Development Index (HDI), with a score of 0.768 (on a scale where 1 denotes high development and 0 low development). Life expectancy at birth in 2012 was estimated at 76.66 years, and the per capita gross domestic product (GDP) in 2011 was estimated at $15,100.

Income distribution in Mexico is relatively unequal: In 2008, the Gini Index (a measure of dispersion, in which perfect equality is denoted by 0 and maximum inequality is denoted by 100) for family income was 51.7, among the 20 highest in the world.

According to the World Economic Forum's *Global Gender Gap Index 2011*, Mexico ranked 89th out of 135 countries on gender equality, with a score of 0.660 (on a scale with a theoretical range of 1 for equality to 0 for inequality and an actual range in 2011 from 0.8530 to 0.4873).

Selected Health Indicators: Mexico Compared With the Organisation for Economic Co-operation and Development (OECD) Country Average

	Mexico	OECD average (2010 or nearest year)
Male life expectancy at birth, 2010	73.2	77
Female life expectancy at birth, 2011	77.9	82.5
Total expenditure on pharmaceuticals and other medical non-durables* (percent total expenditure on health), 2009	27.1	16.6
Total expenditure on pharmaceuticals and other medical non-durables* (per capita, USD purchasing power parity), 2009	249.9	495.4
Doctor consultations (number per capita), 2010	2.9	6.4
Practicing physicians (per 1,000 population), 2010	2.0	3.1
Hospital beds (per 1,000 population), 2010	1.6	4.9
Average length of hospital stay, all causes (days), 2010	3.9	7.1

Source: OECD Health Data 2012 (Organisation for Economic Co-operation and Development, 2012).
*Estimated.

Emergency Health Services

According to the World Health Organization (WHO), as of 2007, Mexico had a formal and publicly available emergency care (prehospital care) system, accessible through regional access numbers, but not a national universal access telephone number.

Insurance

Mexico has a social insurance system covering private-sector employees and members of cooperatives and a social assistance program (the Oportunidades program) for the poor and those without access to social security services (for example, those living in rural areas or marginalized urban areas). The social insurance program, which provides medical benefits and cash sickness and maternity benefits, is funded by contributions from wages, the self-employed, employers, and the government; the Oportunidades program is entirely funded by the government. Medical benefits are provided through the facilities (including hospitals, clinics, and pharmacies) of the Social Security Institute; if a needed service is not available at a Social Security Institute facility, it is reimbursed. Medical benefits provided include hospitalization, convalescent care, surgery, medical care, maternity care, dental care, lab services, and medicines. The Mexican Social Security Institute administers the program.

According to Donald West and colleagues, Mexico has a wide variety of types of insurance, from small private plans to a large social security plan. About 25 percent of Mexicans have public insurance; about 3 million middle- and upper-class Mexicans (2 to 3 percent of the population) have private health insurance. About 40 percent of the population (those working for salaries) belong to the Mexican Institute of Social Security (IMSS), a system funded through employer, employee, and government contributions; about 7 percent of the population is covered through the Institute of Security and Social Services for Civil Servants (ISSSTE), which has its own system of hospitals and clinics. PEMEX, the national petroleum company, has its own hospitals and clinics, and the military has a separate insurance system as well. About 45 million people are insured by the Seguro Popular (PHI) program, which began in 2004 and is being gradually phased in; PHI charges premiums based on family income, with no fee charged to about 20 percent of those in the program. Eventually, PHI will cover basic hospitalization, primary care, and outpatient care.

According to Ke Xu and colleagues, in 2003, 1.5 percent of households in Mexico experienced catastrophic health expenditures annually; "catastrophic" was defined as exceeding 40 percent of household income remaining after basic needs were met.

Costs of Hospitalization

According to Donald West and colleagues, the Mexican system of providing care consists of many separate systems, and thus, the sources of funding for hospitals and other care vary. Those with private insurance (about 3 percent of the population) have access to high-quality private hospitals; the private sector is growing rapidly and includes more than 3,000 facilities, mostly small hospitals. Salaried employees belong to the IMSS, which has its own hospitals and clinics (215 general hospitals, 41 specialty hospitals, and 1,077 primary care clinics); the quality of facilities varies considerably, particularly between urban and rural areas. Civil servants belong to a separate insurance plan (ISSSTE), which has its own network of 95 hospitals, and more than 1,000 health clinics. The national petroleum company, PEMEX, also has its own insurance system and its own system of more than 700 hospitals and clinics. Those not insured by any other system are covered (or will be covered, as the system is still being put into place) by PHI; these patients receive services primarily through hospitals and clinics managed at the state level.

Access to Health Care

According to Donald West and colleagues, from 2010 to 2011, Mexico had 1,107 public hospitals (78,643 beds), 19,103 public health facilities, and 3,082 private hospitals (33,931 beds). IMSS, which covers salaried workers (about 40 percent of the population) has 215 general hospitals, 41 specialty hospitals, and 1,077 primary care clinics. Access to care varies widely according to an individual's circumstances, and the quality of care provided also varies among regions and hospitals. According to Latinobarometer, an annual public opinion survey conducted in Latin America, 57 percent of citizens in Mexico are satisfied with the level of health care available to them (the regional average is 51.9 percent).

According to WHO, in 2007, 93.7 percent of births in Mexico were attended by skilled personnel (for example, physicians, nurses, or midwives). In 2006, 88 percent of pregnant women received at least four prenatal care visits. The 2010 immunization rates for 1-year-olds were 95 percent for diphtheria and pertussis (DPT3), 95 percent for measles (MCV), and 95 percent for Hib (Hib3). In 2010, an estimated 78 percent of persons with advanced human immunodeficiency virus (HIV) infection were receiving antiretroviral therapy in accordance with the 2010 WHO guidelines. According to WHO, in 2010, Mexico had 01.59 magnetic resonance imaging (MRI) machines per 1 million population, 4.12 computer tomography (CT) machines per 1 million, 0.13 positron emission tomography (PET) machines per 1 million, 0.41 telecolbalt units per 1 million, and 0.41 radiotherapy machines per 1 million.

Cost of Drugs

According to Ibis Sanchez-Serrano, in 2009, the pharmaceutical market in Mexico was valued at $13.2 billion, and was projected to reach $17.0 billion by 2014. One reason for the anticipated growth was the government's plan, by 2012, to expand the public health care system to cover 85 percent of the population. According to Douglas Ball, as of 2011, Mexico does not charge the value-added tax (VAT) for medicines (the standard VAT is 15 percent). There is no regulated dispensing fee, and the wholesale and pharmacy markup for medicines is not fixed. Real annual growth in pharmaceutical expenditures in Mexico grew 8.0 percent from 1997 to 2005, much faster than the 4.4 percent growth of total health expenditure (minus pharmaceutical expenditures) over those years. According to Elizabeth Docteur, in 2004, generic drugs represented 15 percent of the market share by value and 20 percent of the market share by volume of the total pharmaceutical market.

Health Care Facilities

In 2007, Mexico had more than 4,000 hospitals, of which just over one-quarter were part of the public health system. In 2004, there were more than 19,695 health units in the country, most of which provided only outpatient care, and of which about 80 percent were public. As of 2010, according to WHO, Mexico had 110.08 health posts per 100,000 population, 3.73 provincial hospitals per 100,000, and 0.06 specialized hospitals per 100,000. In 2008, Mexico had 1.60 hospital beds per 1,000 population.

Major Health Issues

In 2008, WHO estimated that 19 percent of years of life lost in Mexico were due to communicable diseases,

61 percent to noncommunicable diseases, and 20 percent to injuries. In 2008, the age-standardized estimate of cancer deaths was 87 per 100,000 for men and 75 per 100,000 for women; for cardiovascular disease and diabetes, 258 per 100,000 for men and 217 per 100,000 for women; and for chronic respiratory disease, 44 per 100,000 for men and 27 per 100,000 for women. In 2000, an estimated 23.6 percent of adults in Mexico were obese (defined as a body mass index, or BMI, of 30 or greater).

Mexico's maternal mortality rate (death from any cause related to or aggravated by pregnancy) was estimated in 2008 as 85 maternal deaths per 100,000 live births. The infant mortality rate, defined as the number of deaths of infants younger than 1 year, was estimated at 16.77 per 1,000 live births as of 2012. In 2010, tuberculosis incidence was 16.0 per 100,000 population, tuberculosis prevalence 18.0 per 100,000, and deaths due to tuberculosis among HIV-negative people 0.84 per 100,000. As of 2009, an estimated 0.3 percent of adults age 15 to 49 were living with HIV or acquired immune deficiency syndrome (AIDS).

Health Care Personnel

Mexico has more than 50 medical schools. The course of training lasts four to seven years with an additional year of supervised practice required before the degree, Médico Cirjano (physician and surgeon), is granted. The license to practice medicine is granted by the Secretaria de Educación Publica and is regulated by Article 5 of the Constitution. In 2004, Mexico had 2.89 physicians per 1,000 population, 0.76 pharmaceutical personnel per 1,000, 0.46 laboratory health workers per 1,000, 4.17 health management and support workers per 1,000, 1.42 dentistry personnel per 1,000, and 3.98 nurses and midwives per 1,000.

Government Role in Health Care

According to WHO, in 2010, Mexico spent $65 billion on health care, an amount that comes to $604 per capita. Health care funding was provided entirely through domestic sources. Just under half (49 percent) of health care spending was paid for through household expenditures, with the remainder provided through government expenditures (47 percent) and other sources (4 percent). In 2010, Mexico allocated 12 percent of its total government expenditures to health, in the median range for upper-middle-income countries in the Americas region; government expenditures on health came to 3 percent of GDP, in the

low range for upper-middle-income countries in the Americas region. In 2009, according to WHO, official development assistance (ODA) for health in Mexico came to $0.08 per capita.

Public Health Programs

The National Institute of Public Health (INSP) for Mexico is located in Cuernavaca and is headed by Mauricio Hernandez Avila. The INSP has more than 800 employees and is one of the largest public health institutions in the developing world; its departments include the Center for Infectious Disease Research, the Center for Health Systems Research, the Center for Population Health Research, the Center for Nutrition and Health Research, the Center for Assessment and Surveys Research, the Regional Center for Public Health, and the Research Center for Information on Public Health Decisions. The INSP has played a key role in Mexico's expansion of its health system in the last 10 years and also plays a key role in national policies regarding behavioral health, including obesity and tobacco use. The INSP offers a distance education program to help develop Mexico's public health workforce and conducts the National Nutrition and Health Survey. According to the World Higher Education Database (WHED), nine universities in Mexico offer programs in epidemiology or public health.

In 2010, 85 percent of the population of Mexico had access to improved sanitation facilities (79 percent in rural areas and 87 percent in urban), and 96 percent had access to improved sources of drinking water (91 percent in rural areas and 96 percent in urban areas).

MICRONESIA

Micronesia is an island nation in the north Pacific Ocean, made up of about 600 islands. The area of 271 square miles (702 square kilometers) makes Micronesia about four times the size of Washington, D.C.; and the July 2012 population was estimated at 106,487. In 2010, 23 percent of the population lived in urban areas, and the 2010 to 2015 annual rate of urbanization was estimated at 1.3 percent. Palikir is the capital and largest city (with a 2009 population estimated at 7,000). The population growth rate in 2012 was negative 0.3 percent, the net migration rate negative 21.0 residents per 1,000 population (the third-highest emigration rate in the world), the birth rate 23 births per 1,000, and the total fertility rate 1.3 children per woman.

Micronesia was a United Nations (UN) Trust Territory under U.S. administration before becoming independent in 1986. In 2011, Micronesia was classified as a country with medium human development (the second from the lowest of four categories) on the United Nations Development Programme's (UNDP's) Human Development Index (HDI), with a score of 0.636 (on a scale where 1 denotes high development and 0 low development). Life expectancy at birth in 2012 was estimated at 71.80 years, and the estimated gross domestic product (GDP) per capita in 2011 was $2,200. The country suffers from high unemployment, overfishing, and dependence on U.S. aid and is vulnerable to tropical storms and changes in sea level.

Emergency Health Services
According to the World Health Organization (WHO), as of 2007, Micronesia did not have a formal and publicly available system for providing prehospital care (emergency care).

Insurance
Public health services are highly subsidized in Micronesia, although the specific details vary because each state government operates autonomously. As of 2011, most health facilities in the country were public (107 out of 122); private facilities included one hospital, six health clinics, six pharmacies, and two dental clinics.

Costs of Hospitalization
No data available.

Access to Health Care
According to WHO, in 2005, 92 percent of births in Micronesia were attended by skilled personnel (for example, physicians, nurses, or midwives). The 2010 immunization rates for 1-year-olds were 85 percent for diphtheria and pertussis (DPT3), 80 percent for measles (MCV), and 70 percent for Hib (Hib3). According to WHO, in 2010, Micronesia had fewer than 0.01 magnetic resonance imaging (MRI) machines per 1 million population and fewer than 0.01 computer tomography (CT) machines per 1 million.

Cost of Drugs
No data available.

Health Care Facilities
Each state in Micronesia is autonomous in terms of organizing care, but there are some constants. Each state has a hospital providing primary and secondary services, and dispensaries providing primary and referral services are located in outlying islands and municipalities. As of February 2011, the country had five hospitals, five community health centers, and 92 dispensaries. As of 2010, according to WHO, Micronesia had 22.75 health posts per 100,000 population and 0.93 district or rural hospitals per 100,000. In 2009, Micronesia had 3.32 hospital beds per 1,000 population.

Major Health Issues
In 2008, WHO estimated that 41 percent of years of life lost in Micronesia were due to communicable diseases, 49 percent to noncommunicable diseases, and 10 percent to injuries. In 2008, the age-standardized estimate of cancer deaths was 79 per 100,000 for men and 90 per 100,000 for women; for cardiovascular disease and diabetes, 459 per 100,000 for men and 363 per 100,000 for women; and for chronic respiratory disease, 80 per 100,000 for men and 51 per 100,000 for women.

In 2008, the age-standardized death rate from malaria was 0.2 per 100,000 population. The infant

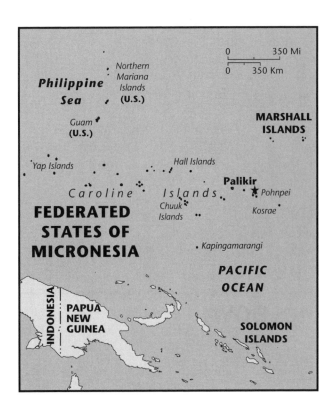

mortality rate, defined as the number of deaths of infants younger than 1 year, was estimated at 23.51 per 1,000 live births as of 2012. No information was available about maternal mortality. In 2010, tuberculosis incidence was 206.0 per 100,000 population, tuberculosis prevalence 320.0 per 100,000, and deaths due to tuberculosis among human immunodeficiency virus (HIV)-negative people 29.00 per 100,000.

Health Care Personnel

The School of Medicine of Pacific Basin University operated temporarily in Pohnpei, Micronesia, but was removed from the WHO World Directory of Medical Schools in 2003 at the request of the government of the Federated States of Micronesia. In 2005, Micronesia had 0.56 physicians per 1,000 population, 0.12 dentistry personnel per 1,000, and 2.26 nurses and midwives per 1,000.

Government Role in Health Care

According to WHO, in 2010, Micronesia spent $583 million on health care, an amount that comes to $449 per capita. More than two-thirds (69 percent) of health care funding was provided from abroad, with 31 percent coming from domestic sources. Almost all (91 percent) of health care spending was paid for through government expenditures, with the remainder provided through household expenditures (9 percent). In 2010, Micronesia allocated 20 percent of its total government expenditures to health, and government expenditures on health came to 13 percent of GDP; both figures are in the high range for lower-middle-income countries in the western Pacific region.

Public Health Programs

According to WHO, in 2008, Micronesia had 0.35 environmental and public health workers per 1,000 population. In 2010, 15 percent of the population had access to improved sanitation facilities (15 percent in rural areas and 61 percent in urban), and 94 percent had access to improved sources of drinking water (94 percent in rural areas and 95 percent in urban).

MOLDOVA

Moldova is a landlocked country in eastern Europe, sharing borders with Ukraine and Romania. The area of

13,070 square miles (33,851 square kilometers) makes Moldova similar in size to Maryland, and the July 2012 population was estimated at 3.7 million. In 2010, 47 percent of the population lived in urban areas, and the 2010 to 2015 annual rate of urbanization was estimated at 0.9 percent. Chisinau is the capital and largest city (with a 2009 population estimated at 650,000). The population growth rate in 2012 was negative 1.0 percent, the net migration rate negative 10.0 migrants per 1,000 population (the 11th-highest emigration rate in the world), the birth rate 12.5 births per 1,000, and the total fertility rate 1.6 children per woman. The United Nations High Commissioner for Refugees (UNHCR) estimated that, in 2010, there were 148 refugees and persons in refugee-like situations in Moldova.

Moldova was incorporated into the Soviet Union after World War II and became independent in 1991; however, Russian forces remain in Moldova, supporting a separatist region east of the Dniester River, where the population is primarily Russian and Ukrainian. Moldova ranked tied for 112th among 183 countries on the *Corruption Perceptions Index 2011*, with a score of 2.9 (on a scale where 0 indicates highly corrupt and 10 very clean). In 2011, Moldova was classified as a country with medium human development (the second from the lowest of four categories) on the United Nations Development Programme's (UNDP's) Human Development Index (HDI), with a score of 0.649 (on a scale

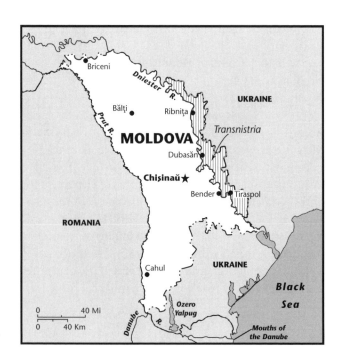

where 1 denotes high development and 0 low development). Life expectancy at birth in 2012 was estimated at 69.51 years, and estimated gross domestic product (GDP) per capita in 2011 was $3,400, making it one of the poorest nations in Europe. In 2008, the Gini Index (a measure of dispersion, in which perfect equality is denoted by 0 and maximum inequality is denoted by 100) for family income was 38. According to the World Economic Forum's *Global Gender Gap Index 2011*, Moldova ranked 39th out of 135 countries on gender equality, with a score of 0.708 (on a scale with a theoretical range of 1 for equality to 0 for inequality and an actual range in 2011 from 0.8530 to 0.4873).

Emergency Health Services

According to the World Health Organization (WHO), as of 2007, Moldova had a formal and publicly available emergency care (prehospital care) system accessible through a national access number.

Insurance

Moldova has a social insurance system, instituted in 2004, providing medical benefits to all residents of Moldova and cash maternity and sickness benefits to broad categories of the employed, self-employed, and unemployed. The medical benefits system is funded out of general government revenues; the cash benefits system is funded through contributions from wages, earnings of the self-employed, and employers and is part of the system that funds pensions. Medical care is provided by the state, with a small copayment by the person receiving services. Hospital care is free up to a specified number of days. The maternity benefit is 100 percent of average earnings, paid for 126 days, with an additional 14 days provided for complications or multiple births. The sickness benefit is 60 to 100 percent of average earnings, depending on the years of employment; medical leave is provided, following the same schedule, for care of a sick child. The National Agency of Health Insurance and local health departments administer medical services under the supervision of the Ministry of Health. As of 2009, according to a WHO report, more than one-quarter (27.6 percent) of the population of Moldova did not have adequate access to health care; the uninsured are mostly rural agricultural workers who must pay out of pocket for care.

Costs of Hospitalization

No data available.

Access to Health Care

According to WHO, in 2005, 100 percent of births in Moldova were attended by skilled personnel (for example, physicians, nurses, or midwives), and 89 percent of pregnant women received at least four prenatal care visits. The 2010 immunization rates for 1-year-olds were 90 percent for diphtheria and pertussis (DPT3), 97 percent for measles (MCV), and 63 percent for Hib (Hib3). In 2010, an estimated 25 percent of persons with advanced human immunodeficiency virus (HIV) infection were receiving antiretroviral therapy in accordance with the 2010 WHO guidelines. According to WHO, in 2010, Moldova had 2.01 magnetic resonance imaging (MRI) machines per 1 million population, 5.52 computer tomography (CT) machines per 1 million, 0.28 telecolbalt units per 1 million, and 0.28 radiotherapy machines per 1 million.

Cost of Drugs

In Moldova, some drugs are provided free through the public health system to children under the age of 5 (25 generic drugs) and pregnant women (three generic drugs). Drugs to treat tuberculosis and human immunodeficiency virus and acquired immune deficiency syndrome (HIV/AIDS) are also provided for free, as are vaccines on WHO's Expanded Programme on Immunization (EPI) list. Both the public health service and private insurance provide at least partial coverage for drugs on the Essential Medicines List (EML). The markup for drugs is controlled by law and limited to 15 percent for wholesalers and 25 percent for retailers; however, Moldova does not actively monitor retail prices.

Health Care Facilities

As of 2010, according to WHO, Moldova had 31.32 health posts per 100,000 population, 0.95 district or rural hospitals per 100,000, 0.59 provincial hospitals per 100,000, and 0.50 specialized hospitals per 100,000. In 2007, Moldova had 6.12 hospital beds per 1,000 population, among the 30 highest ratios in the world.

Major Health Issues

In 2008, WHO estimated that 10 percent of years of life lost in Moldova were due to communicable diseases, 74 percent to noncommunicable diseases, and 16 percent to injuries. In 2008, the age-standardized estimate of cancer deaths was 171 per 100,000 for men and 98 per 100,000 for women; for cardiovascular disease and diabetes, 614 per 100,000 for men and 445 per 100,000 for women; and for chronic respiratory disease, 55 per 100,000 for men and 19 per 100,000 for women.

Compared to other countries at a similar level of development, Moldova ranked close to last (40th out of 43 countries) on the 2011 Mothers' Index, produced by the international nongovernmental organization (NGO) Save the Children, based on a number of health and social factors relating to women, children, and maternal and child care. Moldova's maternal mortality rate (death from any cause related to or aggravated by pregnancy) in 2008 was 32 maternal deaths per 100,000 live births. The infant mortality rate, defined as the number of deaths of infants younger than 1 year, was 13.65 per 1,000 live births as of 2012 data.

In 2010, tuberculosis incidence was 182.0 per 100,000 population, tuberculosis prevalence 277.0 per 100,000, and deaths due to tuberculosis among HIV-negative people 23.00 per 100,000. An estimated 19 percent of new tuberculosis cases and 65 percent of retreatment cases are multidrug resistant. As of 2009, an estimated 0.4 percent of adults age 15 to 49 were living with HIV or AIDS.

Health Care Personnel

As of February 2003, Moldova had two medical schools: the State Medical and Pharmaceutical University "Nicolae Testemitanu" of the Republic of Moldova and the Free International University of Moldova. The basic medical training course lasts six years, and the degree awarded is doctor of medicine. In 2007, Moldova had 2.67 physicians per 1,000 personnel, 0.72 pharmaceutical personnel per 1,000, 0.37 dentistry personnel per 1,000, and 6.65 nurses and midwives per 1,000.

Government Role in Health Care

The right to health, including the right to access to essential medicines and medical technologies, is recognized in national legislation. Moldova has a National Health Policy (NHP), updated in 2007, with an implementation plan written in 2008, and a National Medicines Policy (NMP), updated in 2002, with an implementation plan updated in 2007. The Medicines Agency of the Ministry of Health regularly monitors the implementation of pharmaceutical policies. The NMP covers the selection of medicines for the Essential Medicines List (EML); the financing, pricing, procurement, distribution, and regulation of medicines; pharmacovigilance; the rational use of medicines; human resource development; research; and traditional medicines. The promotion and advertising of prescription medicines is

regulated by the Ministry of Health, and direct advertising to the general public is prohibited.

According to WHO, in 2010, Moldova spent $679 million on health care, an amount that comes to $190 per capita. Most (90 percent) of health care funding came from domestic sources, with 10 percent coming from domestic sources. About half (46 percent) of health care spending was paid for through government expenditures, with the remainder provided through household expenditures (45 percent) and other sources (9 percent). In 2010, Moldova allocated 13 percent of its total government expenditures to health, and government expenditures on health came to 5 percent of GDP; both figures are in the high range for lower-middle-income countries in the European region. In 2009, according to WHO, official development assistance (ODA) for health in Moldova came to $12.59 per capita.

Public Health Programs

The National Center of Public Health (NPHC) for Moldova is located in Chisinau and headed by Ion Bahnarel. The focus of the NPHC is on public health surveillance, capacity building, policy development, and preventive medicine and sanitation. The NPHC has a staff of 320 and is engaged in activities including delivery of vaccinations, monitoring nuclear safety, and creating national programs for health promotions and disease prevention and control. The NPHC played a major role in disease prevention following the floods in Moldova in 2010. In 2010, 85 percent of the population of Moldova had access to improved sanitation facilities (82 percent in rural areas and 89 percent in urban), and 96 percent had access to improved sources of drinking water (93 percent in rural areas and 99 percent in urban). According to the World Higher Education Database (WHED), three universities in Moldova offer programs in epidemiology or public health: Alecu Russo Balti State University in Balti, Nicolae Testemitanu Moldova State University of Medicine and Pharmacy in Chisinau, and the Free International University of Moldova in Chisinau.

MONACO

Monaco is a western European country sharing a border with France and having a coastline on the

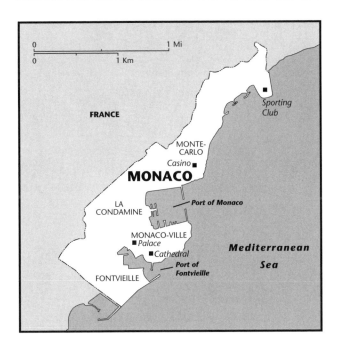

Mediterranean Sea. The area of 0.8 square miles (2 square kilometers) makes Monaco the smallest country in the world; the July 2012 population was estimated at 30,510, and as of 2010, it was 100 percent urban. The population growth rate in 2012 was negative 0.1 percent, the net migration rate 1.0 migrants per 1,000 population, the birth rate 6.9 births per 1,000 (the lowest in the world), and the total fertility rate 1.5 children per woman.

The current ruling family of Monaco, the Grimaldis, assumed power in the 13th century. Monaco is a prosperous country thanks to tourism, aided by the mild climate and the presence of casinos, as well as its status as a tax haven with low business taxes and no income tax. Life expectancy at birth in 2012 was estimated at 89.68 years, the highest in the world, and the infant mortality rate in 2012 was 1.8 deaths per 1,000 live births (the lowest in the world).

Emergency Health Services
The Princess Grace Hospital in Monte Carlo has a 24-hour emergency department. Emergency care is provided without consideration of insurance status.

Insurance
Monaco has a social insurance system for most employed persons; hospital personnel, civil servants, and the self-employed are covered under separate systems. The system is funded through employer contributions (15.2 percent of covered payroll); the same system also finances family, disability, and some social benefits. The medical benefit covers 80 percent of the cost of medical care, up to a ceiling, with 100 percent coverage for pregnancy and some illnesses. Physicians and providers of auxiliary services charge sliding rates based on family size and income. Covered medical services include hospitalization, primary and specialist care, medicines, lab services, transportation, and prostheses. The maternity benefit is 90 percent of average earnings for up to eight weeks before and after the due date (for the first and second child) and eight weeks before and 18 weeks after for the third child and all subsequent children; longer periods are allowed for multiple births. The paternity benefit is 90 percent of average earnings, up to 123.84 euros for up to 12 days, with longer leave for multiple births and large families. The cash sickness benefit is 50 percent of average earnings, up to 123.84 euros for up to 360 days, and may be extended for chronic illness. The program is administered by the Social Services Compensation Fund.

Costs of Hospitalization
No data available.

Access to Health Care
According to the World Health Organization (WHO), the 2010 immunization rates for 1-year-olds were 99 percent for diphtheria and pertussis (DPT3), 99 percent for measles (MCV), and 99 percent for Hib (Hib3). According to WHO, in 2010, Monaco had 152.84 magnetic resonance imaging (MRI) machines per 1 million population, 152.84 computer tomography (CT) machines per 1 million, and 30.57 positron emission tomography (PET) machines per 1 million.

Cost of Drugs
No data available.

Health Care Facilities
Monaco has three hospitals, all in Monte Carlo: the Princess Grace Hospital, the Cardio-Thoracic Center, and the Haemodialysis Center. As of 2010, according to WHO, Monaco had 11.30 provincial hospitals per 100,000.

Major Health Issues
In 2008, WHO estimated that 5 percent of years of life lost in Monaco were due to communicable diseases, 78 percent to noncommunicable diseases, and 16 percent

to injuries. In 2008, the age-standardized estimate of cancer deaths was 166 per 100,000 for men and 78 per 100,000 for women; for cardiovascular disease and diabetes, 139 per 100,000 for men and 76 per 100,000 for women; and for chronic respiratory disease, 21 per 100,000 for men and 10 per 100,000 for women. The infant mortality rate in Monaco was 1.80 per 1,000 live births as of 2012, the lowest in the world.

Health Care Personnel

In 1995, Monaco had 5.81 physicians per 1,000 population, 1.06 dentistry personnel per 1,000, and 14.50 nurses and midwives per 1,000.

Government Role in Health Care

According to WHO, in 2010, Monaco spent $224 million on health care, an amount that comes to $6,236 per capita. Health care funding came entirely from domestic sources. Almost all (88 percent) of health care spending was paid for through government expenditures, with the remainder provided through household expenditures (7 percent) and other sources (5 percent). In 2010, Monaco allocated 19 percent of its total government expenditures to health, in the high range for high-income European countries; government expenditures on health came to 4 percent of gross domestic product (GDP), in the low range for high-income European countries.

Public Health Programs

In 2010, access to improved sanitary facilities and improved sources of drinking water were essentially universal in Monaco.

MONGOLIA

Mongolia is a landlocked northern Asian country sharing borders with China and Russia. The area of 603,909 square miles (1,564,116 square kilometers) makes Mongolia similar in size to Alaska, and the July 2012 population was estimated at 2.6 million. In 2010, 62 percent of the population lived in urban areas, and the 2010 to 2015 annual rate of urbanization was estimated at 1.9 percent. Ulan Bator is the capital and largest city (with a 2009 population estimated at 3.2 million). The population growth rate in 2012 was 1.5 percent, the net migration rate 0.0 migrants per 1,000 population, the

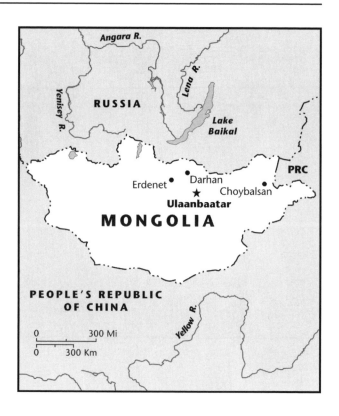

birth rate 20.7 births per 1,000, and the total fertility rate 2.2 children per woman. The United Nations High Commissioner for Refugees (UNHCR) estimated that, in 2010, there were 12 refugees and persons in refugee-like situations in Mongolia.

Mongolia came under Chinese rule in the 17th century and became independent in 1921. Mongolia ranked tied for 120th among 183 countries on the *Corruption Perceptions Index 2011,* with a score of 2.7 (on a scale where 0 indicates highly corrupt and 10 very clean). In 2011, Mongolia was classified as a country with medium human development (the second from the lowest of four categories) on the United Nations Development Programme's (UNDP's) Human Development Index (HDI), with a score of 0.653 (on a scale where 1 denotes high development and 0 low development). Life expectancy at birth in 2012 was estimated at 68.63 years, and estimated gross domestic product (GDP) per capita in 2011 was $4,500. In 2008, the Gini Index (a measure of dispersion, in which perfect equality is denoted by 0 and maximum inequality is denoted by 100) for family income was 36.5.

According to the World Economic Forum's *Global Gender Gap Index 2011,* Mongolia ranked 36th out of 135 countries on gender equality, with a score of 0.714 (on a scale with a theoretical range of 1 for equality to 0 for inequality and an actual range in 2011 from 0.8530 to 0.4873).

Emergency Health Services

According to the World Health Organization (WHO), as of 2007, Mongolia had a formal and publicly available emergency care (prehospital care) system accessible through a national universal access telephone number and regional access numbers.

Insurance

Mongolia implemented a social health insurance program in the mid-1990s, with the goal of universal coverage. The current system is governed by the Citizens Health Insurance Law, which took effect in 2003. Some medical care is also provided free by the government. The health insurance program is part of a broad social insurance program managed by the Ministry of Social Welfare and Labor and covers employees, business owners, children up to age 16 (up to age 18 if enrolled in school), students, pensioners with no other income, mothers with children less than 2 years old (less than 3 years if twins), those serving in the military, prisoners, herdsmen, and various other categories of citizens. The system is funded by employee contributions (the percentage is determined annually but capped at 6 percent) and employer contributions (half of the employee percentage capped at 3 percent), and contributions from other sources (for example, students and herdsmen pay a flat monthly fee; the government pays a flat fee for some covered individuals).

The insurance program covers hospital treatment, outpatient treatment, and half the cost of prescribed drugs from the national Essential Medicines List (EML). Hospitals are paid a set amount to provide care based on the type of hospital but not the number or complexity of cases; a previous system paying a rate per patient-day led to increased use of hospital resources (and thus increased costs) but not discernible improvements in care. Patients are required to make copayments, depending on the level of the hospital (primary, secondary, tertiary). General practice physicians are paid through capitation payments based on the number of insured people registered with them.

According to WHO, although the program is theoretically compulsory and universal, about 78 percent of Mongolia's population was covered by the national health insurance program as of 2005. Mongolia also has additional insurance programs: private insurance and the Revolving Drug Fund (RDF). The RDF was created in 1994 in cooperation with United Nations Children's Fund (UNICEF) in order to increase the supply of essential drugs in rural areas. Currently the RDF, which is independent of the national insurance system, purchases drugs and resells them to hospitals and outpatient consumers; it is financed by community contributions and donor funds. Private insurance plays a small role in Mongolia, with only a few companies in the field; they range from comprehensive programs to those that cover benefits not provided by the national insurance program, including treatment abroad.

Costs of Hospitalization

No data available.

Access to Health Care

According to WHO, in 2007, 100 percent of births in Mongolia were attended by skilled personnel (for example, physicians, nurses, or midwives). The 2010 immunization rates for 1-year-olds were 96 percent for diphtheria and pertussis (DPT3), 97 percent for measles (MCV), and 96 percent for Hib (Hib3). In 2010, an estimated 26 percent of persons with advanced human immunodeficiency virus (HIV) infection were receiving antiretroviral therapy in accordance with the 2010 WHO guidelines.

Cost of Drugs

A 2004 survey found that Mongolia imports most (85 percent) of the drugs used in the country from a state-owned supply company and a number of smaller drug supply companies in the private sector. In 2004, Mongolia spent MNT 78.6 million on pharmaceuticals. Some drugs are provided free in hospitals (for 15 diseases, including cancer, some psychiatric conditions, and dialysis), and 127 medicines are reimbursed through the health insurance fund. Revolving drug funds were established in about three-quarters of Mongolia's *soums* (districts) in 2004, with the remaining soums expected to have revolving drug funds by 2005; the purpose of these funds is to supply medicines to local areas. Prescription drugs are partially subsidized by the national insurance system.

All public pharmacies are supplied by a national system, reducing variation in the medicines available. In the public system, the median availability of medicines on the EML was 72.7 percent. The lowest-priced generics had a median price ratio of 2.6, meaning that they cost on average more than two and a half times as much as the international reference price; there was wide variation among the drugs surveyed, from cephalexin (median price ratio of 0.79) to mebendazole (median price ratio of 55.06). Availability was also good in the private sector: For any generic medicine to treat a condition, the availability was 80 percent, and for the most-sold generic equivalent, 42 percent. Prices were higher on average in the private sector, with a median price ratio for lowest-priced generics of 4.17, with a range from 0.75 (reserpine) to 120.13 (fluconazole). Only one innovator brand was found: ceftriaxone, with a median price ratio of 6.4.

Affordability of drugs required to treat common conditions varied according to the particular disease and the sector within which the drug was purchased; for instance, a month's worth of atenolol to treat hypertension cost on average just over half a day's wages (for the lowest-paid government worker) in the public sector and just over 1 day's wages if purchased in the private sector. A course of treatment with amitriptyline (for depression) cost about 2 days' wages if purchased in the private sector and over 2.5 days' wages if purchased in the private sector. Amoxicillin (to treat pneumonia) costs half a day's wages in the public sector but over 3 days' wages if purchased in the private sector.

Health Care Facilities
As of 2010, according to WHO, Mongolia had 42.27 health posts per 100,000 population, 16.84 health centers per 100,000, 1.27 district or rural hospitals per 100,000, and 1.31 provincial hospitals per 100,000. In 2008, Mongolia had 5.89 hospital beds per 1,000 population, among the 30 highest ratios in the world.

Major Health Issues
In 2008, WHO estimated that 26 percent of years of life lost in Mongolia were due to communicable diseases, 53 percent to noncommunicable diseases, and 21 percent to injuries. In 2008, the age-standardized estimate of cancer deaths was 260 per 100,000 for men and 166 per 100,000 for women; for cardiovascular disease and diabetes, 456 per 100,000 for men and 304 per 100,000 for women; and for chronic respiratory disease, 34 per 100,000 for men and 23 per 100,000 for women.

Mongolia's maternal mortality rate (death from any cause related to or aggravated by pregnancy) was estimated in 2008 as 65 maternal deaths per 100,000 live births. The infant mortality rate, defined as the number of deaths of infants younger than 1 year, was estimated at 36.00 per 1,000 live births in 2012.

In 2010, tuberculosis incidence was 224.0 per 100,000 population, tuberculosis prevalence 331.0 per 100,000, and deaths due to tuberculosis among HIV-negative people 35.00 per 100,000.

Health Care Personnel
Mongolia has four medical schools: Sainshand Medical College, the National Medical University of Mongolia, Darkhan-Uul Medical College, and Ulanbaatar Medical College. The course of training for the basic medical degree lasts five to six years. Government service is obligatory after graduation. The license to practice medicine is granted to graduates of a Mongolian medical school who pass a national exam. Physicians who received their training abroad are not allowed to practice. In 2008, Mongolia had 2.76 physicians per 1,000 population, 0.40 pharmaceutical personnel per 1,000, 0.19 dentistry personnel per 1,000, 0.02 community and traditional health workers per 1,000, and 3.50 nurses and midwives per 1,000.

Government Role in Health Care
According to WHO, in 2010, Mongolia spent $331 million on health care, an amount that comes to $120 per capita. Health care funding came primarily (96 percent) from domestic sources, with 4 percent coming from overseas sources. More than half (55 percent) of health care spending was paid for through government expenditures, with the remainder provided through household expenditures (41 percent) and other sources (4 percent). In 2010, Mongolia allocated 8 percent of its total government expenditures to health, and government expenditures on health came to 3 percent of GDP; both place Mongolia in the low range as compared to other lower-middle-income western Pacific region countries. In 2009, according to WHO, official development assistance (ODA) for health in Mongolia came to $7.37 per capita.

Public Health Programs
The Public Health Institute of the Ministry of Health is located in Ulaanbaatar and is headed (as of 2012) by Janchiv Oyunbileg. According to WHO, in 2002, Mongolia had 0.03 environmental and public health workers per 1,000 population. In 2010, 51 percent of the population had access to improved sanitation facilities (29 percent in rural areas and 64 percent in urban), and 82 percent had access to improved sources of drinking water (53 percent in rural areas and 100 percent in urban). According to the World Higher Education

Database (WHED), one university in Mongolia offers programs in epidemiology or public health: the Health Sciences University of Mongolia in Ulaanbaatar.

MONTENEGRO

Montenegro is a southern European country, sharing borders with Albania, Bosnia and Herzegovina, Croatia, and Serbia and having a coastline on the Adriatic Sea. The area of 5,333 square miles (13,812 square kilometers) makes Montenegro similar in size to Connecticut, and the July 2012 population was estimated at 657,394. In 2010, 61 percent of the population lived in urban areas, and the 2010 to 2015 annual rate of urbanization was estimated at 0.1 percent. Podgorica is the capital and largest city (with a 2009 population estimated at 144,000). The population growth rate in 2012 was negative 0.6 percent and the birth rate 10.9 births per 1,000 population. The United Nations High Commissioner for Refugees (UNHCR) estimated that, in 2010, there were 16,364 refugees and persons in refugee-like situations in Montenegro.

Montenegro was part of Yugoslavia, a country created after World War I; when Yugoslavia dissolved in 1992, Montenegro and Serbia formed the Federal Republic of Yugoslavia. In 2006, voters in Montenegro elected to become independent of Serbia, creating the independent country of Montenegro. Montenegro ranked tied for 66th among 183 countries on the *Corruption Perceptions Index 2011,* with a score of 4.0 (on a scale where 0 indicates highly corrupt and 10 very clean). In 2011, Montenegro was classified as a country with high human development (the second-highest category) on the United Nations Development Programme's (UNDP's) Human Development Index (HDI), with a score of 0.771 (on a scale where 1 denotes high development and 0 low development). Per capita gross domestic product (GDP) in 2011 was estimated at $11,200. Income distribution is among the most equal in the world: In 2010, the Gini Index (a measure of dispersion, in which perfect equality is denoted by 0 and maximum inequality is denoted by 100) for family income was 24.3.

Emergency Health Services

According to the World Health Organization (WHO), as of 2007, Montenegro had a formal and publicly available emergency care (prehospital care) system. Emergency care at general hospitals is free, but proof of insurance or payment is required once the patient is stabilized.

Insurance

Citizens in Montenegro are entitled to health care through a national health fund supported by employer and employee contributions; the program is guided by the Ministry of Health. Certain categories of people, including retired, unemployed, and those on maternity leave or long-term sickness benefit are exempt from making contributions, while the self-employed pay both the employer and employee contributions themselves. Most medical services are covered by the national insurance program, although not all physicians are part of the system; services from those outside the system must be paid out of pocket.

Costs of Hospitalization

No data available.

Access to Health Care

According to WHO, in 2005, 99 percent of births in Montenegro were attended by skilled personnel (for example, physicians, nurses, or midwives). The 2010 immunization rates for 1-year-olds were 94 percent for diphtheria and pertussis (DPT3), 90 percent

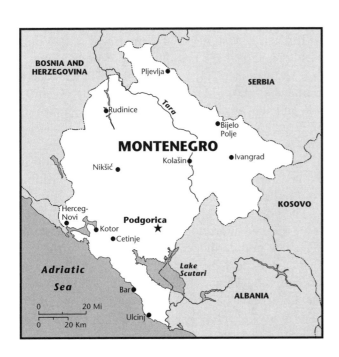

for measles (MCV), and 90 percent for Hib (Hib3). According to WHO, in 2010, Montenegro had 1.61 magnetic resonance imaging (MRI) machines per 1 million population and 9.64 computer tomography (CT) machines per 1 million.

Cost of Drugs

Drugs are sold in both public and private pharmacies throughout the country, and the cost of a drug depends in part on whether it was prescribed by a doctor (the same drug may be cheaper if prescribed than if purchased over the counter). Some costs of prescription drugs are reimbursed by the national insurance system.

Health Care Facilities

Montenegro has a system of 19 health care centers providing both primary care and specialized services, and 10 hospitals. There are also private practice physicians, and most dental care is private. As of 2010, according to WHO, Montenegro had 2.85 health posts per 100,000 population, 1.43 district or rural hospitals per 100,000, 0.48 provincial hospitals per 100,000, and 0.16 specialized hospitals per 100,000. In 2009, Montenegro had 3.98 hospital beds per 1,000 population.

Major Health Issues

In 2008, WHO estimated that 5 percent of years of life lost in Montenegro were due to communicable diseases, 86 percent to noncommunicable diseases, and 9 percent to injuries. In 2008, the age-standardized estimate of cancer deaths was 166 per 100,000 for men and 92 per 100,000 for women; for cardiovascular disease and diabetes, 461 per 100,000 for men and 379 per 100,000 for women; and for chronic respiratory disease, 36 per 100,000 for men and 25 per 100,000 for women. The maternal mortality rate (death from any cause related to or aggravated by pregnancy) in Montenegro in 2008 was 15 maternal deaths per 100,000 live births. In 2010, tuberculosis incidence was 19.0 per 100,000 population, tuberculosis prevalence 23.0 per 100,000, and deaths due to tuberculosis among human immunodeficiency virus (HIV)-negative people 1.40 per 100,000.

Health Care Personnel

In 2007, Montenegro had 1.99 physicians per 1,000 population, 0.17 pharmaceutical personnel per 1,000, 0.40 dentistry personnel per 1,000, and 5.54 nurses and midwives per 1,000.

Government Role in Health Care

According to WHO, in 2010, Montenegro spent $365 million on health care, an amount that comes to $578 per capita. Health care funding came entirely (100 percent) from domestic sources. Two-thirds (67 percent) of health care spending was paid for through government expenditures, with the remainder provided through household expenditures (30 percent) and other sources (3 percent).

In 2010, Montenegro allocated 14 percent of its total government expenditures to health, and government expenditures on health came to 6 percent of GDP; both place Montenegro in the high range as compared to other upper-middle-income European countries. In 2009, according to WHO, official development assistance (ODA) for health in Montenegro came to $5.41 per capita.

Public Health Programs

In 2010, 90 percent of the population of Montenegro had access to improved sanitation facilities (87 percent in rural areas and 92 percent in urban), and 98 percent had access to improved sources of drinking water (96 percent in rural areas and 99 percent in urban).

MOROCCO

Morocco is a north African country, sharing borders with Algeria, Western Sahara, and Spain (Ceuta and Melilla) and having a coastline on the Mediterranean Sea. The area of 172,414 square miles (446,550 square kilometers) makes Morocco a bit larger than California, and the July 2012 population was estimated at 32.3 million. In 2010, 58 percent of the population lived in urban areas, and the 2010 to 2015 annual rate of urbanization was estimated at 2.1 percent. Rabat is the capital and Casablanca the largest city (with a 2009 population estimated at 3.2 million).

The population growth rate in 2012 was 1.0 percent, the net migration rate negative 3.7 migrants per 1,000 population, the birth rate 19.0 births per 1,000, and the total fertility rate 2.2 children per woman. The United Nations High Commissioner for Refugees (UNHCR) estimated that, in 2010, there were 792 refugees and persons in refugee-like situations in Morocco.

Spain occupied parts of Morocco in the 19th century, and France imposed a protectorate in 1912; Morocco became independent in 1956 after a prolonged, armed struggle. According to the Ibrahim Index, in 2011, Morocco ranked 11th among 53 African countries in terms of governance performance, with a score of 58 (out of 100). Morocco ranked tied for 80th among 183 countries on the *Corruption Perceptions Index 2011*, with a score of 3.4 (on a scale where 0 indicates highly corrupt and 10 very clean).

In 2011, Morocco was classified as a country with medium human development (the second from the lowest of four categories) on the United Nations Development Programme's (UNDP's) Human Development Index (HDI), with a score of 0.582 (on a scale where 1 denotes high development and 0 low development). Life expectancy at birth in 2012 was estimated at 76.11 years, and estimated gross domestic product (GDP) per capita in 2011 was $5,100. In 2007, the Gini Index (a measure of dispersion, in which perfect equality is denoted by 0 and maximum inequality is denoted by 100) for family income was estimated as 40.9. According to the World Economic Forum's *Global Gender Gap Index 2011*, Morocco ranked 129th out of 135 countries on gender equality, with a score of 0.580 (on a scale with a theoretical range of 1 for equality to 0 for inequality and an actual range in 2011 from 0.8530 to 0.4873).

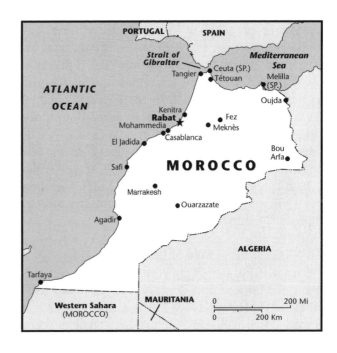

Emergency Health Services

According to the World Health Organization (WHO), as of 2007, Morocco had a formal and publicly available emergency care (prehospital care) system accessible through a national universal access telephone number and regional access numbers. Doctors Without Borders (Médecins Sans Frontières, or MSF) began working in Morocco in 1997 and had 28 staff members in the country at the close of 2010. In Rabat and Oujda, MSF provides health care services to migrants from sub-Saharan Africa and also helps them access the Moroccan health care system. MSF also provides care to victims of sexual violence and included information about their victimization in the report *Sexual Violence and Migration*.

Insurance

Morocco has a social insurance system for many classes of employed people, including salaried workers and apprentices in industry, commerce, forestry, agricultural cooperatives, craftsmen, some fishermen, and some self-employed people; civil servants are covered in a separate system. The system is funded by contributions from employees (2.33 percent of gross monthly earnings) and employers (4.17 percent of gross monthly payroll), with a floor and ceiling on wages used to calculate contributions. Basic medical care is provided through the system, including outpatient and specialist care, surgery, lab services, medicine, and some appliances. The cash maternity benefit is 100 percent of the average daily covered wage for up to 14 weeks; the sickness benefit is 66.7 percent of the average daily covered wage. The National Sickness Insurance Agency supervises the health care system, the National Social Security Fund administers the program, and the Ministry of Employment and Vocational Training supervises the program. According to Ke Xu and colleagues, in 2003, 0.2 percent of households in Morocco experienced catastrophic health expenditures annually; "catastrophic" was defined as exceeding 40 percent of household income remaining after basic needs were met.

Costs of Hospitalization

No data available.

Access to Health Care

According to WHO, in 2004, 62.6 percent of births in Morocco were attended by skilled personnel (for example, physicians, nurses, or midwives), and 31 percent of pregnant women received at least four prenatal care visits. The 2010 immunization rates for 1-year-olds were 99 percent for diphtheria and pertussis (DPT3), 99 percent for measles (MCV), and 98 percent for Hib (Hib3). In 2010, an estimated 30 percent of persons with advanced human immunodeficiency virus (HIV) infection were receiving antiretroviral therapy in accordance with the 2010 WHO guidelines. According to WHO, in 2010, Morocco had 0.38 magnetic resonance imaging (MRI) machines per 1 million population and 1.27 computer tomography (CT) machines per 1 million.

Cost of Drugs

Pharmaceutical prices are regulated by the government of Morocco, and drugs on the Essential Medicines List (EML; it included 270 medicines in 2008) are provided free of charge. Wholesale and retail markups are by law the same for generic and originator brand medications (10 percent for wholesale and 30 percent for retail), and the value-added tax (VAT) is added to the cost of some medicines. According to a study, the public procurement price for a basket of medicines showed that prices were substantially higher than the international reference prices; for the lowest-priced generics, the median price ratio was 2.83 (meaning these drugs in Morocco were purchased at almost three times the international reference price), and for originator brands, the median price ratio was 5.14. In private pharmacies, prices were even higher, although the differential between the lowest-priced generics and originator brands was much smaller: The median price ratio for the lowest-priced generics was 11.07 and, for originator brands, 12.15.

Availability was low in the private sector (only 15 of the 34 medicines surveyed were found in more than half the public facilities), but higher in the public sector, where median availability of generics was 52.5 percent and, of originator brands, 92.5 percent; the fact that drugs were more available in the private rather than the public sector and that originator brands were more available than the lowest-priced generics adds considerably to the cost Moroccans pay for essential medicines. None of the pharmacies surveyed stocked the antiretrovirals included in the study. Because medication is provided for free in the public sector, availability rather than affordability is the main issue in that sector. In the private sector, where medications are more available, affordability varied by condition: For instance, it would cost less

than 1 day's wages for the lowest-paid government worker to treat asthma or a pediatric infection but 2.6 to 4.1 days' wages to treat an ulcer for a month, depending on whether the generic or originator brand or ranitidine were purchased.

Health Care Facilities

In 2009, Morocco had 1.10 hospital beds per 1,000 population.

Major Health Issues

In 2008, WHO estimated that 39 percent of years of life lost in Morocco were due to communicable diseases, 51 percent to noncommunicable diseases, and 10 percent to injuries. In 2008, the age-standardized estimate of cancer deaths was 91 per 100,000 for men and 75 per 100,000 for women; for cardiovascular disease and diabetes, 392 per 100,000 for men and 319 per 100,000 for women; and for chronic respiratory disease, 46 per 100,000 for men and 30 per 100,000 for women.

Morocco's maternal mortality rate (death from any cause related to or aggravated by pregnancy) was estimated in 2008 as 110 maternal deaths per 100,000 live births. The infant mortality rate, defined as the number of deaths of infants younger than 1 year, was estimated at 26.49 per 1,000 live births in 2012.

In 2010, tuberculosis incidence was 91.0 per 100,000 population, tuberculosis prevalence 105.0 per 100,000, and deaths due to tuberculosis among HIV-negative people 6.20 per 100,000. As of 2009, an estimated 0.1 percent of adults age 15 to 49 were living with HIV or acquired immune deficiency syndrome (AIDS).

Health Care Personnel

In 2006, WHO identified Morocco as one of 57 countries with a critical deficit in the supply of skilled health workers. Morocco has two medical schools, the Faculte de Medecine et de Pharmacie de Casablanca and the Faculte de Medecine et de Pharmacie de Rabat. The basic course of training lasts seven years with a one-year internship required before award of the degree Docteur en Médecine (doctor of medicine). Physicians must register with the Conseil National de l'Ordre des Médecins, and the license to practice medicine is granted by the Secrétariat General du Gouvernement. Morocco has agreements with France and Spain. In 2009, Morocco had 0.62 physicians per 1,000 population, 0.27 pharmaceutical personnel per 1,000,

0.08 dentistry personnel per 1,000, and 0.89 nurses and midwives per 1,000. Michael Clemens and Bunilla Petterson estimate that 31 percent of Morocco-born physicians and 15 percent of Morocco-born nurses are working in one of nine developed countries, primarily in France.

Government Role in Health Care

According to WHO, in 2010, Morocco spent $4.7 billion on health care, an amount that comes to $148 per capita. Health care funding came entirely from domestic sources. More than half (54 percent) of health care spending was paid for through household expenditures, with the remainder provided through government expenditures (38 percent) and other sources (8 percent). In 2010, Morocco allocated 7 percent of its total government expenditures to health, in the median range for lower-middle-income eastern Mediterranean region countries; government expenditures on health came to 2 percent of GDP, in the high range as compared to other lower-middle-income eastern Mediterranean region countries. In 2009, according to WHO, official development assistance for health in Morocco came to $3.07 per capita.

Public Health Programs

The National Institute of Hygiene is located in Rabat and headed by Rajae El Aouad. The national institute has a staff of almost 200, organized into seven departments: immunology and virology, medical bacteriology, human genetics, toxicology and hydrology, food microbiology, parasitology, and pathology. Key activities include surveillance of chronic and infectious diseases, monitoring the quality of food and drugs, and accrediting and certifying medical practitioners. The national institute is currently undergoing a merger with the Pasteur Institute of Morocco (IPH), located in Casablanca and headed by Mekki Lalaoui, and the two will ultimately form the National Agency of Public Health. IPH has a staff of more than 250 and carries out research on infectious and parasitic disease, genetics, oncology, and immunology, as well as preparing and importing biological reagents, vaccines, and serums. Currently, the IPH is organized into five departments: clinical biology; water, food, and environmental safety; infectious diseases; immunizations; and genetic diseases.

According to WHO, in 2004, Morocco had 0.02 environmental and public health workers per 1,000 population. In 2010, 70 percent of the population had access to improved sanitation facilities (52 percent in rural areas and 83 percent in urban), and 83 percent had access to improved sources of drinking water (61 percent in rural areas and 98 percent in urban). According to the World Higher Education Database (WHED), two universities in Morocco offer programs in epidemiology or public health: the National Institute of Health Administration in Rabat and Hassan II University in Casablanca.

MOZAMBIQUE

Mozambique is a country on the southeastern coast of Africa, sharing borders with Malawi, South Africa, Swaziland, Tanzania, Zambia, and Zimbabwe and having a coastline on Indian Ocean (the Mozambique Channel between Mozambique and Madagascar). The area of 308,642 square miles (799,380 square kilometers) makes Mozambique about twice the size of California, and the July 2012 population was estimated at 23.5 million. In 2010, 38 percent of the population lived in urban areas, and the 2010 to 2015 annual rate of urbanization was estimated at 4.0 percent. Maputo is the capital and largest city (with a 2009 population estimated at 1.6 million). The population growth rate in 2012 was 2.4 percent, the net

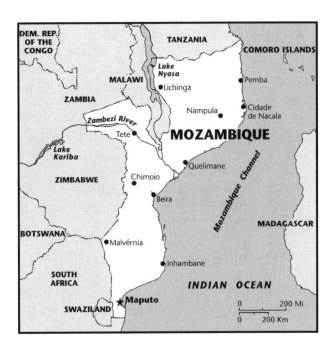

migration rate negative 2.1 migrants per 1,000 population, the birth rate 39.3 births per 1,000 (the 12th-highest in the world), and the total fertility rate 5.4 children per woman (the 12th-highest in the world). The United Nations High Commissioner for Refugees (UNHCR) estimated that, in 2010, there were 2,384 refugees and persons in refugee-like situations in Mozambique.

A former Portuguese colony, Mozambique became independent in 1975. A prolonged civil war came to an end in 1992, with a peace agreement negotiated by the United Nations (UN). According to the Ibrahim Index, in 2011, Mozambique ranked 18th among 53 African countries in terms of governance performance, with a score of 55 (out of 100). Mozambique ranked tied for 120th among 183 countries on the *Corruption Perceptions Index 2011,* with a score of 2.7 (on a scale where 0 indicates highly corrupt and 10 very clean).

In 2011, Mozambique was classified as a country with low human development (the lowest of four categories) on the United Nations Development Programme's (UNDP's) Human Development Index (HDI), with a score of 0.322 (on a scale where 1 denotes high development and 0 low development). In 2011, the International Food Policy Research Institute (IFPRI) classified Mozambique as a country with an "alarming" hunger problem, with a Global Hunger Index (GHI) score of 22.7, the highest in the world (where 0 reflects no hunger and higher scores more hunger). Life expectancy at birth in 2012 was estimated at 52.01 years, among the 10 lowest in the world, and the estimated gross domestic product (GDP) per capita in 2011 was $1,100, among the 20 lowest in the world. In 2008, the Gini Index (a measure of dispersion, in which perfect equality is denoted by 0 and maximum inequality is denoted by 100) for family income was 45.6. Unemployment in 2011 was estimated at 21.0 percent.

According to the World Economic Forum's *Global Gender Gap Index 2011*, Mozambique ranked 26th out of 135 countries on gender equality, with a score of 0.725 (on a scale with a theoretical range of 1 for equality to 0 for inequality and an actual range in 2011 from 0.8530 to 0.4873).

Emergency Health Services

According to the World Health Organization (WHO), as of 2007, Mozambique did not have a formal and publicly available system for providing prehospital care (emergency care). Doctors Without Borders (Médecins Sans Frontières, or MSF) began working in Mozambique in 1984 and had 507 staff members in the country at the close of 2010. In 2001, MSF began offering treatment to human immunodeficiency virus and acquired immune deficiency syndrome (HIV/AIDS) patients, demonstrating the viability of treating HIV/AIDS in remote areas as well as impoverished urban areas. As of August 2010, more than 33,000 persons in Mozambique were receiving antiretroviral treatments from MSF, a substantial portion of the estimated 200,000 receiving such treatments in the country as a whole. After an epidemic of measles in Malawi in September 2010, MSF staff and the Ministry of Health organized a vaccination campaign that resulted in the vaccination of some 250,000 children in Mozambique.

Insurance

Mozambique has a National Health Service that provides services through a system of health posts and health centers, district hospitals, provincial hospitals, and referral hospitals. According to the United States Agency for International Development (USAID), this system reaches less than 60 percent of the population. Private health care has been legal since 1991, but this sector is relatively small and concentrated in Mozambique's cities. About 40 percent of Mozambique's health system is supported by donor funding.

Costs of Hospitalization

No data available.

Access to Health Care

According to USAID, the services of the National Health Service fail to reach about 40 percent of Mozambique's population. A 2004 study found that those who seek care face close to two hours in travel and waiting time in return for limited services, with further barriers crated by the lack of trained personnel, drugs, and medical supplies in many parts of the country. User fees (charged to about half who use the system, according to USAID) constitute another barrier to care. Many citizens use traditional healers in addition to or instead of Western medical care.

According to WHO, in 2008, 55.3 percent of births in Mozambique were attended by skilled personnel (for example, physicians, nurses, or midwives). In 2003, 53 percent of pregnant women received at least four prenatal care visits. The 2010 immunization rates for 1-year-olds were 74 percent for diphtheria and pertussis (DPT3), 70 percent for measles (MCV), and 74 percent for Hib (Hib3). In 2010, an estimated 40 percent of persons with advanced HIV infection were receiving antiretroviral therapy in accordance with the 2010 WHO guidelines.

Cost of Drugs
No data available.

Health Care Facilities
The National Health Service organizes health care delivery into four levels. Level I is basic facilities staffed by clinical officers, nurses, and medical technicians; these facilities deliver at least 40 percent of all care and is frequently the only level accessed by a large proportion of the population. Level II facilities are district hospitals with general practice physicians on their staffs, who deliver basic diagnostic, obstetric, and surgical care. Level III is provincial hospitals, which offer more complex care and more advanced medical equipment and serve as training centers. Level IV is the referral hospitals located in Maputo, Beira, and Nampula. In 2006, Mozambique had 0.8 hospital beds per 1,000 population, one of the 30 lowest rates in the world.

Major Health Issues
In 2008, WHO estimated that 76 percent of years of life lost in Mozambique were due to communicable diseases, 15 percent to noncommunicable diseases, and 8 percent to injuries. In 2008, the age-standardized estimate of cancer deaths was 91 per 100,000 for men and 95 per 100,000 for women; for cardiovascular disease and diabetes, 549 per 100,000 for men and 478 per 100,000 for women; and for chronic respiratory disease, 154 per 100,000 for men and 75 per 100,000 for women.

In 2008, the age-standardized death rate from malaria was 99.7 per 100,000 population, the sixth-highest in the world. According to the United States Agency for International Development (USAID), 95 percent of the population in Mozambique is at risk for malaria. In 2010, tuberculosis incidence was 544.0 per 100,000 population, tuberculosis prevalence 491.0 per 100,000, and deaths due to tuberculosis among HIV-negative people 49.00 per 100,000. WHO estimated that the case detection rate in 2010 was 34 percent. Mozambique has one of the highest HIV/AIDS rates in the world; as of 2009, an estimated 11.5 percent of adults age 15 to 49 were living with HIV or AIDS. As of 2009, an estimated 1.4 million people in Mozambique were living with HIV or AIDS, the fifth-largest number in the world. In 2010, 87 percent of pregnant women tested positive for HIV. The mother-to-child transmission rate for HIV in 2010 was estimated at 31 percent, and in 2009, 10.5 percent of deaths to children under age 5 were attributed to HIV.

Selected Health Indicators: Mozambique Compared With the Global Average (2010)

	Mozambique	Global Average
Male life expectancy at birth* (years)	47	66
Female life expectancy at birth* (years)	51	71
Under-5 mortality rate, both sexes (per 1,000 live births)	135	57
Adult mortality rate, both sexes* (probability of dying between 15 and 60 years per 1,000 population)	493	176
Maternal mortality ratio (per 100,000 live births)	490	210
HIV prevalence* (per 1,000 adults aged 15 to 49)	115	8
Tuberculosis prevalence (per 100,000 population)	491	178

Source: World Health Organization Global Health Observatory Data Repository.
*Data refers to 2009.

Compared to other countries at a similar level of development, Mozambique ranked seventh among 43 least-developed countries on the 2011 Mothers' Index, produced by the international nongovernmental organization (NGO) Save the Children, based on a number of health and social factors relating to women, children, and maternal and child care. Mozambique's maternal mortality rate (death from any cause related to or aggravated by pregnancy) is quite high by global standards, estimated at 550 maternal deaths per 100,000 live births as of 2008. The infant mortality rate, defined as the number of deaths of infants younger than 1 year, also has been high, at 76.85 per 1,000 live births as of 2012. In 2003, 21.2 percent of children under age 5 were underweight (defined as 2 kilograms [kg] below standard weight-for-age at age 1, 3 kg below for ages 2 to 3, and 4 kg below for ages 4 to 5).

Health Care Personnel

Mozambique has a severe shortage of trained medical personnel. In 2006, Mozambique had 0.03 physicians per 1,000 population, 0.04 pharmaceutical personnel per 1,000, 0.04 laboratory health workers per 1,000, 0.02 health management and support workers per 1,000, and 0.31 nurses and midwives per 1,000. Michael Clemens and Bunilla Petterson estimate that 75 percent of Mozambique-born physicians and 19 percent of Mozambique-born nurses are working in one of nine developed countries, primarily in Portugal. Mozambique has one medical school, the Faculdade de Medicine of the Universidade de Eduardo Mondlane, located in Maputo. The course of study for the basic medical degree lasts seven years, and the degree awarded is Licenciatura em Medicine (license in medicine).

Government Role in Health Care

Mozambique has a National Health System, but it reaches only an estimated 60 percent of the population. According to WHO, in 2010, Mozambique spent $499 million on health care, an amount that comes to $21 per capita. Health care funding came primarily (76 percent) from domestic sources, with 24 percent coming from overseas sources. More than two-thirds (72 percent) of health care spending was paid for through government expenditures, with the remainder provided through household expenditures (14 percent) and other sources (15 percent). In 2010, Mozambique allocated 12 percent of its total government expenditures to health, in the median range for low-income African countries; government expenditures on health came to 3 percent of GDP, in the high range for low-income African countries. In 2009, according to WHO, official development assistance (ODA) for health in Mozambique came to $22.06 per capita.

Public Health Programs

The National Institute of Health (NIH), founded in 1991, is located in Maputo and directed by Ilesh Jani. The NIH is located within the Ministry of Health and has the mission of improving the nation's health and promoting scientific and technical solutions to Mozambique's health issues. Major functions of the NIH include training, outbreak investigation, monitoring and evaluation, providing laboratory services, conducting research, and conducting surveys and disease surveillance. The NIH is currently engaged in planning a new public health institute in cooperation with FIOCRUZ (the Oswaldo Cruz Foundation), a public health research institution in Brazil.

According to WHO, in 2004, Mozambique had 0.03 environmental and public health workers per 1,000 population. In 2010, 18 percent of the population had access to improved sanitation facilities (5 percent in rural areas and 38 percent in urban), and 47 percent had access to improved sources of drinking water (29 percent in rural areas and 77 percent in urban). According to C. B. Ijsselmuiden and colleagues, in 2007, Mozambique had one institution offering postgraduate public health programs.

MYANMAR

Myanmar is a southeastern Asian country, sharing borders with Bangladesh, China, India, Laos, and Thailand and having a coastline on the Andaman Sea. The area of 261,228 square miles (676,578 square kilometers) makes Myanmar similar in size to Texas, and the July 2012 population was estimated at 54.6 million (the 24th-largest in the world). In 2010, 34 percent of the population lived in urban areas, and the 2010 to 2015 annual rate of urbanization was estimated at 2.9 percent. Rangoon is the capital and largest city (with a 2009 population estimated at 4.3 million). The population growth rate in 2012 was 1.0 percent, the net migration rate negative 0.3 migrants per 1,000 population, the birth rate 19.1 births per 1,000, and the total fertility rate 2.2 children per woman.

In the 19th century, Great Britain incorporated Myanmar into its Indian Empire; it became a self-governing colony in 1937 and an independent country in 1948. A military junta has ruled the country since 1988 and has used force to suppress the population. The government of Myanmar is considered among the most corrupt in the world, ranking tied for 180th among 183 countries on the *Corruption Perceptions Index 2011*, with a score of 1.5 (on a scale where 0 indicates highly corrupt and 10 very clean).

In 2011, Myanmar was classified as a country with low human development (the lowest of four categories) on the United Nations Development Programme's (UNDP's) Human Development Index (HDI), with a score of 0.483 (on a scale where 1 denotes high development and 0 low development). According to the World Food Programme, in 2012, Myanmar was facing food shortages and high prices due in part to erratic rainfall and decreased agricultural production, resulting in food prices so high that, in Northern Rakhine State, purchasing a basic market basket of food required three-quarters of the wages of a typical laborer. Life expectancy at birth in 2012 was estimated at 65.24 years, and estimated gross domestic (GDP) per capita in 2011 was $1,300, among the 30 lowest in the world.

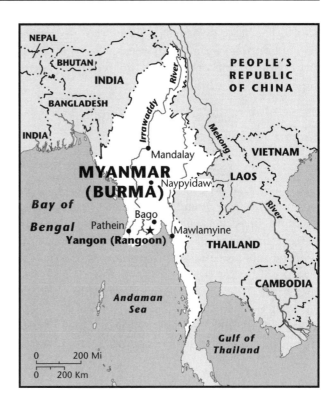

Emergency Health Services

According to the World Health Organization (WHO), as of 2007, Myanmar had a formal and publicly available emergency care (prehospital care) system accessible through regional access numbers but not a national access number.

Doctors Without Borders (Médecins Sans Frontières, or MSF) began working in Myanmar in 1992 and had 1,169 staff members in the country at the close of 2010. MSF provides general health care, human immunodeficiency virus and acquired immune deficiency syndrome (HIV/AIDS) treatment, tuberculosis treatment (including a pilot program to treat drug-resistant tuberculosis), and malaria treatment and provided emergency care after Cyclone Giri hit the Myanmar coast in November 2010. In 2010, MSF staff conducted almost 660,000 general consultations in Myanmar.

Insurance

Myanmar has a social insurance system providing medical benefits and cash maternity and sickness benefits. Many classes of employed people are included in the system, including some civil servants and state enterprise employees and employees of firms with at least five employees and working in commerce or other specified fields; the self-employed, agricultural workers, fishermen, people working in small firms, and construction workers are excluded. The system currently covers only 110 townships but is being expanded to cover the entire country. The system is funded by wage contributions (1.5 percent of monthly earnings, according to a schedule of 15 wage classes) and employer contributions (1.5 percent of monthly payroll, according to a schedule of 15 wage classes); the government provides subsidies as necessary. Medical care is provided directly by dispensaries run by the Social Security board, public hospitals, and larger employer dispensaries. Insured people register with a dispensary and are covered for services from that dispensary (except in cases of referral or emergency); covered benefits include medical care, specialist and lab services, hospitalization, home care, maternity care, and medicines. A single illness is covered for up to 26 weeks, although this may be extended. Pediatric care is provided for up to six months if the child's mother is insured. The maternity benefit is 66 percent of average covered earnings for up to 12 weeks. The sickness benefit is 50 percent of average covered earnings for up to 26 weeks. The Social Security Board administers the program under the general supervision of the Ministry of Labor.

Costs of Hospitalization

No data available.

Access to Health Care

According to WHO, in 2007, 36.9 percent of births in Myanmar were attended by skilled personnel (for example, physicians, nurses, or midwives), and 43 percent of pregnant women received at least four prenatal care visits. The 2010 immunization rates for 1-year-olds were 90 percent for diphtheria and pertussis (DPT3) and 88 percent for measles (MCV). In 2010, an estimated 23 percent of persons with advanced HIV infection were receiving antiretroviral therapy in accordance with the 2010 WHO guidelines.

Cost of Drugs

No data available.

Health Care Facilities

According to the Southeast Asian Regional Office (SEARO) of WHO, in 2008 and 2009, Myanmar had 846 government hospitals, 86 primary and secondary health centers, 348 maternal and child health centers, 1,481 rural health centers, 80 school health teams, 14 traditional medicine hospitals, and 237 traditional medicine clinics. As of 2010, according to WHO, Myanmar had 4.21 health posts per 100,000 population, 1.06 health centers per 100,000, 0.57 district or rural hospitals per 100,000, 0.08 provincial hospitals per 100,000, and 0.06 specialized hospitals per 100,000. In 2006, Myanmar had 0.60 hospital beds per 1,000 population, one of the 20 lowest rates in the world.

Major Health Issues

In 2008, WHO estimated that 41 percent of years of life lost in Myanmar were due to communicable diseases, 21 percent to noncommunicable diseases, and 39 percent to injuries. In 2008, the age-standardized estimate of cancer deaths was 123 per 100,000 for men and 115 per 100,000 for women; for cardiovascular disease and diabetes, 412 per 100,000 for men and 327 per 100,000 for women; and for chronic respiratory disease, 89 per 100,000 for men and 60 per 100,000 for women. In 2007, according to SEARO of WHO, the leading causes of mortality in Myanmar were malaria (6.1 percent), unspecified injuries (5.0 percent), unclassified diseases (4.9 percent), and septicemia (4.8 percent).

Myanmar's maternal mortality rate (death from any cause related to or aggravated by pregnancy) was estimated in 2008 as 240 maternal deaths per 100,000 live births. The infant mortality rate, defined as the number of deaths of infants younger than 1 year, was estimated at 47.74 per 1,000 live births as of 2012. Child malnutrition is a serious problem: In 2003, 29.6 percent of children under age 5 were underweight (defined as 2 kilograms [kg] below standard weight-for-age at age 1, 3 kg below for ages 2 to 3, and 4 kg below for ages 4 to 5), one of the 20 highest rates in the world. In 2010, tuberculosis incidence was 384.0 per 100,000 population, tuberculosis prevalence 525.0 per 100,000, and deaths due to tuberculosis among HIV-negative people 41.00 per 100,000. An estimated 4.2 percent of new tuberculosis cases and 10 percent of retreatment cases are multidrug resistant. WHO estimated that the case detection rate in 2010 was 71 percent. As of 2009, an estimated 0.6 percent of adults age 15 to 49 were living with HIV or AIDS.

Health Care Personnel

In 2006, WHO identified Myanmar as one of 57 countries with a critical deficit in the supply of skilled health workers. Myanmar has three medical schools: the Mandalay Institute of Medicine, which began offering instruction in 1954, the Institute of Medicine I, which began offering instruction in 1923, and the Institute of Medicine II, which began offering instruction in 1962, the latter two both located in Yangon. The course for the basic medical degree lasts 6.5 years, and a one-year internship is required before the license to practice medicine is awarded. The degree is bachelor of medicine or bachelor of surgery. Physicians must register with the Myanmar Medical Council, and foreigners are not allowed to practice medicine in Myanmar. In 2008, Myanmar had 0.46 physicians per 1,000 population, 0.05 dentistry personnel per 1,000, 0.08 community and traditional health workers per 1,000, and 0.80 nurses and midwives per 1,000. According to the Southeast Asian Regional Office (SEARO) of WHO, in 2008 and 2009 Myanmar had 950 traditional medicine practitioners.

Government Role in Health Care

According to WHO, in 2010, Myanmar spent $822 million on health care, an amount that comes to $17 per capita. Health care funding came primarily (91 percent) from domestic sources, with 9 percent coming from overseas sources. Most (81 percent) of health care spending was paid for through household expenditures, with the remainder provided through government expenditures (12 percent) and other sources (7 percent). In 2010, Myanmar allocated 1 percent of its total government expenditures to health, and government expenditures on health came to less than 1 percent of GDP; both place Myanmar in the median range as compared to other low-income southeast Asia region countries. In 2009, according to WHO, official development assistance (ODA) for health in Myanmar came to $1.23 per capita.

Public Health Programs

The National Health Laboratory for Myanmar is located in Yangon and directed by Ne Win. The laboratory is located within the Ministry of Health and is involved in many aspects of public health work, including training, research, quality assurance, laboratory investigations, provision of basic health services, provision of maternal and child health services, environmental sanitation, and provision of school health services. According to WHO, in 2008, Myanmar had 0.04 environmental and public health workers per 1,000 population. In 2010, 76 percent of the population had access to improved sanitation facilities (73 percent in rural areas and 83 percent in urban), and 83 percent had access to improved sources of drinking water (78 percent in rural areas and 93 percent in urban).

NAMIBIA

Namibia is a country in southwestern Africa, sharing borders with Angola, Botswana, South Africa, and Zambia and having a coastline on the south Atlantic Ocean. The area of 318,260 square miles (824,292 square kilometers) makes Namibia the 34th-largest country in the world (about half the size of Alaska); the July 2012 population was estimated at 2.2 million. In 2010, 38 percent of the population lived in urban areas, and the 2010 to 2015 annual rate of urbanization was estimated at 3.3 percent. Windhoek is the capital and largest city (with a 2009 population estimated at 342,000). The population growth rate in 2012 was 0.8

percent, the net migration rate 0.2 migrants per 1,000 population, the birth rate 21.1 births per 1,000, and the total fertility rate 2.4 children per woman. The United Nations High Commissioner for Refugees (UNHCR) estimated that, in 2010, there were 7,254 refugees and persons in refugee-like situations in Namibia.

Namibia became a German colony in the late 19th century and was occupied by South Africa during World War I; after World War II, South Africa annexed the area. In 1990, Namibia became an independent country following a war of independence that began in 1966. According to the Ibrahim Index, in 2011, Namibia ranked sixth among 53 African countries in terms of governance performance, with a score of 70 (out of 100). Namibia ranked tied for 54th among 183 countries on the *Corruption Perceptions Index 2011*, with a score of 4.6 (on a scale where 0 indicates highly corrupt and 10 very clean).

In 2011, Namibia was classified as a country with medium human development (the second from the lowest of four categories) on the United Nations Development Programme's (UNDP's) Human Development Index (HDI), with a score of 0.625 (on a scale where 1 denotes high development and 0 low development). Life expectancy at birth in 2012 was estimated at 52.17 years, among the 20 lowest in the world, and the estimated gross domestic product (GDP) per capita in 2011 was $7,300. Namibia is characterized by income inequality: In 2003, the Gini Index (a measure

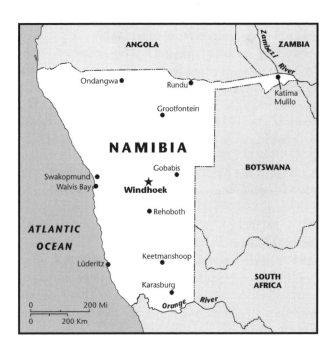

of dispersion, in which perfect equality is denoted by 0 and maximum inequality is denoted by 100) for family income was 70.7, among the highest in the world. Unemployment in 2008 was estimated at 51.2 percent, among the highest rates in the world. According to the World Economic Forum's *Global Gender Gap Index 2011*, Namibia ranked 32nd out of 135 countries on gender equality, with a score of 0.718 (on a scale with a theoretical range of 1 for equality to 0 for inequality and an actual range in 2011 from 0.8530 to 0.4873).

Emergency Health Services

According to the World Health Organization (WHO), as of 2007, Namibia had a formal and publicly available emergency care (prehospital care) system accessible through both regional access numbers and a national access number.

Insurance

According to WHO, less than one-quarter (19.5 percent) of Namibians were covered by public health insurance in 2009, and no information was available about the percentage covered by private insurance. According to Ke Xu and colleagues, in 2003, 0.1 percent of households in Namibia experienced catastrophic health expenditures annually; "catastrophic" was defined as exceeding 40 percent of household income remaining after basic needs were met.

Costs of Hospitalization

No data available.

Access to Health Care

According to WHO, in 2007, 81 percent of births in Namibia were attended by skilled personnel (for example, physicians, nurses, or midwives), and 70 percent of pregnant women received at least four prenatal care visits. The 2010 immunization rates for 1-year-olds were 83 percent for diphtheria and pertussis (DPT3), 75 percent for measles (MCV), and 83 percent for Hib (Hib3). In 2010, an estimated 90 percent of persons with advanced human immunodeficiency virus (HIV) infection were receiving antiretroviral therapy in accordance with the 2010 WHO guidelines. According to WHO, in 2010, Namibia had 0.94 magnetic resonance imaging (MRI) machines per 1 million population, 3.75 computer tomography (CT) machines per 1 million, 0.47 telecolbalt units per 1 million, and 0.47 radiotherapy machines per 1 million.

Cost of Drugs

In 2009, total pharmaceutical expenditures in Namibia were NAD 374.7 million ($57.6 million), and per capita pharmaceutical expenditures were NAD 175.9 ($20.80). Pharmaceutical expenditures represented 18.5 percent of total health expenditures and 0.6 percent of GDP. Certain population groups are entitled to free medications, including children under age 5, pregnant women, the elderly, and the poor. The public health system provides free medications, including those on the Essential Medications List (EML), and those used to treat malaria, tuberculosis, sexually transmitted diseases (STDs), and human immunodeficiency virus and acquired immune deficiency syndrome (HIV/AIDS); vaccines on the Expanded Programme on Immunization (EPI) list, created by WHO, are also provided for free. Private health insurance plans are required to provide EML medications for free.

Health Care Facilities

As of 2010, according to WHO, Namibia had 12.88 health posts per 100,000 population, 2.32 health centers per 100,000, 1.31 district or rural hospitals per 100,000, 0.18 provincial hospitals per 100,000, and 0.44 specialized hospitals per 100,000. In 2009, Namibia had 2.67 hospital beds per 1,000 population.

Major Health Issues

In 2008, WHO estimated that 63 percent of years of life lost in Namibia were due to communicable diseases, 22 percent to noncommunicable diseases, and 15 percent to injuries. In 2008, the age-standardized estimate of cancer deaths was 64 per 100,000 for men and 50 per 100,000 for women; for cardiovascular disease and diabetes, 632 per 100,000 for men and 361 per 100,000 for women; and for chronic respiratory disease, 111 per 100,000 for men and 35 per 100,000 for women.

In 2008, the age-standardized death rate from malaria was 32.4 per 100,000 population. In 2010, tuberculosis incidence was 603.0 per 100,000 population, tuberculosis prevalence 492.0 per 100,000, and deaths due to tuberculosis among HIV-negative people 25.00 per 100,000. Namibia has one of the highest HIV/AIDS rates in the world; as of 2009, an estimated 13.1 percent of adults age 15 to 49 were living with HIV or AIDS. In 2010, 86 percent of pregnant women tested positive for HIV. The mother-to-child transmission rate for HIV in 2010 was estimated at 14 percent, and in 2009, 19.5 percent of deaths to children under age 5 were attributed to HIV.

Namibia's maternal mortality rate (death from any cause related to or aggravated by pregnancy) was estimated in 2008 as 180 maternal deaths per 100,000 live births. The infant mortality rate, defined as the number of deaths of infants younger than 1 year, was estimated at 45.61 per 1,000 live births as of 2012. In 2007, 17.5 percent of children under age 5 were underweight (defined as 2 kilograms [kg] below standard weight-for-age at age 1, 3 kg below for ages 2 to 3, and 4 kg below for ages 4 to 5).

Health Care Personnel

In 2007, Namibia had 0.37 physicians per 1,000 population, 0.18 pharmaceutical personnel per 1,000, 0.08 laboratory health workers per 1,000, 3.87 health management and support workers per 1,000, 0.04 dentistry personnel per 1,000, and 2.78 nurses and midwives per 1,000. Michael Clemens and Bunilla Petterson estimate that 45 percent of Namibia-born physicians and 5 percent of Namibia-born nurses are working in one of nine developed countries, primarily South Africa.

Government Role in Health Care

Namibia has a National Health Policy (NHP), written in 2009, and a National Medicines Policy (NMP), written in 1998. Namibia's NMP addresses selection of essential medicines; financing, pricing, purchase, distribution, and regulation of drugs; pharmacovigilance; rational usage of medicines; human resource development; research; evaluation and monitoring; and traditional medicine. The EML was updated in 2008 and includes about 600 medicines.

According to WHO, in 2010, Namibia spent $825 million on health care, an amount that comes to $361 per capita. Health care funding came primarily (81 percent) from domestic sources, with 19 percent coming from overseas sources. More than half (58 percent) of health care spending was paid for through government expenditures, with the remainder provided through household expenditures (7 percent) and other sources (34 percent). In 2010, Namibia allocated 12 percent of its total government expenditures to health, and government expenditures on health came to 4 percent of GDP; both place Namibia in the high range as compared to other upper-middle-income African countries. In 2009, according to WHO, official development assistance (ODA) for health in Namibia came to $66.64 per capita.

Public Health Programs

According to WHO, in 2008, Namibia had 0.10 environmental and public health workers per 1,000 population. In 2010, 32 percent of the population had access to improved sanitation facilities (17 percent in rural areas and 57 percent in urban), and 93 percent had access to improved sources of drinking water (90 percent in rural areas and 99 percent in urban).

NAURU

Nauru is an island nation in the south Pacific Ocean. The area of 8 square miles (21 square kilometers) makes Nauru about one-tenth the size of Washington, D.C., and is the world's smallest independent republic; the July 2012 population was estimated at 9,378. In 2010, 100 percent of the population lived in urban areas. Nauru does not have an official capital; the government offices are in Yaren district. The population growth rate in 2012 was 0.6 percent, the net migration rate negative 15.0 migrants per 1,000 population (one of the highest emigration rates in the world), the birth

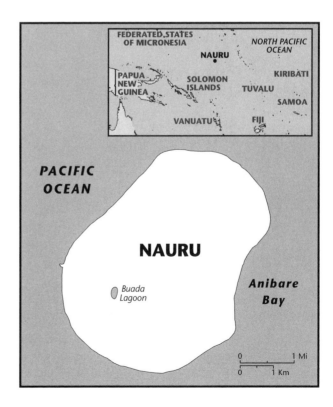

rate 27.1 births per 1,000, and the total fertility rate 3.0 children per woman. Life expectancy at birth in 2012 was estimated at 65.70 years.

Germany annexed Nauru in 1888, and phosphate mining began in the early 20th century. After World War II, Nauru became a United Nations Trust Territory, and in 1968, the country became independent. The country has limited freshwater resources, and the central part of the island has been made a wasteland through intensive phosphate mining. Almost everything needed on the island is imported and the economy is almost entirely based on phosphate, which is running out; unemployment in 2004 was estimated at 90 percent, the second-highest in the world, and estimated gross domestic product (GDP) per capita in 2011 was $5,000.

Emergency Health Services

According to the World Health Organization (WHO), as of 2007, Nauru had a formal and publicly available emergency care (prehospital care) system accessible through a national access number.

Insurance

A 2009 constitutional referendum in Nauru included the right to health for all its citizens, including the right to access a national health system providing quality and affordable health care. Most health care delivery is centralized, with maternal and child health programs based at the community level.

Costs of Hospitalization

No data available.

Access to Health Care

According to WHO, in 2007, 97 percent of births in Nauru were attended by skilled personnel (for example, physicians, nurses, or midwives), and 40 percent of pregnant women received at least four prenatal care visits. The 2010 immunization rates for 1-year-olds were 99 percent for diphtheria and pertussis (DPT3), 99 percent for measles (MCV), and 99 percent for Hib (Hib3). Some tertiary care is available on Nauru (including hemodialysis), with international referrals available for those meeting selection criteria, and some specialist care provided by visiting teams of providers.

Cost of Drugs

No data available.

Health Care Facilities

In 1999, the Republic of Nauru Hospital was formed by the amalgamation of Nauru General Hospital and the National Phosphate Corporation Hospital; the hospital offers medical and surgical care and lab, radiological, and pharmacy services. As of 2010, according to WHO, Nauru had 9.75 provincial hospitals per 100,000 population.

Major Health Issues

In 2008, WHO estimated that 29 percent of years of life lost in Nauru were due to communicable diseases, 56 percent to noncommunicable diseases, and 15 percent to injuries. In 2008, the age-standardized estimate of cancer deaths was 115 per 100,000 for men and 191 per 100,000 for women; for cardiovascular disease and diabetes, 922 per 100,000 for men and 473 per 100,000 for women; and for chronic respiratory disease, 86 per 100,000 for men and 72 per 100,000 for women.

The infant mortality rate, defined as the number of deaths of infants younger than 1 year, was 8.51 per 1,000 live births as of 2012. No information is available from WHO on the maternal mortality rate in Nauru. In 2010, tuberculosis incidence was 40.0 per 100,000 population, tuberculosis prevalence 52.0 per 100,000, and deaths due to tuberculosis among human immunodeficiency virus (HIV)-negative people 3.80 per 100,000.

Health Care Personnel

In 2008, Nauru had 0.71 physicians per 1,000 population, 0.07 pharmaceutical personnel per 1,000, 0.07 dentistry personnel per 1,000, and 4.93 nurses and midwives per 1,000. In 2011, about half of the professional health care staff in Nauru were expatriates.

Government Role in Health Care

According to WHO, in 2010, Nauru spent $7 million on health care, an amount that comes to $713 per capita. About two-thirds (66 percent) of health care funding came from domestic sources, with 34 percent coming from overseas. More than two-thirds (69 percent) of health care spending was paid for through government expenditures, with the remainder provided through household expenditures (5 percent) and other sources (27 percent). In 2010, Nauru allocated 10 percent of its total government expenditures to health, in the low range for upper-middle-income western Pacific region countries; government expenditures on health came to 8 percent of GDP, in the median range for upper-middle-income western Pacific region countries.

Public Health Programs

According to WHO, in 2008, Nauru had 0.71 environmental and public health workers per 1,000 population. In 2010, 65 percent of the population had access to improved sanitation facilities, and 88 percent had access to improved sources of drinking water.

NEPAL

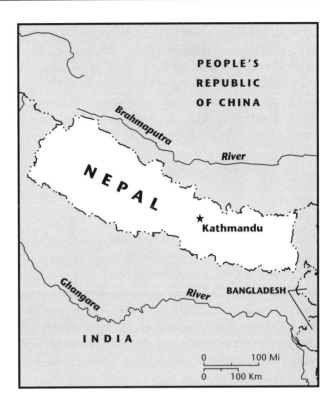

Nepal is a landlocked country in southern Asia sharing borders with China and India. The area of 56,827 square miles (147,181 square kilometers) makes Nepal similar in size to Arkansas, and the July 2012 population was estimated at 29.9 million. In 2010, 19 percent of the population lived in urban areas, and the 2010 to 2015 annual rate of urbanization was estimated at 4.7 percent. Kathmandu is the capital and largest city (with a 2009 population estimated at 990,000). The population growth rate in 2012 was 1.8 percent, the net migration rate 2.6 per 1,000 population (the 31st-highest in the world), the birth rate 21.8 births per 1,000, and the total fertility rate 2.4 children per woman. The United Nations High Commissioner for Refugees (UNHCR) estimated that, in 2010, there were 72,514 refugees and persons in refugee-like situations in Nepal.

Nepal was a monarchy until creation of a cabinet system of government in 1951; in 1990, the country established a multiparty system. A civil war beginning in 1996 lasted until 2006; the monarchy was abolished in 2008. Nepal ranked tied for 152nd among 183 countries on the *Corruption Perceptions Index 2011*, with a score of 2.2 (on a scale where 0 indicates highly corrupt and 10 very clean).

In 2011, Nepal was classified as a country with low human development (the lowest of four categories) on the United Nations Development Programme's (UNDP's) Human Development Index (HDI), with a score of 0.458 (on a scale where 1 denotes high development and 0 low development). Life expectancy at birth in 2012 was estimated at 66.51 years, and the estimated gross domestic product (GDP) per capita in 2011 was $1,300, among the 30 lowest in the world. Income distribution in Nepal is relatively unequal: In 2004, the Gini Index (a measure of dispersion, in

which perfect equality is denoted by 0 and maximum inequality is denoted by 100) for family income was 47.2. Unemployment in 2008 was estimated at 46 percent, among the highest rates in the world.

The status of men and women is highly unequal: According to the World Economic Forum's *Global Gender Gap Index 2011*, Nepal ranked 126th out of 135 countries on gender equality, with a score of 0.589 (on a scale with a theoretical range of 1 for equality to 0 for inequality and an actual range in 2011 from 0.8530 to 0.4873).

Emergency Health Services

According to the World Health Organization (WHO), as of 2007, Nepal did not have a formal and publicly available system for providing prehospital care (emergency care).

Insurance

Nepal has no general social insurance system. Employers in the private sector are required to provide basic medical benefits, under the 1974 Bonus Act, to employees and their dependents. The 1992 Labor Act requires employers to provide sick leave (50 percent of wages for up to 15 days per year) and maternity leave (100 percent of wages for up to 52 days for up to two births) to employees. Government employees are entitled to reimbursement of annual medical expenses (to the limit of the equivalent of 12 to 21 months of salary), and the 1992 Civil Servant Act provides maternity leave for 60 days for up to two births. Government hospitals provide free medical treatment to people age 75 and older.

Costs of Hospitalization
No data available.

Access to Health Care
According to WHO, in 2006, 19 percent of births in Nepal were attended by skilled personnel (for example, physicians, nurses, or midwives), and 29 percent of pregnant women received at least four prenatal care visits. The 2010 immunization rates for 1-year-olds were 82 percent for diphtheria and pertussis (DPT3) and 86 percent for measles (MCV). In 2010, an estimated 18 percent of persons with advanced human immunodeficiency virus (HIV) infection were receiving antiretroviral therapy in accordance with the 2010 WHO guidelines. According to WHO, in 2010, Nepal had 0.35 computer tomography (CT) machines per 1 million population.

Cost of Drugs
In 2008, total pharmaceutical expenditures in Nepal came to NPR 13,089 ($187.6 million), and per capita pharmaceutical expenditures were NPR 45.8 ($7). Total pharmaceutical expenditure represented almost one-third (32.8 percent) of total health expenditures and 1.6 percent of GDP. Some drugs are provided free of charge to certain population groups, including children under the age of 5, pregnant women, the poor, the elderly, and female community health volunteers. Some drugs on the Essential Medicines List (EML, approximately 22 to 45 out of 321 depending on the specific facility) are provided for free at health facilities, as are drugs for malaria, tuberculosis, sexually transmitted diseases (STDs), human immunodeficiency virus and acquired immune deficiency syndrome (HIV/AIDS), filariasis, and control of diarrhea (for children); vaccines listed on the Expanded Programme on Immunization (EPI) list, developed by WHO, are also provided for free.

Health Care Facilities
As of 2010, according to WHO, Nepal had 2.33 health posts per 100,000 population, 0.67 health centers per 100,000, 0.22 district or rural hospitals per 100,000, 0.10 provincial hospitals per 100,000, and 0.04 specialized hospitals per 100,000. In 2008, Nepal had 5.00 hospital beds per 1,000 population, among the 50 highest rates in the world.

Major Health Issues
In 2008, WHO estimated that 60 percent of years of life lost in Nepal were due to communicable diseases, 31 percent to noncommunicable diseases, and 10 percent to injuries. In 2008, the age-standardized estimate of cancer deaths was 114 per 100,000 for men and 119 per 100,000 for women; for cardiovascular disease and diabetes, 400 per 100,000 for men and 301 per 100,000 for women; and for chronic respiratory disease, 86 per 100,000 for men and 55 per 100,000 for women.

Nepal's maternal mortality rate (death from any cause related to or aggravated by pregnancy) is high by global standards, estimated at 380 maternal deaths per 100,000 live births as of 2008. The infant mortality rate, defined as the number of deaths of infants younger than 1 year, was estimated at 43.13 per 1,000 live births as of 2012. Child malnutrition is a serious problem: In 2006, 38.8 percent of children under age 5 were underweight (defined as 2 kilograms [kg] below standard weight-for-age at age 1, 3 kg below for ages 2 to 3, and 4 kg below for ages 4 to 5), one of the highest rates in the world. In 2010, tuberculosis incidence was 163.0 per 100,000 population, tuberculosis prevalence 238.0 per 100,000, and deaths due to tuberculosis among HIV-negative people 21.00 per 100,000. As of 2009, an estimated 0.4 percent of adults age 15 to 49 were living with HIV or AIDS.

Health Care Personnel
In 2006, WHO identified Nepal as one of 57 countries with a critical deficit in the supply of skilled health workers. Nepal has seven medical schools. The basic training course for the medical degree requires 5.5 years to complete, and a one-year internship is also required for a medical license. The degree granted is bachelor of medicine or bachelor of surgery. Physicians must register with the Nepal Medical Council in Kathmandu. Nepal has agreements with Bangladesh, India, Pakistan, and Sri Lanka. In 2004, Nepal had 0.21 physicians per 1,000 population, 0.01 pharmaceutical personnel per 1,000, 0.12 laboratory health workers per 1,000, 0.01 dentistry personnel per 1,000, 0.63 community and traditional health workers per 1,000, and 0.46 nurses and midwives per 1,000.

Government Role in Health Care

The Interim Constitution of 2007 states that every citizen has the right to free basic health services, but this has not yet been put into practice. Nepal has a National Health Policy (NHP), developed in 1991, and a plan for implementation (covering the years 1997 to 2012); this plan includes increased health services, particularly to poor and vulnerable groups. Priority areas for the years 2010 to 2015 include family planning, newborn care, maternal care, reproductive health, oral health, and environmental health; emergency and disaster management and the Ayurvedic system of medicine are also included.

Nepal also has a National Medicines Policy (NMP), developed in 1995, but no implementation plan for it; instead, pharmaceutical policies are addressed by the Ministry of Health and Population. Issues currently monitored and assessed in this regard include selection of essential medicines; pricing, purchase, distribution, and regulation of drugs; rational usage of medicines; human resource development; research; evaluation and monitoring; and traditional medicine.

Before being registered and authorized for sale in Nepal, pharmaceutical products must be assessed according to explicit and publicly available criteria. The government regulates advertising and promotion of prescription drugs, and direct marketing to the general public is forbidden. Nepal is a member of the World Trade Organization (WTO) and has not modified its national law to take advantage of the flexibility offered by the Trade-Related Aspects of Intellectual Property Rights (TRIPS), intended to increase access to medications.

According to WHO, in 2010, Nepal spent $892 million on health care, an amount that comes to $30 per capita. Most (89 percent) of health care funding came from domestic sources, with 1 percent coming from overseas. Almost half (48 percent) of health care spending was paid for through household expenditures, with the remainder provided through government expenditures (33 percent) and other sources (18 percent).

In 2010, Nepal allocated 8 percent of its total government expenditures to health, and government expenditures on health came to 2 percent of GDP; both figures are in the median range for low-income southeast Asian region countries. In 2009, according to WHO, official development assistance (ODA) for health in Nepal came to $3.24 per capita.

Public Health Programs

The School of Public Health and Community Medicine within the B. P. Koirala Institute of Health Sciences (BPKIHS) is located in Sunsari (in eastern Nepal) and headed by Professor Paras K. Pokharel. The BPKIHS was founded in 1993 and, in 1998, was upgraded to the status of an autonomous Health Sciences University. The mission of the BPKIHS includes providing health care, developing the health workforce, engaging in health research, and becoming a center of excellent for infectious diseases and tropical medicine; one example of the latter is the *kala azar* (visceral leishmaniasis) project carried out by the BPKIHS in cooperation with several international bodies.

According to WHO, in 2004, Nepal had 0.01 environmental and public health workers per 1,000 population. In 2010, 31 percent of the population had access to improved sanitation facilities (27 percent in rural areas and 48 percent in urban), and 89 percent had access to improved sources of drinking water (88 percent in rural areas and 93 percent in urban). According to the World Higher Education Database (WHED), one university in Nepal offers programs in epidemiology or public health: Pokhara University.

NETHERLANDS

The Netherlands is a European country, sharing borders with Germany and Belgium and having a coastline on the North Sea. The area of 16,039 square miles (41,543 square kilometers) makes the Netherlands about twice the size of New Jersey, and the July 2012 population was estimated at 16.7 million. In 2010, 83 percent of the population lived in urban areas, and the 2010 to 2015 annual rate of urbanization was estimated at 0.8 percent. Amsterdam is the capital and largest city (with a 2009 population estimated at 1.0 million). The population growth rate in 2012 was 0.4 percent, the net migration rate 2.0 migrants per 1,000 population, the birth rate 10.9 births per 1,000, and the total fertility rate 1.8 children per woman.

The Kingdom of the Netherlands was formed in 1815; Belgium seceded in 1830. The Netherlands is a modern, industrialized country and also a major exporter of agricultural goods. The Dutch government has a reputation for transparency and honesty,

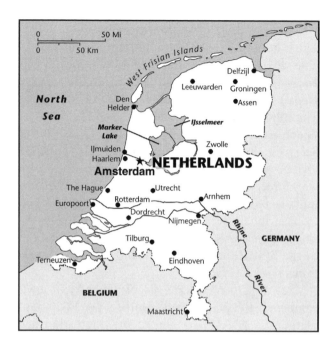

ranking seventh among 183 countries on the *Corruption Perceptions Index 2011,* with a score of 8.9 (on a scale where 0 indicates highly corrupt and 10 very clean). The Netherlands ranked tied for third (with the United States) in 2011 on the United Nations Development Programme's (UNDP's) Human Development Index (HDI), with a score of 0.910 (on a scale where 1 denotes high development and 0 low development).

Life expectancy at birth in 2012 was estimated at 80.91 years, among the highest in the world, and per capita gross domestic product (GDP) in 2011 in the Netherlands was estimated at $42,300. In 2007, the Gini Index (a measure of dispersion, in which perfect equality is denoted by 0 and maximum inequality is denoted by 100) for family income was 30.9. According to the World Economic Forum's *Global Gender Gap Index 2011*, the Netherlands ranked 15th out of 135 countries on gender equality, with a score of 0.747 (on a scale with a theoretical range of 1 for equality to 0 for inequality and an actual range in 2011 from 0.8530 to 0.4873).

Emergency Health Services

The Netherlands's laws governing the emergency health system date from the 2000s, as does recognition of emergency medicine as a medical specialty; by law, free access to hospitals for emergency care is provided for all persons, including the uninsured. Funding for the emergency system is provided by multiple sources.

The Netherlands has only one national telephone number for medical emergencies, 112 (the European Union, or EU, standard); the country has 25 dispatch centers that are interconnected.

Insurance

The Netherlands has a statutory health insurance system (SHI), with coverage mandated and provided through an exchange of private insurers. Insurers provide a standard benefit package including physician and hospital care, dental care up to age 18, and paramedical care, and a national program covers mental health services and long-term care. Since 2006, the purchase of health insurance has been mandatory, with the exception of members of the military and conscientious objectors. In 2007, about 1.5 percent of the Dutch population was uninsured, and from 2009 to 2010, policy was strengthened to police enrollment and payment of premiums. The expenses of asylum seekers and illegal immigrants are covered by the government.

The system is financed through general tax revenues, an earmarked payroll tax, and insurance premiums that are community rated. About 80 percent of citizens buy extra benefits offered through private plans. There is no cap on out-of-pocket expenses, but children are exempt from cost sharing, and about 40 percent of people receive premium assistance based on income. Primary care is paid for through a mix of fee-for-service and capitation payments, while hospital payments are handled through a combination of global budgets and case-based payments; hospital payments include physician costs. Patients are required to register with a general practice physician.

Since 2006, insurers have been required to accept any applicant for basic coverage; in the same year, insurance coverage became mandatory, although there are few effective sanctions against those who do not sign up with a policy or do not pay their premiums. A 2004 study by the World Health Organization (WHO) found that 24.7 percent of the Dutch population had substitutive voluntary health insurance (covering services that would otherwise be available from the state), more than 60 percent had complementary voluntary health insurance (covering services not covered, or not fully covered, by the state), and a marginal proportion had supplementary health insurance (providing increased choice or faster access to services). Most holders of voluntary policies have relatively high incomes.

Costs of Hospitalization

According to Organisation for Economic Co-operation and Development (OECD) data, in 2009, hospital spending per capita in the Netherlands was $1,545 (adjusted for cost of living differences), and hospital spending per discharge was $13,244 in 2011. The average length of stay in acute care was 5.6 days (in 2008), and there were 117 hospital discharges per 1,000 population. About one-third (34 percent) of hospital care is paid for through diagnosis-related groups (DRGs), called in the Netherlands Diagnosis Treatment Combinations (DTCs), which cover hospital and specialist costs. Most reimbursements through DTCs are based on fixed prices, but some are negotiated with insurers.

Access to Health Care

According to WHO, in 2007, 100 percent of births in the Netherlands were attended by skilled personnel (for example, physicians, nurses, or midwives). The 2010 immunization rates for 1-year-olds were 97 percent for diphtheria and pertussis (DPT3), 96 percent for measles (MCV), and 97 percent for Hib (Hib3).

In 2009, according to OECD data, people in the Netherlands had an average of 5.7 physician visits. In 2010, almost three-quarters (72 percent) reported that, when sick, they were able to get a medical appointment the same day or the next day. Only one-third (33 percent) reported it was very or somewhat difficult to get medical care after usual office hours. For those who needed particular types of care, only 16 percent reported they waited two or more months to see a specialist (of those who needed to see a specialist in the prior two years), one in 20 (5 percent) reported waiting four or more months for elective surgery (of those who required elective surgery in the prior two years), and only 5 percent reported they had experienced an access barrier due to cost in the previous two years; an "access barrier" was defined as failing to fill or refill a prescription, failing to visit a physician, or failing to get recommended care. In 2010, just over one in 10 (11 percent) of Dutch people reported experiencing a medical, medication, or lab test error in the previous two years, and only 13 percent of those who needed to visit a specialist in the previous two years reported that the specialist did not have information about their medical history at the

Selected Health Indicators: Netherlands Compared With the Organisation for Economic Co-operation and Development (OECD) Country Average

	Netherlands	OECD average (2010 or nearest year)
Male life expectancy at birth, 2010	78.8	77
Female life expectancy at birth, 2010	82.7	82.5
Public current expenditure on health (per capita, USD purchasing power parity), 2010	4,049.9	2,377.8
Public current expenditure on health (percent total expenditure on health), 2010	85.7	72.2
Tobacco consumption (percent of population 15+ who are daily smokers), 2010	20.9	21.1
Alcohol consumption (liters per capita [age 15+]), 2009	9.4	9.4
Obesity (percent of female population with a BMI>30 kg/m2, self-reported), 2010	12.6	14.8
Obesity (percent of male population with a BMI>30 kg/m2, self-reported), 2010	10.2	15.1

Source: OECD Health Data 2012 (Organisation for Economic Co-operation and Development, 2012).

time of the appointment. Just over half (51 percent) reported experiencing a gap in hospital discharge planning in the previous two years (due to any of the following: did not receive a written plan for care, did not have arrangements made for follow-up visits, did not know who to contact with questions, or did not receive instruction about when to seek further care).

A 2011 Commonwealth Fund Survey compared access to health care for "sicker" adults (those 18 and older, in self-reported poor or fair health, who had been treated for a serious illness or injury in the past year or been hospitalized in the past two years) in 11 OECD countries. This survey found that 15 percent of sicker Dutch people surveyed reported having experienced an access problem related to cost in the previous year; the most common result was failing to fill a prescription, or skipping doses of a prescribed drug, or skipping a medical test, treatment, or follow-up. Other problems reported include having serious problems paying their medical bills (14 percent), waiting six days or longer for needed care (12 percent), having difficulty getting after-hours care except in an emergency room (34 percent), and experiencing coordination gaps in care (37 percent).

Cost of Drugs

In 2009, total pharmaceutical expenditure in the Netherlands was 5.15 billion euros ($7.38 billion) for a per capita pharmaceutical expenditure of 311.80 euros ($446.30). Pharmaceutical expenditures came to 9.6 percent of total health expenditures, and 0.9 percent of GDP. Almost all (99.7 percent) expenditures on pharmaceuticals were provided by the public sector. Generic pharmaceuticals represented 28 percent of the total market, and the growth rate of the pharmaceutical market was 2.1 percent. Real annual growth in pharmaceutical expenditures in the Netherlands grew 4.3 percent from 1997 to 2005, much slower than the 8.2 percent growth of total health expenditure (minus pharmaceutical expenditures) over those years.

Most drugs are reimbursed at least partially through health insurance, and some medications are provided publicly at no cost; these include drugs for tuberculosis, sexually transmitted diseases (STDs), human immunodeficiency virus and acquired immune deficiency syndrome (HIV/AIDS), and vaccines included on the Expanded Programme on Immunization (EPI) list developed by the WHO. According to Elizabeth Docteur, in 2004, generic drugs represented 20 percent of the market share by

value and 49 percent of the market share by volume of the total pharmaceutical market.

Manufacturers must apply for authorization (registration) before selling their drugs in the Netherlands; mutual recognition programs are in place with several EU countries, and 13,686 pharmaceutical products were registered in the Netherlands in 2011. Advertising and promotion of prescription drugs is controlled by the Dutch government, and direct marketing to the public is prohibited. Price controls on pharmaceuticals are applied at the level of retailers and wholesalers: Pharmacists receive discounts from wholesalers, who are then entitled to a 6.8 percent clawback. The government runs an active monitoring system for pharmaceutical prices. Some insurers provide a preference list of medications including lower costs for certain generic medications, as opposed to brand-name or other generic versions of the same drug; if such a list is provided, a pharmacist must dispense the cheaper generic.

According to Douglas Ball, the Netherlands charges a lower value-added tax (VAT) of 6 percent for medicines, as opposed to the standard rate of 19 percent. The pharmacy dispensing fee is fixed at 6.10 euros. The wholesale markup is not fixed by law, but retail pharmacies are allowed a clawback of 6.82 percent, with a ceiling of 6.80 euros, for medicines covered by the Medicines Pricing Act.

Health Care Facilities

Most Dutch hospitals are private and nonprofit. As of 2010, according to WHO, the Netherlands had 0.77 specialized hospitals per 100,000 and, in 2008, had 4.25 hospital beds per 1,000 population, among the 50 highest rates in the world. In 2009, the Netherlands had 11.0 magnetic resonance imaging (MRI) machines per 1 million population, and 43.9 MRI exams were performed per 100,000 population. Almost all (99 percent) of primary care physicians used electronic medical records in 2009.

Major Health Issues

In 2008, WHO estimated that 6 percent of years of life lost in the Netherlands were due to communicable diseases, 86 percent to noncommunicable diseases, and 8 percent to injuries. In 2008, the age-standardized estimate of cancer deaths was 173 per 100,000 for men and 120 per 100,000 for women; for cardiovascular disease and diabetes, 151 per 100,000 for men and 93 per 100,000 for women; and for chronic respiratory disease, 31 per 100,000 for men and 17 per 100,000 for women. The Netherlands ranked ninth among more developed countries in the 2011 Mothers' Index, produced by the international nongovernmental organization (NGO) Save the Children, based on a number of health and social factors relating to women, children, and maternal and child care. The maternal mortality rate (death from any cause related to or aggravated by pregnancy) in the Netherlands in 2008 was nine maternal deaths per 100,000 live births. The infant mortality rate, defined as the number of deaths of infants younger than 1 year, was 3.73 per 1,000 live births as of 2012 data. In 2010, tuberculosis incidence was 7.3 per 100,000 population, tuberculosis prevalence 9.0 per 100,000, and deaths due to tuberculosis among HIV-negative people 0.19 per 100,000. As of 2009, an estimated 0.2 percent of adults age 15 to 49 were living with HIV or AIDS.

Health Care Personnel

The Netherlands has eight medical schools, four of which have been in operation since the 16th or 17th centuries. The basic medical degree course lasts six years, and the degree awarded is Arts (physician). Physicians must register with the Chief Inspector of Health Care, and the license to practice medicine is granted by the Ministry of Health, Welfare and Sport. Graduates of recognized medical schools in the Netherlands or other EU countries are granted the license to practice, while graduates from schools in other countries are licensed at the discretion of the Minister of Health.

The Netherlands, as a member of the EU, cooperates with other countries in recognizing physicians qualified to practice in other EU countries, as specified by Directive 2005/36/EC of the European Parliament. This allows qualified professionals to practice their profession in other EU states on a temporary basis and requires that the host country automatically recognize qualifications for certain professions, including physicians, nurses, dentists, midwives, and pharmacists, if certain conditions have been met (for instance, facility in the language of the host country may be required). In 2007, the Netherlands had 3.92 physicians per 1,000 population and, in 2008, had 0.15 nurses and midwives per 1,000 population.

Government Role in Health Care

National legislation recognizes the right to health, including access to essential medicines and medical technology. The Netherlands has a National Medicines Policy (NMP) and a plan to implement it. The country does not have an Essential Medicines List (EML) but does have policies covering the financing, pricing, distribution, and regulation of drugs; pharmacovigilance; rational usage of medicines; research; and evaluation and monitoring. According to WHO, in 2010, the Netherlands spent $93 billion on health care, an amount that comes to $5,593 per capita. All health care funding came from domestic sources. More than three-quarters (79 percent) of health care spending was paid for through government expenditures, with the remainder provided through household expenditures (5 percent) and other sources (16 percent). In 2010, the Netherlands allocated 18 percent of its total government expenditures to health, and government expenditures on health came to 9 percent of GDP; both figures are in the high range for high-income European countries.

Public Health Programs

The National Institute for Public Health and the Environment (RIVM) for the Netherlands is located in Bilthoven and headed by A. N. van der Zander. It employs more than 1,500 people and is an internationally known center for research in health, nutrition, and environmental protection. The RIVM's responsibilities include research, knowledge accumulation, health promotion, creation of intervention programs, public education, policy support, and coordination at the national level. In 2010, access to improved sanitary facilities and improved sources of drinking water was essentially universal in the Netherlands. According to the World Higher Education Database (WHED), six universities in the Netherlands offer programs in epidemiology or public health: Erasmus University in Rotterdam, the University of Applied Sciences of Henze University Groningen, the Royal Tropical Institute in Amsterdam, Maastricht University, the University of Twente, and Wageningen University and Research Center.

NEW ZEALAND

New Zealand is an island nation in the south Pacific Ocean, consisting of two large islands and numerous smaller islands. The area of 103,363 square miles (267,710 square kilometers) makes New Zealand about the size of Colorado, and the July 2012 population was estimated at 4.3 million. In 2010, 86 percent of the population lived in urban areas, and the 2010 to 2015 annual rate of urbanization is estimated at 0.9 percent. Wellington is the capital and Auckland the largest city (with a 2009 population estimated at 1.4 million); about 90 percent of the population is urban. The population growth rate in 2012 was 0.9 percent, the net migration rate 2.3 migrants per 1,000 population, the birth rate 13.6 births per 1,000, and the total fertility rate 2.1 children per woman.

The islands of New Zealand were settled by the Polynesian Maori around 800 C.E. Great Britain began establishing colonies in 1840 after the Treaty of Waitangi was formalized; the native peoples were defeated in a series of land wars from 1843 to 1872. New Zealand became an independent dominion in 1907. The government has an excellent reputation for transparency and honesty, ranking first among 183 countries on the *Corruption Perceptions Index 2011*, with a score of 9.5 (on a scale where 0 indicates highly corrupt and 10 very clean).

New Zealand ranked fifth in 2011 on the United Nations Development Programme's (UNDP's) Human Development Index (HDI), with a score of 0.908 (on a scale where 1 denotes high development and 0 low development). Life expectancy at birth in 2012 was estimated at 80.71 years, among the highest in the world, and per capita gross domestic product (GDP) in 2011 was estimated at $27,900. In 1997, the Gini Index (a measure of dispersion, in which perfect equality is denoted by 0 and maximum inequality is denoted by 100) for family income was 36.2. According to the World Economic Forum's *Global Gender Gap Index 2011*, New Zealand ranked sixth out of 135 countries on gender equality, with a score of 0.781 (on a scale with a theoretical range of 1 for equality to 0 for inequality and an actual range in 2011 from 0.8530 to 0.4873).

Emergency Health Services

Virtually all emergency care in New Zealand is provided by public hospitals, which are owned and operated by district health boards. According to the World Health Organization (WHO), as of 2007, New Zealand had a formal and publicly available emergency care (prehospital care) system, accessible through a national access number.

Insurance

New Zealand has a national health service financed through general tax revenues. The publicly funded

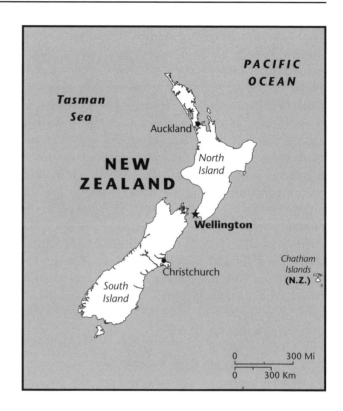

system covers most medical care, including primary health care services, prescription drugs, hospital care, preventive care, disability support services, and dental care for children. Copayments are required for some services, including prescription drugs, specialist care, and adult dental care. About one-third of citizens buy private insurance that provides benefits such as access to private hospitals for elective surgery, access to specialists, and cost sharing.

A subsidy for out-of-pocket expenses begins at 20 prescriptions or 12 doctor visits in the previous year. Young children are primarily exempt from cost sharing, and cost sharing is lower for low-income people, those with certain chronic conditions, and persons of Maori or Pacific Islander heritage. Primary care is paid for with a mix of fee-for-service and capitation payments, and hospital payments are handled through a combination of global budgets and case-based payments; hospital payments include physician costs. Most people (96 percent) are required to register with a general practice physician, whom they are allowed to select.

Costs of Hospitalization

According to Organisation for Economic Co-operation and Development (OECD) data, in 2009, hospital spending per capita in New Zealand was $1,070 (adjusted for differences in the cost of living), and hospital spending per discharge came to $7,160 in 2011. The average length of stay in acute care was 5.9 days (in 2008), and there were 142 hospital discharges per 1,000 population. Hospitals have capped budgets and receive payments that are a mix of case-based and per-diem payments.

Access to Health Care

In 2009, according to OECD data, people in New Zealand had an average of 4.3 physician visits. In 2010, more than three-quarters (78 percent) reported that, when sick, they were able to get a medical appointment the same day or the next day. Just over one-third (38 percent) reported it was very or somewhat difficult to get medical care after usual office hours. For those who needed particular types of care, less than one-quarter (22 percent) reported they waited two or more months to see a specialist (of those who needed to see a specialist in the prior two years), only 8 percent reported waiting four or more months for elective surgery (of those who required elective surgery in the prior two years), and 14 percent reported they had experienced an access barrier due to cost in the previous two years; an access barrier was defined as failing to fill or refill a prescription, failing to visit a physician, or failing to get recommended care.

In 2010, just over one in 10 (12 percent) of people in New Zealand reported experiencing a medical, medication, or lab test error in the previous two years, and 12 percent of those who needed to visit a specialist in the previous two years reported that the specialist did not have information about their medical history at the time of the appointment. Just over half (53 percent) reported experiencing a gap in hospital discharge planning in the previous two years (due to any of the following: did not receive a written plan for care, did not have arrangements made for follow-up visits, did not know who to contact with questions, or did not receive instruction about when to seek further care).

According to WHO, in 2007 95.7 percent of births in New Zealand were attended by skilled personnel (for example, physicians, nurses, or midwives). The 2010 immunization rates for 1-year-olds were 93 percent for diphtheria and pertussis (DPT3), 91 percent for measles (MCV), and 89 percent for Hib (Hib3).

A 2011 Commonwealth Fund Survey compared access to health care for "sicker" adults (those 18 and older, in self-reported poor or fair health, who had been treated for a serious illness or injury in the past year or been hospitalized in the past two years) in 11 OECD countries.

This survey found that 26 percent of sicker residents of New Zealand surveyed reported having experienced an access problem related to cost in the previous year; the most common result was having a medical problem but failing to visit the doctor.

Other problems reported include having serious problems paying their medical bills (11 percent), waiting six days or longer for needed care (5 percent), having difficulty getting after-hours care except in an emergency room (40 percent), and experiencing coordination gaps in care (30 percent).

Cost of Drugs

Under the national health care scheme, there is a copayment of NZD 3.00 per prescription ($2.22). In 2009, according to OECD data, pharmaceutical spending per capita in New Zealand was $254 (adjusted for differences in the cost of living). According to Douglas Ball, New Zealand charges the standard value-added tax (VAT) of 12.5 percent for medicines. For most drugs, the dispensing fee is set at NZD 5.16. The wholesale markup is 10 percent, and the pharmacy markup depends on the price of the drug: It is 4 percent for drugs costing less than NZD 150 and 5 percent for higher-priced drugs. Real annual growth in pharmaceutical expenditures in New Zealand grew 3.9 percent from 1997 to 2005, much slower than the 6.2 percent growth of total health expenditure (minus pharmaceutical expenditures) over those years.

Health Care Facilities

In 2002, New Zealand had 6.18 hospital beds per 1,000 population, among the 30 highest ratios in the world. According to WHO, in 2010, New Zealand had 9.93 magnetic resonance imaging (MRI) machines per 1 million population. Most (97 percent) of primary care physicians used electronic medical records in 2009.

Major Health Issues

In 2008, WHO estimated that 5 percent of years of life lost in New Zealand were due to communicable diseases, 77 percent to noncommunicable diseases, and 77 percent to injuries. In 2008, the age-standardized estimate of cancer deaths was 149 per

100,000 for men and 111 per 100,000 for women; for cardiovascular disease and diabetes, 171 per 100,000 for men and 106 per 100,000 for women; and for chronic respiratory disease, 30 per 100,000 for men and 20 per 100,000 for women. In 2007, an estimated 26.5 percent of adults in New Zealand were obese (defined as a body mass index, or BMI, of 30 or greater).

New Zealand ranked sixth among more developed countries in the 2011 Mothers' Index, produced by the international nongovernmental organization (NGO) Save the Children, based on a number of health and social factors relating to women, children, and maternal and child care. The maternal mortality rate (death from any cause related to or aggravated by pregnancy) in New Zealand in 2008 was 14 maternal deaths per 100,000 live births. The infant mortality rate, defined as the number of deaths of infants younger than 1 year, was 4.72 per 1,000 live births as of 2012.

In 2010, tuberculosis incidence was 7.6 per 100,000 population, tuberculosis prevalence 9.3 per 100,000, and deaths due to tuberculosis among human immunodeficiency virus (HIV)-negative people 0.17 per 100,000. As of 2009, an estimated 0.1 percent of adults age 15 to 49 were living with HIV or acquired immune deficiency syndrome (AIDS).

Health Care Personnel

New Zealand has two medical schools, the Faculty of Medicine and Health Science of the University of Auckland and Otago Medical School of the University of Otago. The basic course of training lasts six years, and the degrees awarded are bachelor of medicine and bachelor of surgery. The license to practice medicine is granted by the Medical Council of New Zealand and is automatically given to graduates of Australian medical schools, while applications of physicians from other countries are individually evaluated.

In 2007, New Zealand had 2.38 physicians per 1,000 population, 0.71 pharmaceutical personnel per 1,000, and 10.87 nurses and midwives per 1,000, and in 2001, had 8.12 community and traditional health workers per 1,000. In 2000, 34.5 percent of practicing physicians in New Zealand were trained in another country. Using Fitzhugh Mullan's methodology, New Zealand has an emigration factor of 22.6, representing a high proportion of New Zealand physicians working abroad.

Government Role in Health Care

According to WHO, in 2010, New Zealand spent $14 million on health care, an amount that comes to $3,279 per capita. All health care funding came from domestic sources. More than three-quarters (83 percent) of health care spending was paid for through government expenditures, with the remainder provided through household expenditures (10 percent) and other sources (6 percent). In 2010, New Zealand allocated 20 percent of its total government expenditures to health, and government expenditures on health came to 8 percent of GDP; both figures are in the high range for high-income western Pacific region countries.

Public Health Programs

In 2010, access to improved sources of drinking water was essentially universal in New Zealand. According to the World Higher Education Database (WHED), three universities in New Zealand offer programs in epidemiology or public health: Auckland University of Technology, the University of Auckland, and the University of Otago.

NICARAGUA

Nicaragua is a Central American country, sharing borders with Costa Rica and Honduras and having coastlines on the north Pacific Ocean and the Caribbean Sea. The area of 50,336 square miles (130,370 square kilometers) makes Nicaragua about the size of New York State, and the July 2012 population was estimated at 5.7 million. In 2010, 57 percent of the population lived in urban areas, and the 2010 to 2015 annual rate of urbanization was estimated at 2.0 percent. Managua is the capital. Nicaragua's population growth rate in 2012 was 1.1 percent, the net migration rate negative 3.4 migrants per 1,000 population, the birth rate 19.1 births per 1,000, and the total fertility rate 2.1 children per woman. The United Nations High Commissioner for Refugees (UNHCR) estimated that, in 2010, there were 11 refugees and persons in refugee-like situations in Nicaragua.

Nicaragua became a Spanish colony in the early 16th century and became independent in 1821. Nicaragua was ruled by the hereditary dictatorship of the Somoza family for much of the 20th century;

opposition to this regime culminated in the Nicaraguan revolution that brought the Sandinista movement to power. Nicaragua's infrastructure was seriously damaged by an earthquake in 1972, and this plus the costs of civil conflict seriously damaged the economy. In 2004, 80 percent of Nicaragua's foreign debt was cancelled through the Heavily Indebted Poor Countries initiatives. Nicaragua ranked tied for 134th among 183 countries on the *Corruption Perceptions Index 2011,* with a score of 2.5 (on a scale where 0 indicates highly corrupt and 10 very clean).

In 2011, Nicaragua was classified as a country with medium human development (the second from the lowest of four categories) on the United Nations Development Programme's (UNDP's) Human Development Index (HDI), with a score of 0.589 (on a scale where 1 denotes high development and 0 low development). Life expectancy at birth in 2012 was estimated at 72.18 years, and estimated gross domestic product (GDP) per capita in 2011 was $3,200. In 2010, the Gini Index (a measure of dispersion, in which perfect equality is denoted by 0 and maximum inequality is denoted by 100) for family income was 40.5. According to the World Economic Forum's *Global Gender Gap Index 2011,* Nicaragua ranked 27th out of 135 countries on gender equality with a score of 0.725

(on a scale with a theoretical range of 1 for equality to 0 for inequality and an actual range in 2011 from 0.8530 to 0.4873).

Emergency Health Services

According to the World Health Organization (WHO), as of 2007, Nicaragua had a formal and publicly available emergency care (prehospital care) system, accessible through both regional access numbers and a national access number. Two-thirds of health centers with beds have means of emergency transport.

Insurance

Nicaragua has a social insurance system providing medical benefits and a cash benefits system covering employed people, with the exclusion of the police and military. The system is funded by contributions from workers (2.25 percent of covered earnings with a floor and ceiling on the amount of earnings subject to this tax), employers (6 percent of covered payroll), and the government (0.25 percent of covered earnings). To receive medical benefits, a person must have contributed to the system for at least nine weeks or be a pensioner or a child younger than 12. Medical benefits are provided directly to patients, depending on availability; pregnant women receive maternity care, and old-age pensioners are covered for specified surgeries and illnesses. The maternity benefit is 60 percent of average earnings, paid four weeks before and eight weeks after the due date; a nursing allowance is also paid for six months after birth. The cash sickness benefit is 60 percent of earnings for up to 52 weeks. The Nicaraguan Institute of Social Security administers the program. According to Ke Xu and colleagues, in 2003, 2.0 percent of households in Nicaragua experienced catastrophic health expenditures annually; "catastrophic" was defined as exceeding 40 percent of household income remaining after basic needs were met.

Costs of Hospitalization

No data available.

Access to Health Care

In 2007, an estimated 40 percent of Nicaraguans lacked access to health services, with the proportion much higher (more than 75 percent) for the indigenous and Afro-descended populations. A 2001 survey found that more than 50 percent of the population did not seek care when sick, and the vast majority of

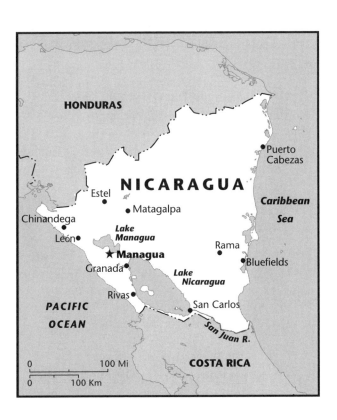

workers were not covered by the social security system. According to the World Health Organization (WHO), in 2007, 74 percent of births in Nicaragua were attended by skilled personnel (for example, physicians, nurses, or midwives), and 78 percent of pregnant women received at least four prenatal care visits. The 2010 immunization rates for 1-year-olds were 98 percent for diphtheria and pertussis (DPT3), 99 percent for measles (MCV), and 98 percent for Hib (Hib3). In 2010, it was estimated that more than 95 percent of persons with advanced human immunodeficiency virus (HIV) infection were receiving antiretroviral therapy in accordance with the 2010 WHO guidelines. According to WHO, in 2010, Nicaragua had 0.18 magnetic resonance imaging (MRI) machines per 1 million population and 0.53 computer tomography (CT) machines per 1 million.

Cost of Drugs

According to WHO, in 2008, the median availability of selected generic drugs in the public sector in Nicaragua was 50.0 percent; in the private sector, the mean availability was 87.1 percent. The median price ratio (comparing the price in Nicaragua to the international reference price) was 5.7 in the private sphere for selected generic medicines, indicating that median prices in the public sphere were almost six times as high as the international reference price.

Health Care Facilities

The Ministry of Health operates a network of 32 hospitals and 1,039 outpatient care units, while a 2001 survey identified 203 private health care establishments, including five hospitals. As of 2010, according to WHO, Nicaragua had 15.38 health posts per 100,000 population, 2.73 health centers per 100,000, 0.45 district or rural hospitals per 100,000, 0.45 provincial hospitals per 100,000, and 0.10 specialized hospitals per 100,000. In 2006, Nicaragua had 0.90 hospital beds per 1,000 population.

Major Health Issues

In 2008, WHO estimated that 33 percent of years of life lost in Nicaragua were due to communicable diseases, 49 percent to noncommunicable diseases, and 17 percent to injuries. In 2008, the age-standardized estimate of cancer deaths was 91 per 100,000 for men and 101 per 100,000 for women; for cardiovascular disease and diabetes, 248 per 100,000 for men and 221 per 100,000 for women; and for chronic respiratory disease, 38 per 100,000 for men and 55 per 100,000 for women. Nicaragua's maternal mortality rate (death from any cause related to or aggravated by pregnancy) was estimated in 2008 as 100 maternal deaths per 100,000 live births. The infant mortality rate, defined as the number of deaths of infants younger than 1 year, was estimated at 21.86 per 1,000 live births as of 2012. In 2010, tuberculosis incidence was 42.0 per 100,000 population, tuberculosis prevalence 47.0 per 100,000, and deaths due to tuberculosis among HIV-negative people 2.60 per 100,000. As of 2009, an estimated 0.2 percent of adults age 15 to 49 were living with HIV or AIDS.

Health Care Personnel

In 2006, WHO identified Nicaragua as one of 57 countries with a critical deficit in the supply of skilled health workers. Nicaragua has four medical schools: the Facultad de Ciencias Medicas of the Universidad Nacional Autonoma de Nicaragua in Leon (began offering instruction in 1893), Facultad de Ciencias Medicas of the Universidad Nacional Autonoma de Nicaragua in Managua (1980), the Facultad de Ciencias of the Universidad American (1994), and the Facultad de Medicina of the Universidad Cátolica Redemptoiris Mater in Managua (2004). The basic medical course lasts six to seven years, and the degree granted is Doctor en Medicine y Cirugia (doctor of medicine and surgery). In 2003, Nicaragua had 0.37 physicians per 1,000 population, 0.04 dentistry personnel per 1,000, and 1.07 nurses and midwives per 1,000.

Government Role in Health Care

According to WHO, in 2010, Nicaragua spent $599 million on health care, an amount that comes to $103 per capita. Most (85 percent) of health care funding came from domestic sources, with 15 percent coming from overseas sources. Just over half (53 percent) of health care spending was paid for through government expenditures, with the remainder provided through household expenditures (43 percent) and other sources (3 percent). In 2010, Nicaragua allocated 17 percent of its total government expenditures to health, and government expenditures on health care came to 5 percent of GDP; both figures are in the high range for lower-middle-income countries in the Americas region.

Public Health Programs

In 2010, 52 percent of the population of Nicaragua had access to improved sanitation facilities (37 percent in rural areas and 63 percent in urban), and 85 percent had access to improved sources of drinking water (68 percent in rural areas and 98 percent in urban).

NIGER

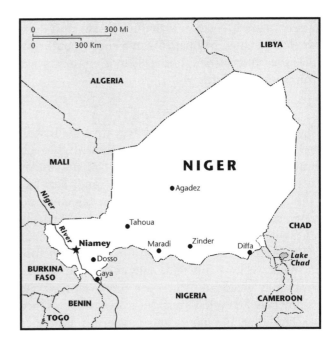

Niger is a landlocked western African country sharing borders with Algeria, Benin, Burkina Faso, Chad, Libya, Mali, and Nigeria. The area of 490,350 square miles (1,270,000 square kilometers) makes Niger the 22nd largest country in the world (about twice the size of Texas), and the July 2012 population was estimated at 17.1 million. In 2010, 17 percent of the population lived in urban areas, and the 2010 to 2015 annual rate of urbanization was estimated at 4.7 percent. Niamey is the capital and largest city (with a 2009 population estimated at 1.0 million). The population growth rate in 2012 was 3.6 percent (the third-highest in the world), the net migration rate 0.0 migrants per 1,000 population, the birth rate 50.1 births per 1,000 (the highest in the world), and the total fertility rate 7.5 children per woman (the highest in the world). The United Nations High Commissioner for Refugees (UNHCR) estimated that, in 2010, there were 314 refugees and persons in refugee-like situations in Niger.

A former French colony, Niger became independent in 1960. The country experienced military and single-party rule until 1993, when multiparty elections were held. Since then, Niger has enjoyed periods of democracy and periods of violent overthrow, including coups in 1996, 1999, and 2010. According to the Ibrahim Index, in 2011, Niger ranked 39th among 53 African countries in terms of governance performance, with a score of 44 (out of 100). Niger ranked tied for 134th among 183 countries on the *Corruption Perceptions Index 2011*, with a score of 2.5 (on a scale where 0 indicates highly corrupt and 10 very clean).

In 2011, Niger was classified as a country with low human development (the lowest of four categories) on the United Nations Development Programme's (UNDP's) Human Development Index (HDI), with a score of 0.295 (on a scale where 1 denotes high development and 0 low development). In 2011, the International Food Policy Research Institute (IFPRI) classified Niger as a country with an "alarming" hunger problem with a Global Hunger Index (GHI) score of 23.0, the highest in the world (where 0 reflects no hunger and higher scores more hunger), and in November 2011, the World Food Programme estimated that 5.4 million people in Niger were food insecure, including 1.3 million who were severely food insecure. Life expectancy at birth in 2012 was estimated at 53.80 years, among the 20 lowest in the world, and estimated gross domestic product (GDP) per capita in 2011 was $800, among the 10 lowest in the world. In 2007, the Gini Index (a measure of dispersion, in which perfect equality is denoted by 0 and maximum inequality is denoted by 100) for family income was 34.0.

Emergency Health Services

According to the World Health Organization (WHO), as of 2007, Niger had a formal and publicly available emergency care (prehospital care) system, accessible through a national access number. Doctors Without Borders (Médecins Sans Frontières, or MSF) began working in Niger in 1985 and had 1,599 staff members in the country at the close of 2010. During the 2010 nutritional crisis, caused by a poor harvest in 2009, MSF treated more than 148,000 children for malnutrition. In addition, MSF runs a preventive malnutrition program in which children at risk for malnutrition are provided with supplementary food. In Zinder, Maradi, and Tahoua, MSF treated more than 216,330 children for malaria and organized meningitis vaccination campaigns in

Zinder, Maradi, Agadez, Madaoua, Dosso, and Boboye. MSF treated 249 patients in a cholera outbreak in Zinder and cleaned four wells to keep the disease from spreading further.

Insurance

Niger has a social insurance system covering maternity benefits only. The system is funded through employer contributions (8.4 percent of payroll) and is part of the same system that provides Family Benefits. Employers are required to provide certain medical services, but there are no statutory medical benefits other than maternity care. The cash maternity benefit is 100 percent of earnings, paid for six weeks before and eight weeks after the due date; an additional three weeks may be added if there are complications. The Family Benefits system provides a prenatal allowance of CFAR 1,000 per month and a maternity allowance paid as a lump sum of CFAR 10,000, and a birth allowance of CFAR 10,000 is paid for the first three births; receipt of these benefits requires that the woman undergo prescribed medical exams. The Family Benefits system also pays a family allowance of CFAR 1,000 per month per child until the child is 14 (extended to 18 for an apprentice and 21 if disabled or a student). The system is administered by the National Social Security Fund under the general supervision of the Ministry of Public Administration and Labor.

Costs of Hospitalization

No data available.

Access to Health Care

According to WHO, in 2006, 33 percent of births in Niger were attended by skilled personnel (for example, physicians, nurses, or midwives), and 15 percent of pregnant women received at least four prenatal care visits. The 2010 immunization rates for 1-year-olds were 70 percent for diphtheria and pertussis (DPT3), 71 percent for measles (MCV), and 70 percent for Hib (Hib3). In 2010, an estimated 29 percent of persons with advanced human immunodeficiency virus (HIV) infection were receiving antiretroviral therapy in accordance with the 2010 WHO guidelines.

Cost of Drugs

Total pharmaceutical expenses in 2009 in Niger came to XOF 32,747 million ($70.3 million), or XOF 2,153.30 ($4.60) per capita. Pharmaceutical expenditures constituted 32.9 percent of total health spending,

and 1.3 percent of GDP. Most pharmaceutical expenditures were paid for privately, with public expenditures forming 5.6 percent of the total. Niger's National Medicines Policy (NMP) includes selection of drugs for placement on the Essential Medicines List (EML), and the right to access essential medicines and medical technologies is specified in national legislation as part of the right to health.

Medications are provided for free to children under the age of 5, pregnant women, and the poor. Medications to treat tuberculosis and human immunodeficiency virus and acquired immune deficiency syndrome (HIV/AIDS) are provided for free, as are the vaccines included on WHO's Expanded Programme for Immunization (EPI) list.

Health Care Facilities

As of 2010, according to WHO, Niger had 16.07 health posts per 100,000 population, 5.71 health centers per 100,000, 0.50 district or rural hospitals per 100,000, 0.07 provincial hospitals per 100,000, and 0.06 specialized hospitals per 100,000. In 2005, Niger had 0.31 hospital beds per 1,000 population, one of the 10 lowest rates in the world.

Major Health Issues

In 2008, WHO estimated that 90 percent of years of life lost in Niger were due to communicable diseases, 8 percent to noncommunicable diseases, and 3 percent to injuries. In 2008, the age-standardized estimate of cancer deaths was 74 per 100,000 for men and 89 per 100,000 for women; for cardiovascular disease and diabetes, 351 per 100,000 for men and 412 per 100,000 for women; and for chronic respiratory disease, 95 per 100,000 for men and 56 per 100,000 for women. In 2008, the age-standardized death rate from malaria was 79.6 per 100,000 population, the 10th-highest in the world. In 2010, tuberculosis incidence was 185.0 per 100,000 population, tuberculosis prevalence 33.0 per 100,000, and deaths due to tuberculosis among HIV-negative people 37.00 per 100,000. As of 2009, an estimated 0.8 percent of adults age 15 to 49 were living with HIV or AIDS.

Compared to other countries at a similar level of development, Niger ranked next to last among 43 least-developed countries on the 2011 Mothers' Index, produced by the international nongovernmental organization (NGO) Save the Children, based on a number of health and social factors relating to women, children, and maternal and child care. Niger's maternal mortality rate (death from any cause related to or aggravated by pregnancy) has been quite high by global standards, estimated at 820 maternal deaths per 100,000 live births as of 2008. A 2006 survey estimated the prevalence of female genital mutilation at 2.2 percent. The infant mortality rate, defined as the number of deaths of infants younger than 1 year, is second-highest in the world at 109.98 per 1,000 live births as of 2012. Child malnutrition is a serious problem: In 2006, 36.9 percent of children under age 5 were underweight (defined as 2 kilograms [kg] below standard weight-for-age at age 1, 3 kg below for ages 2 to 3, and 4 kg below for ages 4 to 5), one of the highest rates in the world.

Health Care Personnel

Niger has one medical school, the Faculté des Sciences de la Santé of the University of Niamey, which began offering instruction in 1974. The course of training lasts seven years, and the degree awarded is Docteur en Médecine (Diplôme d'État), or doctor of medicine (state diploma). In 2008, Niger had 0.02 physicians per 1,000 population, 0.02 laboratory health workers per 1,000, 0.19 health management and support workers per 1,000, and 0.14 nurses and midwives per 1,000. Michael Clemens and Bunilla Petterson estimate that 9 percent of Niger-born physicians and 2 percent of Niger-born nurses are working in one of nine developed countries, primarily in France (physicians) and France and the United States (nurses).

Government Role in Health Care

The right to health is recognized in national legislation. Niger has a National Health Policy (NHP), written in 2002, and a National Medicines Policy (NMP), written in 1995; the NMP covers selection of essential medicines; financing, pricing, purchase, distribution, and regulation of drugs; pharmacovigilance; rational usage of medicines; human resource development; research; evaluation and monitoring; and traditional medicine.

According to WHO, in 2010, Niger spent $284 million on health care, an amount that comes to $18 per capita. More than two-thirds (71 percent) of health care funding came from domestic sources, with 29 percent coming from overseas sources. Just over half (51 percent) of health care spending was paid for through government expenditures, with the remainder provided through household expenditures (41 percent) and other sources (8 percent). In 2010, Niger allocated 11 percent of its total government expenditures to health, and government expenditures on health came to 3 percent of GDP; both figures are in the median range for low-income African countries. In 2009, according to WHO, official development assistance (ODA) for health in Niger came to $4.88 per capita.

Public Health Programs

According to WHO, in 2008, Niger had 0.01 environmental and public health workers per 1,000 population. In 2010, only 9 percent of the population had access to improved sanitation facilities (4 percent in rural areas and 34 percent in urban), and 49 percent had access to improved sources of drinking water (39 percent in rural areas and 10 percent in urban). According to the World Higher Education Database (WHED), one university in Niger offers programs in epidemiology or public health: Abdou Moumouni University of Niamey.

NIGERIA

Nigeria is a west African country, sharing borders with Benin, Cameroon, Chad, and Niger and having a coastline on the Gulf of Guinea. The area of 356,669 square miles (923,768 square kilometers) makes Nigeria the 32nd-largest county in the world (about twice the size of California). Nigeria is the

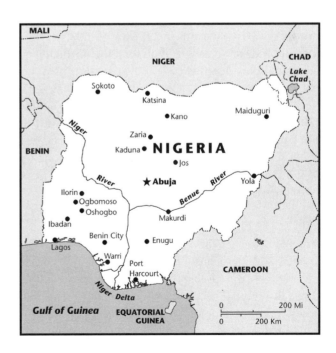

seventh-most populous country in the world, and the most populous in Africa, with an estimated population of 170.1 million as of July 2012. Abuja is the capital and Lagos the largest city (with a 2009 population estimated at 10.2 million). The population growth rate in 2012 was 2.6 percent (the 27th highest in the world), the net migration rate negative 0.2 migrants per 1,000 population, the birth rate 39.2 births per 1,000 (the 14th highest in the world), and the total fertility rate 5.4 children per woman (the 13th highest in the world).

Nigeria became a British protectorate in 1901 and became independent in 1960. Nigeria has experienced a series of dictatorships and military governments along with periods of democracy; the elections in April 2007 constituted the first civilian-to-civilian transfer of power since independence. According to the Ibrahim Index, in 2011, Nigeria ranked 41st among 53 African countries in terms of governance performance, with a score of 41 (out of 100). Nigeria ranked tied for 143rd among 183 countries on the *Corruption Perceptions Index 2011*, with a score of 2.4 (on a scale where 0 indicates highly corrupt and 10 very clean).

In 2011, Nigeria was classified as a country with low human development (the lowest of four categories) on the United Nations Development Programme's (UNDP's) Human Development Index (HDI), with a score of 0.459 (on a scale where 1 denotes high development and 0 low development). Life expectancy at birth in 2012 was estimated at 52.05 years, among the 20 lowest in the world, and estimated gross domestic product (GDP) per capita in 2011 was $2,600. In 2003, the Gini Index (a measure of dispersion, in which perfect equality is denoted by 0 and maximum inequality is denoted by 100) for family income was 43.7. According to the World Economic Forum's *Global Gender Gap Index 2011*, Nigeria ranked 120th out of 135 countries on gender equality, with a score of 0.601 (on a scale with a theoretical range of 1 for equality to 0 for inequality and an actual range in 2011 from 0.8530 to 0.4873).

Emergency Health Services

According to the World Health Organization (WHO), as of 2007, Nigeria had a formal and publicly available emergency care (prehospital care) system accessible through regional access numbers but not a national access number. Doctors Without Borders (Médecins Sans Frontières, or MSF) began working in Nigeria

in 1996 and had 954 staff members in the country at the close of 2010. After flooding in Sokoto (northeast Nigeria), MSF treated more than 9,000 patients for cholera and also treated victims of outbreaks of measles and meningitis. In Lagos, MSF provides a health center and mobile clinics providing emergency, reproductive, and general health care. In northern Nigeria, MSF provides maternal and child health care, including treatment for child malnutrition and has provided surgery for fistula repair. In Zamfara, MSF treated more than 400 children for lead poisoning and educated villagers about the dangers of lead contamination in small-scale gold mining.

Insurance

Firms with 10 or more workers are entitled to medical benefits financed by salary contributions; public sector employees are covered by a similar plan. Employers are required to provide employees with maternity leave for six weeks before and after the due date of at least 50 percent of wages and 12 days of paid sick leave. According to Nigeria's *Pharmaceutical Country Report*, about one-third (31.3 percent) of Nigerians are covered by a private health plan and (0.8 percent) by a public plan. Limited medical care in Nigeria is also available through public clinics and hospitals, but according to a 2004 survey sponsored by WHO, due to the low quality of care, many Nigerians prefer to use the private care system; only 38 percent of households reported using the public care system.

Costs of Hospitalization

No data available.

Access to Health Care

A 2004 survey conducted by WHO and Health Action International found that generic medicines were more available in the Nigerian public sector than brand-name medicines (21.4 percent versus 1.2 percent), and availability was higher for both in the private sector (30.7 percent availability for generics and 14.8 percent for brand names). As of 2004, medicines were largely paid for out of pocket, creating a burden in particular on low-income Nigerians.

According to WHO, in 2008, 38.9 percent of births in Nigeria were attended by skilled personnel (for example, physicians, nurses, or midwives), and 45 percent of pregnant women received at least four prenatal care visits. The 2010 immunization rates for 1-year-olds were 69 percent for diphtheria and pertussis

(DPT3) and 71 percent for measles (MCV). In 2010, an estimated 26 percent of persons with advanced human immunodeficiency virus (HIV) infection were receiving antiretroviral therapy in accordance with the 2010 WHO guidelines. In 2010, 14 percent of pregnant women tested positive for HIV. The mother-to-child transmission rate for HIV in 2010 was estimated at 33 percent, and in 2009, 4.1 percent of deaths to children under 5 were attributed to HIV.

Cost of Drugs

Total pharmaceutical expenditures in 2007 in Nigeria came to NGN 72.2 billion ($573.9 million) for per capita pharmaceutical expenditures of NGN 488 ($3.90). Pharmaceutical expenditures accounted for 5.4 percent of total health expenditures and 0.4 percent of GDP. Nigeria has a National Medicines Policy (NMP) covering topics such as selecting medicines for the Essential Medicines List (EML) and the financing, distribution, and regulation of medicines. Pricing of medicines is not covered by any law or regulatory provision, and the government has no price monitoring system.

Nigeria has no national program to provide medications for free to certain sectors of the population, but some states do offer medications free to groups such as children under 5, pregnant women, the elderly, and the poor. The public health system provides free medications to treat certain conditions, including malaria, tuberculosis, and human immunodeficiency virus and acquired immune deficiency syndrome (HIV/AIDS); the vaccines listed on WHO's Expanded Programme on Immunization (EPI) list are also provided for free. Some private insurance plans offer medication coverage but are not required to cover the medicines included on the EML.

According to a 2004 survey conducted by WHO and Health Action International, prices for drugs in Nigeria are high relative to international reference levels. Median prices for a market basket of pharmaceuticals were far above the national reference price: For the public sector, the median price was more than three times as high for generics and four times as high for brand-name drugs, while in the private sector, the median price was more than four times as high for generics and more than 14 times as high for brand-name drugs. Generic medication (co-trimaxazole) to treat a child's respiratory infection represented about 1 day's wages for the lowest-paid government worker (0.5 day's wages if purchased in the public sector and 0.6 in the private), while the brand-name medicine equivalent cost 1.3 or 1.5 days' wages in the public and private sectors, respectively. Availability was also a problem: Less than half (46 percent) of a basket of essential medicines were found in the health care facilities surveyed.

Health Care Facilities

In 2004, Nigeria had 0.53 hospital beds per 1,000 population, one of the 20 lowest rates in the world.

Major Health Issues

In 2008, WHO estimated that 81 percent of years of life lost in Nigeria were due to communicable diseases, 14 percent to noncommunicable diseases, and 5 percent to injuries. In 2008, the age-standardized estimate of cancer deaths was 89 per 100,000 for men and 99 per 100,000 for women; for cardiovascular disease and diabetes, 436 per 100,000 for men and 476 per 100,000 for women; and for chronic respiratory disease, 119 per 100,000 for men and 72 per 100,000 for women.

In 2008, the age-standardized death rate from malaria was 79.3 per 100,000 population. In 2010, tuberculosis incidence was 133.0 per 100,000 population, tuberculosis prevalence 199.0 per 100,000, and deaths due to tuberculosis among HIV-negative people 21.00 per 100,000. An estimated 2.2 percent of new tuberculosis cases and 9.4 percent of retreatment cases are multidrug resistant. WHO estimates that the case detection rate in 2010 was 4 percent. As of 2009, an estimated 3.6 percent of adults age 15 to 49, and an estimated 3.3 million people in Nigeria, were living with HIV or AIDS, the second-largest number in the world. Polio remains endemic in Nigeria, and it is the only country in the world in which all three serotypes continue to be transmitted. Most cases are in the northern region of the country, where some leaders have opposed vaccination campaigns. In 2011, 43 cases of polio were reported versus 11 in 2010.

Compared to other countries at a similar level of development, Nigeria ranked next to last among 80 less-developed countries on the 2011 Mothers' Index, produced by the international nongovernmental organization (NGO) Save the Children, based on a number of health and social factors relating to women, children, and maternal and child care. Nigeria's maternal mortality rate (death from any cause related to or aggravated by pregnancy) is the ninth-highest in the world, estimated at 850 per 100,000 live births as of 2008. A 2008 survey estimated the prevalence of female genital mutilation at 29.6 percent. The infant mortality rate, defined as the number of deaths of infants younger than 1 year, has also been also high, at 74.36 per 1,000 live births as of 2012. In 2008, 26.8 percent of children under age 5 were underweight (defined as 2 kilograms [kg] below standard weight-for-age at age 1, 3 kg below for ages 2 to 3, and 4 kg below for ages 4 to 5).

Health Care Personnel

Nigeria has 16 medical schools. The course of training for a basic medical school lasts five to six years, and graduates must work for one year in a rotating internship in an accredited hospital before receiving a medical license. The degrees awarded are bachelor of medicine and bachelor of surgery. Nigerian medical graduates must serve in the National Year Service after graduation. Graduates of foreign medical schools must pass an exam and work as an intern in Nigeria for one year. In 2008, Nigeria had 0.40 physicians per 1,000 population, 0.13 pharmaceutical personnel per 1,000, 0.17 laboratory health workers per 1,000, 2.51 health management and support workers per 1,000, 0.03 dentistry personnel per 1,000, 0.14 community and traditional health workers per 1,000, and 1.61 nurses and midwives per 1,000. Michael Clemens and Bunilla Petterson estimate that 14 percent of Nigeria-born physicians and 12 percent of Nigeria-born nurses are working in one of nine developed countries, primarily in the United States and the United Kingdom.

Government Role in Health Care

National legislation recognizes the right to health. Nigeria has a National Health Policy (NHP), updated in 2004, and a National Medicines Policy (NMP), updated in 2005; however, there is no implementation plan for the NMP. According to WHO, in 2010, Nigeria spent $9.9 million on health care, an amount that comes to $63 per capita. Most (91 percent) of health care funding came from domestic sources, with 9 percent coming from overseas sources. More than half (59 percent) of health care spending was paid for through household expenditures, with the remainder provided through government expenditures (38 percent) and other sources (3 percent). In 2010, Nigeria allocated 4 percent of its total government expenditures to health, and government expenditures on health came to 2 percent of GDP; both figures are in the low range for lower-middle-income African countries. In 2009, according to WHO, official development assistance (ODA) for health in Nigeria came to $6.88 per capita.

Nigeria is a member of the World Trade Organization (WTO) and has not implemented any of the Trade-Related Aspects of Intellectual Property Rights (TRIPS) flexibilities and safeguards. Nigeria requires registration (marketing authorization) for all pharmaceutical products sold in the country but waives the registration process for donated health products; as of 2010, Nigeria had 1,870 pharmaceutical products registered.

Public Health Programs

The National Primary Health Care Development Agency, located in Abuja and headed by Dr. Emmanuel Abanida, was founded in 1992 to promote and implement high-quality primary health care, including developing community infrastructure and promoting childhood immunization. The Nigerian Institute of Medical Research (NIMR), located in Yaba (a suburb of Nigeria), is headed by Innocent Ujah, the primary coordinator of health research for Nigeria. The NIMR has five research divisions: biochemistry, clinical sciences, microbiology, molecular biology and genetics, and public health and is focused on research into diseases of public significance and improving health care delivery.

According to WHO, in 2008, Nigeria had 0.03 environmental and public health workers per 1,000 population. In 2010, 31 percent of the population had access to improved sanitation facilities (27 percent in rural areas and 35 percent in urban), and 58 percent had access to improved sources of drinking water (43 percent in rural areas and 74 percent in urban). According to the World Higher Education Database (WHED), 12 universities in Nigeria offer programs in epidemiology or public health.

NORTH KOREA

North Korea is a country in northeastern Asia, sharing borders with China, South Korea, and Russia and having coastlines on the East China Sea and the Sea of Japan. The area of 46,540 square miles (120,538 square kilometers) makes North Korea about the size of Mississippi, and the July 2012 population was estimated at 24.6 million. In 2010, 60 percent of the population lived in urban areas, and the 2010 to 2015 annual rate of urbanization was estimated at 0.6 percent. Pyongyang is the capital. The population growth rate in 2012 was 0.4 percent, the net migration rate 0.0 migrants per 1,000 population, the birth rate 14.51 births per 1,000, and the total fertility rate 2.0 children per woman.

The Korean Peninsula was annexed by Japan in 1910, and after World War II, the northern part of the peninsula was controlled by the Soviet Union, and the southern part by the United States; in 1948, North Korea became an independent state. Although the Korean War (1950–53) ended with an armistice, North and South Korea remain hostile toward each other. North Korea has been a single-party state since independence and was ruled by Kim Il-sung from 1948 to 1994, by his son Kim Jong-Il from 1994 to 2011, and by Kim Jong-Il's son Kim Jong-un since 2011. The government is considered extremely corrupt, ranking second-lowest among 183 countries on the *Corruption Perceptions Index 2011,* with a score of 1.0 (on a scale where 0 indicates highly corrupt and 10 very clean). North Korea is a secretive country, and up-to-date information on health and safety matters is often difficult to obtain. The infrastructure is underdeveloped, and shortages of food and fuel are common; in 1995, international aid was necessary to prevent widespread famine.

The per capita gross domestic product (GDP) in 2011 was estimated at $1,800 per capita, among the lowest in Asia, and life expectancy at birth in 2012 was estimated at 69.20 years. According to the World Food Programme, as of 2011, about 16 million people (two-thirds of the population) of North Korea are chronically food insecure.

Emergency Health Services

In urban areas, large health care centers often have ambulances, but as of 2010, they are seldom used due to fuel shortages, according to a 2010 report by Amnesty International.

Insurance

Theoretically, North Korea provides free health care for all through a network of government-run health care facilities. However, a 2010 Amnesty International report said that care was often substandard (hospitals lacking essential medicines, hypodermic needles

being reused with sterilization, surgery performed without anesthesia) and that unofficial payments (in cash or goods, for example, alcohol or cigarettes) were often required in order for patients to receive medical services.

Costs of Hospitalization

Although hospital care is theoretically provided to North Koreans without charge, a 2010 Amnesty International report claims that, in reality, patients have to pay for care, either with cash or with goods such as cigarettes or alcohol.

Access to Health Care

North Korea provides health care through a system of state-run facilities. However, a 2010 report from Amnesty International stated that the care provided was often not up to modern expectations and that patients were required to pay for services. Even in the best of circumstances, the necessity to travel to a health facility for care can prove to be an insurmountable barrier. Theoretically, the North Korean government provides transportation for health care or reimburses patients for their costs, but a 2010 Amnesty International report says this does not happen in practice. Despite these difficulties, North Korea

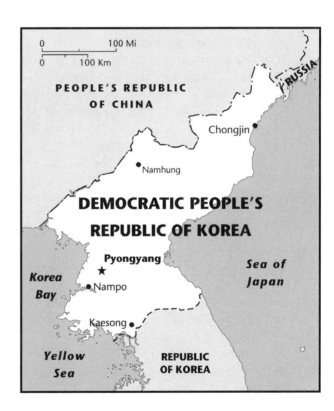

has some accomplishments in terms of the delivery of essential health services. According to the World Health Organization (WHO), in 2004, 97 percent of births in North Korea were attended by skilled personnel (for example, physicians, nurses, or midwives). In 2004, 95 percent of pregnant women received at least four prenatal care visits. The 2010 immunization rates for 1-year-olds were 93 percent for diphtheria and pertussis (DPT3), 99 percent for measles (MCV), and 63 percent for Hib (Hib3).

Cost of Drugs

Prescribed medicines in North Korea are supposed to be provided without charge through clinics and hospitals, but according to a 2010 report by Amnesty International, medicines are often in short supply, and patients often must pay in order to receive them. Unofficially, medicines imported from China or South Korea are sometimes sold in the marketplaces, including addictive drugs such as morphine.

Health Care Facilities

As of 2010, according to WHO, North Korea had 25.72 health posts per 100,000 population, 4.00 health centers per 100,000, 6.47 district or rural hospitals per 100,000, and 0.55 provincial hospitals per 100,000. In 2002, North Korea had 13.20 hospital beds per 1,000 population, the second-highest ratio in the world.

Major Health Issues

In 2008, WHO estimated that 39 percent of years of life lost in North Korea were due to communicable diseases, 52 percent to noncommunicable diseases, and 10 percent to injuries. In 2008, the age-standardized estimate of cancer deaths was 123 per 100,000 for men and 98 per 100,000 for women; for cardiovascular disease and diabetes, 345 per 100,000 for men and 262 per 100,000 for women; and for chronic respiratory disease, 79 per 100,000 for men and 47 per 100,000 for women.

The health status of many people in North Korea is compromised by the country's recurring food shortages. North Korea's maternal mortality rate (death from any cause related to or aggravated by pregnancy) was estimated in 2008 as 250 maternal deaths per 100,000 live births. The infant mortality rate, defined as the number of deaths of infants younger than 1 year, was estimated at 26.21 per 1,000 live births in 2012. In 2004, 20.6 percent of children under age 5 were underweight (defined as 2 kilograms [kg] below

standard weight-for-age at age 1, 3 kg below for ages 2 to 3, and 4 kg below for ages 4 to 5). In 2010, tuberculosis incidence was 345.0 per 100,000 population, tuberculosis prevalence 399.0 per 100,000, and deaths due to tuberculosis among human immunodeficiency virus (HIV)-negative people 23.00 per 100,000. In 2010, 13,393 cases of malaria were reported.

Health Care Personnel

North Korea has 10 medical schools. The basic course of training lasts six years, after which the degree of doctor is awarded. In 2003, North Korea had 3.29 physicians per 1,000 population, 0.60 pharmaceutical personnel per 1,000, 0.04 laboratory health workers per 1,000, 0.37 dentistry personnel per 1,000, and 4.12 nurses and midwives per 1,000.

Government Role in Health Care

In 2009, according to WHO, official development assistance (ODA) for health in North Korea came to $0.35 per capita, extremely low by international standards.

Public Health Programs

In 2010, 80 percent of the North Korean population had access to improved sanitation facilities (71 percent in rural areas and 86 percent in urban), and 98 percent had access to improved sources of drinking water (97 percent in rural areas and 99 percent in urban). According to WHO, in 2003, North Korea had 0.12 environmental and public health workers per 1,000 population. According to the World Higher Education Database (WHED), no university in North Korea offers programs in epidemiology or public health.

NORWAY

Norway is a northern European country, sharing borders with Finland, Sweden, and Russia and having coastlines on the North Sea and north Atlantic Oceans. The area of 125,021 square miles (323,802 square kilometers) makes Norway about twice the size of New Mexico, and the July 2012 population was estimated at 4.7 million. In 2010, 79 percent of the population lived in urban areas, and the 2010 to 2015 annual rate of urbanization was estimated at 1.2 percent. Oslo is the capital and largest city (with a 2009 population estimated at 875,000). The population growth rate in 2012 was 0.3 percent, the net migration rate 1.7 migrants per 1,000 population, the birth rate 10.8 births per 1,000, and the total fertility rate 1.8 children per woman.

Norway became independent from Sweden in 1905. Oil and natural gas was discovered in 1960, boosting Norway's economy. The government has a reputation for transparency and honesty, ranking sixth among 183 countries on the *Corruption Perceptions Index 2011,* with a score of 9.0 (on a scale where 0 indicates highly corrupt and 10 very clean). Norway ranked first in 2011 on the United Nations Development Programme's (UNDP's) Human Development Index (HDI), with a score of 0.943 (on a scale where 1 denotes high development and 0 low development). Life expectancy at birth in 2012 was estimated at 80.32 years, among the highest in the world, and per capita gross domestic product (GDP) in 2011 in Norway was estimated at $53,300, among the highest in the world. Income distribution is among the most equal in the world: In 2008 the Gini Index (a measure of dispersion, in which perfect equality is denoted by 0 and maximum inequality is denoted by 100) for family income was 25.0. Gender equality is also high in Norway: According to the World Economic Forum's *Global Gender Gap Index 2011,* Norway ranked second out of 135 countries on gender equality with a score of 0.840 (on a scale with a theoretical range of 1 for equality to 0 for inequality and an actual range in 2011 from 0.8530 to 0.4873).

Emergency Health Services

According to the World Health Organization (WHO), as of 2007, Norway had a formal and publicly available emergency care (prehospital care) system accessible through a national access number.

Insurance

Norway has a national health service with universal coverage paid for out of general tax revenues. It is legal to buy private insurance, but less than 5 percent do; private insurance is usually provided by employers. The health service includes some cost sharing (for example, for prescription drugs, physician consultations, and lab tests), and in 2007, about 15 percent of total spending on health care came from out-of-pocket payments. However, there is a cap on out-of-pocket expenses of NOK 1,880 ($339), and there are some exemptions on cost sharing for young children, pregnant women, and disabled persons. Primary care is paid for through a mix of fee-for-service and capitation payments, while hospital payments are handled through a combination of global budgets and case-based payments; hospital payments include physician costs. Patients are required to register with a general practice physician. According to Ke Xu and colleagues, in 2003, 0.3 percent of households in Norway experienced catastrophic health expenditures annually; "catastrophic" was defined as exceeding 40 percent of household income remaining after basic needs were met.

Costs of Hospitalization

According to Organisation for Economic Co-operation and Development (OECD) data, in 2009, hospital spending per capita in Norway was $1,800 (adjusted for differences in the cost of living), and hospital spending per discharge came to $10,441 in 2011. The average length of stay in acute care was 4.6 days (in 2008), and there were 177 hospital discharges per 1,000 population.

In 2008, according to the OECD, hospital spending in Norway represented 38.2 percent of total spending on health, and per capita spending was $1,613; hospitals were paid based on a prospective global budget (60 percent) and payment per procedure (40 percent).

Access to Health Care

In 2009, according to OECD data, people in Norway had an average of 4.3 physician visits. In 2010, just

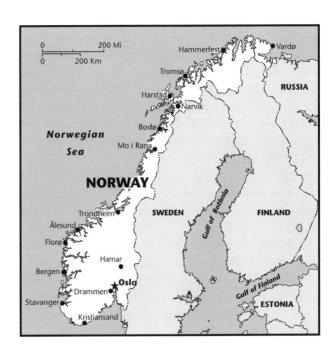

Selected Health Indicators: Norway Compared With the Organisation for Economic Co-operation and Development (OECD) Country Average

	Norway	OECD average (2010 or nearest year)
Total expenditure on health (percent of GDP), 2011	9.2	9.5
Total expenditure on health (per capita, USD purchasing power parity), 2011	5,235.6	3,265
Public expenditure on health (per capita, USD purchasing power parity), 2011	4,483.9	2,377.8
Public expenditure on health (percent total expenditure on health), 2011	85.6	72.2
Doctor consultations (number per capita), 2009	5.2	6.4
Hospital beds (per 1,000 population), 2010	3.3	4.9
Curative (acute) care beds (per 1,000 population), 2010	2.4	3.4

Source: OECD Health Data 2012 (Organisation for Economic Co-operation and Development, 2012).

under half (45 percent) reported that, when sick, they were able to get a medical appointment the same day or the next day. The same percentage (45 percent) reported it was very or somewhat difficult to get medical care after usual office hours. For those who needed particular types of care, about one-third (34 percent) reported they waited two or more months to see a specialist (of those who needed to see a specialist in the prior two years), about one in 10 (11 percent) reported waiting four or more months for elective surgery (of those who required elective surgery in the prior two years), and the same percentage (11 percent) reported they had experienced an access barrier due to cost in the previous two years; an "access barrier" was defined as failing to fill or refill a prescription, failing to visit a physician, or failing to get recommended care. In 2010, just over one in five (21 percent) of Norwegians reported experiencing a medical, medication, or lab test error in the previous two years. The 2010 immunization rates for 1-year-olds were 93 percent for diphtheria and pertussis (DPT3), 93 percent for measles (MCV), and 94 percent for Hib (Hib3).

A 2011 Commonwealth Fund Survey compared access to health care for "sicker" adults (those 18 and older, in self-reported poor or fair health, who had been treated for a serious illness or injury in the past year or been hospitalized in the past two years) in 11 OECD countries. This survey found that 14 percent of sicker Norwegians surveyed reported having experienced an access problem related to cost in the previous year; the most common result was having a medical problem and failing to visit the doctor. Other problems reported include having serious problems paying their medical bills (7 percent), waiting six days or longer for needed care (14 percent), having difficulty getting after-hours care except in an emergency room (35 percent), and experiencing coordination gaps in care (43 percent).

Cost of Drugs

The national health care system in Norway includes copayments for prescription drugs up to a maximum of $85; however, some are exempt from these copayments, including children age 6 or younger, pregnant women, and those on disability pensions. The price for a specific drug is set at the average of the three lowest market prices for the drug in comparison countries in western Europe and Scandinavia, and new drugs expected to increase costs must be approved by the Norwegian parliament before being eligible for reimbursement. Norway encourages the use of generic drugs by setting their prices as a decreasing percentage of the prices for the comparable branded drugs so that the cost of the generic drugs decreases over time. In 2009, according to OECD data, pharmaceutical spending per capita in Norway was $391 (adjusted for differences in the cost of living).

According to Douglas Ball, Norway has kept its drug costs lower than those of many OECD countries: Norway spends 0.7 percent of GDP on drugs versus the OECD average of 1.5 percent, and total pharmaceutical expenditures in Norway are about 9 percent of total health expenditures versus the OECD average of 17 percent. Until 1994, Norway restricted the number of drugs available by assessing each new drug on the basis of health priorities; this regulation was dropped when Norway joined the European Economic Area in 1994, resulting in more medicines registered for sale in Norway. Norway was a leader in publishing information about drug sales that included information about regional differences and, since 2004, has tracked all outpatient medicine use through a national system. Norway charges the standard value-added tax (VAT) rate of 25 percent on medicines, and the prescription dispensing fee is set at NOK 21.50 (2.70 euros). The wholesale markup is unregulated but averages 5 to 7 percent for patented medicines and higher for other drugs; pharmacy markups are set at 8 percent for drugs costing less than 25 euros and 5 percent for those more than 25 euros. Real annual growth in pharmaceutical expenditures in Norway grew 3.4 percent from 1997 to 2005, about the same as the 3.3 percent growth of total health expenditure (minus pharmaceutical expenditures) over those years.

Health Care Facilities

Norway introduced a pilot scheme testing a combination of fixed grants and patient and diagnosis-related group (DRG)-based payments; in 1997, 30 percent of funding was based on DRGs. In 2008, Norway had 3.80 hospital beds per 1,000 population. Most (97 percent) of primary care physicians in Norway used electronic medical records in 2009.

Major Health Issues

In 2008, WHO estimated that 6 percent of years of life lost in Norway were due to communicable diseases, 80 percent to noncommunicable diseases, and 14 percent to injuries. In 2008, the age-standardized estimate of cancer deaths was 151 per 100,000 for men and 108 per 100,000 for women; for cardiovascular disease and diabetes, 158 per 100,000 for men and 91 per 100,000 for women; and for chronic respiratory disease, 31 per 100,000 for men and 20 per 100,000 for women.

Norway ranked first among more-developed countries in the 2011 Mothers' Index, produced by the international nongovernmental organization (NGO) Save the Children, based on a number of health and social factors relating to women, children, and maternal and child care. The maternal mortality rate (death from any cause related to or aggravated by pregnancy) in Norway in 2008 was seven maternal deaths per 100,000 live births, among the lowest in the world. The infant mortality rate, defined as the number of deaths of infants younger than 1 year, was 3.50 per 1,000 live births in 2012, also among the lowest in the world. In 2010, tuberculosis incidence was 6.0 per 100,000 population, tuberculosis prevalence 7.5 per 100,000, and deaths due to tuberculosis among human immunodeficiency virus (HIV)-negative people 0.18 per 100,000. As of 2009, an estimated 0.1 percent of adults age 15 to 49 were living with HIV or acquired immune deficiency syndrome (AIDS).

Health Care Personnel

Norway has four medical schools, located in Bergen, Oslo, Trondheim, and Tromso. The course of training lasts six to 6.5 years for the basic medical degree, Candidatus medicinae (cand. med.), and an additional 1.5 years medical practice is required before licensing. Graduates must work for 1.5 years in government service. Graduates of foreign medical schools wishing to be licensed in Norway must have their degrees approved and pass a series of exams on medical subjects, while foreigners must also pass a language exam. Norway has agreements with other countries of the European Union (EU) and the other Scandinavian countries.

Norway, as a member of the EU, cooperates with other countries in recognizing physicians qualified to practice in other EU countries, as specified by Directive 2005/36/EC of the European Parliament. This allows qualified professionals to practice their profession in other EU states on a temporary basis and requires that the host country automatically recognize qualifications for certain professions, including physicians, nurses, dentists, midwives, and pharmacists, if certain conditions have been met (for instance, facility in the language of the host country may be required). In 2008, Norway had 4.08 physicians per 1,000 population, 0.76 pharmaceutical personnel per 1,000, 0.89 dentistry personnel per 1,000, and 14.76 nurses and midwives per 1,000. In 2001, 11.1 percent of practicing physicians in Norway were trained in another country, primarily Germany, Sweden, and Denmark.

Government Role in Health Care

All Norwegians are covered under a statutory health care system, but the specific details of health care delivery are organized at the local and regional levels. The organization of primary, preventive, and nursing care is handled by Norway's 430 municipalities, and the budgets for this care are also determined at this local level, but many services are mandated. Norway has four regional health authorities that organize specialty care; they are mandated to provide equal access to care within their boundaries.

Each December, the Norwegian government sets an overall budget for health care for the coming year. Norway's per capita health care expenditures are among the highest in the world, although health care spending as a percentage of GDP is lower than in many OECD countries. According to WHO, in 2010 Norway spent $40 billion on health care, an amount that comes to $8,091 per capita. All health care funding came from domestic sources. Most (84 percent) of health care spending was paid for through government expenditures, with the remainder provided through household expenditures (16 percent) and other sources (1 percent). In 2010, Norway allocated 17 percent of its total government expenditures to health, and government expenditures on health came to 8 percent of GDP; both figures are in the high range for high-income European countries.

Public Health Programs

The Norwegian Institute of Public Health (NIPH), located in Oslo and directed by Geir Stene-Larsen, is located within the Ministry of Health and Care Services. The NIPH is dedicated to the improvement of public health, including gathering data, preparing for disease outbreaks, performing laboratory-based research, and monitoring disease; particular areas of concern include health inequalities and issues relating to aging, drug abuse, and mental health. The NIPH has approximately 1,000 staff members organized into departments of epidemiology, environmental medicine, infectious disease control, forensic toxicology and drug abuse research, and mental health. The NIPH has recently been involved in several disease outbreak investigations, including a multinational outbreak of *Salmonella typhimurium*, an outbreak of influenza, and an outbreak of Legionnaire's Disease. In 2010, access to improved sanitation facilities and improved sources of drinking water was essentially universal in Norway. According to the World Higher Education Database (WHED), three universities in Norway offer programs in epidemiology or public health: Bergen University College, Narvik University College, and the University of Tromso.

OMAN

Oman is a Middle Eastern country, sharing borders with Yemen, the United Arab Emirates, and Saudi Arabia and having a coastline on the Arabia Sea, the Gulf of Oman, and the Persian Gulf. The area of 119,499 square miles (309,500 square kilometers) makes Oman about the size of Kansas, and the July 2012 population was estimated at 3.1 million. In 2010, 73 percent of the population lived in urban areas, and the 2010 to 2015 annual rate of urbanization was estimated at 2.3 percent. Muscat is the capital and largest city (with a 2009 population estimated at 634,000). The population growth rate in 2012 was 2.0 percent, the net migration rate negative 0.5 migrants per 1,000 population, the birth rate 24.3 births per 1,000, and the total fertility rate 2.9 children per woman. The United Nations High Commissioner for Refugees (UNHCR) estimated that, in 2010, there were 78 refugees and persons in refugee-like situations in Oman.

In the 18th century, the sultanate of Oman signed a friendship treaty with Great Britain; Oman relied on Britain for military and political advice but was never a British colony. Qaboos bin Said al-Said has ruled the country since 1970 and has implemented an extensive modernization plan. Oman ranked tied for 50th among 183 countries on the *Corruption Perceptions Index 2011*, with a score of 4.8 (on a scale where 0 indicates highly corrupt and 10 very clean). In 2011, Oman was classified as a country with high human development (the second-highest category) on the United Nations Development Programme's (UNDP's) Human Development Index (HDI), with a score of 0.728 (on a scale where 1 denotes high development and 0 low development). Life expectancy at birth in 2012 was estimated at 74.47 years, and per capita gross domestic product (GDP) in 2011 was estimated at $26,200.

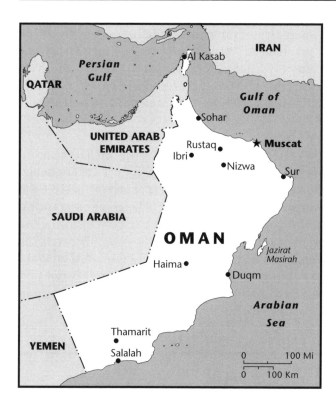

According to the World Economic Forum's *Global Gender Gap Index 2011*, Oman ranked 127th out of 135 countries on gender equality, with a score of 0.587 (on a scale with a theoretical range of 1 for equality to 0 for inequality and an actual range in 2011 from 0.8530 to 0.4873).

Emergency Health Services

According to the World Health Organization (WHO), as of 2007, Oman had a formal and publicly available emergency care (prehospital care) system accessible through a national access number.

Insurance

Oman provides health services to employees in the public sector under the direction of the Ministry of Health; this coverage includes free medicines.

Costs of Hospitalization

No data available.

Access to Health Care

According to WHO, in 2009, 99.9 percent of births in Oman were attended by skilled personnel (for example, physicians, nurses, or midwives), and 100 percent of pregnant women received at least one prenatal care visit. The 2010 immunization rates for 1-year-olds were 99 percent for diphtheria and pertussis (DPT3), 97 percent for measles (MCV), and 99 percent for Hib (Hib3). In 2010, an estimated 44 percent of persons with advanced human immunodeficiency virus (HIV) infection were receiving antiretroviral therapy in accordance with the 2010 WHO guidelines. According to WHO, in 2010, Oman had 4.31 magnetic resonance imaging (MRI) machines per 1 million population and 8.62 computer tomography (CT) machines per 1 million.

Cost of Drugs

Oman provides drugs free to employees in the public sector, while the prices of drugs in the private sector are regulated by the Directorate-General of Pharmaceutical Affairs and Drug Control. Drugs are procured, stored, and distributed under the direction of the Directorate-General of Medical Supply; the same agency is responsible for providing public pharmacies with approved medicines. A 2009 survey found that, for a market basket of drugs, generic drugs were procured for the public sector at a median price ratio slightly below the international reference price (0.95), meaning that, on average, they were obtained a bit more cheaply than the international reference price; however, a few had high median price ratios (meaning they were more expensive relative to the international reference prices), including diazepam (13.8) and fluoxetine (8.7). The mean availability of generic drugs was 83 percent in the public sector; for originator brands, the mean availability was 13 percent. In the private sector, drugs were more expensive: The median price ratio for the lowest-priced generics was 7.4, while for originator brands, it was 22.4. The mean availability was 55.3 for generics and 51 percent for originator brands in the private sector. A low-wage private-sector employee could purchase a course of treatment for most common illnesses for less than 1 day's wages using generic drugs, with a few exceptions, including ulcers (3.1 days' wages for omeprazole) and depression (5.2 days' wages).

Health Care Facilities

As of 2010, according to WHO, Oman had 3.63 health posts per 100,000 population, 2.66 health centers per 100,000, 1.26 district or rural hospitals per 100,000, 0.36 provincial hospitals per 100,000, and 0.14 specialized hospitals per 100,000. In 2008, Oman had 1.90 hospital beds per 1,000 population.

Major Health Issues

In 2008, WHO estimated that 13 percent of years of life lost in Oman were due to communicable diseases, 67 percent to noncommunicable diseases, and 20 percent to injuries. In 2008, the age-standardized estimate of cancer deaths was 81 per 100,000 for men and 72 per 100,000 for women; for cardiovascular disease and diabetes, 546 per 100,000 for men and 333 per 100,000 for women; and for chronic respiratory disease, 31 per 100,000 for men and 19 per 100,000 for women.

The maternal mortality rate (death from any cause related to or aggravated by pregnancy) in Oman in 2008 was 20 maternal deaths per 100,000 live births. The infant mortality rate, defined as the number of deaths of infants younger than 1 year, was 14.95 per 1,000 live births as of 2012. In 2010, tuberculosis incidence was 13.0 per 100,000 population, tuberculosis prevalence 16.0 per 100,000, and deaths due to tuberculosis among HIV-negative people 0.99 per 100,000. As of 2009, an estimated 0.1 percent of adults age 15 to 49 were living with HIV or acquired immune deficiency syndrome (AIDS).

Health Care Personnel

Oman has one medical school, the College of Medicine of Sultan Qaboos University in Muscat. The course of study is seven years with an additional year of supervised practice required. The degree awarded is doctor of medicine (MD). Physicians must register with the Ministry of Health, and graduates of foreign medical schools must pass a qualifying exam. Oman has an agreement with the General Medical Council of the United Kingdom for limited registration. In 2008, Oman had 1.90 physicians per 1,000 population, 0.81 pharmaceutical personnel per 1,000, 0.75 laboratory health workers per 1,000, 1.60 health management and support workers per 1,000, 0.20 dentistry personnel per 1,000, and 4.11 nurses and midwives per 1,000.

Government Role in Health Care

According to WHO, in 2010, Oman spent $1.6 billion on health care, an amount that comes to $574 per capita. All health care funding came from domestic sources. More than three-quarters (80 percent) of health care spending was paid for through government expenditures, with the remainder provided through household expenditures (12 percent) and other sources (8 percent). In 2010, Oman allocated 6 percent of its total government expenditures to health, in the low range for high-income eastern Mediterranean region countries; government expenditures on health came to 2 percent of GDP, in the median range for high-income eastern Mediterranean region countries. In 2009, according to WHO, official development assistance (ODA) for health in Oman came to $0.16 per capita.

Public Health Programs

According to WHO, in 2008, Oman had 0.08 environmental and public health workers per 1,000 population. In 2010, 99 percent of the population had access to improved sanitation facilities (95 percent in rural areas and 81 percent in urban), and 89 percent had access to improved sources of drinking water (79 percent in rural areas and 93 percent in urban). According to the World Higher Education Database (WHED), one university in Oman offers programs in epidemiology or public health: Sultan Qaboos University in Muscat.

PAKISTAN

Pakistan is a south Asian country, sharing borders with Afghanistan, China, India, and Iran and having a coastline on the Arabian Sea. The area of 307,374 square miles (796,095 square kilometers) makes Pakistan about twice the size of California, and the July 2012 population was estimated at 190.3 million, making Pakistan the sixth-most populous country in the world. In 2010, 36 percent of the population lived in urban areas, and the 2010 to 2015 annual rate of urbanization was estimated at 3.1 percent. Islamabad is the capital. The population growth rate in 2012 was 1.6 percent, the net migration rate negative 2.0 migrants per 1,000 population, the birth rate 24.3 births per 1,000, and the total fertility rate 3.1 children per woman. The United Nations High Commissioner for Refugees (UNHCR) estimated that, in 2010, there were 1.9 million refugees and persons in refugee-like situations in Pakistan and 1.2 million internally displaced persons and persons in internally displaced-person-like situations.

Pakistan became part of British India in the 18th century; in 1947, India and Pakistan became two independent countries, and in 1971, East Pakistan separated to become Bangladesh. Pakistan ranked tied for 134th among 183 countries on the *Corruption Perceptions Index 2011,* with a score of 2.5 (on a scale where 0 indicates highly corrupt and 10 very clean). In 2011, Pakistan was classified as a country with low human

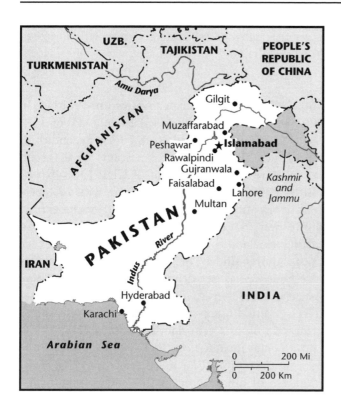

development (the lowest of four categories) on the United Nations Development Programme's (UNDP's) Human Development Index (HDI), with a score of 0.504 (on a scale where 1 denotes high development and 0 low development). In 2011, the International Food Policy Research Institute (IFPRI) classified Pakistan as a country with an "alarming" hunger problem, with a Global Hunger Index (GHI) score of 20.7 (where 0 reflects no hunger and higher scores more hunger). Life expectancy at birth in 2012 was estimated at 66.35 years, and the estimated gross domestic product (GDP) per capita in 2011 was $2,800. In fiscal year 2007 to 2008, the Gini Index (a measure of dispersion, in which perfect equality is denoted by 0 and maximum inequality is denoted by 100) for family income was 30.6. According to the World Economic Forum's *Global Gender Gap Index 2011*, Pakistan ranked 133rd out of 135 countries on gender equality with a score of 0.558 (on a scale with a theoretical range of 1 for equality to 0 for inequality and an actual range in 2011 from 0.8530 to 0.4873).

Emergency Health Services

According to the World Health Organization (WHO), as of 2007, Pakistan had a formal and publicly available emergency care (prehospital care) system accessible through a national access number. Doctors Without Borders (Médecins Sans Frontières, or MSF) began working in Pakistan in 2000 and had 1,177 staff members in the country at the close of 2010. More than 1,600 MSF staff responded to the monsoon floods in Pakistan in 2010, providing medical care and general emergency assistance, including the provision of clean drinking water; MSF provided more than 100,000 consultations during the emergency. In northern Pakistan, MSF provided emergency care to those affected by fighting between government troops and armed opposition. MSF is one of the few providers of emergency obstetric care outside urban areas, and more than 7,100 births (including 482 cesarean sections) took place in MSF facilities in Pakistan in 2010.

Pakistan experienced catastrophic flooding in August 2010, affecting more than 20 million people and leaving an estimated 8 million in need of assistance; risks caused by the flooding included destruction of sanitary and water supply systems, leading to outbreaks of water-borne diseases, and the presence of large pools of stagnant water, increasing the risk of vector-borne diseases including malaria and dengue fever. The Ministry of Health and WHO coordinated emergency response efforts involving more than 100 organizations, including public health experts from the Centers for Disease Control and Prevention (CDC) and the International Centre for Diarrhoeal Disease Research (Bangladesh). Most (80 percent) of those affected by the floods were able to return home by January 2011, and efforts now focus on restoring primary health care in the affected areas and providing essential medical services to those still displaced. The International Federation of Red Cross and Red Crescent Societies (IFRC) deployed 11 emergency response units (ERUs) in response to the catastrophic flooding in July 2010 and also raised more than CHF 78.8 million to aid victims of the flooding. The IFRC operation was planned to continue for two years. The Pakistan Red Crescent also deployed more than 1,400 volunteers in response to the crisis.

Insurance

Pakistan has a social insurance system providing cash and medical benefits. Employees earning less than PRK 10,000 per month and working for establishments with five or more employees are covered; the self-employed are excluded. Separate systems cover railway employees, public sector employees, members of the military, the police, and local authority employees.

The system is financed by employer contributions (6 percent of monthly payroll, with a cap on maximum earnings used to calculate this contribution). Medical benefits are provided through social security facilities and include general and specialist care, maternity care, hospitalization, medicines, and transportation. The maternity benefit is 100 percent of earnings for 12 weeks. The sickness benefit is 75 percent of earnings for up to 121 days, with more generous benefits for cancer and tuberculosis. Provincial Employees' Social Security Institutions in each province administer the program and either provide their own dispensaries and hospitals or contract with public and private agencies to provide these services. The Provincial Labour Department provides general supervision.

Costs of Hospitalization

No data available.

Access to Health Care

A survey conducted in 2004 by WHO and Health Action International found that many medicines were unavailable; in the public sector, the median availability of generic medicines was 3.3 percent and 0.0 percent for brand-name medications, while in the private sector, availability was higher, at 31.3 percent for generic drugs and 54.2 percent for brand-name drugs. Surveys indicate that cost is a minor barrier for most Pakistanis when it comes to following drug regimens: 91.2 percent of adult patients reported taking all medicines prescribed, as did 89.4 percent of adult patients from poor households. For children with acute conditions from poor households, 85.5 percent reported taking all medicines prescribed. For adult patients with chronic conditions, 83.8 percent reported taking all medicines prescribed, as did 70.5 percent of adult patients from poor households. For those who did not take all medications prescribed, cost was cited as the reason by 68 percent of adult patients with acute conditions.

According to WHO, in 2007, 39 percent of births in Pakistan were attended by skilled personnel (for example, physicians, nurses, or midwives), and 28 percent of pregnant women received at least four prenatal care visits. The 2010 immunization rates for 1-year-olds were 88 percent for diphtheria and pertussis (DPT3), 86 percent for measles (MCV), and 88 percent for Hib (Hib3). In 2010, an estimated 9 percent of persons with advanced human immunodeficiency virus (HIV) infection were receiving antiretroviral therapy in accordance with the 2010 WHO guidelines.

Cost of Drugs

Total pharmaceutical expenditures in Pakistan in 2007 were PKR 112 billion ($1.84 billion), or PKR 683 ($11.30) per capita. Pharmaceutical expenditures represented almost half (47.3 percent) of all health expenditures, and 1.3 percent of GDP. Most expenditures came from the private sector, with 27.1 percent being public expenditures; most private expenditures were out of pocket, including the purchase of medicines. Public programs provide drugs free to the poor, children under age 5, pregnant women, and the elderly, as well as free drugs for conditions including malaria, tuberculosis, sexually transmitted diseases (STDs), and human immunodeficiency virus and acquired immune deficiency syndrome (HIV/AIDS), and vaccines included on the Expanded Programme for Immunizations (EPI) list, created by WHO. However, lack of funding means that such programs are not always implemented. The public health services provide some coverage for medicines on the Essential Medicines List (EML); private health insurance plans also provide coverage for medicines but are not obliged to cover those on the EML.

In 2004, a survey by WHO and Health Action International found the price of medicines varied considerably within Pakistan. The median price ratio for a basket of generic medications was 0.57 as compared to the international reference price (meaning that the median price in Pakistan was about half of the reference price), while the median price ratio for brand-name drugs in the public sector in Pakistan was 2.24 (more than twice as high as the international reference price). In the private sector, the median price ratio for generics was 2.26 and, for brand-name drugs, was 3.4. Using the wage of the lowest-paid government worker as a standard, generic medication for a child's respiratory infection (co-trimoxazole) would require 0.3 day's wages to purchase on the private market, and brand-name medication purchased on the private market would require 0.4 day's wages; in the public sector, this drug is provided for free.

As a member of the World Trade Organization (WTO), Pakistan observes patent law, but Pakistan is also eligible for the transitional period to 2016, and national law also includes some elements of the Trade-Related Aspects of Intellectual Property Rights (TRIPS), which provide exceptions to patent

Health Expenditures: Pakistan Compared With the Global Average (2009)

	Pakistan	Global Average
Out-of-pocket expenditure as percent of private expenditure on health	81.9	50.2
Private prepaid plans as percent of private expenditure on health	0.4	38.9
Per capita total expenditure on health at average exchange rate (USD)	20	900
Per capita total expenditure on health (purchasing power parity, international dollars)	57	990
Per capita government expenditure on health at average exchange rate (USD)	7	549
Per capita government expenditure on health (purchasing power parity, international dollars)	20	584

Source: 2011 World Health Organization Global Health Expenditure Atlas.

law. In Pakistan, these exceptions include compulsory licensing for reasons of public health, the Bolar exception that allows manufacturers to perform research and testing to create generic drugs before a patent has expired, and parallel importing provisions (allowing import of drugs created for sale in a different country). Promotion and advertising of pharmaceuticals is regulated by law, and direct advertising to the public of prescription medicines is forbidden.

Health Care Facilities

As of 2010, according to WHO, Pakistan had 3.13 health posts per 100,000 population, 0.87 health centers per 100,000, 0.37 district or rural hospitals per 100,000, 0.09 provincial hospitals per 100,000, and 0.10 specialized hospitals per 100,000. In 2009, Pakistan had 0.60 hospital beds per 1,000 population, one of the 20 lowest rates in the world.

Major Health Issues

In 2008, WHO estimated that 64 percent of years of life lost in Pakistan were due to communicable diseases, 26 percent to noncommunicable diseases, and 9 percent to injuries. In 2008, the age-standardized estimate of cancer deaths was 95 per 100,000 for men and 94 per 100,000 for women; for cardiovascular disease and diabetes, 455 per 100,000 for men and 388 per 100,000 for women; and for chronic respiratory

disease, 89 per 100,000 for men and 71 per 100,000 for women.

In 2008, the age-standardized death rate from malaria was 0.5 per 100,000 population. In 2010, tuberculosis incidence was 231.0 per 100,000 population, tuberculosis prevalence 364.0 per 100,000, and deaths due to tuberculosis among HIV-negative people 34.00 per 100,000. As estimated, 3.4 percent of new tuberculosis cases and 21 percent of retreatment cases are multidrug resistant. WHO estimated that the case detection rate in 2010 was 65 percent. As of 2009, an estimated 0.1 percent of adults age 15 to 49 were living with HIV or AIDS. Polio remains endemic in Pakistan, but persistent transmission is restricted to 11 of Pakistan's 152 districts in the city of Karachi, some districts in Balochistan Province, and some districts in the Federally Administered Tribal Areas and the Pesahawar District of the North-West Frontier Province.

Pakistan's maternal mortality rate (death from any cause related to or aggravated by pregnancy) was estimated in 2008 as 260 maternal deaths per 100,000 live births. The infant mortality rate, defined as the number of deaths of infants younger than 1 year, also has been high, at 61.27 per 1,000 live births as of 2012. Child malnutrition is a serious problem: In 2001, 31.3 percent of children under age 5 were underweight (defined as 2 kilograms [kg] below standard weight-for-age at age 1, 3 kg below for ages 2 to 3, and 4 kg below for ages 4 to 5), one of the 20 highest rates in the world.

Health Care Personnel

In 2006, WHO identified Pakistan as one of 57 countries with a critical deficit in the supply of skilled health workers. Pakistan has 20 medical schools. The duration of the basic medical degree course is five years with one year of work in government service obligatory after graduation. The degrees awarded are bachelor of medicine and bachelor of surgery. Physicians must register with the Pakistan Medical and Dental Council, and graduates of foreign medical schools must pass a qualifying exam. Foreigners may be granted licenses to practice medicine on a year-to-year basis for institutional service only. In 2009, Pakistan had 0.81 physicians per 1,000 population, 0.06 dentistry personnel per 1,000, 0.06 community and traditional health workers per 1,000, and 0.56 nurses and midwives per 1,000.

Government Role in Health Care

The right to health, including access to essential medicines and medical technologies, is recognized in national legislation. Pakistan has a National Health Policy (NHP), updated in 2001, and a National Medicines Policy (NMP), updated in 1997. The NMP includes selection of essential medicines; pricing, purchase, distribution, and regulation of drugs; pharmacovigilance; rational usage of medicines; human resource development; research; evaluation and monitoring; and traditional medicine.

According to WHO, in 2010, Pakistan spent $3.8 billion on health care, an amount that comes to $22 per capita. Almost all (95 percent) of health care funding came from domestic sources, with 5 percent coming from overseas sources. Half (50 percent) of health care spending was paid for through government expenditures, with the remainder provided through household expenditures (38 percent) and other sources (11 percent). In 2010, Pakistan allocated 4 percent of its total government expenditures to health, and government expenditures on health came to 1 percent of GDP; both figures are in the low range for lower-middle-income eastern Mediterranean region countries. In 2009, according to WHO, official development assistance (ODA) for health in Pakistan came to $2.21 per capita.

Public Health Programs

Pakistan's Institute of Public Health is located in Karachi and headed by M. Amanullah Khan. It is affiliated with the University of Health Sciences in Lahore and has a staff of more than 100. The institute's original focus was prevention of communicable disease, but it is currently in the process of transforming itself into a training and research institution as well and also partners with international organizations (for example, United Nations Children's Fund, or UNICEF, and WHO) to address public health matters such as infant mortality and maternal health.

According to WHO, in 2004, Pakistan had fewer than 0.01 environmental and public health workers per 1,000 population. In 2010, 48 percent of the population had access to improved sanitation facilities (34 percent in rural areas and 72 percent in urban), and 92 percent had access to improved sources of drinking water (89 percent in rural areas and 96 percent in urban). According to the World Higher Education Database (WHED), three universities in Pakistan offer programs in epidemiology or public health: Kyber Medical University in Peshawar, Liaquat University and Health Sciences in Jamshoro, and the University of Veterinary and Animal Sciences in Lahore.

PALAU

Palau is an island country in the north Pacific Ocean. The area of 177 square miles (459 square kilometers) makes Palau about 2.5 times as large as Washington, D.C., and the July 2012 population was estimated at 21,032. In 2010, 83 percent of the population lived in urban areas, and the 2010 to 2015 annual rate of urbanization was estimated at 1.4 percent. Melekeok is the capital. The population growth rate in 2012 was 0.4 percent, the net migration rate 0.7 migrants per 1,000 population, the birth rate 10.8 births per 1,000, and the total fertility rate 1.7 children per woman.

Palau was administered by the United States as part of the United Nations Trust Territory of the Pacific after World War II; the country became independent in 1978. In 2011, Palau was classified as a country with high human development (the second-highest category) on the United Nations Development Programme's (UNDP's) Human Development Index (HDI), with a score of 0.782 (on a scale where 1 denotes high development and 0 low development). Life expectancy at birth in 2012 was estimated at 72.06 years, and gross domestic product (GDP) per capita in 2008 was $8,100.

Emergency Health Services

According to the World Health Organization (WHO), as of 2007, Palau had a formal and publicly available emergency care (prehospital care) system accessible through a national access number.

Insurance

Palau's government intends to provide health care for citizens through the country's main hospital in Koror and community-based care in outlying areas. Health care services in Palau are heavily subsidized by the U.S. government and United Nations (UN) agencies.

Costs of Hospitalization

No data available.

Access to Health Care

According to WHO, in 2007, 100 percent of births in Palau were attended by skilled personnel (for example, physicians, nurses, or midwives). The 2010 immunization rates for 1-year-olds were 49 percent for diphtheria and pertussis (DPT3), 75 percent for measles (MCV), and 66 percent for Hib (Hib3).

Cost of Drugs

No data available.

Health Care Facilities

In 2009, Palau had five hospital beds per 1,000 population, among the 50 highest rates in the world.

Major Health Issues

In 2008, WHO estimated that 24 percent of years of life lost in Palau were due to communicable diseases, 65 percent to noncommunicable diseases, and 11 percent to injuries. In 2008, the age-standardized estimate of cancer deaths was 91 per 100,000 for men and 105 per 100,000 for women; for cardiovascular disease and diabetes, 470 per 100,000 for men and 215 per 100,000 for women; and for chronic respiratory disease, 79 per 100,000 for men and 28 per 100,000 for women.

The infant mortality rate, defined as the number of deaths of infants younger than 1 year, was 12.10 per 1,000 live births as of 2012. No information is available from WHO about the maternal mortality ratio in Palau. In 2010, tuberculosis incidence was 124.0 per 100,000 population, tuberculosis prevalence 179.0 per 100,000, and deaths due to tuberculosis among human immunodeficiency virus (HIV)-negative people 15.0 per 100,000.

Health Care Personnel

Palau has no medical school. Physicians must register with the Ministry of Health, and the license to practice is granted to persons who have graduated from a recognized medical school and hold a current medical license. In 2006, Palau had 1.30 physicians per 1,000 population, 0.05 pharmaceutical personnel per 1,000, and 5.90 nurses per 1,000, and in 2007, had 0.25 dentistry personnel per 1,000 and 0.05 pharmaceutical personnel per 1,000.

Government Role in Health Care

According to WHO, in 2010, Palau spent $17 million on health care, an amount that comes to $850 per capita. About two-thirds (61 percent) of health care funding came from domestic sources, with 39 percent coming from overseas sources. More than three-quarters (77 percent) of health care spending was paid for through government expenditures, with the remainder provided through household expenditures (9 percent) and other sources (14 percent). In 2010, Palau allocated 14 percent of its total government expenditures to health, and government expenditures on health came to 8 percent of GDP; both figures are in the high range for upper-middle-income western Pacific region countries.

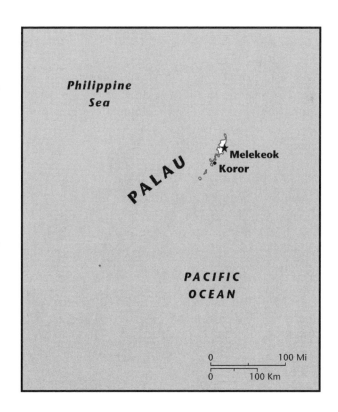

Public Health Programs

According to WHO, in 2000 (the most recent year for which data is available), Palau had 0.07 environmental and public health workers per 1,000 population. In 2010, access to improved sanitation facilities was essentially universal, while 85 percent of the population had access to improved sources of drinking water (96 percent in rural areas and 83 percent in urban).

PANAMA

Panama is a Central American country, sharing borders with Costa Rica and Colombia and having coastlines on the Caribbean Sea and the north Pacific Ocean. The area of 29,120 square miles (75,420 square kilometers) makes Panama about the size of South Carolina, and the July 2012 population was estimated at 3.5 million. In 2010, 75 percent of the population lived in urban areas, and the 2010 to 2015 annual rate of urbanization was estimated at 2.3 percent. Panama City is the capital and largest city (with a 2009 population estimated at 1.3 million). The population growth rate in 2012 was 1.4 percent, the net migration rate negative 0.4 migrants per 1,000 population, the birth rate 19.2 births per 1,000, and the total fertility rate 12.4 children per woman. The United Nations High Commissioner for Refugees (UNHCR) estimated that, in 2010, there were 3,967 refugees and persons in refugee-like situations in Panama. Panama was colonized by Spain in the 16th century. In 1821, Panama joined the Union of Gran Colombia (with Colombia, Ecuador, and Venezuela) and remained part of Colombia when the union dissolved in 1830. Panama seceded from Colombia in 1903 and signed a treaty allowing the United States to construct the Panama Canal; the Panama Canal Zone, the area around the Panama Canal, was U.S. territory until it was transferred back to Panama in 1999. Panama ranked tied for 86th among 183 countries on the *Corruption Perceptions Index 2011*, with a score of 3.3 (on a scale where 0 indicates highly corrupt and 10 very clean).

In 2011, Panama was classified as a country with high human development (the second-highest category) on the United Nations Development Programme's (UNDP's) Human Development Index (HDI), with a score of 0.768 (on a scale where 1 denotes high development and 0 low development).

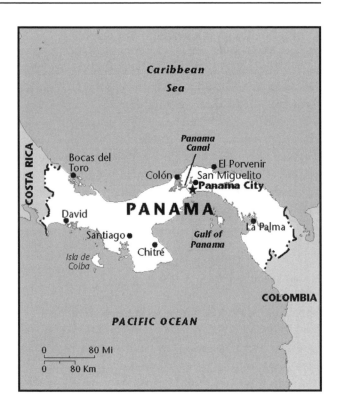

Life expectancy at birth in 2012 was estimated at 77.96 years, and per capita gross domestic product (GDP) in 2011 was estimated at $13,600. Income distribution in Panama is relatively unequal: In 2010, the Gini Index (a measure of dispersion, in which perfect equality is denoted by 0 and maximum inequality is denoted by 100) for family income was estimated at 51.9, among the 20 highest in the world. According to the World Economic Forum's *Global Gender Gap Index 2011*, Panama ranked 40th out of 135 countries on gender equality with a score of 0.704 (on a scale with a theoretical range of 1 for equality to 0 for inequality and an actual range in 2011 from 0.8530 to 0.4873).

Emergency Health Services

According to the World Health Organization (WHO), as of 2007, Panama had a formal and publicly available emergency care (prehospital care) system accessible through regional access numbers, but not a national access number. All public and private institutions provide first aid at no cost. Panama City has an integrated system of ambulances whose services are provided free to the public, while in other parts of the country, different operating units provide emergency care; however, there are no unified protocols for emergency management and referral.

Insurance

Panama has a social insurance system covering employees, including voluntary and household workers and public-sector employees, the self-employed, and pensioners. The system is financed by contributions from wages (0.5 percent of gross earnings), earnings of the self-employed (8.5 percent of declared earnings), pensioners (a percentage of the monthly pension), employers (8 percent of gross payroll), and the government (10 percent of income from the sale of rights to fiber optic businesses). Medical services are provided by facilities of the Social Insurance Fund or Ministry of Health, with most provided at no cost; if a needed facility is not available, private care will be reimbursed. Benefits include hospitalization, surgery, general and specialist care, lab services, maternity care, dental care, medicines, appliances, and limited reimbursement for eyeglasses and dental prostheses. Eligible dependents include the spouse, parents, and children of the insured; children are eligible to age 18, to age 25 if a student, and with no limit if disabled. The maternity benefit is 100 percent of average earnings for six weeks before and eight weeks after birth. The sickness benefit is 70 percent of average earnings for up to 26 weeks, with possible extension to 52 weeks. The program is managed by the Social Insurance Fund. According to Ke Xu and colleagues, in 2003, 2.4 percent of households in Panama experienced catastrophic health expenditures annually; "catastrophic" was defined as exceeding 40 percent of household income remaining after basic needs were met.

Costs of Hospitalization

No data available.

Access to Health Care

According to Latinobarometer, an annual public opinion survey conducted in Latin America, 60 percent of citizens in Panama are satisfied with the level of health care available to them (the regional average is 51.9 percent). According to WHO, in 2009, 88.5 percent of births in Panama were attended by skilled personnel (for example, physicians, nurses, or midwives). The 2010 immunization rates for 1-year-olds were 94 percent for diphtheria and pertussis (DPT3), 95 percent for measles (MCV), and 94 percent for Hib (Hib3). In 2010, an estimated 36 percent of persons with advanced human immunodeficiency virus (HIV) infection were receiving antiretroviral therapy in accordance with the 2010 WHO guidelines.

Cost of Drugs

Medicines and medical supplies in Panama are regulated by Law 1 of 2003 and Law 54 of 2005; topics covered include maintaining a list of essential medications, updating it regularly, providing a registration process for medications and medical equipment, and having clear rules for the interchangeability of generic medications. A 2003 survey found that the largest category of out-of-pocket medical expenditures were for drugs (53.9 percent); in indigenous areas, 32 percent was spent on medications.

Health Care Facilities

As of 2010, according to WHO, Panama had 13.65 health posts per 100,000 population, 11.03 health centers per 100,000, 0.43 district or rural hospitals per 100,000, 0.37 provincial hospitals per 100,000, and 0.20 specialized hospitals per 100,000. In 2009, Panama had 2.20 hospital beds per 1,000 population.

Major Health Issues

In 2008, WHO estimated that 30 percent of years of life lost in Panama were due to communicable diseases, 48 percent to noncommunicable diseases, and 22 percent to injuries. In 2008, the age-standardized estimate of cancer deaths was 111 per 100,000 for men and 98 per 100,000 for women; for cardiovascular disease and diabetes, 202 per 100,000 for men and 145 per 100,000 for women; and for chronic respiratory disease, 29 per 100,000 for men and 21 per 100,000 for women.

Panama's maternal mortality rate (death from any cause related to or aggravated by pregnancy) was estimated in 2008 as 71 maternal deaths per 100,000 live births. The infant mortality rate, defined as the number of deaths of infants younger than 1 year, was 11.32 per 1,000 live births as of 2012. In 2010, tuberculosis incidence was 48.0 per 100,000 population, tuberculosis prevalence 52.0 per 100,000, and deaths due to tuberculosis among HIV-negative people 8.60 per 100,000. As of 2009, an estimated 0.9 percent of adults age 15 to 49 were living with HIV or acquired immune deficiency syndrome (AIDS).

Health Care Personnel

Panama has four medical schools: the Facultad de Medicina of the University of Panama, the Facultad de Ciencias Medicas y de la Salud of the Universidad Latina de Panama, the Faculty of Medicine of Columbus University, and the Facultad de Ciencias Medicas y de la Salud of the Universidad Latinoamericana de Ciencia y Tecnologia (affiliated with Laureate International Universities). The basic medical degree course lasts six years, and the degree awarded is Doctor en Medicina (doctor of medicine). The medical license requires a two-year internship as well. Physicians must register with the Ministry of Education, and graduates of foreign medical must have their degrees certified. Foreigners are not entitled to practice medicine in Panama. In 2000, Panama had 1.50 physicians per 1,000 population, 0.86 pharmaceutical personnel per 1,000, 2.33 health management and support workers per 1,000, 0.76 dentistry personnel per 1,000, 0.46 community and traditional health workers per 1,000, and 2.77 nurses and midwives per 1,000.

Government Role in Health Care

According to WHO, in 2010, Panama spent $2.2 billion on health care, an amount that comes to $616 per capita. All health care funding came from domestic sources. Three-quarters (75 percent) of health care spending was paid for through government expenditures, with the remainder provided through household expenditures (20 percent) and other sources (5 percent).

In 2010, Panama allocated 15 percent of its total government expenditures to health, and government expenditures on health came to 6 percent of GDP; both figures are in the high range for upper-middle-income Americas region countries. In 2009, according to WHO, official development assistance (ODA) for health in Panama came to $4.83 per capita.

Public Health Programs

The Instituto Commemorativo Gorgas de Estudios de la Salud, located in Panama City and with Nestor Sosa as the acting director general, is the primary public health institute in Panama. The Gorgas Institute is named to honor the physician who led the effort to eradicate yellow fever in Panama, Dr. William Gorgas, and was founded in 1921. Today, the Gorgas Institute includes departments of epidemiology, entomology, parasitology, genomics, virology, and reproductive health along with several labs and an education and training center. In 2008, the Gorgas Institute began a national survey of renal disease and risk factors for cardiovascular disease and completed a national survey of reproductive health.

According to WHO, in 2001, Panama had 0.32 environmental and public health workers per 1,000

population. In 2005, 68 percent of the population of Panama had access to improved sanitation facilities (51 percent in rural areas and 75 percent in urban), and 93 percent had access to improved sources of drinking water (83 percent in rural areas and 93 percent in urban).

PAPUA NEW GUINEA

Papua New Guinea occupies the eastern half of the island of New Guinea in the south Pacific Ocean, sharing a border with Indonesia. The area of 178,704 square miles (462,840 square kilometers) makes Papua New Guinea about the size of California, and the July 2012 population was estimated at 6.3 million. In 2010, 13 percent of the population lived in urban areas, and the 2010 to 2015 annual rate of urbanization was estimated at 2.9 percent. Port Moresby is the capital and largest city (with a 2009 population estimated at 314,000). The population growth rate in 2012 was 1.9 percent, the net migration rate 0.0 migrants per 1,000 population, the birth rate 25.9 births per 1,000, and the total fertility rate 3.4 children per woman. The United Nations High Commissioner for Refugees (UNHCR) estimated that, in 2010, there were 2,639 refugees and persons in refugee-like situations in Papua New Guinea.

Colonial dominion over Papua New Guinea was divided between Germany and the United Kingdom in 1885; the British area was transferred to Australia in 1902. Papua New Guinea became independent in 1975. Papua New Guinea ranked tied for 152nd among 183 countries on the *Corruption Perceptions Index 2011,* with a score of 2.2 (on a scale where 0 indicates highly corrupt and 10 very clean).

In 2011, Papua New Guinea was classified as a country with low human development (the lowest of four categories) on the United Nations Development Programme's (UNDP's) Human Development Index (HDI), with a score of 0.466 (on a scale where 1 denotes high development and 0 low development). Life expectancy at birth in 2012 was estimated at 66.46 years, and estimated gross domestic product (GDP) per capita in 2011 was $2,500. Income distribution in Papua New Guinea is relatively unequal: In 1996, the Gini Index (a measure of dispersion, in which perfect equality is denoted by 0 and maximum inequality is denoted by 100) for family income was 50.9, among the 20 highest in the world.

Emergency Health Services

According to the World Health Organization (WHO), as of 2007, Papua New Guinea had a formal and publicly available emergency care (prehospital care) system accessible through a national access number. Doctors Without Borders (Médecins Sans Frontières, or MSF) began working in Papua New Guinea in 2009 and had 133 staff members in the country at the close of 2010. MSF provides care to victims of sexual and domestic violence in several locations in Papua New Guinea and published a report on the problem, *Hidden and Neglected: The Medical and Emotional Needs of Survivors of Family and Sexual Violence in Papua New Guinea* in December 2010 based on this experience. MSF runs a Family Support Center in Lae, Papua New Guinea's second-largest city, providing social and psychological support and medical care to about 200 new patients each month; a second MSF Family Support Center is located in Tari, a rural town in the southern highlands; MSF staff provided more than 5,400 mental health consultations and more than 13,000 general consultations in Tari and Lae. MSF responded to a cholera outbreak in November 2010 in the Fly River region while also wrapping up its care for victims of a cholera outbreak in East Sepik in mid-2010.

Insurance

In 2010, premiums for private health insurance plans constituted 6.5 percent of total private expenditures on health. Employers are required to provide sick leave and maternity leave under the 1981 Employment Act. Limited medical services are available in government clinics and hospitals at no or nominal cost.

Costs of Hospitalization

No data available.

Access to Health Care

According to WHO, in 2006, 53 percent of births in Papua New Guinea were attended by skilled personnel (for example, physicians, nurses, or midwives), and 55 percent of pregnant women received at least four prenatal care visits. The 2010 immunization rates for 1-year-olds were 56 percent for diphtheria and pertussis (DPT3), 55 percent for measles (MCV), and 56 percent for Hib (Hib3). In 2010, an estimated 54 percent of persons with advanced human immunodeficiency virus

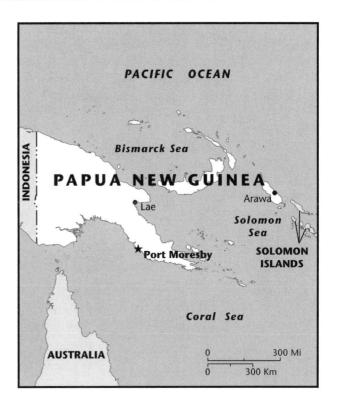

(HIV) infection were receiving antiretroviral therapy in accordance with the 2010 WHO guidelines. According to WHO, in 2010, Papua New Guinea had fewer than 0.01 magnetic resonance imaging (MRI) machines per 1 million population, 1.12 computer tomography (CT) machines per 1 million, 0.15 telecolbalt units per 1 million, and 0.15 radiotherapy machines per 1 million.

Cost of Drugs

Public pharmaceutical expenditures in Papua New Guinea in 2010 came to PNG Kina 94 million ($40 million), and per capita expenditures to PNG Kina 14.0 ($6.00). Papua New Guinea is a member of the World Trade Organization (WTO) and has implemented some flexibilities within the Trade-Related Aspects of Intellectual Property Rights (TRIPS), including compulsory licensing for reasons of public health. Drugs must be registered before being sold in Papua New Guinea, and as of 2011, 37 drugs were registered. Children under age 5 and the elderly are eligible to receive medications for free, and reduced fees are sometimes charged to those who cannot afford the full price. Public health programs provide free medications for tuberculosis, sexually transmitted diseases (STDs), and human immunodeficiency virus and acquired immune deficiency syndrome (HIV/AIDS), and vaccines on the Expanded Programme on Immunization (EPI) list, developed by WHO, are also free.

Health Care Facilities
As of 2010, according to WHO, Papua New Guinea had 37.91 health posts per 100,000 population, 9.87 health centers per 100,000, 1.30 district or rural hospitals per 100,000, 0.38 provincial hospitals per 100,000, and 0.10 specialized hospitals per 100,000.

Major Health Issues
In 2008, WHO estimated that 62 percent of years of life lost in Papua New Guinea were due to communicable diseases, 28 percent to noncommunicable diseases, and 11 percent to injuries. In 2008, the age-standardized estimate of cancer deaths was 152 per 100,000 for men and 107 per 100,000 for women; for cardiovascular disease and diabetes, 460 per 100,000 for men and 395 per 100,000 for women; and for chronic respiratory disease, 100 per 100,000 for men and 74 per 100,000 for women.

Papua New Guinea's maternal mortality rate (death from any cause related to or aggravated by pregnancy) was estimated in 2008 as 250 maternal deaths per 100,000 live births. The infant mortality rate, defined as the number of deaths of infants younger than 1 year, was estimated at 42.05 per 1,000 live births as of 2012. In 2005, 18.1 percent of children under age 5 were underweight (defined as 2 kilograms [kg] below

standard weight-for-age at age 1, 3 kg below for ages 2 to 3, and 4 kg below for ages 4 to 5). In 2010, tuberculosis incidence was 303.0 per 100,000 population, tuberculosis prevalence 465.0 per 100,000, and deaths due to tuberculosis among HIV-negative people 34.0 per 100,000. As of 2009, an estimated 0.9 percent of adults age 15 to 49 were living with HIV or AIDS.

Health Care Personnel
In 2006, WHO identified Papua New Guinea as one of 57 countries with a critical deficit in the supply of skilled health workers. Papua New Guinea has one medical school, the Faculty of Medicine of the University of Papua New Guinea in Boroko, which began offering instruction in 1959. The basic medical degree course lasts six years, and the degrees awarded are bachelor of medicine and bachelor of surgery. In 2008, Papua New Guinea had 0.05 physicians per 1,000 population, 0.01 dentistry personnel per 1,000, 0.62 community and traditional health workers per 1,000, and 0.51 nurses and midwives per 1,000.

Government Role in Health Care
The right to health, including access to essential medicines and medical technologies, is recognized by national legislation in Papua New Guinea. The country has a National Health Policy (NHP), and an implementation plan for the NHP was created in 2010. Papua New Guinea also has a National Medicines Plan

Selected Health Indicators: Papua New Guinea Compared With the Global Average (2010)

	Papua New Guinea	Global Average
Male life expectancy at birth* (years)	62	66
Female life expectancy at birth* (years)	65	71
Under-5 mortality rate, both sexes (per 1,000 live births)	61	57
Adult mortality rate, both sexes* (probability of dying between 15 and 60 years per 1,000 population)	248	176
Maternal mortality ratio (per 100,000 live births)	230	210
HIV prevalence* (per 1,000 adults aged 15 to 49)	9	8
Tuberculosis prevalence (per 100,000 population)	465	178

Source: World Health Organization Global Health Observatory Data Repository.
*Data refers to 2009.

(NMP), which covers selection of essential medicines; financing, pricing, purchase, distribution, and regulation of drugs; pharmacovigilance; rational usage of medicines; human resource development; and evaluation and monitoring; however, policy implementation is not regularly monitored. Papua New Guinea has an Essential Medicines List (EML) including 323 medications.

According to WHO, in 2010, Papua New Guinea spent $339 million on health care, an amount that comes to $49 per capita. More than three-quarters (76 percent) of health care funding came from domestic sources, with 24 percent coming from overseas sources. Almost three-quarters (72 percent) of health care spending was paid for through government expenditures, with the remainder provided through household expenditures (16 percent) and other sources (13 percent). In 2010, Papua New Guinea allocated 8 percent of its total government expenditures to health, and government expenditures on health came to 3 percent of GDP; both figures are in the low range for lower-middle-income western Pacific region countries. In 2009, according to WHO, official development assistance (ODA) for health in Papua New Guinea came to $9.23 per capita.

Public Health Programs

The National Department of Health for Papua New Guinea is located in Waigani (a suburb of Port Moresby) and is headed by Paison Dakulala. Its role is to provide leadership on health priorities, help develop affordable and effective programs and strategies, and assist in their implementation at the district and local levels. Current programs address food and water sanitation, control of communicable disease, nutrition, dental care, mental health, public education about health, and development of human resources. In 2010, 45 percent of the population of Papua New Guinea had access to improved sanitation facilities (41 percent in rural areas and 71 percent in urban), and 40 percent had access to improved sources of drinking water (33 percent in rural areas and 87 percent in urban).

PARAGUAY

Paraguay is a landlocked South American country sharing borders with Argentina, Bolivia, and Brazil.

The area of 157,048 square miles (406,752 square kilometers) makes Paraguay about the size of California, and the July 2012 population was estimated at 6.5 million. In 2010, 61 percent of the population lived in urban areas, and the 2010 to 2015 annual rate of urbanization was estimated at 2.5 percent. Asuncion is the capital and largest city (with a 2009 population estimated at 2.0 million). The population growth rate in 2012 was 1.3 percent, the net migration rate negative 0.1 migrants per 1,000 population, the birth rate 17.2 births per 1,000, and the total fertility rate 2.1 children per woman. The United Nations High Commissioner for Refugees (UNHCR) estimated that, in 2010, there were 94 refugees and persons in refugee-like situations in Paraguay.

A former Spanish colony, Paraguay became independent in 1811; an estimated two-thirds of all adult males in Paraguay were killed in the War of the Triple Alliance from 1865 to 1870, and Paraguay also lost considerable territory as a result of this war. Paraguay ranked tied for 152nd among 183 countries on the *Corruption Perceptions Index 2011*, with a score of 2.2 (on a scale where 0 indicates highly corrupt and 10 very clean). In 2011, Paraguay was classified as a country with medium human development (the second from the lowest of four categories) on the United Nations

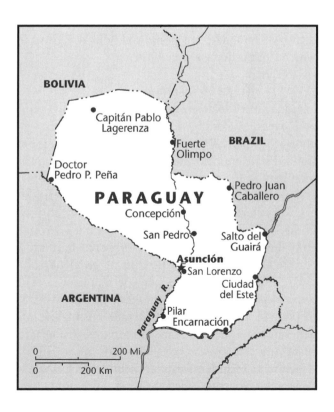

Development Programme's (UNDP's) Human Development Index (HDI), with a score of 0.665 (on a scale where 1 denotes high development and 0 low development). Life expectancy at birth in 2012 was estimated at 76.40 years, and estimated gross domestic product (GDP) per capita in 2011 was $5,500. Income distribution in Paraguay is relatively unequal: In 2009, the Gini Index (a measure of dispersion, in which perfect equality is denoted by 0 and maximum inequality is denoted by 100) for family income was 53.2, among the 20 highest in the world. According to the World Economic Forum's *Global Gender Gap Index 2011*, Paraguay ranked 67th out of 135 countries on gender equality with a score of 0.682 (on a scale with a theoretical range of 1 for equality to 0 for inequality and an actual range in 2011 from 0.8530 to 0.4873).

Emergency Health Services

According to the World Health Organization (WHO), as of 2007, Paraguay had a formal and publicly available emergency care (prehospital care) system accessible through regional access numbers, but not a national access number. The private nonprofit care system includes 15 emergency services. Doctors Without Borders (Médecins Sans Frontières, or MSF) began working in Paraguay in 2010 and had six staff members in the country at the close of 2010. MSF established diagnosis and treatment for Chagas disease in Boquerón department, part of the Gran Chaco region of Paraguay, Argentina, and Bolivia, an area in which Chagas disease is endemic.

Insurance

Paraguay has a social insurance system covering most employees, including teachers and employees of enterprises partially owned by the state or of decentralized state entities; public-sector employees, police, members of the military, railroad and bank employees, and household workers are excluded. Pensioners, war veterans, and household workers are covered under separate systems. The system is funded through contributions from employees (9 percent of gross earnings), employers (14 percent of gross payroll), and the government (1.5 percent of income). The Social Insurance Institute provides services directly to patients; covered benefits include hospitalization, generalist and specialist care, lab services, dental care, maternity care, medications, and prostheses. Eligible dependents include wives and unemployed husbands, dependent parents older than 60, and unmarried

children younger than 18 (no age limit if the child is disabled). The maternity benefit is 50 percent of average earnings for three weeks before and six weeks after the due date. The sickness benefit is 50 percent of average earnings for up to 26 weeks and may be extended for 24 more weeks. The program is administered by the Social Insurance Institute. According to Ke Xu and colleagues, in 2003, 3.5 percent of households in Paraguay experienced catastrophic health expenditures annually; "catastrophic" was defined as exceeding 40 percent of household income remaining after basic needs were met.

Costs of Hospitalization

No data available.

Access to Health Care

As of 2007, an estimated 18.4 percent of the population of Paraguay had health insurance (7 percent in rural areas). According to WHO, in 2008, 96.7 percent of births in Paraguay were attended by skilled personnel (for example, physicians, nurses, or midwives), and 91 percent of pregnant women received at least four prenatal care visits. The 2010 immunization rates for 1-year-olds were 90 percent for diphtheria and pertussis (DPT3), 94 percent for measles (MCV), and 98 percent for Hib (Hib3). In 2010, an estimated 66 percent of persons with advanced human immunodeficiency virus (HIV) infection were receiving antiretroviral therapy in accordance with the 2010 WHO guidelines. According to Latinobarometer, an annual public opinion survey conducted in Latin America, 36 percent of citizens in Paraguay are satisfied with the level of health care available to them (the regional average is 51.9 percent).

Cost of Drugs

Paraguay has had a National Drug Policy since 2001, providing a system for registering drugs and pharmacies, oversight for establishments that manufacture or dispense drugs, and implementation of a quality-control program for drugs. Vaccines are obtained through the Pan American Health Organization's (PAHO) Revolving Fund for Vaccine Procurement.

Health Care Facilities

In 2004, Paraguay's Ministry of Public Health and Social Welfare operated 23 district hospitals, 18 specialized hospitals, 50 dispensaries, 130 health centers, and 670 health posts, while the Institute of Public Welfare operated one general hospital, one specialized hospital, 10 regional hospitals, five outlying clinics, and 60 first-level units. The National University of Asuncion has a teaching hospital, providing care primarily for low-income people, and the Police Clinic in Asuncion provides the most complex hospital care available in Paraguay. The private nonprofit sector operates 30 care facilities, and the private for-profit sector operate a number of hospitals, emergency services, pharmacies, laboratories, physician offices, and other care facilities. As of 2010, according to WHO, Paraguay had 10.18 health posts per 100,000 population, 1.83 health centers per 100,000, 2.17 district or rural hospitals per 100,000, 0.12 provincial hospitals per 100,000, and 0.26 specialized hospitals per 100,000. In 2009, Paraguay had 1.30 hospital beds per 1,000 population. As of 2007, 26 outpatient facilities plus the Psychiatric Hospital provide mental health services.

Major Health Issues

In 2008, WHO estimated that 35 percent of years of life lost in Paraguay were due to communicable diseases, 45 percent to noncommunicable diseases, and 21 percent to injuries. In 2008, the age-standardized estimate of cancer deaths was 133 per 100,000 for men and 98 per 100,000 for women; for cardiovascular disease and diabetes, 269 per 100,000 for men and 228 per 100,000 for women; and for chronic respiratory disease, 24 per 100,000 for men and 10 per 100,000 for women.

Paraguay's maternal mortality rate (death from any cause related to or aggravated by pregnancy) was estimated in 2008 as 95 maternal deaths per 100,000 live births. The infant mortality rate, defined as the number of deaths of infants younger than 1 year, was estimated at 22.24 per 1,000 live births as of 2012. In 2010, tuberculosis incidence was 46.0 per 100,000 population, tuberculosis prevalence 64.0 per 100,000, and deaths due to tuberculosis among HIV-negative people 4.20 per 100,000. As of 2009, an estimated 0.3 percent of adults age 15 to 49 were living with HIV or acquired immune deficiency syndrome (AIDS).

Health Care Personnel

As of 2007, Paraguay had four medical schools. The basic medical degree course lasts six years, and the degree awarded is Médico Cirujano (physician and surgeon). In 2002, Paraguay had 1.11 physicians per 1,000 population, 0.33 pharmaceutical personnel per 1,000, 0.55 dentistry personnel per 1,000, 1.15

community and traditional health workers per 1,000, and 1.79 nurses and midwives per 1,000.

Government Role in Health Care

According to WHO, in 2010, Paraguay spent $1.1 billion on health care, an amount that comes to $163 per capita. Most (98 percent) health care funding came from domestic sources, with 2 percent coming from sources from abroad. More than half (57 percent) of health care spending was paid for through household expenditures, with the remainder provided through government expenditures (36 percent) and other sources (7 percent). In 2010, Paraguay allocated 11 percent of its total government expenditures to health, and government expenditures on health came to 2 percent of GDP; both figures are in the low range for lower-middle-income Americas region countries. In 2009, according to WHO, official development assistance (ODA) for health in Paraguay came to $3.63 per capita.

Public Health Programs

According to WHO, in 2002, Paraguay had 0.02 environmental and public health workers per 1,000 population. In 2010, 71 percent of the population had access to improved sanitation facilities (40 percent in rural areas and 90 percent in urban), and 86 percent had access to improved sources of drinking water (66 percent in rural areas and 99 percent in urban). According to the World Higher Education Database (WHED), two universities in Paraguay offer programs in epidemiology or public health: the National University of Asuncion, and the University of the Integration of the Americas in Asuncion.

PERU

Peru is a northwestern South American country, sharing borders with Bolivia, Brazil, Chile, Colombia, and Ecuador and having a coastline on the south Pacific Ocean. The area of 496,225 square miles (1,285,216 square kilometers) makes Peru the 20th-largest country in the world (similar in size to Alaska), and the July 2012 population was estimated at 29.5 million. In 2010, 77 percent of the population lived in urban areas, and the 2010 to 2015 annual rate of urbanization was estimated at 1.6 percent. Lima is the capital and largest city (with a 2009 population estimated at 8.8 million). The population growth rate in 2012 was 1.0 percent, the net migration rate negative 3.0 migrants per 1,000 population, the birth rate 19.1 births per 1,000, and the total fertility rate 2.3 children per woman. The United Nations High Commissioner for Refugees (UNHCR) estimated that, in 2010, there were 136 refugees and persons in refugee-like situations in Peru.

Peru became a Spanish colony in the 16th century and became an independent country in 1824. Peru ranked tied for 80th among 183 countries on the *Corruption Perceptions Index 2011,* with a score of 3.4 (on a scale where 0 indicates highly corrupt and 10 very clean). In 2011, Peru was classified as a country with high human development (the second-highest category) on the United Nations Development Programme's (UNDP's) Human Development Index (HDI), with a score of 0.725 (on a scale where 1 denotes high development and 0 low development). Life expectancy at birth in 2012 was estimated at 72.73 years, and per capita gross domestic product (GDP) in 2011 was estimated at $10,000. In 2010, the Gini Index (a measure of dispersion, in which perfect equality is denoted by 0 and maximum inequality is denoted by 100) for family income was 46.0. According to the World Economic Forum's *Global Gender Gap Index 2011*, Peru ranked 73rd out of 135 countries on gender equality with a score of 0.680 (on a scale with a theoretical range of 1 for equality to 0 for inequality and an actual range in 2011 from 0.8530 to 0.4873).

Emergency Health Services

According to the World Health Organization (WHO), as of 2007, Peru did not have a formal and publicly available system for providing prehospital care (emergency care). However, all medical facilities are required to provide emergency care without regard for the patient's ability to pay.

Insurance

Peru has a social insurance (ESSALUD) system that requires monthly contributions and a number of private insurance plans (EPS); those covered by the social system can opt out and contract with the private system. The private plans are required to provide at least the level of care provided by ESSALUD. The Integrated Health Insurance System (SIS) provides free care for the extremely poor. The social insurance system covers many categories of workers and their dependents, including employees in the public

and private sectors; the self-employed; those working in cooperative and worker-owned and cooperative enterprises; and professional artists. Employees whose employers provide health services are excluded. Pensioners are covered for health benefits, nursing, and the funeral grant only. Employees not covered under the national system, including fishermen and dock workers, are covered under separate systems.

The systems are funded through contributions from the self-employed (the amount depends on the system chosen), pensioners (4 percent of the pension), and employers (9 percent of payroll; those who provide medical benefits directly, or contract with EPS to provide them, receive a 25 percent credit on contributions). Employees can choose to have medical benefits from EPS or ESSALUD; to join EPS, at least 51 percent of the employees must agree. Medical services covered include hospitalization; lab services; medicines; rehabilitation; preventative care; immunization; and general, specialist, dental, and maternity care. Medical benefits from an EPS provider require a copayment of 2 percent of monthly income up to 10 percent of income. The maternity benefit is 100 percent of average earnings, with a ceiling, paid for 45 days before and after the due date, with an additional 30 days for multiple births. The sickness benefit is 100 percent

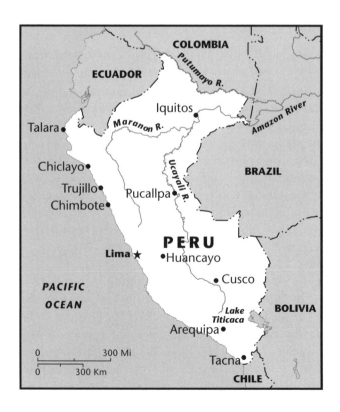

of average earnings for up to 18 months. The nursing allowance is a lump sum of PEN 820; the funeral grant is up to six times the monthly wage. ESSALUD administers the program, the Superintendent of Private Health Providers authorizes and supervises private health providers, and the Comptroller General of the Republic provides general supervision. According to Ke Xu and colleagues, in 2003, 3.2 percent of households in Peru experienced catastrophic health expenditures annually; "catastrophic" was defined as exceeding 40 percent of household income remaining after basic needs were met.

Costs of Hospitalization

Users must pay for hospital care, including drugs and lab tests, with the exception of services provided under the ESSALUD system.

Access to Health Care

According to Latinobarometer, an annual public opinion survey conducted in Latin America, 26 percent of citizens in Peru are satisfied with the level of health care available to them (the regional average is 51.9 percent). According to WHO, in 2009, 82.9 percent of births in Peru were attended by skilled personnel (for example, physicians, nurses, or midwives), and 93 percent of pregnant women received at least four prenatal care visits. The 2010 immunization rates for 1-year-olds were 93 percent for diphtheria and pertussis (DPT3), 94 percent for measles (MCV), and 93 percent for Hib (Hib3). In 2010, an estimated 57 percent of persons with advanced human immunodeficiency virus (HIV) infection were receiving antiretroviral therapy in accordance with the 2010 WHO guidelines.

Cost of Drugs

Drugs marketed in Peru must be registered, but the approval process is straightforward, and more than 12,000 pharmaceutical products were registered by 2002. An Essential Medicines List (EML) specifies which drugs are used in public-sector outlets; the EML included over 360 active substances as of 2006. A centralized process procures drugs used in the public sector. Some drugs are exempt from the import tax (12 percent) and the sales tax (19 percent), including cancer drugs and antiretrovirals. According to a 2006 Health Action International survey of the price and availability of a market basket of drugs, in the public sector drugs were procured and distributed to patients at prices somewhat above international norms.

The median price ratio for procurement prices (the ratio of the price in Peru to the international reference price) for generics was 1.28, and the median price ratio for the prices paid by patients was 1.40; only a few originator brands were found in the public sector. Median availability was 61.5 percent for generics, with a range of 11 percent to 100 percent for medicines on the EML. Prices were higher in the private sector, with a median price ratio of 5.61 for the lowest-priced generics, with a range of 0.4 to 40.0, and 27.79 for originator brands, with a range of 2.0 to 181.0. The median availability for the lowest-priced generics was 60.9 percent versus 14.6 percent for originator brands.

In the 2006 survey, medicines were found to be generally affordable, using the wages of the lowest-paid government worker as a standard, if generics were available in the public sector; for instance, an adult respiratory infection could be treated with generic amoxicillin for 0.2 day's wages if public-sector generics were used, while purchase of the equivalent originator brand drugs in the private sector would cost 1.9 days' wages or 0.4 day's wages for generic drugs purchased in the private sector. To treat a urinary tract infection with generic ciprofloxacin purchased in the private sector would cost 0.1 day's wages; generics purchased in the private sector would cost 0.5 day's wages, and originator brand drugs purchased in the private sector would cost 11.0 days' wages.

Health Care Facilities

In 2009, Peru had 1.50 hospital beds per 1,000 population.

Major Health Issues

In 2008, WHO estimated that 37 percent of years of life lost in Peru were due to communicable diseases, 46 percent to noncommunicable diseases, and 17 percent to injuries. In 2008, the age-standardized estimate of cancer deaths was 109 per 100,000 for men and 119 per 100,000 for women; for cardiovascular disease and diabetes, 148 per 100,000 for men and 121 per 100,000 for women; and for chronic respiratory disease, 33 per 100,000 for men and 20 per 100,000 for women.

In 2008, the age-standardized death rate from malaria was 0.1 per 100,000 population. Peru's maternal mortality rate (death from any cause related to or aggravated by pregnancy) was estimated in 2008 as 88 maternal deaths per 100,000 live births. The infant mortality rate, defined as the number of deaths of infants younger than 1 year, was estimated at 21.50 per 1,000 live births as of 2012.

In 2010, tuberculosis incidence was 106.0 per 100,000 population, tuberculosis prevalence 118.0 per 100,000, and deaths due to tuberculosis among HIV-negative people 6.10 per 100,000. As of 2009, an estimated 0.4 percent of adults age 15 to 49 were living with HIV or acquired immune deficiency syndrome (AIDS).

Health Care Personnel

In 2006, WHO identified Peru as one of 57 countries with a critical deficit in the supply of skilled health workers. As of 2007, Peru had 18 medical schools. The basic medical degree course lasts six to eight years with a further year of supervised practice required for the degree Médico Cirujano (physician and surgeon). One year of service in a rural area is required after graduation. Physicians must register with the Colegio Médico del Perú. In 2009, Peru had 0.92 physicians per 1,000 population, 0.06 pharmaceutical personnel per 1,000, 0.04 laboratory health workers per 1,000, 2.90 health management and support workers per 1,000, 0.12 dentistry personnel per 1,000, and 1.27 nurses and midwives per 1,000.

Government Role in Health Care

According to WHO, in 2010, Peru spent $7.8 billion on health care, an amount that comes to $269 per capita. Most (98 percent) health care funding came from domestic sources, with 2 percent of funding coming from abroad. Just over half (54 percent) of health care spending was paid for through government expenditures, with the remainder provided through household expenditures (39 percent) and other sources (7 percent). In 2010, Panama allocated 14 percent of its total government expenditures to health, in the median range for upper-middle-income countries in the Americas; government expenditures on health came to 3 percent of GDP, in the low range for upper-middle-income countries in the Americas. In 2009, according to WHO, official development assistance (ODA) for health in Peru came to $3.38 per capita.

Public Health Programs

The National Institute of Health (INS) is located in Lima and headed by Percy Minaya. Its chief responsibility is to control the spread of communicable disease, improve occupational health, and monitor and improve nutritional health. The INS staff of more than 700 is organized into seven departments, with specialties including research and technology transfer, biologics production, food and nutrition, public health, intercultural health, occupation health, environmental health, and quality control. The INS completed modern labs in Lima and Iquitos in 2008 in order to better track disease outbreaks and epidemics. In the same year, the INS produced the first antivenom for the bite of the Bothrop snake, and it also produces antivenom to treat other snake and spider bites and produces the antirabies vaccine.

According to WHO, in 2009, Peru had fewer than 0.01 environmental and public health workers per 1,000 population. In 2010, 71 percent of the population had access to improved sanitation facilities (37 percent in rural areas and 81 percent in urban), and 85 percent had access to improved sources of drinking water (65 percent in rural areas and 91 percent in urban).

According to the World Higher Education Database (WHED), three universities in Peru offer programs in epidemiology or public health: Daniel Alcides Carrion National University in Cerro de Pasco, Cayetano Heredia Peruvian University in Lima, and Peruvian Union University in Lima.

PHILIPPINES

The Philippines is an island nation in the north Pacific Ocean, consisting of more than 7,000 islands. The area of 115,831 square miles (300,000 square kilometers) makes the Philippines about the size of Arizona, and the July 2012 population was estimated at 103.8 million. In 2010, 49 percent of the population lived in urban areas, and the 2010 to 2015 annual rate of urbanization was estimated at 2.3 percent. Manila is the capital and largest city (with a 2009 population estimated at 11.5 million). The population growth rate in 2012 was 1.9 percent, the net migration rate negative 1.3 migrants per 1,000 population, the birth rate 25.0 births per 1,000, and the total fertility rate 3.2 children per woman. The United Nations High Commissioner for Refugees (UNHCR) estimated that, in 2010, there were 65 refugees and persons in refugee-like situations in the Philippines.

The Philippines became a Spanish colony in the 16th century and were ceded to the United States in

1898; in 1946, the Philippines became an independent country. The United States maintained a military presence on the islands until 1992, when the last U.S. military bases in the Philippines were closed. The Philippines ranked tied for 129th among 183 countries on the *Corruption Perceptions Index 2011,* with a score of 2.6 (on a scale where 0 indicates highly corrupt and 10 very clean). In 2011, the Philippines was classified as a country with medium human development (the second from the lowest of four categories) on the United Nations Development Programme's (UNDP's) Human Development Index (HDI), with a score of 0.644 (on a scale where 1 denotes high development and 0 low development). The Philippines experienced severe typhoons in the last quarter of 2011, and as of March 2012, 38 percent of households in the affected areas were food insecure, according to the World Food Programme. Life expectancy at birth in 2012 was estimated at 71.94 years, and estimated gross domestic product (GDP) per capita in 2011 was $4,100. In 2006, the Gini Index (a measure of dispersion, in which perfect equality is denoted by 0 and maximum inequality is denoted by 100) for family income was 45.8. Gender equality is high: According to the World Economic Forum's *Global Gender Gap Index 2011*, the Philippines ranked eighth out of 135

countries on gender equality with a score of 0.769 (on a scale with a theoretical range of 1 for equality to 0 for inequality and an actual range in 2011 from 0.8530 to 0.4873).

Emergency Health Services

According to the World Health Organization (WHO), as of 2007, the Philippines had a formal and publicly available emergency care (prehospital care) system accessible through regional access numbers, but not a national access number. Doctors Without Borders (Médecins Sans Frontières, or MSF) began working in the Philippines in 2008 and had 51 staff members in the country at the close of 2010. MSF first began working in the Philippines in Mindanao, providing basic health care. In 2010, MSF also provided health care to persons displaced by violence; MSF provided more than 27,500 consultations in this context, including providing care for 267 severely malnourished children and 3,455 pregnant women. MSF operations have been reduced in the Philippines following the presidential election in May 2010 as conflicts reduced and many people were able to return home; as a result, MSF reduced medical services and transferred most of its work to local authorities in October 2010.

Insurance

The Philippines has a social insurance system providing cash and medical benefits. Employees in the private sector, the self-employed, and household workers are covered to age 60, if they earn at least PHP 1,000 per month. Pensioners are also covered if they are 60 or older and have made at least 120 contributions since 1972. Sickness benefits are provided to government employees through a separate system. The system is funded through contributions from employed people, the self-employed, and employers; the government makes up deficits and covers the costs of people with low or no income. Medical benefits are provided by accredited providers who are paid by the health fund; cost sharing is required for some types of care, and inpatient care is limited to 45 days annually. The maternity benefit is 100 percent of average earnings for 60 days; the sickness benefit is 90 percent of average earnings for up to 120 days annually. The Philippine Health Insurance Corporation (PHIC, also called PhilHealth) collects contributions and administers benefits; the Department of Health provides policy coordination and guidance.

A 2005 study by WHO estimated that 55 percent of the total population had coverage through the PhilHealth National Health Insurance Programme. According to Donald West and colleagues, by 2009, 76 percent of the population was covered through the PHIC, but many do not use the system because they don't understand how it works. In addition, benefits are limited mainly to inpatient care and are capped, so out-of-pocket spending constitutes almost 60 percent of total health care spending. According to Ke Xu and colleagues, in 2003, 0.8 percent of households in the Philippines experienced catastrophic health expenditures annually; "catastrophic" was defined as exceeding 40 percent of household income remaining after basic needs were met.

Costs of Hospitalization

The Philippines has about 700 public hospitals and between 595 and 1,180 private hospitals. About two-thirds of hospital payments by PhilHealth went to private hospitals, and most of the top users of PhilHealth funds are private, tertiary-care facilities. In addition, private hospitals are required to provide emergency treatment to the poor (stable patients can be transferred to public facilities).

Access to Health Care

According to Donald West and colleagues, as of 2011, the Philippines has many problems providing access to health care to many of its citizens. Although most (76 percent) are covered by PHIC, it leaves many expenses uncovered, and many citizens do not understand how to use the system. The Philippines has a national network of public health care facilities supported by local governments, but financing is insufficient and many lack up-to-date technology. Shortages of professional personnel are another problem: The country's medical schools graduate about 2,000 physicians annually, but the number has been declining, while many nurses emigrate to work in other countries, particularly the United States, where nurses from the Philippines constitute 76 percent of foreign nursing graduates. About 5,000 to 8,000 nurses leave the Philippines annually, with about 4,000 of these being physicians who are retraining in order to emigrate; most (70 percent) of the nurses who pass the licensure exam leave the Philippines.

Pay is so low in public facilities that recruiting personnel can be a problem; in March 2010, it was reported that 200 hospitals were closed due to lack of staff, and 800 are only partially operating; many of the hospitals affected were located in the poorest areas of the Philippines. An estimated 70 percent of health care personnel work in the private sector, serving 20 to 30 percent of the population. Private health care facilities are located primarily in major metropolitan areas (Manila, Cebu, and Davos), and half of the members of the Philippine College of Physicians work in the Manila Metropolitan area; about 90 percent of physicians, dentists, and pharmacists work in urban areas, as do 35 percent of nurses and 20 percent of medical technicians. Firm figures are not available on the number of private hospitals in the Philippines—estimates range from more than 1,000 to less than 600.

According to WHO, in 2008, 62.2 percent of births in the Philippines were attended by skilled personnel (for example, physicians, nurses, or midwives), and 78 percent of pregnant women received at least four prenatal care visits. The 2010 immunization rates for 1-year-olds were 87 percent for diphtheria and pertussis (DPT3) and 88 percent for measles (MCV). In 2010, an estimated 51 percent of persons with advanced human immunodeficiency virus (HIV) infection were receiving antiretroviral therapy in accordance with the 2010 WHO guidelines. According to WHO, in 2010, the Philippines had 0.3 magnetic resonance imaging (MRI) machines per 1 million population and 1.18 computer tomography (CT) machines per 1 million.

Cost of Drugs

According to WHO, less than 30 percent of the population of the Philippines has regular access to essential medicines. The price of medicines has increased faster than the rate of inflation since 1985, and drugs are generally more expensive than in neighboring countries. Generic medicines are not commonly used, accounting for about 5 percent of sales. In 2002, the value of the pharmaceutical market in the Philippines was about PHP 65.7 million ($1.34 million). A 2005 survey by a team from Ateneo de Manila examined the price and availability of a market basket of drugs. This survey found that, even in the private sector, originator brand drugs were favored and that costs for both generics and originator brands were high.

The median price ratio for the lowest-priced generics was 5.14, meaning the price in the Philippines was on average more than five times as high as the international reference price for the drugs in question. For originator brands, the median price ratio was even higher, at 14.19. Patient prices, which included an average 22 percent markup, were even higher, with a median price ratio of 6.4 for the lowest-priced generics and 15.31 for originator brands. Availability was also low in the public sector, with median availability of 15.4 percent for the lowest-priced generic medicines and 7.7 percent for originator brands. Availability was somewhat higher in the private sector, at 26.5 percent for the lowest-priced generics and 33.3 percent for originator brands, but prices were also high; the median price ratio for the lowest-priced generic was 5.64 and 17.28 for originator brands. Affordability was a problem, particularly given the low availability of generics and drugs in general in the public sector; most courses of treatments would cost more than one day's wages (using the standard of the income of the lowest-paid government worker), and some would cost more than 20 days' wages.

Health Care Facilities
As of 2010, according to WHO, the Philippines had 1.56 district or rural hospitals per 100,000, 0.23 provincial hospitals per 100,000, and 0.13 specialized hospitals per 100,000. In 2006, the Philippines had 0.50 hospital beds per 1,000 population, one of the 20 lowest rates in the world.

Major Health Issues
In 2008, WHO estimated that 42 percent of years of life lost in the Philippines were due to communicable diseases, 45 percent to noncommunicable diseases, and 13 percent to injuries. In 2008, the age-standardized estimate of cancer deaths was 99 per 100,000 for men and 75 per 100,000 for women; for cardiovascular disease and diabetes, 395 per 100,000 for men and 295 per 100,000 for women; and for chronic respiratory disease, 81 per 100,000 for men and 33 per 100,000 for women.

In 2008, the age-standardized death rate from malaria was 0.2 per 100,000 population. In 2010, tuberculosis incidence was 275.0 per 100,000 population, tuberculosis prevalence 502.0 per 100,000, and deaths due to tuberculosis among HIV-negative people 33.00 per 100,000. As estimated, 4 percent of new tuberculosis cases and 21 percent of retreatment cases are multidrug resistant. WHO estimated the 2010 case detection rate at 65 percent. As of 2009, an estimated 0.1 percent of adults age 15 to 49 were living with HIV or acquired immune deficiency syndrome (AIDS).

The maternal mortality rate (death from any cause related to or aggravated by pregnancy) in the Philippines was estimated in 2008 as 94 maternal deaths per 100,000 live births. The infant mortality rate, defined as the number of deaths of infants younger than 1 year, was estimated at 18.75 per 1,000 live births as of 2012. In 2003, 20.7 percent of children under age 5 were underweight (defined as 2 kilograms [kg] below standard weight-for-age at age 1, 3 kg below for ages 2 to 3, and 4 kg below for ages 4 to 5).

Health Care Personnel
As of 2007, the Philippines had 30 medical schools. The basic course of training lasts four to seven years, and the degree awarded is Manggagamot (doctor of medicine). Physicians must also do a one-year internship and pass a licensing exam before receiving their medical licenses. Graduates of foreign medical schools and foreigners may practice in the Philippines only if the country in question has a reciprocal arrangement with the Philippines. In 2004, the Philippines had 1.15 physicians per 1,000 population, 0.61 pharmaceutical personnel per 1,000, 0.56 dentistry personnel per 1,000, and 6.00 nurses and midwives per 1,000. Using Fitzhugh Mullan's methodology, the Philippines has an emigration factor of 16.7, representing a high proportion of Filipino physicians working abroad.

Government Role in Health Care
According to WHO, in 2010, the Philippines spent $7.2 billion on health care, an amount that comes to $77 per capita. Almost all (99 percent) of health care funding came from domestic sources, with 1 percent coming from abroad. Just over half (54 percent) of health care spending was paid for through household expenditures, with the remainder provided through government expenditures (35 percent) and other sources (11 percent). In 2010, the Philippines allocated 8 percent of its total government expenditures to health, and government expenditures on health came to 1 percent of GDP; both figures are in the low range for lower-middle-income western Pacific region countries. In 2009, according to WHO, official development assistance (ODA) for health in the Philippines came to $1.05 per capita.

Public Health Programs
In 2010, 74 percent of the population of the Philippines had access to improved sanitation facilities (69 percent in rural areas and 79 percent in urban), and

92 percent had access to improved sources of drinking water (92 percent in rural areas and 93 percent in urban). According to the World Higher Education Database (WHED), 23 universities in the Philippines offer programs in epidemiology or public health.

POLAND

Poland is a central European country, sharing borders with Belarus, the Czech Republic, Germany, Lithuania, Russia (Kaliningrad), Slovakia, and Ukraine and having a coastline on the Baltic Sea. The area of 120,728 square miles (312,685 square kilometers) makes Poland about the size of New Mexico, and the July 2012 population was estimated at 38.4 million. In 2010, 61 percent of the population lived in urban areas, and the 2010 to 2015 annual rate of urbanization was estimated at negative 0.1 percent. Warsaw is the capital and largest city (with a 2009 population estimated at 1.7 million). The population growth rate in 2012 was negative 0.1 percent, the net migration rate negative 0.5 migrants per 1,000 population, the birth rate 10.0 births per 1,000, and the total fertility rate 1.3 children per woman (one of the 20th lowest in the world).

Poland became independent in 1918 but became a Soviet satellite after World War II. Poland held free elections in 1989 and 1990, with the Solidarity trade union movement winning control of the parliament and presidency. Poland ranked tied for 39th among 183 countries on the *Corruption Perceptions Index 2011*, with a score of 5.6 (on a scale where 0 indicates highly corrupt and 10 very clean). In 2011, Poland was classified as a country with very high human development (the highest of four categories) on the United Nations Development Programme's (UNDP's) Human Development Index (HDI), with a score of 0.813 (on a scale where 1 denotes high development and 0 low development). Life expectancy at birth in 2012 was estimated at 76.25 years, and per capita gross domestic product (GDP) in 2011 was estimated at $20,100. In 2008, the Gini Index (a measure of dispersion, in which perfect equality is denoted by 0 and maximum inequality is denoted by 100) for family income was 34.2.

According to the World Economic Forum's *Global Gender Gap Index 2011*, Poland ranked 42nd out of 135 countries on gender equality with a score of 0.704 (on a scale with a theoretical range of 1 for equality to 0 for inequality and an actual range in 2011 from 0.8530 to 0.4873).

Emergency Health Services

Poland's laws governing the emergency health system date from the 2000s, as does recognition of emergency medicine as a medical specialty; by law, free access to hospitals for emergency care is provided for all persons, including the uninsured. Funding for outpatient care in the emergency system is provided entirely by the state budget, while funding for inpatient emergency care is provided from public sources. Poland has two national telephone numbers for medical emergencies, 112 (the European Union, or EU, standard) and 999; the country has 290 dispatch centers that are interconnected.

Insurance

Poland has a social insurance system that provides medical benefits to a broad category of people and cash sickness and maternity benefits to employees. People eligible for the medical benefits system include the employed and self-employed, those receiving an unemployment allowance, students, persons in rehabilitation, pensioners, artists, authors, and family members of insured persons. The police, military, and farmers are covered under special systems. The system is funded through contributions from the employed and self-employed (2.45 percent for the cash benefits system, 9 percent for the medical benefits system, from gross earnings and declared earnings respectively); the government provides subsidies for medical benefits. Health care is provided by private providers under contract to the National Health Fund; covered services include hospitalization, specified surgeries, general and specialist care, lab services, eye and dental care, rehabilitation, some prescription drugs, and transportation.

Patients are allowed to select the physician and hospital for care. Most care is provided free, with cost sharing for prescription drugs. The maternity benefit is 100 percent of average earnings for 20 weeks (31 to 37 weeks for multiple births); the sickness benefit is 80 percent of average earnings for up to 90 days. A care allowance of 80 percent of average earnings is paid for up to 60 days if the person misses work to care for a sick family member or a well child younger than age 8. The National Health Fund contracts for medical services and administers public health funds,

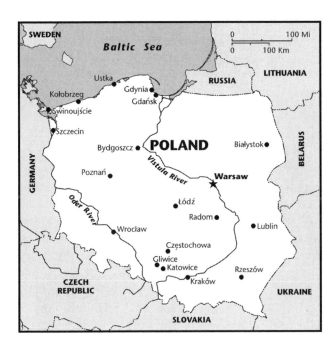

the Ministry of Health supervises medical benefits, and the Social Service Institution administers cash benefits under the supervision of the Ministry of Labor and Social Policy.

Costs of Hospitalization

In 2008, according to the Organisation for Economic Co-operation and Development (OECD), hospital spending in Poland represented 34.5 percent of total spending on health, and per capita spending was $391; hospitals were paid on a per case or diagnosis-related group (DRG) basis.

Access to Health Care

According to the World Health Organization (WHO), in 2006, 100 percent of births in Poland were attended by skilled personnel (for example, physicians, nurses, or midwives). The 2010 immunization rates for 1-year-olds were 99 percent for diphtheria and pertussis (DPT3), 98 percent for measles (MCV), and 99 percent for Hib (Hib3). In 2010, an estimated 34 percent of persons with advanced human immunodeficiency virus (HIV) infection were receiving antiretroviral therapy in accordance with the 2010 WHO guidelines. According to WHO, in 2010, Poland had 3.28 magnetic resonance imaging (MRI) machines per 1 million population, 10.63 computer tomography (CT) machines per 1 million, and 0.34 positron emission tomography (PET) machines per 1 million.

Cost of Drugs

According to Douglas Ball, Poland charges a lower value-added tax (VAT) of 7 percent for medicines as opposed to the standard VAT rate of 22 percent. There is no set pharmacy dispensing fee. The wholesale markup for reimbursed drugs is capped at 9.78 percent of ex-factory price (the manufacturer's list price before discounts), while the wholesale markup for nonreimbursed drugs is not regulated but averages 12 to 14 percent. The pharmacy markup for reimbursed medicines ranges from 12 to 40 percent of the wholesale price, with a cap of PLN 12; the markup for nonreimbursed drugs is not regulated but averages 25 percent. According to Elizabeth Docteur, in 2004, Poland ranked first among OECD countries in terms of the use of generic drugs in relation to the total use of pharmaceuticals; generics represented 65 percent of the market share in Poland as measured by value and 87 percent of the market share as measured by volume.

Health Care Facilities

As of 2010, according to WHO, Poland had 0.18 district or rural hospitals per 100,000, 0.61 provincial hospitals per 100,000, and 0.15 specialized hospitals per 100,000. In 2008, Poland had 6.62 hospital beds per 1,000 population, among the 20 highest ratios in the world.

Major Health Issues

In 2008, WHO estimated that 5 percent of years of life lost in Poland were due to communicable diseases, 80 percent to noncommunicable diseases, and 15 percent to injuries. In 2008, the age-standardized estimate of cancer deaths was 229 per 100,000 for men and 121 per 100,000 for women; for cardiovascular disease and diabetes, 366 per 100,000 for men and 205 per 100,000 for women; and for chronic respiratory disease, 29 per 100,000 for men and eight per 100,000 for women.

The maternal mortality rate (death from any cause related to or aggravated by pregnancy) in Poland in 2008 was six maternal deaths per 100,000 live births, among the lowest in the world. The infant mortality rate, defined as the number of deaths of infants younger than 1 year, was 6.42 per 1,000 live births as of 2012. In 2010, tuberculosis incidence was 23.0 per 100,000 population, tuberculosis prevalence 29.0 per 100,000, and deaths due to tuberculosis among HIV-negative people 2.0 per 100,000. As of 2009, an estimated 0.1 percent of adults age 15 to 49 were living with HIV or acquired immune deficiency syndrome (AIDS).

Health Care Personnel

As of 2007, Poland had 14 medical schools. The basic medical degree course lasts four or six years and the degree awarded is Lekarz (doctor of medicine). A one-year internship is also required for medical licensure. A foreigner wishing to practice in Poland must hold a residence permit and must have an adequate command of the Polish language.

Poland, as a member of the EU, cooperates with other countries in recognizing physicians qualified to practice in other EU countries, as specified by Directive 2005/36/EC of the European Parliament. This allows qualified professionals to practice their profession in other EU states on a temporary basis and requires that the host country automatically recognize qualifications for certain professions, including physicians, nurses, dentists, midwives, and pharmacists, if certain conditions have been met (for instance, facility in the language of the host country may be required). In 2008, Poland had 2.14 physicians per 1,000 population, 0.61 pharmaceutical personnel per 1,000, 0.34 dentistry personnel per 1,000, and 5.73 nurses and midwives per 1,000.

Government Role in Health Care

According to WHO, in 2010, Poland spent $35 billion on health care, an amount that comes to $917 per capita. All health care funding came from domestic sources. Almost three-quarters (73 percent) of health care spending was paid for through government expenditures, with the remainder provided through household expenditures (22 percent) and other sources (5 percent). In 2010, Poland allocated 12 percent of its total government expenditures to health, and government expenditures on health came to 5 percent of GDP; both figures are in the low range for high-income European countries.

Public Health Programs

The National Institute of Public Health for Poland is located in Warsaw and directed by Miroslaw J. Wysocki. It has been in operation for more than 90 years and has as its primary goals monitoring and surveillance of infectious diseases, along with a few noncommunicable diseases, and training public health workers. The institute also monitors pharmaceutical products, vaccines, and blood products. It has more than 300 staff

members organized in three divisions: epidemiology and microbiology, public health, and environmental health. One notable recent achievement was the publication, in 2008, of a national health survey comparing Poland to other European countries; future directions for planned research include health inequalities and public health genomics.

In 2010, 96 percent of the population of Poland had access to improved sanitation facilities, and 100 percent had access to improved sources of drinking water. According to the World Higher Education Database (WHED), eight universities in Poland offer programs in epidemiology or public health: the Academy of Medicine "Piastow Slaskich" in Wroclaw, the Academy of Medicine in Gdansk, the Silesian University of Medicine in Katowice, the Warsaw University of Life Science, Jagiellonian University in Krakow, the Poznan University of Medical Sciences, the University of Medicine in Bialystok, and the Medical University of Lodz.

PORTUGAL

Portugal is a western European country, sharing a border with Spain and having a coastline on the north Atlantic Ocean. The area of 35,556 square miles (92,090 square kilometers) makes Portugal about twice the size of Indiana, and the July 2012 population was estimated at 10.8 million. In 2010, 61 percent of the population lived in urban areas, and the 2010 to 2015 annual rate of urbanization was estimated at 0.1 percent. Lisbon is the capital and largest city (with a 2009 population estimated at 2.8 million). The population growth rate in 2012 was 0.2 percent, the net migration rate 2.9 migrants per 1,000 population, the birth rate 9.8 births per 1,000, and the total fertility rate 1.5 children per woman.

Portugal was a maritime and colonial power in the 15th to 19th centuries, with major colonies including Brazil, Goa (India), and Angola and Mozambique (Africa); the Portuguese empire was gradually disbanded in the 19th and 20th centuries, and the country also lost wealth due to a severe earthquake in Lisbon in 1755 and occupation during the Napoleonic Wars in the early 19th century. In 1910, the Portuguese monarchy was deposed, and a military government ran the county until 1974, when democratic reforms were instituted. Portugal ranks tied for 32nd among 183 countries on the *Corruption Perceptions Index 2011,* with a score of 6.1 (on a scale where 0 indicates highly corrupt and 10 very clean).

In 2011, Portugal was classified as a country with very high human development (the highest of four categories) on the United Nations Development Programme's (UNDP's) Human Development Index (HDI), with a score of 0.809 (on a scale where 1 denotes high development and 0 low development). Life expectancy at birth in 2012 was estimated at 78.70 years, and per capita gross domestic product (GDP) in 2011 was estimated at $23,200. In 2007, the Gini Index (a measure of dispersion, in which perfect equality is denoted by 0 and maximum inequality is denoted by 100) for family income was 38.5. According to the World Economic Forum's *Global Gender Gap Index 2011*, Portugal ranked 35th out of 135 countries on gender equality with a score of 0.704 (on a scale with a theoretical range of 1 for equality to 0 for inequality and an actual range in 2011 from 0.8530 to 0.4873).

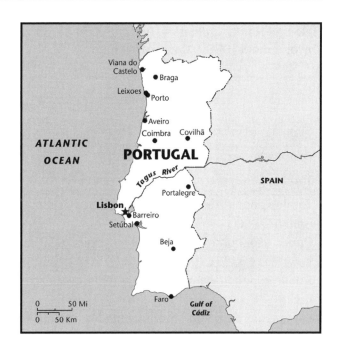

Emergency Health Services

Portugal's laws governing the emergency health system date from the 2000s; by law, free access to hospitals for emergency care is provided for all persons, including the uninsured. Funding for inpatient care in the emergency system is provided entirely by public sources, while funding for emergency outpatient care is funded entirely by the state budget. Portugal has two national telephone numbers for medical emergencies, 112 (the European Union, or EU, standard) and 03; the country has four dispatch centers that are interconnected.

Insurance

Portugal has a universal medical benefits system and a social insurance and social assistance system for cash benefits. All Portuguese citizens are covered under the medical benefits system, as are foreign citizens residing in Portugal from countries that have reciprocal agreements with Portugal. Employed people are eligible for the cash sickness benefit, and employed and self-employed people are eligible for cash maternity, paternity, and adoption benefits. The systems are funded by contributions from wages and earnings, employers, and the government. Medical benefits are provided directly at health centers and hospitals; services covered include hospitalization, surgery, general and specialist care, maternity care, some medicines, and long-term care; some benefits require cost sharing.

The maternity and paternity benefits are 100 percent of average earnings for a total of 120 days (shared between the mother and father) or 150 days at 80 percent of average earnings. The adoption benefit is 100 percent of average daily earnings for 120 days following adoption of a child age 14 or younger or 150 days at 80 percent of average earnings. The disabled or sick child allowance is 65 percent of average daily earnings paid to care for a child at home, with the number of days depending on the child's age and illness or disability.

Medical benefits are administered by regional health administrations and cash benefits by the Social Security Institute, and the program is supervised by the Ministry of Labor and Social Solidarity.

More than three-quarters (77.0 percent) of Portugal's population is covered by public health insurance, and 17.9 percent are covered by private health insurance. A 2004 study by the World Health Organization (WHO) found that none of the Portuguese population had substitutive voluntary health insurance (covering services that would otherwise be available from the state), and 12 percent had complementary voluntary health insurance (covering services not covered or not fully covered by the state) or supplementary health insurance (providing increased choice or faster access to services). The typical holder of a voluntary policy is between the ages of 25 and 54, is a professional or is self-employed, has a relatively high income, and lives

Selected Health Indicators: Portugal Compared With the Organisation for Economic Co-operation and Development (OECD) Country Average

	Portugal	OECD average (2010 or nearest year)
Male life expectancy at birth, 2010	76.7	77
Female life expectancy at birth, 2010	82.8	82.5
Total expenditure on health (percent of GDP), 2010	10.7	9.5
Total expenditure on health (per capita, USD purchasing power parity), 2010	2,727.7	3,265
Public expenditure on health (per capita, USD purchasing power parity), 2010	1,794.8	2,377.8
Public expenditure on health (percent total expenditure on health), 2010	65.8	72.2
Total expenditure on pharmaceuticals and other medical non-durables (percent total expenditure on health), 2010	18.6	16.6
Total expenditure on pharmaceuticals and other medical non-durables (per capita, USD purchasing power parity), 2010	508.1	495.4
Hospital beds (per 1,000 population), 2009	3.4	4.9
Average length of hospital stay, all causes (days), 2009	5.9	7.1

Source: OECD Health Data 2012 (Organisation for Economic Co-operation and Development, 2012).

in an urban area. According to Ke Xu and colleagues, in 2003, 2.7 percent of households in Portugal experienced catastrophic health expenditures annually; "catastrophic" was defined as exceeding 40 percent of household income remaining after basic needs were met.

Costs of Hospitalization

In 2008, according to the Organisation for Economic Co-operation and Development (OECD), hospital spending in Portugal represented 37.5 percent of total spending on health, and per capita spending was $796; hospitals were paid based on a prospective global budget. In 1990, Portugal began applying case-mix adjustment to the global hospital budget model, making it the first European country to do so.

Access to Health Care

According to WHO, in 2001, 100 percent of births in Portugal were attended by skilled personnel (for example, physicians, nurses, or midwives). The 2010 immunization rates for 1-year-olds were 98 percent for diphtheria and pertussis (DPT3), 96 percent for measles (MCV), and 97 percent for Hib (Hib3). According to WHO, in 2010, Portugal had 9.83 magnetic resonance imaging (MRI) machines per 1 million population, 27.25 computer tomography (CT) machines per 1 million, 0.56 positron emission tomography (PET) machines per 1 million, 0.56 telecolbalt units per 1 million, and 0.56 radiotherapy machines per 1 million.

Cost of Drugs

In 2005, total pharmaceutical expenditure in Portugal came to 3.31 billion euros ($4.10 billion), for a per capita expenditure of 311.20 euros ($440.90). Pharmaceutical expenditures made up 20 percent of total health expenditures, and 1.5 percent of GDP. About two-thirds (63.2 percent) of pharmaceutical expenditures were in the public sector. Generic pharmaceuticals constituted 19.1 percent of the market and have become more important: The annual growth rate for the total pharmaceutical market is negative 2.5 percent, while for generics alone, it is 4.5 percent. Some medications are provided publicly at no cost, including insulin, cancer drugs used in inpatient treatment, drugs for human immunodeficiency virus and acquired immune deficiency syndrome (HIV/AIDS), and contraceptives; vaccines on WHO's Expanded Programme on Immunization (EPI) list are provided free of charge. Drugs for treating some conditions are fully reimbursed: These include cystic fibrosis, lupus, hemophilia, paramyloidosis, rheumatoid arthritis, thalassemia, and Turner's syndrome. Private health insurance plans include some drug coverage, but what is covered is not mandated.

Drugs provided during hospital care are generally provided free of charge. Drugs provided for outpatient care are divided into four categories, with different levels of reimbursement for each. Category A drugs are reimbursed at 95 percent; these include life-saving or essential pharmaceuticals to treat chronic disease. Category B drugs are reimbursed at 69 percent; these include essential pharmaceuticals to treat serious illnesses such as asthma and cardiovascular disease. Category C drugs are reimbursed at 37 percent; these include drugs with proven therapeutic value but which are not priorities, such as vaccines not included in the National Vaccination Plan. Category D drugs are reimbursed at 15 percent; these include drugs whose therapeutic value is uncertain. Drugs that will be reimbursed for outpatient care are listed on a positive list of medicines, while medicines eligible for use within hospitals are listed on the National Hospital Pharmaceutical Formulary.

As a member of the World Trade Organization (WTO), Portugal observes patent law, but national law also includes some elements of the Trade-Related Aspects of Intellectual Property Rights (TRIPS), which provide exceptions to patent law. In Portugal, this includes the Bolar exception, which allows manufacturers to perform research and testing to create generic drugs before a patent has expired, and parallel importing provisions (allowing import of drugs created for sale in a different country). Drugs sold in Portugal must be approved and registered; as of 2011, there were 14,655 drugs registered in Portugal. According to Elizabeth Docteur, in 2004, generic drugs represented 9 percent of the market share by value and 5 percent of the market share by volume of the total pharmaceutical market.

Drug prices for prescription-only and reimbursed over-the-counter medicines are regulated at several levels within Portugal. At the manufacturer level, maximum prices are set. At the wholesale level and retail levels, the profit margin is set by law. The Portuguese government has systems to monitor retail prices, and prices for medicines are available through a publicly available database. According to Douglas Ball, Portugal charges a lower value-added tax (VAT) for medicines (5 percent of the manufacturer's price) than for other goods (the standard VAT is 22 percent). There is no set pharmacy dispensing fee. The wholesale markup is 6.87 percent of the retail price (without VAT) for reimbursed medicines and 8 percent of the retail price without VAT for nonreimbursed medicines. The pharmacy markup is 18.27 percent of the retail price without VAT for reimbursed medicines and 20 percent of the retail price without VAT for reimbursed medicines. Real annual growth in pharmaceutical expenditures in Portugal grew 4.0 percent from 1997 to 2005, slower than the 5.4 percent growth of total health expenditure (minus pharmaceutical expenditures) over those years.

Health Care Facilities

As of 2010, according to WHO, Portugal had 3.06 health posts per 100,000 population and 0.18 health centers per 100,000. In 2008, Portugal had 3.37 hospital beds per 1,000 population.

Major Health Issues

In 2008, WHO estimated that 10 percent of years of life lost in Portugal were due to communicable diseases, 81 percent to noncommunicable diseases, and 9 percent to injuries. In 2008, the age-standardized estimate of cancer deaths was 182 per 100,000 for men and 89 per 100,000 for women; for cardiovascular disease and diabetes, 185 per 100,000 for men and 125 per 100,000 for women; and for chronic respiratory disease, 35 per 100,000 for men and 15 per 100,000 for women.

The maternal mortality rate (death from any cause related to or aggravated by pregnancy) in Portugal in 2008 was seven maternal deaths per 100,000 live births, among the lowest in the world. The infant mortality rate, defined as the number of deaths of infants younger than 1 year, was 4.60 per 1,000 live births as of 2012. In 2010, tuberculosis incidence was 29.0 per 100,000 population, tuberculosis prevalence 32.0 per 100,000, and deaths due to tuberculosis among HIV-negative people 1.50 per 100,000. As of 2009, an estimated 0.6 percent of adults age 15 to 49 were living with HIV or AIDS.

Health Care Personnel

Portugal has five medical schools, the oldest of which, the Faculty of Medicine of the University of Coimbra, has been offering instruction since 1290. The basic course of study lasts six years with an additional 18 months of supervised practice required before licensure. The degree awarded is Licenciatura em Medicina (license in medicine). Registration is required with the Ordem dos Médicos in Lisbon.

Portugal, as a member of the EU, cooperates with other countries in recognizing physicians qualified to practice in other EU countries, as specified by Directive 2005/36/EC of the European Parliament. This allows qualified professionals to practice their profession in other EU states on a temporary basis and requires that the host country automatically recognize qualifications for certain professions, including physicians, nurses, dentists, midwives, and pharmacists, if certain conditions have been met (for instance, facility in the language of the host country may be required). In 2009, Portugal had 3.76 physicians per 1,000 population and, in 2008, had 0.65 pharmaceutical personnel per 1,000, 0.67 dentistry personnel per 1,000, and 5.33 nurses and midwives per 1,000.

Government Role in Health Care

The right to health, including the right to essential medicines and medical technologies, is recognized in the 2005 constitution. Portugal has a National Health Policy (NHP), updated in 2010, and a plan to implement it; a new national health plan for 2011 to 2016 is being drafted. Portugal also has a National Medicines Policy (NMP), updated in 2005, and policy implementation is monitored by the National Authority of Medicines and Health Products. The NMP does not include selection of essential medicines but does cover the financing, pricing, procurement, distribution and regulation of medicines; pharmacovigilance; the rational use of medicines; human resource development; research; and monitoring and evaluation. Promotion and advertising of prescription drugs is controlled by law in Portugal, and direct advertising to the public is prohibited.

According to WHO, in 2010, Portugal spent $25 billion on health care, an amount that comes to $2,367 per capita. All health care funding came from domestic sources. More than two-thirds (68 percent) of health care spending was paid for through government expenditures, with the remainder provided through household expenditures (25 percent) and

other sources (7 percent). In 2010, Portugal allocated 15 percent of its total government expenditures to health, and government expenditures on health came to 7 percent of GDP; both figures are in the median range for high-income European countries.

Public Health Programs

The Institute of Hygiene and Tropical Medicine (IHMT) is located within the New University of Lisbon and is supervised by the Ministry of Science and Higher Education Innovation; Paulo Ferrinho is the director. The IHMT, founded in 1902, focuses primarily on tropical medicine and health care in developing countries; it is involved in many cooperative projects with international organizations such as the World Bank, WHO, and the European School of Tropical Medicine. The National Health Institute (INSA), also located in Lisbon, focuses on public health within Portugal; the INSA was founded in 1899 and is directed by Jose Pereira Miguel. The primary responsibilities of INSA are organizing and promoting research, monitoring population health and conducting epidemiological surveys, and providing training to researchers and technicians. The INSA has more than 600 employees and is organized into six departments: food and nutrition, epidemiology, infectious diseases, genetics, environmental health, and health promotion and chronic disease. In 2010, access to improved sanitation facilities was essentially universal in Portugal, as was access to improved sources of drinking water.

According to the World Higher Education Database (WHED), eight universities in Portugal offer programs in epidemiology or public health: the Instituto Politecnico de Saude do Norte, the Egas Moniz School of Health, the Ribeiro Sanches School of Health, the Polytechnic Institute of Coimbra, the Institute of Health Studies of Alto Ave, the University of Oporto, the Lusophone University of Humanities and Technologies, and the New University of Lisbon.

QATAR

Qatar is a Middle Eastern country, sharing a border with Saudi Arabia and having a coastline on the Persian Gulf. The area of 4,473 square miles (11,586 square kilometers) makes Qatar about the size of Connecticut, and the July 2012 population was estimated

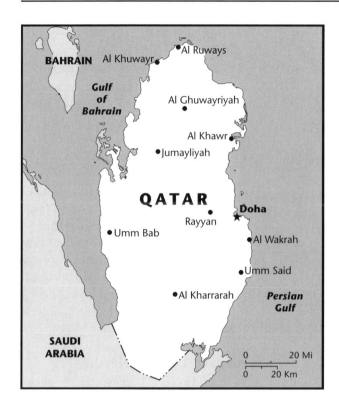

(UNDP's) Human Development Index (HDI), with a score of 0.831 (on a scale where 1 denotes high development and 0 low development). Life expectancy at birth in 2012 was estimated at 78.09 years, and per capita gross domestic product (GDP) in 2011 in Qatar was estimated at \$102,700, the second-highest in the world. In 2007, the Gini Index (a measure of dispersion, in which perfect equality is denoted by 0 and maximum inequality is denoted by 100) for family income was 41.1. According to the World Economic Forum's *Global Gender Gap Index 2011*, Qatar ranked 111th out of 135 countries on gender equality with a score of 0.623 (on a scale with a theoretical range of 1 for equality to 0 for inequality and an actual range in 2011 from 0.8530 to 0.4873).

Emergency Health Services

According to the World Health Organization (WHO), as of 2007, Qatar had a formal and publicly available emergency care (prehospital care) system accessible through a national access number.

Insurance

Public spending on health care has greatly increased in Qatar since 1991, and although currently Qatar does not have national health insurance, health care services are heavily subsidized by the government. Private and public health care institutions exist side by side, with private institutions and insurance sometimes chosen for reasons of convenience. One of the goals of Qatar's National Health Strategy (NHS) from 2011 to 2016 was to introduce a national health insurance scheme as part of the country's efforts to create a high-quality, sustainable health system.

Costs of Hospitalization

Costs for hospital treatment are heavily subsidized by the government.

Access to Health Care

Hamad Medical Corporation was established in Qatar in 1979 to improve health care services. Besides managing eight hospitals, it is responsible for the national ambulance services, home health care services, and residential services. Although the availability of specialty care in Qatar has increased, some services are not available in the country, and then citizens seek care abroad. One of the goals of the 2011 to 2016 National Health Strategy is to bring this process under closer control by establishing a

at 16.7 million. In 2010, 96 percent of the population lived in urban areas, and the 2010 to 2015 annual rate of urbanization was estimated at 1.6 percent. Doha is the capital and largest city (with a 2009 population estimated at 427,000). The population growth rate in 2012 was 0.4 percent, the net migration rate 2.0 migrants per 1,000 population, the birth rate 10.9 births per 1,000, and the total fertility rate 1.8 children per woman. The United Nations High Commissioner for Refugees (UNHCR) estimated that, in 2010, there were 51 refugees and persons in refugee-like situations in Qatar.

Qatar has been ruled by the Al Thani family since the mid-19th century; Ami Hamad bin Kalifa Al Thani became the ruler in 1995, deposing his father in a bloodless coup. Oil and natural gas resources have helped to make Qatar a prosperous country, and the country is also well known for the Al Jazirah news network based in Doha. The current government has a reputation for transparency and honesty, ranking tied for 22nd among 183 countries on the *Corruption Perceptions Index 2011,* with a score of 7.2 (on a scale where 0 indicates highly corrupt and 10 very clean).

In 2011, Qatar was classified as a country with very high human development (the highest of four categories) on the United Nations Development Programme's database of preferred providers, negotiating costs, making clear rules for eligibility to seek treatment abroad, and using an organized system to make travel arrangements. According to WHO, in 2009, 100 percent of births in Qatar were attended by skilled personnel (for example, physicians, nurses, or midwives). The 2010 immunization rates for 1-year-olds were 97 percent for diphtheria and pertussis (DPT3), 99 percent for measles (MCV), and 97 percent for Hib (Hib3).

Cost of Drugs

The National Health Strategy for Qatar from 2011 to 2016 includes development of a community pharmacy network, ensuring that the full range of drugs will be available at these pharmacies and encouraging medical providers to use them. Currently, in Qatar, only public-sector hospital pharmacies carry the full range of drugs, leading to inefficiencies.

Health Care Facilities

Hamad Medical Corporation is the primary non-profit health care provider in Qatar. Established in 1979, it now manages eight hospitals: Hamad General Hospital, Rumallah Hospital, the Women's Hospital, the National Center for Cancer Care and Research, Al Khor Hospital, the Heart Hospital, Al Wakra Hospital, and the Cuban Hospital; all these hospitals are accredited by the Joint Commission International. Several additional facilities are currently under construction, including a children's hospital, a new women's hospital, and facilities to provide skilled nursing care and physical medicine and rehabilitation. In 2008, Qatar had 1.40 hospital beds per 1,000 population.

Major Health Issues

In 2008, WHO estimated that 11 percent of years of life lost in Qatar were due to communicable diseases, 55 percent to noncommunicable diseases, and 34 percent to injuries. In 2008, the age-standardized estimate of cancer deaths was 101 per 100,000 for men and 84 per 100,000 for women; for cardiovascular disease and diabetes, 180 per 100,000 for men and 239 per 100,000 for women; and for chronic respiratory disease, 26 per 100,000 for men and 31 per 100,000 for women.

The maternal mortality rate (death from any cause related to or aggravated by pregnancy) in Qatar in 2008 was eight maternal deaths per 100,000 live births, among the lowest in the world. The infant mortality rate, defined as the number of deaths of infants younger than 1 year, was 6.81 per 1,000 live births as of 2012. In 2010, tuberculosis incidence was 38.0 per 100,000 population, tuberculosis prevalence 45.0 per 100,000, and deaths due to tuberculosis among human immunodeficiency virus (HIV)-negative people 2.10 per 100,000. As of 2009, an estimated 0.1 percent of adults age 15 to 49 were living with HIV or acquired immune deficiency syndrome (AIDS).

Health Care Personnel

In 2006, Qatar had 2.76 physicians per 1,000 population, 1.26 pharmaceutical personnel per 1,000, 0.58 dentistry personnel per 1,000, and 7.37 nurses and midwives per 1,000. Weill Cornell Medical College in Qatar, established in 2001 and affiliated with Weill Cornell Medical College in the United States, began classes with 25 students in 2002 and grew to enroll 265 students in 2012.

Government Role in Health Care

Qatar has a National Health Strategy (NHS) whose goals include providing world-class health care services to its citizens, creating a skilled workforce, conducting high-caliber research, and providing preventive health care. Health care in Qatar is regulated by the Supreme Council of Health, but most services are provided by private and public care providers. The Qatar Preventive Health Department focuses on communicable diseases and provides immunization services, education for maternal and child health, and services related to environmental health safety; it also has units focused on tobacco control, chronic diseases, accidents, statistics, and nutrition.

According to WHO, in 2010, Qatar spent $2.6 billion on health care, an amount that comes to $1,489 per capita. All health care funding came from domestic sources. More than three-quarters (77 percent) of health care spending was paid for through government expenditures, with the remainder provided through household expenditures (16 percent) and other sources (7 percent). In 2010, Qatar allocated 6 percent of its total government expenditures to health, and government expenditures on health came to 1 percent of GDP; both figures are in the low range for high-income eastern Mediterranean region countries.

Public Health Programs

In 2010, access to improved sanitary facilities and improved sources of drinking water was essentially universal in Qatar. Part of Qatar's 2011 to 2016

National Health Strategy addressed disease prevention and public health, including programs focusing on tobacco cessation, nutritional and physical activity, and prevention of communication diseases; a national screening program for diseases such as diabetes, breast cancer, and cardiovascular disease; and consanguinity risk reduction.

ROMANIA

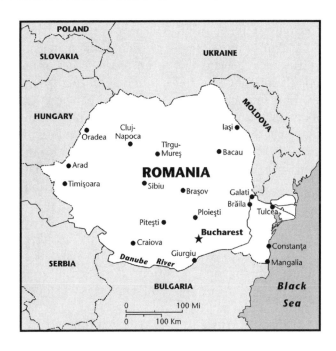

Romania is a country in southeastern Europe, sharing borders with Bulgaria, Hungary, Moldova, Serbia, and Ukraine and having a coastline on the Black Sea. The area of 92,043 square miles (238,391 square kilometers) makes Romania about the size of Oregon, and the July 2012 population was estimated at 21.8 million. In 2010, 57 percent of the population lived in urban areas, and the 2010 to 2015 annual rate of urbanization was estimated at 0.6 percent. Bucharest is the capital and largest city (with a 2009 population estimated at 1.9 million). The population growth rate in 2012 was negative 0.3 percent, the net migration rate negative 0.3 migrants per 1,000 population, the birth rate 9.5 births per 1,000, and the total fertility rate 1.8 children per woman. The United Nations High Commissioner for Refugees (UNHCR) estimated that, in 2010, there were 270 refugees and persons in refugee-like situations in Romania.

Romania was formed in 1862 by the union of Wallachia and Moldavia and achieved recognition of its independence in 1878. After World War II, Romania was occupied by the Soviet Union, and the king abdicated in 1947. Nicolae Ceausescu ruled as head of a police state from 1965 until 1989, when he was overthrown and executed. The country has operated as a democracy since the 1990s and joined the European Union (EU) in 2007. Romania ranked tied for 75th among 183 countries on the *Corruption Perceptions Index 2011,* with a score of 3.6 (on a scale where 0 indicates highly corrupt and 10 very clean).

In 2011, Romania was classified as a country with high human development (the second-highest category) on the United Nations Development Programme's (UNDP's) Human Development Index (HDI), with a score of 0.781 (on a scale where 1 denotes high development and 0 low development). Life expectancy at birth in 2012 was estimated at 74.22

years, and per capita gross domestic product (GDP) in 2011 was estimated at $12,300. In 2010, the Gini Index (a measure of dispersion, in which perfect equality is denoted by 0 and maximum inequality is denoted by 100) for family income was 33.3. According to the World Economic Forum's *Global Gender Gap Index 2011,* Romania ranked 68th out of 135 countries on gender equality with a score of 0.681 (on a scale with a theoretical range of 1 for equality to 0 for inequality and an actual range in 2011 from 0.8530 to 0.4873).

Emergency Health Services

Romania's laws governing the emergency health system date from the 2000s, while recognition of emergency medicine as a medical specialty dates from the 1990s; by law, free access to hospitals for emergency care is provided for all persons, including the uninsured. Funding for the emergency system is provided by multiple sources. Romania has only one national telephone number for medical emergencies, 112 (the EU standard); the country has 42 dispatch centers that are interconnected. In 2003, a team from the University of Toronto's International Emergency Medicine Fellowship program traveled to Romania to help plan improvement of the emergency medicine system.

Insurance

Romania has a social insurance system providing medical benefits to everyone residing in Romania (including foreign nationals who are not citizens) and a social insurance program providing cash maternity and sickness benefits that covers broad classes of the population. Those included in the cash benefits program include civil servants, employed persons with individual labor contracts, those receiving unemployment benefits, the self-employed, members of craft cooperatives, and some officials working for the legislative, executive, and judicial authorities. The medical benefits program is funded by contributions from wages (5.2 percent), the earnings of the self-employed (5.2 percent), and employers (5.5 percent of covered payroll); the government subsidizes deficits in the program. The cash benefits system is funded by contributions from the self-employed (0.85 percent of earnings) and employers (0.85 percent of covered payroll).

Medical benefits are provided directly through providers contracted with local health insurance funds. Covered benefits include hospitalization, general and specialist care, preventive care, maternity care, medicines, appliances, rehabilitation, and transportation. The maternity benefit is 85 percent of average monthly earnings paid for up to 126 days. The child care benefit is 85 percent of average monthly earnings for up to 45 days annually for a child age 6 or younger (age 17 or younger if the child is disabled); the benefit may be extended for serious conditions or contagious diseases (for example, emergency surgery, acquired immune deficiency syndrome, or AIDS, and tuberculosis). The cash sickness benefit is 75 percent of average monthly earnings for up to 183 days, with an extension possible; payment is 100 percent of average monthly earnings for contagious illnesses or emergency surgery.

The system is administered by the National Health Insurance Fund. According to Ke Xu and colleagues, in 2003, less than 0.1 percent of households in Romania experienced catastrophic health expenditures annually; "catastrophic" was defined as exceeding 40 percent of household income remaining after basic needs were met.

Costs of Hospitalization
No data available.

Access to Health Care
According to the World Health Organization (WHO), in 2008, 98.7 percent of births in Romania were attended by skilled personnel (for example,

physicians, nurses, or midwives). In 2004, 76 percent of pregnant women received at least four prenatal care visits. The 2010 immunization rates for 1-year-olds were 97 percent for diphtheria and pertussis (DPT3) and 95 percent for measles (MCV). In 2010, an estimated 69 percent of persons with advanced human immunodeficiency virus (HIV) infection were receiving antiretroviral therapy in accordance with the 2010 WHO guidelines.

Cost of Drugs
No data available.

Health Care Facilities
As of 2010, according to WHO, Romania had 0.02 health posts per 100,000 population, 0.06 health centers per 100,000, 0.43 district or rural hospitals per 100,000, 0.51 provincial hospitals per 100,000, and 0.76 specialized hospitals per 100,000. In 2008, Romania had 6.54 hospital beds per 1,000 population, among the 20 highest ratios in the world.

Major Health Issues
In 2008, WHO estimated that 8 percent of years of life lost in Romania were due to communicable diseases, 80 percent to noncommunicable diseases, and 12 percent to injuries. In 2008, the age-standardized estimate of cancer deaths was 189 per 100,000 for men and 100 per 100,000 for women; for cardiovascular disease and diabetes, 477 per 100,000 for men and 323 per 100,000 for women; and for chronic respiratory disease, 30 per 100,000 for men and 10 per 100,000 for women.

Romania's maternal mortality rate (death from any cause related to or aggravated by pregnancy) in 2008 was 27 maternal deaths per 100,000 live births. The infant mortality rate, defined as the number of deaths of infants younger than 1 year, was 10.73 per 1,000 live births as of 2012. In 2010, tuberculosis incidence was 116.0 per 100,000 population, tuberculosis prevalence 159.0 per 100,000, and deaths due to tuberculosis among HIV-negative people 7.0 per 100,000. As of 2009, an estimated 0.1 percent of adults age 15 to 49 were living with HIV or AIDS.

Health Care Personnel
As of December 2007, Romania had 12 medical schools. The course of training for the basic medical degree lasts six years, and the degree awarded is Doctor-medic (doctor of medicine). The Ministry of

Health grants the license to practice medicine, and foreigners are allowed to practice only if they are from a country with which Romania has a reciprocal agreement.

Romania, as a member of the EU, cooperates with other countries in recognizing physicians qualified to practice in other EU countries, as specified by Directive 2005/36/EC of the European Parliament. This allows qualified professionals to practice their profession in other EU states on a temporary basis and requires that the host country automatically recognize qualifications for certain professions, including physicians, nurses, dentists, midwives, and pharmacists, if certain conditions have been met (for instance, facility in the language of the host country may be required). In 2006, Romania had 1.92 physicians per 1,000 population, 0.08 pharmaceutical personnel per 1,000, 0.20 dentistry personnel per 1,000, and 4.19 nurses and midwives per 1,000.

Government Role in Health Care

According to WHO, in 2010, Romania spent $9.2 billion on health care, an amount that comes to $428 per capita. All health care funding came from domestic sources. More than three-quarters (78 percent) of health care spending was paid for through government expenditures, with the remainder provided through household expenditures (21 percent) and less than 1 percent coming from other sources. In 2010, Romania allocated 11 percent of its total government expenditures to health, and government expenditures on health came to 4 percent of GDP; both figures are in the median range for upper-middle-income European countries.

Public Health Programs

In 2005, 73 percent of the population of Romania had access to improved sanitation facilities (54 percent in rural areas and 88 percent in urban), and 89 percent had access to improved sources of drinking water (76 percent in rural areas and 99 percent in urban). According to the World Higher Education Database (WHED), four universities in Romania offer programs in epidemiology or public health: the Carol Davila University of Medicine and Pharmacy of Bucharest, the Iuliu Hatieganu University of Medicine and Pharmacy of Cluj-Napoca, the Victor Babes University of Medicine and Pharmacy of Timisoara, and the University of Agricultural Sciences and Veterinary Medicine of Cluj-Napoca.

RUSSIA

Russia is a northern European country sharing borders with 14 other countries and having coastlines (23,396 miles or 37,653 kilometers total) on the Arctic Sea, the north Pacific Ocean, and the Black Sea. The area of 8,801,668 square miles (17,098,242 square kilometers) makes Russia the largest country in the world, about 1.8 times the size of the United States. The July 2012 population was estimated at 138.0 million, the ninth-largest in the world. Moscow is the capital and largest city (with a 2009 population estimated at 10.5 million). In 2010, 73 percent of the population lived in urban areas, and the 2010 to 2015 annual rate of urbanization was estimated at negative 0.2 percent. The population growth rate in 2012 was negative 0.5 percent, the net migration rate 0.3 migrants per 1,000 population, the birth rate 10.9 births per 1,000, and the total fertility rate 1.4 children per woman. The United Nations High Commissioner for Refugees (UNHCR) estimated that, in 2010, there were 4,922 refugees and persons in refugee-like situations in Russia and 758 internally displaced persons and persons in internally displaced-person-like situations.

The Russian Empire was formed in the 17th and 18th centuries. In 1917, the imperial family was overthrown and executed, and the Union of Soviet

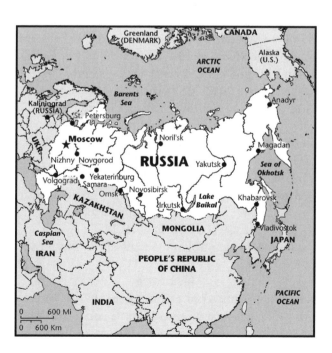

Socialist Republics (Soviet Union) was formed under Vladimir Lenin. The Soviet Union expanded during the 20th century, annexing some territories and exerting influence over others; in 1991, the Soviet Union split up, and many of the former Soviet republics became independent countries. Russia ranked tied for 143rd among 183 countries on the *Corruption Perceptions Index 2011,* with a score of 2.4 (on a scale where 0 indicates highly corrupt and 10 very clean).

In 2011, Russia was classified as a country with high human development (the second-highest category) on the United Nations Development Programme's (UNDP's) Human Development Index (HDI), with a score of 0.755 (on a scale where 1 denotes high development and 0 low development). Life expectancy at birth in 2012 was estimated at 66.46 years, and per capita gross domestic product (GDP) in 2011 was estimated at $16,700. In 2010, the Gini Index (a measure of dispersion, in which perfect equality is denoted by 0 and maximum inequality is denoted by 100) for family income was 42.0. According to the World Economic Forum's *Global Gender Gap Index 2011*, Russia ranked 43rd out of 135 countries on gender equality with a score of 0.704 (on a scale with a theoretical range of 1 for equality to 0 for inequality and an actual range in 2011 from 0.8530 to 0.4873).

Emergency Health Services

According to the World Health Organization (WHO), as of 2007, Russia had a formal and publicly available emergency care (prehospital care) system accessible through a national access number. Doctors Without Borders (Médecins Sans Frontières, or MSF) began working in Russia in 1988 and in the North Caucasus in 1995 and had 192 staff members in the country at the close of 2010. MSF provides psychological services to support victims of violence in Ingushetia and Chechnya, including in mountainous areas where violence is more frequent, and provides general medical care and counseling to migrants and other displaced persons in Khasavyurt, Dagestan. MSF has operated pediatric and gynecological clinics in Grozny, Chechnya, since 2005 and, in 2010, opened two similar clinics in northern Chechnya. In 2010, MSF began working to improve control of tuberculosis in Chechnya.

Insurance

Russia has a universal medical benefits system covering all citizens and refugees and a social insurance system providing cash sickness and maternity benefits to employed persons. The medical benefits system is partially funded out of general tax revenues by the federal and local governments and by an employer payroll tax (5.1 percent of payroll; this also partially funds the family allowance system). The cash benefits program is funded by employer contributions (2.9 percent of payroll). Individuals may also choose to belong to a supplementary medical and maternity insurance plan, with costs varying according to the plan chosen.

Medical benefits are provided through direct service provision by public and private health care providers. Services covered include hospitalization, preventive care, emergency care, general medical care, lab services, maternity care, dental care, vaccinations, and transportation. Medicines require payment, although they are provided free during hospitalization, and are also free or at reduced cost to some population categories, including the elderly, the disabled, war veterans, and people with certain illnesses.

The maternity benefit is 100 percent of earnings for 70 days before and after childbirth, with possible extension of up to an additional 40 days; the ceiling for the benefit is RUB 25,390. A pregnancy registration supplement of RUB 374.62 is paid (the woman must register the pregnancy in the first 12 weeks), along with a childbirth grant of RUB 9,989.86. The child care benefit (also available to unemployed parents) is 40 percent of the average wage until the child is 18 months old; the minimum benefit is RUB 1,873 for the first child and RUB 3,746.20 for all subsequent children. The sickness benefit depends on the length of employment and ranges from 60 to 100 percent of current earnings. The sickness benefit is also paid for the care of a sick child or family member, and the length of the benefit ranges from seven to 60 days per year, depending on the age of the sick person.

Health care programs are developed and state health care policy implemented by the Ministry of Health and Social Development and regional health departments, and the Federal Compulsory Medical Insurance Fund administers the financing of medical insurance and implements health care policy within the social insurance system.

Costs of Hospitalization

As of 2002, different methods of paying for hospital care were in use in Russia's 89 administrative regions; per-case payments were the most common (about 35 percent), followed by bed days (about 24 percent), with line-item funding, global budgets, and other methods also in use.

Access to Health Care

According to WHO, in 2008, 99.6 percent of births in Russia were attended by skilled personnel (for example, physicians, nurses, or midwives). The 2010 immunization rates for 1-year-olds were 97 percent for diphtheria and pertussis (DPT3) and 98 percent for measles (MCV).

Cost of Drugs

According to Ibis Sanchez-Serrano, in 2009, the pharmaceutical market in Russia was valued at $7.9 billion and was projected to reach $13.6 billion in 2014. Although most drug costs are currently paid out of pocket, the country intends to institute universal coverage for prescription drugs in the future.

Health Care Facilities

In 2006, Russia had 9.66 hospital beds per 1,000 population, the fifth-highest ratio in the world and reflective of the hospital-centered model of health care typical of the Soviet Union.

Major Health Issues

In 2008, WHO estimated that 11 percent of years of life lost in Russia were due to communicable diseases, 64 percent to noncommunicable diseases, and 25 percent to injuries. In 2008, the age-standardized estimate of cancer deaths was 194 per 100,000 for men and 89 per 100,000 for women; for cardiovascular disease and diabetes, 772 per 100,000 for men and 414 per 100,000 for women; and for chronic respiratory disease, 41 per 100,000 for men and nine per 100,000 for women. Russia's maternal mortality rate (death from any cause related to or aggravated by pregnancy) in 2008 was 39 maternal deaths per 100,000 live births. The infant mortality rate, defined as the number of deaths of infants younger than 1 year, was 9.88 per 1,000 live births as of 2012.

In 2010, tuberculosis incidence was 106.0 per 100,000 population, tuberculosis prevalence 136.0 per 100,000, and deaths due to tuberculosis among human immunodeficiency virus (HIV)-negative people 18.0 per 100,000. As estimated, 18 percent of new tuberculosis cases and 46 percent of retreatment cases are multidrug resistant. WHO estimated the 2010 case detection rate at 73 percent. As of 2009, an estimated 1.0 percent of adults age 15 to 49 were living with HIV

or acquired immune deficiency syndrome (AIDS). As of 2009, an estimated 980,000 people in Russia were living with HIV or AIDS, the 10th-largest number in the world.

Health Care Personnel

Russia has more than 50 medical schools. The basic medical degree course lasts six to seven years, and one to five years of work in government service is required after graduation. The degree awarded is doctor of medicine. Russia has agreements with more than 60 countries. In 2006, Russia had 4.31 physicians per 1,000 population, 0.08 pharmaceutical personnel per 1,000, 0.32 dentistry personnel per 1,000, and 8.52 nurses and midwives per 1,000.

Government Role in Health Care

According to WHO, in 2010, Russia spent $75 billion on health care, an amount that comes to $525 per capita. All health care funding came from domestic sources. A little less than two-thirds (62 percent) of health care spending was paid for through government expenditures, with the remainder provided through household expenditures (31 percent) and other sources (2 percent). In 2010, Russia allocated 8 percent of its total government expenditures to health, and government expenditures on health came to 3 percent of GDP; both figures are in the low range for upper-middle-income European countries.

Public Health Programs

Russia's National Research Center for Preventive Medicine is located in Moscow and directed by Sergej A. Boytsov. Its primary roles are to improve health standards within the country, improve the registry process, and help prevent noncommunicable disease. The National Center has a staff of more than 800 organized into seven departments: primary prevention, secondary prevention, epidemiology, biochemistry, lab standardization, genetics, and coordination.

According to WHO, in 2001, Russia had 0.50 environmental and public health workers per 1,000 population. In 2010, 70 percent of the population had access to improved sanitation facilities (59 percent in rural areas and 74 percent in urban), and 97 percent had access to improved sources of drinking water (92 percent in rural areas and 99 percent in urban). According to the World Higher Education Database (WHED), 13 universities in Russia offer programs in epidemiology or public health.

RWANDA

Rwanda is a landlocked central African country sharing borders with Burundi, the Democratic Republic of the Congo, Tanzania, and Uganda. The area of 10,169 square miles (26,338 square kilometers) makes Rwanda about the size of Maryland, and the July 2012 population was estimated at 11.7 million. In 2010, 19 percent of the population lived in urban areas, and the 2010 to 2015 annual rate of urbanization was estimated at 4.4 percent. Kigali is the capital and largest city (with a 2009 population estimated at 909,000). The population growth rate in 2012 was 2.8 percent (the 18th-highest in the world), the net migration rate 1.0 migrants per 1,000 population, the birth rate 36.1 births per 1,000, and the total fertility rate 4.8 children per woman (the 24th-highest in the world). The United Nations High Commissioner for Refugees (UNHCR) estimated that, in 2010, there were 55,398 refugees and persons in refugee-like situations in Rwanda.

Germany was granted colonial dominion over Rwanda in 1890, and Belgium became the colonial power after World War I. Rwanda achieved independence in 1962. Ethnic strife between the Hutus (the majority group) and the Tutsis began while Belgium was in charge of the country and surfaced again in a civil war in 1990 and a genocide in 1994; the latter

resulted in the death of about three-quarters of the Tutsi population. Many Hutu fled the country, fearing retribution; some formed an insurgency in the Democratic Republic of the Congo.

According to the Ibrahim Index, in 2011, Rwanda ranked 24th among 53 African countries in terms of governance performance, with a score of 52 (out of 100). Rwanda ranked 49th among 183 countries on the *Corruption Perceptions Index 2011,* with a score of 5.0 (on a scale where 0 indicates highly corrupt and 10 very clean).

In 2011, Rwanda was classified as a country with low human development (the lowest of four categories) on the United Nations Development Programme's (UNDP's) Human Development Index (HDI), with a score of 0.429 (on a scale where 1 denotes high development and 0 low development). In 2011, the International Food Policy Research Institute (IFPRI) classified Rwanda as a country with an "alarming" hunger problem, with a Global Hunger Index (GHI) score of 21.0 (where 0 reflects no hunger and higher scores more hunger), and the World Food Programme estimated in 2011 that more than one-third of rural households in Rwanda suffered from food shortages.

Life expectancy at birth in 2012 was estimated at 58.44 years, among the 30 lowest in the world, and the estimated gross domestic product (GDP) per capita in 2011 was $1,300, among the 30 lowest in the world. Income distribution in Rwanda is relatively unequal: In 2000, the Gini Index (a measure of dispersion, in which perfect equality is denoted by 0 and maximum inequality is denoted by 100) for family income was 46.8.

Compared to other countries at a similar level of development, Rwanda ranked second among 43 least-developed countries on the 2011 Mothers' Index, produced by the international nongovernmental organization (NGO) Save the Children, based on a number of health and social factors relating to women, children, and maternal and child care.

Emergency Health Services

According to the World Health Organization (WHO), as of 2007, Rwanda did not have a formal and publicly available system for providing prehospital care (emergency care).

Insurance

According to the *2010 World Health Report* published by WHO, Rwanda has three health insurance

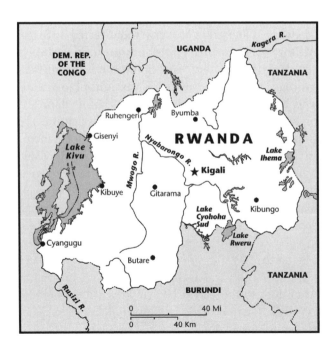

Selected Health Indicators: Rwanda Compared With the Global Average (2010)

	Rwanda	Global Average
Male life expectancy at birth[*] (years)	57	66
Female life expectancy at birth[*] (years)	60	71
Under-5 mortality rate, both sexes (per 1,000 live births)	64	57
Adult mortality rate, both sexes[*] (probability of dying between 15 and 60 years per 1,000 population)	279	176
Maternal mortality ratio (per 100,000 live births)	340	210
HIV prevalence[*] (per 1,000 adults aged 15 to 49)	29	8
Tuberculosis prevalence (per 100,000 population)	128	178

Source: World Health Organization Global Health Observatory Data Repository.
[*]Data refers to 2009.

schemes that together cover 91 percent of the country's population. Rwandaise d'Assurance Maladie is a compulsory social health insurance plan for government employees; private-sector employees may join the plan voluntarily. The Military Medical Insurance plan covers military personnel. The Assurances maladies communautaires are a system of mutual insurance schemes covering primarily people who work in the informal sector in rural settings; these plans are funded about equally by member premiums and government donations from general tax revenues and cover more than 80 percent of the population.

These schemes do not cover all medical services, and out-of-pocket payments are still required, but they have greatly increased access to health services across the country, corresponding with improvements in outcomes such as lowered child mortality. Rwanda is in the process of creating a national legal framework to govern health insurance. In 2007, 55 percent of health expenditures were provided by donor organizations.

Costs of Hospitalization

In 2003, 16 percent of out-of-pocket health care expenditures in Rwanda went for treatment in private, for-profit hospitals; 25 percent for treatment in public hospitals and health centers; and 15 percent for treatment in government-assisted, not-for-profit health centers and hospitals.

Access to Health Care

In 2001, according to United States Agency for International Development (USAID), 85 percent of the population lived within 1.5 hours' travel time of a primary care unit. However, many units are poorly equipped and lack basics such as electricity and a dependable water supply. High out-of-pocket expenditures (estimated at 42 percent of all health care expenditures in 2003, according to USAID) also constitute a barrier to care.

According to WHO, in 2008, 52 percent of births in Rwanda were attended by skilled personnel (for example, physicians, nurses, or midwives), and 24 percent of pregnant women received at least four prenatal care visits. The 2010 immunization rates for 1-year-olds were 80 percent for diphtheria and pertussis (DPT3), 82 percent for measles (MCV), and 80 percent for Hib (Hib3). In 2010, an estimated 88 percent of persons with advanced human immunodeficiency virus (HIV) infection were receiving antiretroviral therapy in accordance with the 2010 WHO guidelines.

Cost of Drugs

No data available.

Health Care Facilities

In 2001, Rwanda's public health care sector included 11 provincial health offices, 30 district health offices, and 365 peripheral health facilities; in 1999, Rwanda had 329 private health facilities, more than half of which were located in Kigali. In 2007, Rwanda had 1.60 hospital beds per 1,000 population.

Major Health Issues

In 2008, WHO estimated that 77 percent of years of life lost in Rwanda were due to communicable diseases, 15 percent to noncommunicable diseases, and 8 percent to injuries. In 2008, the age-standardized estimate of cancer deaths was 110 per 100,000 for men and 115 per 100,000 for women; for cardiovascular disease and diabetes, 405 per 100,000 for men and 410 per 100,000 for women; and for chronic respiratory disease, 110 per 100,000 for men and 60 per 100,000 for women.

In 2008, the age-standardized death rate from malaria was 10.2 per 100,000 population. In 2010, tuberculosis incidence was 106.0 per 100,000 population, tuberculosis prevalence 128.0 per 100,000, and deaths due to tuberculosis among HIV-negative people 1.0 per 100,000. As of 2009, an estimated 2.9 percent of adults age 15 to 49 were living with HIV or acquired immune deficiency syndrome (AIDS). As of December 2010, an estimated 96 percent of adults and 45 percent of children who needed antiretroviral therapy were receiving it.

Rwanda's maternal mortality rate (death from any cause related to or aggravated by pregnancy) has been quite high by global standards, estimated at 540 maternal deaths per 100,000 live births as of 2008. The infant mortality rate, defined as the number of deaths of infants younger than 1 year, also has been high, at 62.51 per 1,000 live births as of 2012. In 2005, 18.0 percent of children under age 5 were underweight (defined as 2 kilograms [kg] below standard weight-for-age at age 1, 3 kg below for ages 2 to 3, and 4 kg below for ages 4 to 5).

Health Care Personnel

Rwanda has one medical school, the Faculté de Médecine of the Université Nationale de Rwanda, which began offering instruction in 1963. The basic medical course lasts seven years, and the degree awarded is Docteur en Médecine (doctor of medicine). In 2005, Rwanda had 0.02 physicians per 1,000 population, 0.06 laboratory health workers per 1,000, and 0.45 nurses and midwives per 1,000, and in 2004, had 0.10 health management and support workers per 1,000 and 1.48 community and traditional health workers per 1,000. Michael Clemens and Bunilla Petterson

estimate that 43 percent of Rwanda-born physicians and 14 percent of Rwanda-born nurses are working in one of nine developed countries, primarily Belgium and the United States.

Government Role in Health Care

According to WHO, in 2010, Rwanda spent $590 million on health care, an amount that comes to $56 per capita. Just over half (53 percent) of health care funding came from domestic sources, with 47 percent coming from abroad. Half (50 percent) of health care spending was paid for through government expenditures, with the remainder provided through household expenditures (22 percent) and other sources (28 percent). In 2010, Rwanda allocated 20 percent of its total government expenditures to health, and government expenditures on health came to 5 percent of GDP; both figures are in the high range for low-income African countries. In 2009, according to WHO, official development assistance (ODA) for health in Rwanda came to $25.87 per capita.

Public Health Programs

According to WHO, in 2005, Rwanda had fewer than 0.01 environmental and public health workers per 1,000 population. In 2010, 55 percent of the population had access to improved sanitation facilities (56 percent in rural areas and 52 percent in urban), and 65 percent had access to improved sources of drinking water (63 percent in rural areas and 76 percent in urban). According to the World Higher Education Database (WHED), two universities in Rwanda offer programs in epidemiology or public health: the Kigali Health Institute and the National University of Rwanda.

SAINT KITTS AND NEVIS

Saint Kitts and Nevis is an island nation in the Caribbean Sea. The area of 101 square miles (261 square kilometers) makes Saint Kitts and Nevis about 1.5 times the size of Washington, D.C., and the July 2012 population was estimated at 50,726. In 2010, 32 percent of the population lived in urban areas, and the 2010 to 2015 annual rate of urbanization was estimated at 1.8 percent. Basseterre is the capital and largest city (with a 2009 population estimated at 13,000).

The population growth rate in 2012 was 0.8 percent, the net migration rate 1.2 migrants per 1,000 population, the birth rate 13.9 births per 1,000, and the total fertility rate 1.8 children per woman.

Britain began establishing colonies in Saint Kitts and Nevis in 1623; the country became autonomous in 1967 and independent in 1998. Anguilla seceded from Saint Kitts and Nevis in 1971, and there is also a separatist movement in Nevis, although a referendum to separate failed in 1998.

In 2011, Saint Kitts and Nevis was classified as a country with high human development (the second-highest category) on the United Nations Development Programme's (UNDP's) Human Development Index (HDI), with a score of 0.735 (on a scale where 1 denotes high development and 0 low development). Life expectancy at birth in 2012 was estimated at 74.84 years, and per capita gross domestic product (GDP) in 2011 was estimated at $16,400.

Emergency Health Services

The Joseph N. France Hospital in Basseterre has an emergency department.

Insurance

Saint Kitts and Nevis has a social insurance system, as specified in the 1977 Social Security Act, providing cash benefits only. The system covers employed and self-employed people ages 16 to 62. The system is funded by wage contributions (5 percent of covered earnings), contributions from the earnings of the self-employed (10 percent of earnings, according to earnings category), and employer contributions (5 percent of covered payroll); the same system funds old-age, disability, and survivor benefits. The maternity benefit is 65 percent of average covered earnings for 13 weeks, and a maternity grant of XCD 450 is paid for each birth. The sickness benefit is 65 percent of average weekly earnings paid for up to 26 weeks.

There are no statutory medical benefits provided in the system, but medical care is provided at public health centers and hospitals. The system is administered by the Social Security Board under the supervision of the Ministry of Foreign Affairs, National Security, Labour, Immigration and Social Security.

Costs of Hospitalization

Sixty percent of the health budget of Saint Kitts and Nevis is devoted to operating hospitals and other institutions; the country has a cost recovery plan for hospital services, but some categories of citizens are exempt, including schoolchildren and senior citizens.

Access to Health Care

Although there is no public health insurance in St. Kitts and Nevis, the government provides a basic package of services at a sustainable cost. Community services are provided without charge, and government expenditures finance most health care on the islands. According to the World Health Organization (WHO), in 2008, 100 percent of births in St. Kitts and Nevis were attended by skilled personnel (for example, physicians, nurses, or midwives). The 2010 immunization rates for 1-year-olds were 95 percent for diphtheria and pertussis (DPT3), 99 percent for measles (MCV), and 96 percent for Hib (Hib3).

According to WHO, in 2010, Saint Kitts and Nevis had fewer than 0.01 magnetic resonance imaging (MRI) machines per 1 million population and 19.58 computer tomography (CT) machines per 1 million.

Cost of Drugs

Essential drugs are provided at low cost through public-sector pharmacies, and antiretrovirals are provided to human immunodeficiency virus and acquired immune deficiency syndrome (HIV/AIDS)

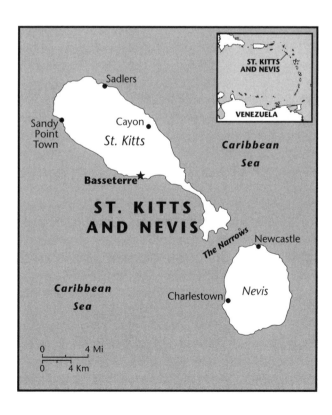

patients through an international partner. All drugs and medical supplies are imported, and medications for the public sector are obtained through the Organization of Eastern Caribbean States Pharmaceutical Procurement Service.

Health Care Facilities

As of 2010, according to WHO, Saint Kitts and Nevis had 32.44 health centers per 100,000 population, 3.82 district or rural hospitals per 100,000, and 3.82 provincial hospitals per 100,000. In 2009, Saint Kitts and Nevis had 6.00 hospital beds per 1,000 population, among the 30 highest ratios in the world.

Major Health Issues

In 2008, WHO estimated that 14 percent of years of life lost in Saint Kitts and Nevis were due to communicable diseases, 63 percent to noncommunicable diseases, and 23 percent to injuries. In 2008, the age-standardized estimate of cancer deaths was 161 per 100,000 for men and 123 per 100,000 for women; for cardiovascular disease and diabetes, 307 per 100,000 for men and 331 per 100,000 for women; and for chronic respiratory disease, 17 per 100,000 for men and 10 per 100,000 for women.

The infant mortality rate, defined as the number of deaths of infants younger than 1 year, was 9.43 per 1,000 live births as of 2012. No information is available from WHO about the maternal mortality rate in Saint Kitts and Nevis.

In 2010, tuberculosis incidence was 7.6 per 100,000 population, tuberculosis prevalence 11.0 per 100,000, and deaths due to tuberculosis among HIV-negative people 4.7 per 100,000.

Health Care Personnel

Saint Kitts and Nevis has three medical schools: the Medical University of the Americas (which began offering instruction in 1998), the International University of the Health Sciences (1998), and the Windsor University Medical School (2000). St. Theresa's Medical University began operation in 2005 and closed in 2009. In 2000, Saint Kitts and Nevis had 1.10 physicians per 1,000 population, 0.50 pharmaceutical personnel per 1,000, 0.40 laboratory health workers per 1,000, 0.40 dentistry personnel per 1,000, 1.55 community and traditional health workers per 1,000, and 4.71 nurses and midwives per 1,000. Alok Bhargava and colleagues place Saint Kitts and Nevis fourth among countries most affected by the

international medical " "brain drain" " (emigration of skilled personnel) in 2004. Many of the students who attend medical school in St. Kitts are from the United States or other foreign countries and intend to return home for their medical careers.

Government Role in Health Care

According to WHO, in 2010, Saint Kitts and Nevis spent $35 billion on health care, an amount that comes to $669 per capita. All health care funding came from domestic sources. More than three-fifths (61 percent) of health care spending was paid for through government expenditures, with the remainder provided through household expenditures (37 percent) and other sources (2 percent). In 2010, Saint Kitts and Nevis allocated 8 percent of its total government expenditures to health, in the low range for upper-middle-income Americas region countries; government expenditures on health came to 4 percent of GDP, in the median range for upper middle-income Americas region countries.

Public Health Programs

According to WHO, in 2001, Saint Kitts and Nevis had 0.40 environmental and public health workers per 1,000 population. In 2010, 96 percent of the population had access to improved sanitation facilities, and 99 percent had access to improved sources of drinking water. According to the World Higher Education Database (WHED), one university in Saint Kitts and Nevis offers programs in epidemiology or public health: the Medical University of the Americas, located in Charlestown, Nevis.

SAINT LUCIA

Saint Lucia is an island nation in the Caribbean Sea. The area of 238 square miles (616 square kilometers) makes Saint Lucia about 3.5 times the size of Washington, D.C., and the July 2012 population was estimated at 162,178. In 2010, 28 percent of the population lived in urban areas, and the 2010 to 2015 annual rate of urbanization was estimated at 1.6 percent. Castries is the capital and largest city (with a 2009 population estimated at 150,000). The population growth rate in 2012 was 0.4 percent, the net migration rate negative 3.5 migrants per 1,000 population, the birth rate 14.4 births per 1,000, and the total fertility rate 1.8 children per woman. Saint Lucia was a colony of both France and Great Britain at different points in its history, with Britain taking control in 1814; it became self-governing in 1967 and independent in 1979. Saint Lucia ranked tied for 25th among 183 countries on the *Corruption Perceptions Index 2011,* with a score of 7.0 (on a scale where 0 indicates highly corrupt and 10 very clean). In 2011, Saint Lucia was classified as a country with high human development (the second-highest category) on the United Nations Development Programme's (UNDP's) Human Development Index (HDI), with a score of 0.723 (on a scale where 1 denotes high development and 0 low development). Life expectancy at birth in 2012 was estimated at 77.04 years, and per capita gross domestic product (GDP) in 2011 was estimated at $12,000.

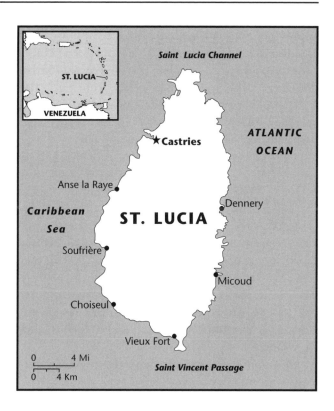

Emergency Health Services
According to the World Health Organization (WHO), as of 2007, Saint Lucia had a formal and publicly available emergency care (prehospital care) system accessible through a national access number. General hospitals provide emergency care through their casualty or emergency departments; in 2002, four health professionals in Saint Lucia specialized in accident and emergency care.

Insurance
Saint Lucia has a social insurance system providing cash benefits and covering the employed, the self-employed, and apprentices. Those who were civil servants prior to February 1, 2003, are covered under a separate system. The system is funded through contributions from wages (5 percent of covered earnings), earnings of the self-employed (varies according to wage category), and employers (5 percent of covered payroll); the same funds finance the system of old-age, survivor, and disability pensions. The maternity benefit is 65 percent of average earnings for up to three months; the sickness benefit is 65 percent of average earnings. Those who receive a cash sickness benefit are eligible for medical treatment and hospitalization at approved hospitals. The National Insurance Corporation administers the program under the supervision of the Ministry of Finance.

Costs of Hospitalization
In 2002 and 2003, secondary care services accounted for 53 percent of the total health budget, with Golden Hope Hospital (a mental health institution) receiving 5 percent of the total.

Access to Health Care
According to WHO, in 2007, 100 percent of births in Saint Lucia were attended by skilled personnel (for example, physicians, nurses, or midwives). The 2010 immunization rates for 1-year-olds were 97 percent for diphtheria and pertussis (DPT3), 95 percent for measles (MCV), and 97 percent for Hib (Hib3). According to WHO, in 2010, Saint Lucia had 11.74 magnetic resonance imaging (MRI) machines per 1 million population and 11.74 computer tomography (CT) machines per 1 million.

Cost of Drugs
Drugs in Saint Lucia are obtained through the Eastern Caribbean Drug Services, and vaccines used in the public sector are obtained by the Pan American Health Organization (PAHO) Revolving Fund.

Health Care Facilities
Saint Lucia's main hospital is Victoria Hospital, located in Castries and managed by the Ministry of Health; St. Jude's hospital is a quasi-public institution, and Taipon Hospital is a private facility in Castries. Outpatient care

is provided through medical clinics at health centers and district hospitals. Tertiary care is provided in other countries, primarily Trinidad, Martinique, and Barbados. As of 2010, according to WHO, Saint Lucia had 19.51 health posts per 100,000 population and 1.72 specialized hospitals per 100,000. In 2009, Saint Lucia had 1.40 hospital beds per 1,000 population.

Major Health Issues

In 2008, WHO estimated that 20 percent of years of life lost in Saint Lucia were due to communicable diseases, 60 percent to noncommunicable diseases, and 20 percent to injuries. In 2008, the age-standardized estimate of cancer deaths was 155 per 100,000 for men and 84 per 100,000 for women; for cardiovascular disease and diabetes, 312 per 100,000 for men and 246 per 100,000 for women; and for chronic respiratory disease, 47 per 100,000 for men and 17 per 100,000 for women.

The infant mortality rate, defined as the number of deaths of infants younger than 1 year, was 12.39 per 1,000 live births as of 2012. No information is available from WHO about the maternal mortality rate in Saint Lucia. In 2010, tuberculosis incidence was 7.9 per 100,000 population, tuberculosis prevalence 12.0 per 100,000, and deaths due to tuberculosis among human immunodeficiency virus (HIV)-negative people 1.80 per 100,000.

Health Care Personnel

As of 2007, three medical schools were operating in Saint Lucia: the School of Medicine of Spartan Health Sciences University (founded in 1980), the College of Medicine and Health Sciences (founded in 2001 in Saint Lucia), and the College of Medicine of International American University (founded in 2004). Many of the students who attend these schools are not from St. Lucia and intend to practice elsewhere. In 2002, Saint Lucia had 0.47 physicians per 1,000 population and 0.05 dentistry personnel per 1,000, and in 2000, had 1.55 community and traditional health workers per 1,000 and 4.71 nurses and midwives per 1,000.

Despite the location of a medical school on St. Lucia, the country has a relative undersupply of physicians because most of the students are foreigners who do not stay to practice in St. Lucia. Alok Bhargava and colleagues place St. Lucia third among countries most affected by medical "brain drain" (emigration of skilled personnel) in 2004.

Government Role in Health Care

According to WHO, in 2010, Saint Lucia spent $81 million on health care, an amount that comes to $465 per capita. Most (97 percent) of health care funding came from domestic sources, with 3 percent coming from abroad. Three-fifths (60 percent) of health care spending was paid for through government expenditures, with the remainder provided through household expenditures (39 percent) and other sources (1 percent). In 2010, Saint Lucia allocated 13 percent of its total government expenditures to health, in the median range for upper-middle-income Americas region countries; government expenditures on health came to 5 percent of GDP, in the high range for upper-middle-income Americas region countries.

Public Health Programs

Preventive care is provided at 34 health centers, two hospitals, and a polyclinic. The Bureau of Health Education of the Ministry of Health provides health promotion and education, and the Environmental Health Department monitors food and water safety, sanitation, and vector control. In 2010, 65 percent of the population Saint Lucia had access to improved sanitation facilities (63 percent in rural areas and 71 percent in urban), and 96 percent had access to improved sources of drinking water (95 percent in rural areas and 98 percent in urban).

SAINT VINCENT AND THE GRENADINES

Saint Vincent and the Grenadines (SVG) is an island nation in the Caribbean, consisting of one large island and an archipelago of smaller islands. The area of 150 square miles (389 square kilometers) makes SVG about twice the size of Washington, D.C., and the July 2012 population was estimated at 103,537. In 2010, 49 percent of the population lived in urban areas, and the 2010 to 2015 annual rate of urbanization was estimated at 0.1 percent. Kingstown is the capital and largest city (with a 2009 population estimated at 28,000). The population growth rate in 2012 was negative 0.3 percent, the net migration rate negative 10.5 migrants per 1,000 population (the 12th-highest emigration rate in the world), the birth rate 10.9 births

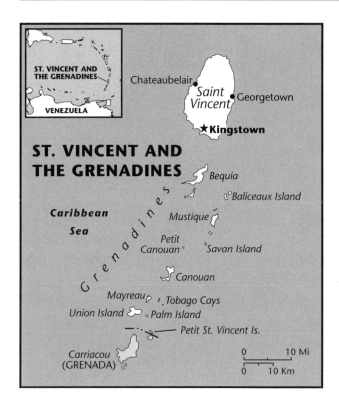

Milton Cato Memorial Hospital in Kingstown has an accident and emergency department.

Insurance

SVG has a social insurance system providing cash benefits and covering the employed and self-employed aged 16 to 59 years; voluntary coverage is available for citizens who have lost their coverage or live abroad. Some categories of civil servants are included in a separate system. The system is funded through contributions from wages (3.5 percent of covered earnings and 3.29 percent for some government workers), earnings of the self-employed (7.5 percent, according to income category), the voluntarily insured (6.84 percent of declared income), employers (4.5 percent of covered payroll), and the government (4.25 percent or 4.5 percent of payroll; the percentage paid depends on the work category); these funds also finance the system of old-age, survivor, and disability pensions. The maternity benefit is 65 percent of average earnings for up to 13 weeks; the sickness benefit is 65 percent of average earnings for up to 26 weeks. The National Insurance Board administers the program.

Costs of Hospitalization

No data available.

Access to Health Care

The Ministry of Health has the responsibility of providing equitable and sustainable primary, secondary, and tertiary health care to SVG's population. Thirty-nine health centers provide primary care to catchment areas averaging 2,900 persons, some also offer dental care, and mental health services are offered on a visiting basis. According to WHO, in 2008, 99.2 percent of births in SVG were attended by skilled personnel (for example, physicians, nurses, or midwives). The 2010 immunization rates for 1-year-olds were 99 percent for diphtheria and pertussis (DPT3), 99 percent for measles (MCV), and 99 percent for Hib (Hib3).

Cost of Drugs

The Central Pharmacy procures, prepares, dispenses, and distributes drugs for the national health system. Most pharmaceuticals are purchased through the Organization of Eastern Caribbean States' Pharmaceutical Procurement Services. Drugs are supplied to the public health system through 39 district pharmacies; there are also 13 registered private pharmacies in SVG. The two greatest categories of expense for

per 1,000, and the total fertility rate 1.9 children per woman.

SVG was both a French and British colony at different times in its history; Great Britain took possession in 1793. SVG became part of the Federation of the West Indies in 1960, became autonomous in 1969, and became independent in 1979. SVG ranks tied for 36th among 183 countries on the *Corruption Perceptions Index 2011,* with a score of 5.8 (on a scale where 0 indicates highly corrupt and 10 very clean). In 2011, SVG was classified as a country with high human development (the second-highest category) on the United Nations Development Programme's (UNDP's) Human Development Index (HDI), with a score of 0.717 (on a scale where 1 denotes high development and 0 low development). Life expectancy at birth in 2012 was estimated at 74.39 years, and per capita gross domestic product (GDP) in 2011 was estimated at $11,700.

Emergency Health Services

According to the World Health Organization (WHO), as of 2007, SVG did not have a formal and publicly available system for providing prehospital care (emergency care). However, each of the 39 health centers in SVG is equipped to provide emergency care, and pharmaceuticals in SVG in 2004 were medications for diabetes ($407,154) and medications for hypertension ($230,032), representing 20 percent of the annual public pharmaceutical budget.

Health Care Facilities
Primary care is provided through a network of 39 health centers staffed with a district nurse, nursing assistant, and community health aide; no citizen lives further than three miles from a health center. More advanced support is provided through district health personnel and visiting staff, including a district medical officer, nursing supervisor, nurse practitioner, nutrition officer, and social worker. Milton Cato Memorial Hospital (211 beds) in Kingstown provides specialist care in seven departments (accident and emergency, outpatient, surgery, medicine, operating theater, pediatric services, and obstetrics and gynecology) and is the country's only public referral hospital. In the public sector, SVG also has five rural hospitals (a total of 58 beds), a 186-bed Mental Health Centre, and the Lewis Punnett Care Home for the indigent elderly; in the private sector, the Maryfield Hospital (10 beds) provides acute care, and five private institutions (55 beds total) offer residential elderly care. As of 2010, according to WHO, SVG had 35.67 health posts per 100,000 population, and 0.91 health centers per 100,000. In 2007, SVG had 3.00 hospital beds per 1,000 population.

Major Health Issues
In 2008, WHO estimated that 24 percent of years of life lost in SVG were due to communicable diseases, 60 percent to noncommunicable diseases, and 17 percent to injuries. In 2008, the age-standardized estimate of cancer deaths was 135 per 100,000 for men and 100 per 100,000 for women; for cardiovascular disease and diabetes, 355 per 100,000 for men and 324 per 100,000 for women; and for chronic respiratory disease, 31 per 100,000 for men and 11 per 100,000 for women.

The infant mortality rate, defined as the number of deaths of infants younger than 1 year, was 13.86 per 1,000 live births as of 2012. No information is available from WHO about the maternal mortality rate in SVG. In 2010, tuberculosis incidence was 24.0 per 100,000 population, tuberculosis prevalence 33.0 per 100,000, and deaths due to tuberculosis among human immunodeficiency virus (HIV)-negative people 2.00 per 100,000. Dengue fever and leptospirosis are endemic to SVG.

Health Care Personnel
SVG has one medical school, Kingstown Medical College, which began offering instruction in 1979. The basic medical training course lasts 4.5 years with an addition two years of supervised clinical practice required for the degree (doctor of medicine). Two years of government service is required after graduation. Physicians must register with the Medical Board of the Ministry of Health, and graduates of foreign medical schools must be registered to practice in the country in which they were trained. In 2000, SVG had 0.75 physicians per 1,000 population, 0.04 dentistry personnel per 1,000, 0.38 community and traditional health workers per 1,000, and 3.79 nurses and midwives per 1,000.

Government Role in Health Care
According to WHO, in 2010, SVG spent $30 million on health care, an amount that comes to $278 per capita. Most (94 percent) of health care funding came from domestic sources, with 6 percent coming from abroad. Most (86 percent) of health care spending was paid for through government expenditures, with the remainder provided through household expenditures (14 percent). In 2010, SVG allocated 8 percent of its total government expenditures to health, in the low range for upper-middle-income Americas region countries; government expenditures on health came to 4 percent of GDP, in the median range for upper-middle-income Americas region countries.

Public Health Programs
In 2010, 96 percent of the population of SVG had access to improved sanitation facilities. However, squatting (living in unregulated settlements on public land) is widespread and poses a number of public health problems, including lack of access to clean water and sanitary facilities and crowding into substandard housing, which promote the spread of communicable disease.

SAMOA

Samoa is an island nation in the south Pacific Ocean. The area of 1,093 square miles (2,831 square kilometers) makes Samoa about twice the size of Rhode

Island, and the July 2012 population was estimated at 194,320. In 2010, 20 percent of the population lived in urban areas, and the 2010 to 2015 annual rate of urbanization is estimated at 0.0 percent. Apia is the capital and largest city (with a 2009 population estimated at 36,000). The population growth rate in 2012 was 0.6 percent, the net migration rate negative 10.8 migrants per 1,000 population (the 10th-highest in the world), the birth rate 122.1 births per 1,000, and the total fertility rate 3.1 children per woman.

Samoa was a German protectorate and then was administered by New Zealand from 1914 to 1962, when it became the first country in Polynesia to become independent in the 20th century. Samoa's infrastructure was severely damaged by an earthquake and tsunami in 2009.

Samoa ranked tied for 69th among 183 countries on the *Corruption Perceptions Index 2011,* with a score of 3.9 (on a scale where 0 indicates highly corrupt and 10 very clean). In 2011, Samoa was classified as a country with medium human development (the second from the lowest of four categories) on the United Nations Development Programme's (UNDP's) Human Development Index (HDI), with a score of 0.688 (on a scale where 1 denotes high development and 0 low development). Life expectancy at birth in 2012 was estimated at 72.66 years, and estimated gross domestic product (GDP) per capita in 2011 was $6,000.

Emergency Health Services

According to the World Health Organization (WHO), as of 2007, Samoa had a formal and publicly available emergency care (prehospital care) system accessible through a national access number.

Insurance

Samoa has no universal medical benefit or cash benefit system. Some free medical services are provided in government health centers, and senior citizens and those with work injuries are also entitled to some medical services. Cash benefits for disability are provided for both work-related and other injuries in a system funded by wage and payroll contributions; an earmarked tax on motor fuel provides benefits for people injured in boat and motor vehicle accidents. Samoa also has a private sector providing health care services; the private sector includes 14 medical clinics, four private pharmacies, and the MedCEN private hospital. Several religious organizations are also important providers of health care services.

Costs of Hospitalization

No data available.

Access to Health Care

According to WHO, in 2009, 80.8 percent of births in Samoa were attended by skilled personnel (for example, physicians, nurses, or midwives). In 2009, 58 percent of pregnant women received at least four prenatal care visits. Most specialized medical care is not available on Samoa and must be sought overseas; the Samoan and New Zealand governments both have programs to assist those seeking overseas care. The 2010 immunization rates for 1-year-olds were 87 percent for diphtheria and pertussis (DPT3), 61 percent for measles (MCV), and 87 percent for Hib (Hib3). Samoa also has an estimated 900 traditional healers providing health care services and 119 traditional birth attendants.

Cost of Drugs

No data available.

Health Care Facilities

As of 2010, according to WHO, Samoa had 1.64 health centers per 100,000, 03.28 district or rural hospitals per 100,000, 0.55 provincial hospitals per 100,000,

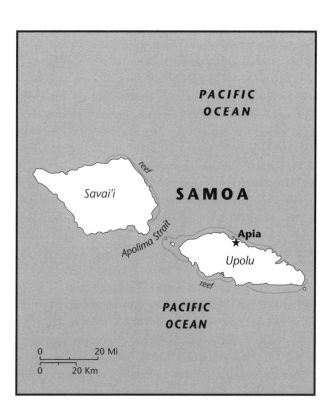

and 0.55 specialized hospitals per 100,000. In 2005, Samoa had 0.97 hospital beds per 1,000 population.

Major Health Issues

In 2008, WHO estimated that 34 percent of years of life lost in Samoa were due to communicable diseases, 55 percent to noncommunicable diseases, and 10 percent to injuries. In 2008, the age-standardized estimate of cancer deaths was 69 per 100,000 for men and 40 per 100,000 for women; for cardiovascular disease and diabetes, 477 per 100,000 for men and 374 per 100,000 for women; and for chronic respiratory disease, 83 per 100,000 for men and 50 per 100,000 for women.

In 2008, the age-standardized death rate from malaria was 0.6 per 100,000 population. Typhoid, dengue fever, and lymphatic filariasis are all endemic to the country. In 2010, tuberculosis incidence was 11.0 per 100,000 population, tuberculosis prevalence 16.0 per 100,000, and deaths due to tuberculosis among human immunodeficiency virus (HIV)-negative people 1.3 per 100,000. The infant mortality rate, defined as the number of deaths of infants younger than 1 year, was estimated at 21.85 per 1,000 live births as of 2012.

Health Care Personnel

Samoa has one medical school, Oceania University of Medicine in Apia, which began offering instruction in 2002. The course of study typically lasts four years (18 blocks of eight weeks). The degrees granted are bachelor of medicine and bachelor of surgery. The curriculum was developed by professors from Australia, and many students do their internships in Australia. Samoan students who receive scholarships to Oceania University of Medicine are required to work in the country's health system for four years after graduation. Foreign graduates wishing to practice in Samoa must apply to the Ministry of Health and meet immigration requirements. In 2005, Samoa had 0.27 physicians per 1,000 population, 0.02 pharmaceutical personnel per 1,000, 0.03 dentistry personnel per 1,000, and 0.94 nurses and midwives per 1,000.

Government Role in Health Care

According to WHO, in 2010, Samoa spent $37 million on health care, an amount that comes to $204 per capita. Most (87 percent) of health care funding came from domestic sources, with 13 percent coming from abroad. Most (88 percent) of health care spending was paid for through government expenditures, with the

remainder provided through household expenditures (8 percent) and other sources (5 percent). In 2010, Samoa allocated 23 percent of its total government expenditures to health, in the high range for lower-middle-income western Pacific region countries; government expenditures on health came to 6 percent of GDP, in the median range for lower-middle-income western Pacific region countries.

Public Health Programs

According to WHO, in 2008, Samoa had 0.12 environmental and public health workers per 1,000 population. In 2010, 98 percent of the population had access to improved sanitation facilities, and 96 percent had access to improved sources of drinking water.

SAN MARINO

San Marino is a landlocked southern European country sharing a border with Italy. The area of 24 square miles (61 square kilometers) makes San Marino about one-third the size of Washington, D.C., and the July 2012 population was estimated at 32,140. In 2010, 94 percent of the population lived in urban areas, and the 2010 to 2015 annual rate of urbanization was estimated at 0.6 percent. San Marino is the capital. The population

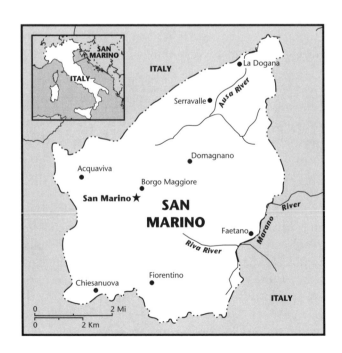

growth rate in 2012 was 1.0 percent, the net migration rate 9.0 migrants per 1,000 population (the 13th-highest in the world), the birth rate 9.0 births per 1,000, and the total fertility rate 1.5 children per woman.

San Marino's economy is heavily dependent on banking and tourism, and citizens enjoy a high standard of living. Life expectancy at birth in 2012 was estimated at 83.07 years, the fifth-highest in the world. Per capita gross domestic product (GDP) in 2009 was estimated at $36,200.

Emergency Health Services

According to the World Health Organization (WHO), as of 2007, San Marino had a formal and publicly available emergency care (prehospital care) system accessible through a national access number.

Insurance

San Marino has a universal medical benefits system covering everyone residing in the country and a social insurance system providing cash benefits to the employed and self-employed. The system is funded by tax revenues, employer contributions (5 percent of payroll), and contributions from the self-employed (up to 4 percent of gross earnings). Medical care is provided by state hospitals and doctors from the national Social Security Institute; benefits covered include hospitalization, medicine, all medical services, and maternity care. There is no cost sharing in the medical system. Dental care is free for children 13 and younger and pensioners; others must pay nominal fees (for example, 12.91 euros for an extraction).

The maternity benefit is 100 percent of earnings for five months; leave can be continued for another six months at 20 to 30 percent of earnings, and mothers are entitled to two hours per day of leave at full pay until their children turn 1. The sickness benefit is 86 percent of pay for 15 days, 100 percent through six months, then 86 percent through 12 months. The National Social Security Institute administers the program.

Costs of Hospitalization

No data available.

Access to Health Care

The 2010 immunization rates for 1-year-olds were 92 percent for diphtheria and pertussis (DPT3), 93 percent for measles (MCV), and 92 percent for Hib (Hib3). According to WHO, in 2010, San Marino had

64.14 magnetic resonance imaging (MRI) machines per 1 million population and 32.07 computer tomography (CT) machines per 1 million.

Cost of Drugs

No data available.

Health Care Facilities

As of 2010, according to WHO, San Marino had 9.51 health posts per 100,000 population and 3.17 provincial hospitals per 100,000.

Major Health Issues

In 2008, WHO estimated that 7 percent of years of life lost in San Marino were due to communicable diseases, 86 percent to noncommunicable diseases, and 7 percent to injuries. As of 2005, the leading causes of death were cardiovascular disease (40.1 percent of all deaths), cancer (37.2 percent), and respiratory diseases (5.8 percent). The infant mortality rate, defined as the number of deaths of infants younger than 1 year, was 4.65 per 1,000 live births as of 2012. No information on maternal mortality rates is available. In 2008, the age-standardized estimate of cancer deaths was 162 per 100,000 for men and 70 per 100,000 for women; for cardiovascular disease and diabetes, 136 per 100,000 for men and 169 per 100,000 for women; for chronic respiratory disease, three per 100,000 for men and three per 100,000 for women.

Health Care Personnel

In 1990, San Marino had 47.35 physicians per 1,000 population and 95.48 nurses and midwives per 1,000. The University of the Republic of San Marino includes a Department of Biomedical Studies, which offers a degree program for nursing personnel and special courses for physicians.

Government Role in Health Care

According to WHO, in 2010, San Marino spent $115 million on health care, an amount that comes to $3,655 per capita. All health care funding came from domestic sources. Most (85 percent) of health care spending was paid for through government expenditures, with the remainder provided through household expenditures (14 percent) and other sources (1 percent). In 2010, San Marino allocated 14 percent of its total government expenditures to health, in the low range for high-income European countries; government expenditures on health came to 6 percent of GDP, in the low range for high-income European countries.

Public Health Programs

No data available.

SÃO TOMÉ AND PRÍNCIPE

São Tomé and Príncipe is an island nation in the Gulf of Guinea (north Atlantic Ocean) just off the coast of Africa. The area of 372 square miles (964 square kilometers) makes São Tomé and Príncipe about five times the size of Washington, D.C., and the July 2012 population was estimated at 183,176. In 2010, 62 percent of the population lived in urban areas, and the 2010 to 2015 annual rate of urbanization was estimated at 2.8 percent. São Tomé is the capital and largest city (with a 2009 population estimated at 60,000). In 2012, São Tomé and Príncipe had one of the highest emigration rates (negative 9.14 net migrants per 1,000 population); it also had one of the 20 highest total fertility rates in the world (4.94 children per woman), and birth rates were 37.0 births per 1,000 population.

São Tomé and Príncipe was colonized by Portugal in the 15th century, and slave labor was used to cultivate crops on plantations into the 20th century. São Tomé and Príncipe became independent in 1975 but did not hold free elections until 1991. According to the Ibrahim Index, in 2011, São Tomé and Príncipe ranked 12th among 53 African countries in terms of governance performance, with a score of 58 (out of 100). São Tomé and Príncipe ranked tied for 100th among 183 countries on the *Corruption Perceptions Index 2011,* with a score of 3.0 (on a scale where 0 indicates highly corrupt and 10 very clean). In 2011, São Tomé and Príncipe was classified as a country with low human development (the lowest of four categories) on the United Nations Development Programme's (UNDP's) Human Development Index (HDI), with a score of 0.509 (on a scale where 1 denotes high development and 0 low development). Life expectancy at birth in 2012 was estimated at 63.49 years, and estimated gross domestic product (GDP) per capita in 2011 was $2,000.

Emergency Health Services

According to the World Health Organization (WHO), as of 2007, São Tomé and Príncipe did not have a formal and publicly available system for providing prehospital care (emergency care).

Insurance

São Tomé and Príncipe has a national Health System (NHS) organized into two levels: The central level provides secondary care and the district level primary care. Tertiary care is generally not available in the country and requires evacuation to Portugal. Access to care improved substantially in the 21st century thanks to the project Health for All, financed in part by the Portuguese Development Institute. As of 2008, São Tomé and Príncipe had two hospitals, six district health centers, and 28 health posts, providing care across the country.

São Tomé and Príncipe has a social insurance system providing cash benefits and covering the employed, including military and civil servants; the self-employed are excluded. The system is funded through contributions from the employed (4 percent of gross earnings) and employers (6 percent of gross payroll); these funds also finance the system of old-age, survivor, and disability pensions.

The maternity benefit is 100 percent of average earnings for 30 days before and after the due date (with an additional 15 days for multiple births); mothers are also entitled to special leave at 60 percent of earnings for up to 360 days following the birth of a child. The sickness benefit is 60 percent of average earnings for up to 365 days. The National Institute of Social Security administers the program, with general supervision from the Ministry of Health, Labor, and Social Security.

Costs of Hospitalization

No data available.

Access to Health Care

According to WHO, in 2009, 81.7 percent of births in São Tomé and Príncipe were attended by skilled personnel (for example, physicians, nurses, or midwives), and 72 percent of pregnant women received at least four prenatal care visits. The 2010 immunization rates for 1-year-olds were 98 percent for diphtheria and pertussis (DPT3), 92 percent for measles (MCV), and 98 percent for Hib (Hib3). In 2010, an estimated 34 percent of persons with advanced human immunodeficiency virus (HIV) infection were receiving antiretroviral therapy in accordance with the 2010 WHO guidelines.

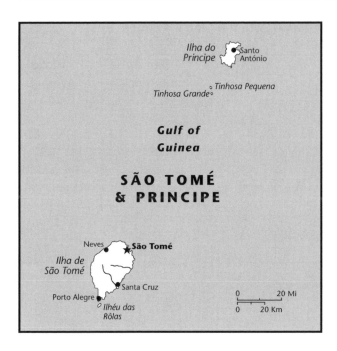

Cost of Drugs

Essential medicines for the public sector are procured and distributed primarily by the Fundo Nacional de Medicamentos, a semiautonomous government organization; two other organizations, the nongovernmental organization (NGO) Instituto Marques de Valle Flor (Portugal) and the Cooperative of Taiwan, also procure and distribute medicines in the public sector. There are nine private pharmacies in the country (as of 2008) but only one pharmacist, and little control is exerted over the quality of drugs sold in the private sector. Most medicines must be paid for by the patients, even in the public sector, although in theory, a 1996 law in São Tomé and Príncipe provides for free medications to be supplied to pregnant women and children under the age of 5; those with conditions such as malaria, tuberculosis, and human immunodeficiency virus/acquired immune deficiency syndrome (HIV/AIDS); as well as the vaccines on WHO's Expanded Programme on Immunization (EPI) list. However, there is no mechanism to monitor the application of this law.

A 2008 survey of the price and availability of a market basket of medicines found that availability was generally low and prices high and that there were significant disparities in different regions of the country. Public procurement prices were generally just above the international reference price for the lowest-priced generic drugs. For the Cooperative of Taiwan, the median price ratio (comparing the price to the international reference price) was 1.06; for the Instituto Marques de Valle Flor, the median price ratio was 1.02; and for the Fundo Nacional de Medicamentos, it was 1.13. Drugs were priced much higher for patients, however: The median price ratio for the patient price in the public sector was 2.36 (more than twice as high as the international reference price) for the lowest-priced generics and 2.90 for originator brands (almost three times as high as the international reference price). These public-sector prices include a markup of more than 100 percent. In the private sector, drugs were much more expensive: The median price ratio for the lowest-priced generics was 13.76 and, for originator brands, 53.27. In the NGO sector, the median price ratio for the lowest-priced generics was 2.50.

The most reliable source for drugs was the NGO sector, with a mean availability of 82 percent for lowest-priced generics; however, this was based on a single outlet. This NGO outlet did not carry any originator brands. In the public sector, the mean availability of the lowest-priced generic drugs was 55.1 percent, and the mean availability of originator brands was 2.0 percent. In the private sector, the mean availability of the lowest-priced generic drugs was 24.3 percent, with 9.8 percent mean availability of originator brands.

Affordability of medicines, expressed as the number of days' wages of the lowest-paid government worker required to purchase a course of treatment for various common diseases, varied according to the disease; whether the drugs were purchased in a public, NGO, or private facility; and whether generics or branded medicines were purchased. For instance, diabetes could be treated for 30 days with glibenclamide costing half a day's wages if the drug was purchased in the public or NGO sector; in the private sector, it would cost 6.6 days' wages for the lowest-priced generic, and 16.5 days' wages for the originator brand. Asthma could be treated for 30 days with a salbutamol inhaler for 2.0 days' wages if the lowest-priced generic was purchased in either the public or NGO sector but would cost 7.2 days' wages if the originator brand was purchased in the private sector.

Health Care Facilities

As of 2010, according to WHO, São Tomé and Príncipe had 16.93 health posts per 100,000 population and 2.42 health centers per 100,000. In 2006, São Tomé and Príncipe had 3.20 hospital beds per 1,000 population.

Selected Health Indicators: São Tomé and Príncipe Compared With the Global Average (2010)

	São Tomé and Príncipe	Global Average
Male life expectancy at birth* (years)	66	66
Female life expectancy at birth* (years)	70	71
Under-5 mortality rate, both sexes (per 1,000 live births)	80	57
Adult mortality rate, both sexes* (probability of dying between 15 and 60 years per 1,000 population)	130	176
Maternal mortality ratio (per 100,000 live births)	70	210
Tuberculosis prevalence (per 100,000 population)	141	178

Source: World Health Organization Global Health Observatory Data Repository.
*Data refers to 2009.

Major Health Issues

In 2008, WHO estimated that 67 percent of years of life lost in São Tomé and Príncipe were due to communicable diseases, 25 percent to noncommunicable diseases, and 8 percent to injuries. In 2008, the age-standardized estimate of cancer deaths was 175 per 100,000 for men and 131 per 100,000 for women; for cardiovascular disease and diabetes, 302 per 100,000 for men and 313 per 100,000 for women; and for chronic respiratory disease, 85 per 100,000 for men and 47 per 100,000 for women.

In 2008, the age-standardized death rate from malaria was 11.5 per 100,000 population. In 2010, tuberculosis incidence was 96.0 per 100,000 population, tuberculosis prevalence 141.0 per 100,000, and deaths due to tuberculosis among HIV-negative people 13.0 per 100,000. The infant mortality rate, defined as the number of deaths of infants younger than 1 year, was estimated at 51.83 per 1,000 live births as of 2012. Data on maternal mortality was not available. In 2009, 13.1 percent of children under age 5 were underweight (defined as 2 kilograms [kg] below standard weight-for-age at age 1, 3 kg below for ages 2 to 3, and 4 kg below for ages 4 to 5).

Health Care Personnel

In 2004, São Tomé and Príncipe had 0.49 physicians per 1,000 population, 0.15 pharmaceutical personnel per 1,000, 0.31 laboratory health workers per 1,000, 1.75 health management and support workers per 1,000, 0.07 dentistry personnel per 1,000, 2.27 community and traditional health workers per 1,000, and 1.87 nurses and midwives per 1,000. Michael Clemens and Bunilla Petterson estimate that 61 percent of São Tomé and Príncipe–born physicians and 46 percent of São Tomé and Príncipe–born nurses are working in one of nine developed countries, primarily in Portugal.

Government Role in Health Care

The right to health, including the right to access essential medicines and medical devices, is recognized in the 1990 constitution. São Tomé and Príncipe has a National Health Policy (NHP), written in 1999, and a plan for implementation of it, written in 2000. It does not have a National Medicines Policy (NMP). According to WHO, in 2010, São Tomé and Príncipe spent $15 million on health care, an amount that comes to $90 per capita. More than three-quarters (79 percent) of health care funding came from domestic sources, with 21 percent coming from abroad. The majority (54 percent) of health care spending was paid for through household expenditures, with the remainder provided through government expenditures (38 percent) and other sources (8 percent). In 2010, São Tomé and Príncipe allocated 13 percent of its total government expenditures to health, in the high range for lower-middle-income African countries; government expenditures on health came to 3 percent of GDP, in the median range for lower-middle-income African countries.

Public Health Programs

According to WHO, in 2004, São Tomé and Príncipe had 0.12 environmental and public health workers per 1,000 population. In 2010, 26 percent of the population of São Tomé and Príncipe had access to improved sanitation facilities (19 percent in rural areas and 30 percent in urban), and 89 percent had access to improved sources of drinking water (88 percent in rural areas and 89 percent in urban).

SAUDI ARABIA

Saudi Arabia is a Middle Eastern country, sharing borders with Iraq, Jordan, Kuwait, Oman, Qatar, the United Arab Emirates, and Yemen and having coastlines on the Red Sea, the Arabian Sea, and the Persian Gulf. The area of 830,000 square miles (2,149,690 square kilometers) makes Saudi Arabia about one-fifth the size of the United States, and the July 2012 population was estimated at 26.5 million. In 2010, 82 percent of the population lived in urban areas, and the 2010 to 2015 annual rate of urbanization was estimated at 2.2 percent. Riyadh is the capital and largest city (with a 2009 population estimated at 4.7 million). The population growth rate in 2012 was 1.5 percent, the net migration rate negative 0.6 migrants per 1,000 population, the birth rate 19.2 births per 1,000, and the total fertility rate 2.3 children per woman. The United Nations High Commissioner for Refugees (UNHCR) estimated that, in 2010, there were 582 refugees and persons in refugee-like situations in Saudi Arabia.

The modern state of Saudi Arabia was founded in 1932. Saudi Arabia ranked tied for 54th among 183 countries on the *Corruption Perceptions Index 2011,* with a score of 4.6 (on a scale where 0 indicates highly corrupt and 10 very clean). In 2011, Saudi Arabia was classified as a country with high human development (the second-highest category) on the United Nations Development Programme's (UNDP's) Human Development Index (HDI), with a score of 0.770 (on a scale where 1 denotes high development and 0 low development). Life expectancy at birth in 2012 was estimated at 74.35 years, and per capita gross domestic product (GDP) in 2011 was estimated at $24,000. According to the World Economic Forum's *Global Gender Gap Index 2011*, Saudi Arabia ranked 131st out of 135 countries on gender equality with a score of 0.575 (on a scale with a theoretical range of 1 for equality to 0 for inequality and an actual range in 2011 from 0.8530 to 0.4873).

Emergency Health Services

According to the World Health Organization (WHO), as of 2007, Saudi Arabia had a formal and publicly available emergency care (prehospital care) system accessible through a national access number.

Insurance

According to Donald West and colleagues, Saudi Arabia has what is in effect a national health care system but one that is managed through a number of separate national agencies. The Ministry of Health is the overall authority for the system and manages a public network of 220 hospitals and 1,925 health centers; large hospitals (with 150 to 350 beds) are built to standard design in population centers, with smaller clinics (with 20 to 50 beds) built in small towns. Three additional systems have their own hospitals and provide comprehensive health care services to their members: the Ministry of Defense and Aviation, the Ministry of the Interior, and the National guard. Smaller programs exist to cover other population sectors, including students, universities, ARAMCO (the national oil company), and airline employees. The entire health system is supported by the national government through the sale of natural resources. A system of mandatory health insurance for expatriate workers (about 28 percent of the population) has been gradually expanded since 2004. Private insurance is legal, and the market is expanding.

Costs of Hospitalization

No data available.

Access to Health Care

According to WHO, in 2008, 100 percent of births in Saudi Arabia were attended by skilled personnel (for example physicians, nurses, or midwives). The 2010 immunization rates for 1-year-olds were 98 percent for diphtheria and pertussis (DPT3), 98 percent for measles (MCV), and 98 percent for Hib (Hib3). According to WHO, in 2010, Saudi Arabia had 1.11 magnetic resonance imaging (MRI) machines per 1 million population and 4.36 computer tomography (CT) machines per 1 million.

Cost of Drugs

No data available.

Health Care Facilities

As of 2010, according to WHO, Saudi Arabia had 0.22 district or rural hospitals per 100,000, 0.86 provincial hospitals per 100,000, and 0.01 specialized hospitals per 100,000. In 2008, Saudi Arabia had 2.20 hospital beds per 1,000 population. According to Donald West and colleagues, as of 2011, Saudi Arabia had the largest health care sector in the Middle East, with 220 public hospitals (64 percent of total beds) operated by the Ministry of Health, 87 private hospitals, and 1,925 health centers. The system is expected to continue to expand, with up to 92 additional hospitals constructed and upgrades and expansions to the primary care network as well. Several smaller hospital and health care systems exist to serve members of the military and security forces, including the Ministry of Defense and Aviation (8 percent of total beds), the Ministry of the Interior (7 percent of beds), and the National Guard (3 percent of beds). The National Guard system includes the 1,000-bed King Abdulaziz teaching hospital, and the government also finances two famous referral hospitals, the King Khalid Eye Specialist Hospital and the King Faisal Specialist Hospital and Research Center.

The private sector also plays a role in Saudi health care. As of 2000, there were 97 private, investor-owned hospitals in Saudi Arabia (about 19 percent of total beds), and 622 private dispensaries, 785 private clinics, 45 private laboratories, and 11 private physiotherapy centers.

Major Health Issues

In 2008, WHO estimated that 20 percent of years of life lost in Saudi Arabia were due to communicable diseases, 55 percent to noncommunicable diseases, and 25 percent to injuries. In 2008, the age-standardized estimate of cancer deaths was 79 per 100,000 for men and 66 per 100,000 for women; for cardiovascular disease and diabetes, 541 per 100,000 for men and 348 per 100,000 for women; and for chronic respiratory disease, 31 per 100,000 for men and 20 per 100,000 for women. Saudi Arabia has one of the highest adult obesity rates in the world, estimated at 35.6 percent in 2000; obesity is defined as a body mass index (BMI) of 30 or above.

In 2010, tuberculosis incidence was 18.0 per 100,000 population, tuberculosis prevalence 24.0 per 100,000, and deaths due to tuberculosis among human immunodeficiency virus (HIV)-negative people 1.4 per 100,000. The maternal mortality rate (death from any cause related to or aggravated by pregnancy) in Saudi Arabia in 2008 was 24 maternal deaths per 100,000 live births. The infant mortality rate, defined as the number of deaths of infants younger than 1 year, was 15.61 per 1,000 live births as of 2012.

Health Care Personnel

As of 2007, Saudi Arabia had 10 medical schools. The course of training for the basic medical degree lasts six years with an additional year of supervised clinical practice required. The degrees awarded are bachelor of medicine and bachelor of surgery. The Ministry of Health in Riyadh grants medical licenses to graduates of recognized medical schools who have completed a one-year internship, and foreigners must be authorized to practice. In 2008, Saudi Arabia had 0.94 physicians per 1,000 population, 0.06 pharmaceutical personnel per 1,000, 2.42 health management and support workers per 1,000, and 2.10 nurses and midwives per 1,000.

Government Role in Health Care

According to WHO, in 2010, Saudi Arabia spent $19 billion on health care, an amount that comes to $680 per capita. All health care funding came from domestic sources. Almost two-thirds (63 percent) of health care spending was paid for through government

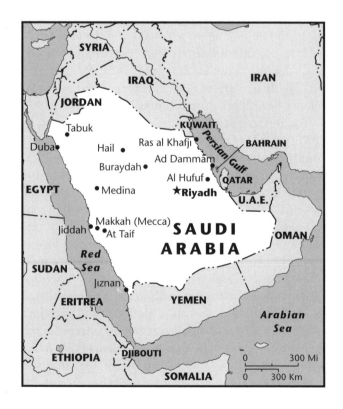

expenditures, with the remainder provided through household expenditures (19 percent) and other sources (19 percent). In 2010, Saudi Arabia allocated 7 percent of its total government expenditures to health, in the median range for high-income eastern Mediterranean region countries; government expenditures on health came to 3 percent of GDP, in the median range for high-income eastern Mediterranean region countries.

Public Health Programs

The formal practice of public health in Saudi Arabia dates back to 1925, when King Abdul Aziz established a Public Health Department in Makkah, which focused on health and the environment and also governed medical and pharmacological practice. Today, the Ministry of Health for Saudi Arabia is located in Riyadh and is directed by Dr. Ziad A. Memish. The focus of the Ministry of Health is to provide health care in line with medical ethics and Islamic principles, to provide public education about health issues, to provide training for people working in medicine and public health, and to ensure that the same standard of care is provided throughout the country. In 2010, 100 percent of the population of Saudi Arabia had access to improved sanitation facilities, and 97 percent had access to improved sources of drinking water (76 percent in rural areas and 94 percent in urban). According to the World Higher Education Database (WHED), four universities in Saudi Arabia offer programs in epidemiology or public health: King Faisal University in Al-Hassa, King Khalid University in Abha, King Saud bin Abdulaziz University for Health Sciences in Riyadh, and Qassim University in Qassim.

SENEGAL

Senegal is a west African country, sharing borders with The Gambia, Guinea, Guinea-Bissau, Mali, and Mauritania and having a coastline on the north Atlantic Ocean. The area of 75,955 square miles (196,722 square kilometers) makes Senegal about the size of South Dakota, and the July 2012 population was estimated at 13.0 million. In 2010, 42 percent of the population lived in urban areas, and the 2010 to 2015 annual rate of urbanization was estimated at 3.3 percent. Dakar is the capital and largest city (with a 2009

population estimated at 2.8 million). The population growth rate in 2012 was 2.5 percent, the net migration rate negative 1.8 migrants per 1,000 population, the birth rate 36.2 births per 1,000 (the 23rd-highest in the world), and the total fertility rate 1.8 children per woman (the 25th-highest in the world). The United Nations High Commissioner for Refugees (UNHCR) estimated that, in 2010, there were 20,672 refugees and persons in refugee-like situations in Senegal.

Senegal was a French colony before achieving independence (along with French Sudan) as the Mali federation in 1960; the federation broke up in a few months. In 1982, Senegal formed the confederation of Senegambia in 1982 with The Gambia, but that union was dissolved in 1989. According to the Ibrahim Index, in 2011, Senegal ranked 15th among 53 African countries in terms of governance performance, with a score of 57 (out of 100). Senegal ranked tied for 112th among 183 countries on the *Corruption Perceptions Index 2011*, with a score of 2.9 (on a scale where 0 indicates highly corrupt and 10 very clean).

In 2011, Senegal was classified as a country with low human development (the lowest of four categories) on the United Nations Development Programme's (UNDP's) Human Development Index (HDI), with a score of 0.459 (on a scale where 1 denotes high development and 0 low development). In 2012, the World Food Programme estimated that 806,000 people in Senegal were food insecure due to a below-average harvest, fewer remittances from abroad, and increases in food prices. Life expectancy at birth in 2012 was estimated at 60.18 years, and estimated gross domestic product (GDP) per capita in 2011 was $1,900; unemployment in 2007 was estimated at 48 percent, among the highest rates in the world. In 2001, the Gini Index (a measure of dispersion, in which perfect equality is denoted by 0 and maximum inequality is denoted by 100) for family income was 41.3. According to the World Economic Forum's *Global Gender Gap Index 2011*, Senegal ranked 92nd out of 135 countries on gender equality with a score of 0.657 (on a scale with a theoretical range of 1 for equality to 0 for inequality and an actual range in 2011 from 0.8530 to 0.4873).

Emergency Health Services

According to the World Health Organization (WHO), as of 2007, Senegal had a formal and publicly available emergency care (prehospital care) system accessible through a national access number.

Insurance

Senegal has a social insurance system providing medical benefits and cash maternity benefits. The medical benefits system covers employed people, including seasonal workers, apprentices, and some temporary workers; the self-employed are excluded. In some areas, workers in the informal sector received medical benefits from health mutual insurance companies. The cash maternity benefits are provided to women who are insured or married to a man who is insured. Military and civil servants are covered under a separate system. Companies with more than 100 employees are required to participate by joining a health institute that provides medical benefits, and smaller firms may band together to join one.

The medical system is funded through contributions from wages (up to 3 percent) and employers (up to 3 percent of payroll); the specific percentage depends on the health institute. The maternity benefit is funded through the Family Allowance system, funded by employer contributions (7 percent of payroll); the same system provides a prenatal and maternity allowance and family allowances. The prenatal allowance, which requires the woman to undergo prescribed medical exams, is WFA 2,400 monthly for up to nine months; the maternity allowance is WFA 2,400, paid monthly for the first two years of the child's life, which requires the mother and child to undergo prescribed medical exams. The family allowance is XFA 2,500 per month for each of the first six children. All family allowances may be adjusted due to availability of funds.

Medical benefits are provided on a cost sharing basis, according to the availability of funds; covered benefits include physician visits, medicines, and hospitalization. Dependents are covered on the same basis as the insured; eligible dependents are the spouse of the insured and his or her dependent children (from age 2 through age 14, through age 18 if an apprentice, and through age 21 if disabled or a student). Recipients of survivor and old-age pensions receive medical benefits directly through the Social Insurance Institute. The maternity benefit is 100 percent of earnings paid six weeks before and eight weeks after the due date, with a possible three-week extension for complications. According to Ke Xu and colleagues, in 2003, 0.6 percent of households in Senegal experienced catastrophic health expenditures annually; "catastrophic" was defined as exceeding 40 percent of household income remaining after basic needs were met.

Costs of Hospitalization

No data available.

Access to Health Care

According to WHO, in 2005, 52 percent of births in Senegal were attended by skilled personnel (for example, physicians, nurses, or midwives). In 2005, 40 percent of pregnant women received at least four prenatal care visits. The 2010 immunization rates for 1-year-olds were 70 percent for diphtheria and pertussis (DPT3), 60 percent for measles (MCV), and 70 percent for Hib (Hib3). In 2010, an estimated 50 percent of persons with advanced human immunodeficiency virus (HIV) infection were receiving antiretroviral therapy in accordance with the 2010 WHO guidelines. According to WHO, in 2010, Senegal had 0.16 magnetic resonance imaging (MRI) machines per 1 million population, 0.41 computer tomography (CT) machines per 1 million, 0.08 telecolbalt units per 1 million, and 0.08 radiotherapy machines per 1 million.

Cost of Drugs

In 2005, total expenditures for pharmaceuticals in Senegal came to XOF 72.1 billion ($156.6 million) and per capita pharmaceutical expenditures to XOF 5,924 ($12.90). Pharmaceutical expenditures made up 28.4 percent of all health expenditures, and 1.2 percent of GDP. Most pharmaceutical expenses were paid privately, as public pharmaceutical expenditures constituted only 14.2 percent of the total. Medicines are provided free of charge to pregnant women, the elderly, and the poor. Free medications are also provided for some illnesses, including malaria, tuberculosis, and human immunodeficiency virus/acquired immune deficiency syndrome (HIV/AIDS), and vaccines on WHO's Expanded Programme on Immunization (EPI) list are also provided free.

Health Care Facilities

As of 2010, according to WHO, Senegal had 7.81 health posts per 100,000 population, 0.61 provincial hospitals per 100,000, and 0.18 district/rural hospitals per 100,000. In 2008, Senegal had 0.34 hospital beds per 1,000 population, one of the 10 lowest rates in the world.

Major Health Issues

In 2008, WHO estimated that 77 percent of years of life lost in Senegal were due to communicable diseases, 17 percent to noncommunicable diseases, and 6 percent to injuries. In 2008, the age-standardized estimate of cancer deaths was 105 per 100,000 for men and 101 per 100,000 for women; for cardiovascular disease and diabetes, 357 per 100,000 for men and 368 per 100,000 for women; and for chronic respiratory disease, 98 per 100,000 for men and 56 per 100,000 for women.

In 2008, the age-standardized death rate from malaria was 42.0 per 100,000 population. In 2010, tuberculosis incidence was 288.0 per 100,000 population, tuberculosis prevalence 542.0 per 100,000, and deaths due to tuberculosis among HIV-negative people 62.00 per 100,000. As of 2009, an estimated 0.9 percent of adults age 15 to 49 were living with HIV or AIDS.

Senegal's maternal mortality rate (death from any cause related to or aggravated by pregnancy) is high by global standards, estimated at 410 maternal deaths per 100,000 live births as of 2008. A 2005 survey estimated the prevalence of female genital mutilation at 28.2 percent. The infant mortality rate, defined as the number of deaths of infants younger than 1 year, is also high, at 55.16 per 1,000 live births as of 2012. In 2005, 14.5 percent of children under age 5 were underweight (defined as 2 kilograms [kg] below standard weight-for-age at age 1, 3 kg below for ages 2 to 3, and 4 kg below for ages 4 to 5).

Health Care Personnel
Senegal has two medical schools: the Faculté de Médecine et de Pharmacie of the University of Dakar and St. Christopher Iba Mar Diop College of Medicine (formerly St. Christopher's College of Medicine), although degrees from the latter are not recognized in the United Kingdom and in some U.S. states. The basic medical degree training course lasts eight years, and the degree awarded is Doctorat d'Etat en Médecine (doctor of medicine). Physicians must register with the Conseil National de l'Ordre des Médecins du Sénégal. Senegal recognizes medical degrees from approved universities in France and has an agreement with other countries in the Conseil Africain et Malagache de l'Enseignement Supérieur.

In 2008, Senegal had 0.06 physicians per 1,000 population, 0.01 pharmaceutical personnel per 1,000, 0.02 laboratory health workers per 1,000, 0.79 health management and support workers per 1,000, 0.01 dentistry personnel per 1,000, and 0.42 nurses and midwives per 1,000. Michael Clemens and Bunilla Petterson estimate that 51 percent of Senegal-born physicians and 27 percent of Senegal-born nurses are working in one of nine developed countries, primarily in France.

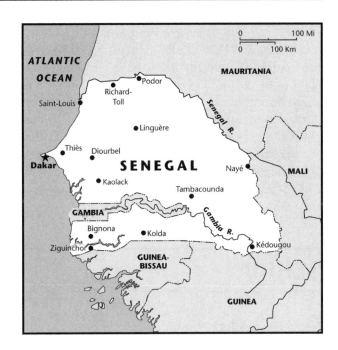

Government Role in Health Care
The right to health, including the right to access essential medicines and health care technology, is recognized in the 2001 Senegalese constitution. Senegal has a National Health Policy (NHP) and a plan to implement it, both written in 2009. It also has a National Medicines Policy (NMP), written in 2006. The NMP covers selection of essential medicines; financing, pricing, purchase, distribution, and regulation of drugs; pharmacovigilance; rational usage of medicines; human resource development; research; evaluation and monitoring; and traditional medicine.

According to WHO, in 2010, Senegal spent $727 million on health care, an amount that comes to $59 per capita. Most (82 percent) of health care funding came from domestic sources, with 18 percent coming from abroad. Just over half (55 percent) of health care spending was paid for through government expenditures, with the remainder provided through household expenditures (35 percent) and other sources (10 percent).

In 2010, Senegal allocated 12 percent of its total government expenditures to health, in the median range for lower-middle-income African countries; government expenditures on health came to 3 percent of GDP, in the high range for lower-middle-income African countries. In 2009, according to WHO, official development assistance (ODA) for health in Senegal came to $8.72 per capita.

Public Health Programs

According to WHO, in 2008, Senegal had 0.10 environmental and public health workers per 1,000 population. In 2010, 52 percent of the population had access to improved sanitation facilities (39 percent in rural areas and 70 percent in urban), and 76 percent had access to improved sources of drinking water (56 percent in rural areas and 93 percent in urban). According to C. B. Ijsselmuiden and colleagues, in 2007, Senegal had one institution offering postgraduate public health programs.

SERBIA

Serbia is a landlocked southeastern European nation sharing borders with Bosnia and Herzegovina, Bulgaria, Croatia, Hungary, Kosovo, Macedonia, Montenegro, and Romania. The area of 29,913 square miles (77,474 square kilometers) makes Serbia about twice the size of New Jersey, and the July 2012 population was estimated at 16.7 million. In 2010, 56 percent of the population lived in urban areas, and the 2010 to 2015 annual rate of urbanization is estimated at 0.6 percent. Belgrade is the capital and largest city (with a 2009 population estimated at 1.1 million). The population growth rate in 2012 was negative 0.5 percent, the net migration rate 0.0 migrant per 1,000 population, the birth rate 9.2 births per 1,000, and the total fertility rate 1.4 children per woman. The United Nations High Commissioner for Refugees (UNHCR) estimated that, in 2010, there were 73,608 refugees and persons in refugee-like situations in Serbia, and 1,803 internally displaced persons and persons in internally displaced-person-like situations.

Serbia was part of the country of Yugoslavia, formed in 1918. Slobodan Milosevic was elected president of the Republic of Serbia in 1989, and his calls for Serbian dominance led Croatia, Slovenia, Macedonia, and Bosnia to declare their independence in 1991 and 1992; Montenegro declared its independence from Serbia in 2006. Several brutal wars fought in the 1990s among the countries once part of Yugoslavia brought the term *ethnic cleansing* into common speech; several government and military leaders, including Milosevic, were charged with war crimes and crimes against humanity for their parts in these wars. Serbia ranked tied for 86th among 183 countries on the *Corruption*

Perceptions Index 2011, with a score of 3.3 (on a scale where 0 indicates highly corrupt and 10 very clean).

In 2011, Serbia was classified as a country with high human development (the second-highest category) on the United Nations Development Programme's (UNDP's) Human Development Index (HDI), with a score of 0.766 (on a scale where 1 denotes high development and 0 low development). Life expectancy at birth in 2012 was estimated at 74.56 years, per capita gross domestic product (GDP) in 2011 was estimated at $10,700, and unemployment in 2011 was estimated at 23.7 percent. Income distribution in Serbia is among the most equal in the world: In 2008, the Gini Index (a measure of dispersion, in which perfect equality is denoted by 0 and maximum inequality is denoted by 100) for family income was 28.2.

Emergency Health Services

According to the World Health Organization (WHO), as of 2007, Serbia had a formal and publicly available emergency care (prehospital care) system accessible through both a national access number and regional access numbers.

Insurance

According to the European Commission, in 2011, most health care in Serbia was a governmental responsibility, provided through a network of 345 public institutions. Primary care is provided by several types of institutions, some attached to hospitals, while secondary and tertiary care is provided by general and specialized hospitals. This public care system was financed primarily by health insurance contributions (70 percent), with the remainder coming from budget transfers and other sources. About 93 percent of the population is covered by compulsory governmental health insurance; those not covered are primarily members of minority groups (for example, Roma), asylum seekers, and refugees and internally displaced people. The National Health Accounts for 2010 attest that more than 35 percent of the costs of health care were borne by private individuals as out-of-pocket expenses, largely for drugs not covered by the state. The national health system gives citizens the right to health care treatment, income compensation when an individual is unable to work, and a travel allowance if it is necessary to travel to receive care.

Costs of Hospitalization

No data available.

Access to Health Care

According to WHO, in 2005, 99 percent of births in Serbia were attended by skilled personnel (for example, physicians, nurses, or midwives). The 2010 immunization rates for 1-year-olds were 95 percent for diphtheria and pertussis (DPT3), 91 percent for measles (MCV), and 95 percent for Hib (Hib3). In 2010, an estimated 34 percent of persons with advanced human immunodeficiency virus (HIV) infection were receiving antiretroviral therapy in accordance with the 2010 WHO guidelines. Also in 2010, Serbia had 7.96 magnetic resonance imaging (MRI) machines per 1 million population, 17.53 computer tomography (CT) machines per 1 million, 0.99 positron emission tomography (PET) machines per 1 million, 0.50 telecolbalt units per 1 million, and 0.50 radiotherapy machines per 1 million.

Cost of Drugs

In 2011, the third-largest expense in the public health care system was the cost of medical devices and medicines (14 percent), followed by the cost of prescription drugs (12 percent). Serbia has a positive medicines list, and those drugs not on the list must be purchased out of pocket.

Health Care Facilities

In 2011, according to the European Commission, most health care in Serbia was provided through a network of 345 public institutions, including health centers and hospitals. There were also more than 5,000 private care facilities, primarily pharmacies and dental surgeries; more than one-third of the private care facilities were located in Belgrade. Although Serbia has an accreditation process for health care facilities carried out since 2009 by the Agency for the Accreditation of Health Care, it is voluntary, and there are no sanctions for facilities that do not meet minimum standards. As of 2010, according to WHO, Serbia had 7.81 health posts per 100,000 population, 0.61 health centers per 100,000, and 0.18 district or rural hospitals per 100,000. In 2007, Serbia had 5.40 hospital beds per 1,000 population, among the 50 highest rates in the world.

Major Health Issues

In 2008, WHO estimated that 4 percent of years of life lost in Serbia were due to communicable diseases, 88 percent to noncommunicable diseases, and 8 percent to injuries. In 2008, the age-standardized estimate of cancer deaths was 211 per 100,000 for men and 129 per 100,000 for women; for cardiovascular disease and diabetes, 463 per 100,000 for men and 381 per 100,000 for women; and for chronic respiratory disease, 37 per 100,000 for men and 16 per 100,000 for women.

Serbia's maternal mortality rate (death from any cause related to or aggravated by pregnancy) was estimated at eight per 100,000 live births in 2008. The infant mortality rate, defined as the number of deaths of infants younger than 1 year, was 6.40 per 1,000 live births as of 2012. In 2010, tuberculosis incidence was 18.0 per 100,000 population, tuberculosis prevalence 22.0 per 100,000, and deaths due to tuberculosis among HIV-negative people 1.4 per 100,000. As of 2009, an estimated 0.1 percent of adults age 15 to 49 were living with HIV or acquired immune deficiency syndrome (AIDS).

Health Care Personnel

Serbia has one medical school, the Faculty of Medicine of the University of Kragujevac, which began offering instruction in 1986. In 2007, Serbia had 2.04 physicians per 1,000 population, 0.19 pharmaceutical personnel per 1,000, 0.25 dentistry personnel per 1,000, and 4.43 nurses and midwives per 1,000.

Government Role in Health Care

According to WHO, in 2010, Serbia spent $4.0 billion on health care, an amount that comes to $546 per capita. Almost all (99 percent) of health care funding came from domestic sources, with 1 percent coming

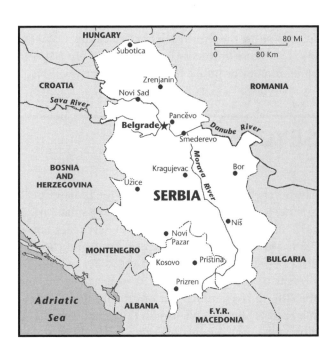

from abroad. More than three-fifths (62 percent) of health care spending was paid for through government expenditures, with the remainder provided through household expenditures (36 percent) and other sources (2 percent). In 2010, Serbia allocated 14 percent of its total government expenditures to health, in the high range for upper-middle-income European countries; government expenditures on health came to 6 percent of GDP, in the high range for upper-middle-income European countries. In 2009, according to WHO, official development assistance (ODA) for health in Serbia came to $3.06 per capita.

Public Health Programs

Serbia's Institute of Public Health was created in 1919 as the Ministerial Commission for Epidemiology; it assumed its current form in 2006 and is located in Belgrade and directed by Tanja Knezevic. The institute has more than 240 employees whose tasks include collecting and making available data about the health of the Serbian population; promoting public health through education and community health activities and providing care for vulnerable groups; improving emergency preparedness; preventing and controlling disease; monitoring environmental risk factors to health, including enforcing sanitation and water safety laws; and performing clinical and public health microbiology. In 2010, 92 percent of the population of Serbia had access to improved sanitation facilities (88 percent in rural areas and 96 percent in urban), and 99 percent had access to improved sources of drinking water (98 percent in rural areas and 99 percent in urban). According to the World Higher Education Database (WHED), one university in Serbia offers programs in epidemiology or public health: the University of Nis.

SEYCHELLES

The Seychelles is an island nation in the Indian Ocean northeast of Madagascar. The area of 176 square miles (455 square kilometers) makes the Seychelles about 2.5 times the size of Washington, D.C., and the July 2012 population was estimated at 90,024. In 2010, 55 percent of the population lived in urban areas, and the 2010 to 2015 annual rate of urbanization was estimated at 1.3 percent. Victoria is the capital and largest city (with a 2009 population estimated at 26,000). The

population growth rate in 2012 was 0.9 percent, the net migration rate 1.0 migrants per 1,000 population, the birth rate 15.1 births per 1,000, and the total fertility rate 1.9 children per woman.

The Seychelles became a possession of Great Britain in 1814 and became independent in 1976. According to the Ibrahim Index, in 2011, the Seychelles is among the best-governed countries in Africa, ranking fourth among 53 African countries in terms of governance performance, with a score of 73 (out of 100). The Seychelles ranked tied for 50th among 183 countries on the *Corruption Perceptions Index 2011,* with a score of 4.8 (on a scale where 0 indicates highly corrupt and 10 very clean).

In 2011, the Seychelles was classified as a country with high human development (the second-highest category) on the United Nations Development Programme's (UNDP's) Human Development Index (HDI), with a score of 0.773 (on a scale where 1 denotes high development and 0 low development). Life expectancy at birth in 2012 was estimated at 73.77 years, and per capita gross domestic product (GDP) in 2011 was estimated at $24,700. Income distribution in the Seychelles is relatively unequal: In 2007, the Gini Index (a measure of dispersion, in which perfect equality is denoted by 0 and maximum inequality is denoted by 100) for family income was 65.8, among the highest in the world.

Emergency Health Services

According to the World Health Organization (WHO), as of 2007, Seychelles had a formal and publicly available emergency care (prehospital care) system accessible through a national access number.

Insurance

Seychelles has a social insurance system covering employed and self-employed people and providing cash maternity and sickness benefits. The system is funded through contributions from wages, earnings of the self-employed, and employer payroll contributions; the same funds finance the system of old-age, disability, and survivor's pensions. The National Health Plan (NHP) provides free medical services. The maternity benefit is 100 percent of salary for two weeks before and eight weeks after birth. The sickness benefit in Seychelles is 100 percent of salary for two months (paid 80 percent by the sickness fund and 20 percent by the employer), then 1,800 rupees per month (paid by the sickness fund) for up to 130 working days.

A means-tested dependent's supplement is paid: SCR 900 monthly for an adult and SCR 800 monthly for each child. Benefits are regularly adjusted according to changes in the cost of living. Income-tested benefits are administered by the Social Welfare Agency, and the social security fund is administered by the Ministry of Finance.

Costs of Hospitalization

No data available.

Access to Health Care

According to WHO, in 2010, Seychelles had 11.93 magnetic resonance imaging (MRI) machines per 1 million population and 11.93 computer tomography (CT) machines per 1 million. The 2010 immunization rates for 1-year-olds were 99 percent for diphtheria and pertussis (DPT3), 99 percent for measles (MCV), and 99 percent for Hib (Hib3).

Cost of Drugs

Total pharmaceutical expenditures in Seychelles in 2009 came to SCR 11.2 million ($0.9 million) and per capita pharmaceutical expenditures to SCR 129.20 ($10.00). Pharmaceutical expenditures constituted 3.1 percent of total health expenditures and 0.1 percent of GDP. Just over one-quarter (26.4 percent) of pharmaceutical expenditures were funded by the public sector. Medicines are provided free of charge to children under the age of 5, pregnant women, elderly people, and the poor. The public health system provides some drugs for free, including drugs on the Essential Medicines List (EML) and drugs to treat malaria, tuberculosis, sexually transmitted diseases (STDs), and human immunodeficiency virus/ acquired immune deficiency syndrome (HIV/AIDS); vaccines on WHO's Expanded Programme on Immunization (EPI) list are also provided free.

Health Care Facilities

As of 2010, according to the World Health Organization, the Seychelles had 21.96 health posts per 100,000 population, 5.78 health centers per 100,000, and 1.16 specialized hospitals per 100,000. In 2009, the Seychelles had 3.94 hospital beds per 1,000 population.

Major Health Issues

In 2008, WHO estimated that 21 percent of years of life lost in the Seychelles were due to communicable diseases, 66 percent to noncommunicable diseases, and 14 percent to injuries. In 2008, the age-standardized estimate of cancer deaths was 227 per 100,000 for men and 96 per 100,000 for women; for cardiovascular disease and diabetes, 323 per 100,000 for men and 230 per 100,000 for women; and for chronic respiratory disease, 53 per 100,000 for men and 21 per 100,000 for women. In 2004, an estimated 26.0 percent of adults in the Seychelles were obese (defined as a body mass index, or BMI, of 30 or greater).

In 2010, tuberculosis incidence was 31.0 per 100,000 population, tuberculosis prevalence 48.0 per 100,000, and deaths due to tuberculosis among HIV-negative people 1.70 per 100,000. The infant mortality rate, defined as the number of deaths of infants younger than 1 year, was 11.35 per 1,000 live births in 2012. No information is available from WHO on the maternal mortality rate in Seychelles.

Health Care Personnel

Seychelles has one medical school, the University of Seychelles-American Institute of Medicine in Victoria. The basic degree course requires four years with the curriculum modeled on the U.S. medical curriculum, and students are prepared for the U.S. Medical Licensing Exam. In 2004, Seychelles had 1.51 physicians per 1,000 population, 0.76 pharmaceutical personnel per 1,000, 0.74 laboratory health workers per 1,000, 1.18 dentistry personnel per 1,000, and 7.93 nurses and midwives per 1,000. Michael Clemens and Bunilla

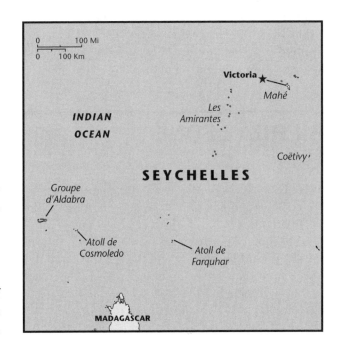

Petterson estimate that 29 percent of Seychelles-born physicians and 29 percent of Seychelles-born nurses are working in one of nine developed countries, primarily in the United Kingdom.

Government Role in Health Care

The right to health, including access to essential medicines and medical technology, is recognized by national legislation. The Seychelles has a National Health Policy (NHP) and a plan to implement it, both written in 2010; it also has a National Medicines Policy (NMP), written in 2010. The NMP covers the selection of medicines for the Essential Medicines List (EML); financing, procurement and regulation of medicines; and rational use of medicines. According to WHO, in 2010, Seychelles spent $32 million on health care, an amount that comes to $368 per capita. Most (96 percent) of health care funding came from domestic sources, with 4 percent coming from abroad. Most (92 percent) of health care spending was paid for through government expenditures, with the remainder provided through household expenditures (6 percent) and other sources (3 percent). In 2010, Seychelles allocated 9 percent of its total government expenditures to health, in the median range for upper-middle-income African countries; government expenditures on health came to 3 percent of GDP, in the median range for upper-middle-income African countries.

Public Health Programs

According to WHO, in 2004, Seychelles had 0.96 environmental and public health workers per 1,000 population. In 2010, 98 percent of the population had access to improved sanitation facilities, and 100 percent had access to improved sources of drinking water.

SIERRA LEONE

Sierra Leone is a west African country, sharing borders with Guinea and Liberia and having a coastline on the north Atlantic Ocean. The area of 27,699 square miles (71,740 square kilometers) makes Sierra Leone about the size of South Carolina, and the July 2012 population was estimated at 5.5 million. In 2010, 38 percent of the population lived in urban areas, and the 2010 to 2015 annual rate of urbanization was estimated at 3.3 percent. Freetown is the capital and largest city (with

a 2009 population estimated at 875,000). The population growth rate in 2012 was 2.3 percent, the net migration rate negative 3.8 migrants per 1,000 population, the birth rate 38.1 births per 1,000 (the 16th-highest in the world), and the total fertility rate 4.9 children per woman (the 22nd-highest in the world). The United Nations High Commissioner for Refugees (UNHCR) estimated that, in 2010, there were 8,341 refugees and persons in refugee-like situations in Sierra Leone.

Sierra Leone was used as a trading point by Europeans from the 15th century and became the home of escaped or freed slaves from the Americas in the 18th and 19th centuries. Sierra Leone was a British colony from the mid-19th century to 1961, when it became an independent country. The country was the site of a brutal civil war from 1991 to 2002 that displaced about one-third of the population. According to the Ibrahim Index, in 2011, Sierra Leone ranked 30th among 53 African countries in terms of governance performance, with a score of 48 (out of 100). Sierra Leone ranked tied for 134th among 183 countries on the *Corruption Perceptions Index 2011*, with a score of 2.5 (on a scale where 0 indicates highly corrupt and 10 very clean).

In 2011, Sierra Leone was classified as a country with low human development (the lowest of four categories) on the United Nations Development Programme's (UNDP's) Human Development Index (HDI), with a score of 0.336 (on a scale where 1 denotes high

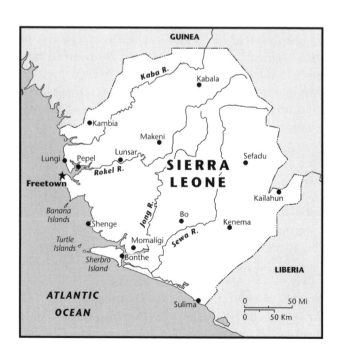

development and 0 low development). In 2011, the International Food Policy Research Institute (IFPRI) classified Sierra Leone as a country with an "alarming" hunger problem, with a Global Hunger Index (GHI) score of 25.2, the highest in the world (where 0 reflects no hunger and higher scores more hunger).

Life expectancy at birth in 2012 was estimated at 56.55 years, among the 30 lowest in the world, and estimated gross domestic product (GDP) per capita in 2011 was $800, among the 10 lowest in the world. Income distribution in Sierra Leone is relatively unequal: In 1989, the Gini Index (a measure of dispersion, in which perfect equality is denoted by 0 and maximum inequality is denoted by 100) for family income was 62.9, among the highest in the world. Unemployment in 2002 was estimated at 45 percent, among the highest rates in the world.

Emergency Health Services

According to the World Health Organization (WHO), as of 2007, Sierra Leone did not have a formal and publicly available system for providing prehospital care (emergency care). Doctors Without Borders (Médecins Sans Frontières, or MSF) began working in Sierra Leone in 1986 and had 439 staff members in the country at the close of 2010. MSF is a major provider of maternal and child care outside the national capital of Freetown and runs a hospital in Bo (Sierra Leone's second-largest city) focusing on maternal and child health. MSF also trains local workers to diagnose and treat malaria and has improved the system of transporting emergency cases to hospitals. In 2010, MSF provided more than 210,000 consultations and treated more than 14,000 patients in Sierra Leone.

Insurance

Sierra Leone began a policy of providing free medical care for pregnant and breast-feeding women and children under age 5 in April 2010, although shortages of physicians and other medical staff have hampered implementation of this policy. Employers provide medical care, through cooperative agreements, for employees and their dependents.

Costs of Hospitalization

No data available.

Access to Health Care

According to WHO, in 2008, 42 percent of births in Sierra Leone were attended by skilled personnel (for example, physicians, nurses, or midwives), and 56 percent of pregnant women received at least four prenatal care visits. The 2010 immunization rates for 1-year-olds were 90 percent for diphtheria and pertussis (DPT3), 82 percent for measles (MCV), and 90 percent for Hib (Hib3). In 2010, an estimated 31 percent of persons with advanced human immunodeficiency virus (HIV) infection were receiving antiretroviral therapy in accordance with the 2010 WHO guidelines.

Cost of Drugs

By government policy, medications in Sierra Leone are provided free of charge to children under 5, pregnant women, elderly people, and the poor. The public health system provides (through the Global Fund) medications to treat malaria, tuberculosis, sexually transmitted diseases (STDs), and human immunodeficiency virus/acquired immune deficiency syndrome (HIV/AIDS) for free; vaccines on WHO's Expanded Programme on Immunization (EPI) list are also available for free.

Health Care Facilities

As of 2010, according to WHO, Sierra Leone had 1.26 health centers per 100,000 population. In 2006, Sierra Leone had 0.40 hospital beds per 1,000 population, one of the 10 lowest rates in the world.

Major Health Issues

In 2008, WHO estimated that 85 percent of years of life lost in Sierra Leone were due to communicable diseases, 10 percent to noncommunicable diseases, and 5 percent to injuries. In 2008, the age-standardized estimate of cancer deaths was 101 per 100,000 for men and 101 per 100,000 for women; for cardiovascular disease and diabetes, 421 per 100,000 for men and 459 per 100,000 for women; and for chronic respiratory disease, 117 per 100,000 for men and 70 per 100,000 for women.

In 2008, the age-standardized death rate from malaria was 132.5 per 100,000 population, the highest in the world. In 2008, the age-standardized death rate from childhood-cluster diseases (pertussis, polio, diphtheria, measles, and tetanus) was 30.8 per 100,000 population, the third-highest in the world. In 2010, tuberculosis incidence was 682.0 per 100,000 population, tuberculosis prevalence 1,282.0 per 100,000, and deaths due to tuberculosis among HIV-negative people 146.0 per 100,000. As of 2009, an estimated 1.8 percent of adults age 15 to 49 were living with HIV or AIDS.

Sierra Leone's maternal mortality rate (death from any cause related to or aggravated by pregnancy) is the sixth-highest in the world, estimated at 970 per 100,000 live births as of 2008. A 2006 survey estimated the prevalence of female genital mutilation at 94.0 percent. The infant mortality rate, defined as the number of deaths of infants younger than 1 year, also has been high, at 76.64 per 1,000 live births as of 2012. In 2008, 21.3 percent of children under age 5 were underweight (defined as 2 kilograms [kg] below standard weight-for-age at age 1, 3 kg below for ages 2 to 3, and 4 kg below for ages 4 to 5).

Health Care Personnel

Sierra Leone has one medical school, the College of Medicine and Allied Health Sciences of the University of Sierra Leone in Freetown, which began offering instruction in 1988. The basic medical degree course lasts 5.5 years, and the degrees awarded are the bachelor of medicine and bachelor of surgery. In 2008, Sierra Leone had 0.02 physicians per 1,000 population, 0.03 pharmaceutical personnel per 1,000, 0.01 laboratory health workers per 1,000, 0.28 health management and support workers per 1,000, 0.02 community and traditional health workers per 1,000, and 0.17 nurses and midwives per 1,000. Michael Clemens and Bunilla Petterson estimate that 42 percent of Sierra Leone-born physicians and 49 percent of Sierra Leone-born nurses are working in one of nine developed countries, primarily in the United Kingdom and the United States.

Government Role in Health Care

Sierra Leone has both a National Health Policy (NHP) and a National Medicine Policy (NMP). The NMP includes the selection of essential medicines; financing, procurement, distribution, and regulation of medicines; the rational use of medicines; research; monitoring and evaluation; and traditional medicine. According to WHO, in 2010, Sierra Leone spent $250 million on health care, an amount that comes to $43 per capita. More than three-quarters (79 percent) of health care funding came from domestic sources, with 21 percent coming from abroad. More than three-quarters (79 percent) of health care spending was paid for through household expenditures, with the remainder provided through government expenditures (11 percent) and other sources (9 percent). In 2010, Sierra Leone allocated 6 percent of its total government expenditures to health, in the low range for low-income African countries; government expenditures on health came to 1 percent of GDP, in the low range for low-income African countries. In 2009, according to WHO, official development assistance (ODA) for health in Sierra Leone came to $9.19 per capita.

Public Health Programs

According to WHO, in 2008, Sierra Leone had 0.02 environmental and public health workers per 1,000 population. In 2010, only 13 percent of the population

Health Expenditures: Sierra Leone Compared With the Global Average (2009)

	Sierra Leone	Global Average
Out-of-pocket expenditure as percent of private expenditure on health	89.5	50.2
Private prepaid plans as percent of private expenditure on health	1	38.9
Per capita total expenditure on health at average exchange rate (USD)	45	900
Per capita total expenditure on health (purchasing power parity, international dollars)	110	990
Per capita government expenditure on health at average exchange rate (USD)	5	549
Per capita government expenditure on health (purchasing power parity, international dollars)	12	584

Source: 2011 World Health Organization Global Health Expenditure Atlas.

had access to improved sanitation facilities (6 percent in rural areas and 23 percent in urban), and 55 percent had access to improved sources of drinking water (35 percent in rural areas and 87 percent in urban). According to the World Higher Education Database (WHED), one university in Sierra Leone offers programs in epidemiology or public health: Njala University, located in Freetown.

SINGAPORE

Singapore is an island nation in southeast Asia just off the coast of Malaysia. The area of 269 square miles (697 square kilometers) makes Singapore about 3.5 times the size of Washington, D.C., and the July 2012 population was estimated at 5.4 million; the population is entirely urban. The population growth rate in 2012 was 2.0 percent, the net migration rate 15.6 migrants per 1,000 population (the sixth-highest in the world), the birth rate 7.7 births per 1,000 (the second-lowest in the world), and the total fertility rate 0.8 children per woman (the lowest in the world). The United Nations High Commissioner for Refugees (UNHCR) estimated that, in 2010, there were seven refugees and persons in refugee-like situations in Singapore.

Singapore was founded in 1819 as a British trading colony, joined the Malaysian Federation in 1963, and became an independent country in 1965. The government has a reputation for transparency and honesty, ranking fifth among 183 countries in terms on the *Corruption Perceptions Index 2011,* with a score of 9.2 (on a scale where 0 indicates highly corrupt and 10 very clean). In 2011, Singapore was classified as a country with very high human development (the highest of four categories) on the United Nations Development Programme's (UNDP's) Human Development Index (HDI), with a score of 0.866 (on a scale where 1 denotes high development and 0 low development). Life expectancy at birth in 2012 was estimated at 83.75 years, the fourth-highest in the world, and per capita gross domestic product (GDP) in 2011 in Singapore was estimated at $59,900, among the highest in the world. Income distribution in Singapore is relatively unequal: In 2011, the Gini Index (a measure of dispersion, in which perfect equality is denoted by 0 and maximum inequality is denoted by 100) for family income was

47.3. According to the World Economic Forum's *Global Gender Gap Index 2011,* Singapore ranked 57th out of 135 countries on gender equality with a score of 0.691 (on a scale with a theoretical range of 1 for equality to 0 for inequality and an actual range in 2011 from 0.8530 to 0.4873).

Emergency Health Services

Singapore had dual emergency medical systems from 1960 to 1976: the Central Ambulance Service affiliated with Singapore General Hospital and the second run by the Singapore Fire Brigade. In 1977, the two services were integrated as the Emergency Ambulance Services, and in 1989, this service was absorbed into the Singapore Civil Defence Force (SCDF). In 1992, a motorcycle-based response force was created to respond to traffic accidents in order to work around the problem that ambulances were frequently delayed in traffic. As of 2000, the SCDF worked out of 13 fire stations and answered 60,000 to 70,000 calls annually. Six acute-care public hospitals have emergency departments, and there are also specialized units for burns, neurosurgery, and pediatric trauma.

Insurance

Singapore provides medical benefits through a provident fund (MediSave) and social assistance program and cash sickness and maternity benefits through an employer-liability system. Employed and self-employed people with annual net incomes over SGD 6,000 are covered under the medical benefits system; those unable to pay for medical treatment are eligible for financial assistance through the MediFund program. People with no sources of income may be provided free medical treatment at government clinics and hospitals. Some public-sector employees are covered under a separate system. The cash benefit system covers employed persons. The cash benefit system is funded by employer contributions. The social assistance system is funded entirely through tax revenues. Under the medical benefit provident fund, each insured person has an individual Medisave account, funded through contributions from employed and self-employed people and employers; a complex system prescribing the amount of contribution (depending on earnings and age) and distribution of the contribution into various accounts, including the Medisave account, covers the cost of hospitalization and medical care. The government subsidizes some hospital care.

Medical and hospital care is provided through approved private hospitals and institutions and government hospitals; the cost of approved treatments is deducted from an individual's Medisave account. There are maximum limits to the charges for different types of services (for example, SGD 450 per day for hospitalization). Singaporean patients can receive subsidies of up to 80 percent for treatment in government hospitals. Insured members can use their Medisave accounts to pay for the care of dependents, including children, parents, spouses, and grandparents (the latter must be permanent residents or citizens of Singapore).

The maternity benefit is 100 percent of pay for up to 16 weeks, with the cost split between the employer and government. The Singapore government pays up to SGD 20,000 for the first two births and SGD 40,000 for subsequent births. The Ministry of Health provides and contracts for health services, the Central Provident Fund administers the program, and the Ministry of Manpower provides policy direction, law enforcement, and general supervision.

Costs of Hospitalization

Most patients pay a percentage of the cost of treatment in hospitals, which can range from private or semi-private rooms (where the patient pays 100 percent of the cost) to four-bed rooms (where the patient pays 80 percent), to open dormitories (where the patient pays 20 percent). The government caps prices on all procedures and services provided in public (but not private) hospitals and promotes competition based on price by publishing the costs of common treatments at different facilities. Foreigners working in Singapore are excluded from the national system but generally (at least, those in white-collar professions) have health care through their employers.

Access to Health Care

Most Singaporeans (85 percent) are covered under the mandatory MediSave program, and MediFund provides a safety net for the poor. However, the insurance policies have high copayments and high deductibles, so middle- and upper-income people often purchase private insurance to cover these costs, while those with lower incomes may be left with large out-of-pocket expenses. According to the World Health Organization (WHO), in 2007, 99.7 percent of births in Singapore were attended by skilled personnel (for example, physicians, nurses, or midwives). The 2010 immunization rates for 1-year-olds were 97 percent for diphtheria and pertussis (DPT3) and 95 percent for measles (MCV).

Cost of Drugs

No data available.

Health Care Facilities

As of 2010, according to WHO, Singapore had 63.01 health posts per 100,000 population and 0.53 provincial hospitals per 100,000. In 2008, Singapore had 3.14 hospital beds per 1,000 population, and as of 2011, had 13 public hospitals (75 percent of total beds), 16 private hospitals, and 1,400 private ambulatory clinics.

Most (80 percent) of acute care in Singapore is provided at public hospitals, while most (80 percent) of primary care is provided by private providers, with government clinics providing the rest. The public hospital network includes six national specialty centers clustered in Singapore General Hospital and the National University Hospital. Singapore also has a well-developed network of community and residential-based services that care for the elderly, including nursing homes, inpatient hospices, day care centers, community hospitals, and rehabilitation homes. Due

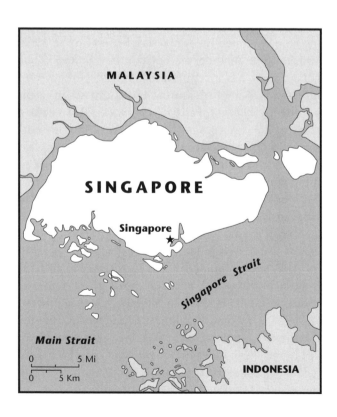

to the high quality of care, Singapore is becoming a popular medical tourism destination: More than 400,000 foreigners came to Singapore for medical care in 2006.

Major Health Issues

In 2008, WHO estimated that 11 percent of years of life lost in Singapore were due to communicable diseases, 78 percent to noncommunicable diseases, and 11 percent to injuries. In 2008, the age-standardized estimate of cancer deaths was 142 per 100,000 for men and 91 per 100,000 for women; for cardiovascular disease and diabetes, 171 per 100,000 for men and 109 per 100,000 for women; and for chronic respiratory disease, 23 per 100,000 for men and seven per 100,000 for women.

The maternal mortality rate (death from any cause related to or aggravated by pregnancy) in Singapore in 2008 was nine maternal deaths per 100,000 live births. The infant mortality rate was 3.17 per 1,000 live births as of 2012, the fourth lowest in the world. In 2010, tuberculosis incidence was 35.0 per 100,000 population, tuberculosis prevalence 44.0 per 100,000, and deaths due to tuberculosis among human immunodeficiency virus (HIV)-negative people 2.3 per 100,000. As of 2009, an estimated 0.1 percent of adults age 15 to 49 were living with HIV or acquired immune deficiency syndrome (AIDS).

Health Care Personnel

Singapore has one medical school, the Faculty of Medicine of the National University of Singapore, which has been offering instruction since 1905. The basic medical course lasts five years, and the degrees awarded are bachelor of medicine and bachelor of surgery. One year of work in government service is required after graduation. The license to practice is granted by the Singapore Medical Council to graduates of a recognized medical school who have completed a one-year internship, but graduates of foreign medical schools receive only temporary licensure.

In 2009, Singapore had 1.83 physicians per 1,000 population, 0.37 pharmaceutical personnel per 1,000, 0.32 dentistry personnel per 1,000, and 5.90 nurses and midwives per 1,000. Using Fitzhugh Mullan's methodology, Singapore has an emigration factor of 11.5, representing a moderate ratio of Singapore physicians working outside the country (in the United States, the United Kingdom, Canada, or Australia) relative to those working in Singapore.

Government Role in Health Care

According to WHO, in 2010, Singapore spent $8.8 billion on health care, an amount that comes to $1,733 per capita. All health care funding came from domestic sources. Just over half (54 percent) of health care spending was paid for through household expenditures, with the remainder provided through government expenditures (36 percent) and other sources (10 percent). In 2010, Singapore allocated 8 percent of its total government expenditures to health, in the low range for high-income western Pacific region countries; government expenditures on health came to 1 percent of GDP, in the low range for high-income western Pacific region countries.

Public Health Programs

In 2010, access to improved sanitation facilities and access to improved sources of drinking water was essentially universal in Singapore.

SLOVAKIA

Slovakia is a landlocked central European country sharing borders with Austria, the Czech Republic, Hungary, Poland, and Ukraine. The area of 18,933 square miles (49,035 square kilometers) makes Slovakia about twice the size of New Hampshire, and the July 2012 population was estimated at 5.5 million. In 2010, 55 percent of the population lived in urban areas, and the 2010 to 2015 annual rate of urbanization was estimated at 0.1 percent. Bratislava is the capital and largest city (with a 2009 population estimated at 428,000). The population growth rate in 2012 was 0.1 percent, the net migration rate 0.3 migrants per 1,000 population, the birth rate 10.4 births per 1,000, and the total fertility rate 1.8 children per woman.

After the Austro-Hungarian Empire was dissolved following World War I, Slovakia became part of the new nation of Czechoslovakia; the country came under Soviet influence after World War II, but Soviet influence ended in 1989. In 1993, Slovakia and the Czech Republic became separate countries by mutual agreement.

Slovakia ranked tied for 66th among 183 countries on the *Corruption Perceptions Index 2011*, with a score of 4.0 (on a scale where 0 indicates highly corrupt and 10 very clean).

In 2011, Slovakia was classified as a country with very high human development (the highest of four categories) on the United Nations Development Programme's (UNDP's) Human Development Index (HDI), with a score of 0.834 (on a scale where 1 denotes high development and 0 low development). Life expectancy at birth in 2012 was estimated at 76.03 years. Per capita gross domestic product (GDP) in 2011 was estimated at $23,400. Income distribution is among the most equal in the world: In 2005, the Gini Index (a measure of dispersion, in which perfect equality is denoted by 0 and maximum inequality is denoted by 100) for family income was 26.0. According to the World Economic Forum's *Global Gender Gap Index 2011*, Slovakia ranked 72nd out of 135 countries on gender equality, with a score of 0.580 (on a scale with a theoretical range of 1 for equality to 0 for inequality and an actual range in 2011 from 0.8530 to 0.4873).

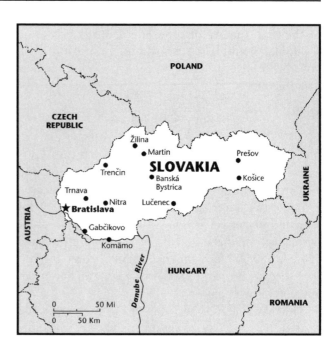

Emergency Health Services

Slovakia's laws governing its emergency health system date from the 2000s, as does recognition of emergency medicine as a medical specialty; by law, free access to hospitals for emergency care is provided for all persons, including the uninsured. Funding for the emergency system is provided by multiple sources. Slovakia has only one national telephone number for medical emergencies, 155 (not 112, the European Union, or EU, standard); the country has eight dispatch centers, which are not interconnected.

Insurance

Slovakia has a social insurance system providing universal coverage for medical benefits (with the exception of persons insured abroad and some non-Slovaks working in Slovakia) and cash sickness and maternity benefits for the employed and self-employed. Some workers are covered under separate systems, including those working in the military, policemen, firemen, and some intelligence, customs, and security personnel. The system is financed through contributions from wages (1.4 percent of covered monthly earnings for the cash benefits system and 4 percent for the medical benefits system), contributions from the self-employed (4.4 percent of declared monthly earnings for the cash benefits system and 14 percent for the medical benefits system), and employer contributions (1.4 percent of covered payroll for the cash benefits system and 10 percent for the medical benefits

system); the government covers deficits and contributes for people who are nonactive.

Medical benefits include preventive treatment, medical treatment, maternity care, hospitalization, medicines, treatment at a sanitarium or spa, some convalescent stays, and vaccinations. There is some cost sharing required, but some people are exempt, including children age 5 and younger, blood donors, the disabled, those receiving maternity care, the mentally disabled, and those being treated for cancer or renal or cardiac disease. Some drugs require cost sharing. The maternity benefit is 55 percent of earnings for a total of 28 weeks (longer for multiple births or a single mother); a nursing benefit of 55 percent of earnings is paid for up to the first 10 days of nursing. The cash benefit for sickness is 25 percent of wages for three days and then 55 percent for up to 52 weeks. Those caring for a family member may receive a benefit of 55 percent of earnings for up to 10 days.

The Ministry of Health and the Health Care Supervision Authority administer medical benefits through health centers and clinics, the Social Insurance Agency administers the cash benefit program, and the Ministry of Labor, Social Affairs, and the Family provides supervision. According to Ke Xu and colleagues, in 2003, less than 0.1 percent of households in Slovakia experienced catastrophic health expenditures annually; "catastrophic" was defined as exceeding 40 percent of household income remaining after basic needs were met.

Costs of Hospitalization

In 2008, according to the Organisation for Economic Co-operation and Development (OECD), hospital spending in Slovakia represented 26.7 percent of total spending on health (a considerable reduction from 45 percent reported in 2002), and per capita spending was $442; hospitals were paid based on payment per case or a diagnosis-related group (DRG). Medical staff in hospitals are salaried. In 1999, the government changed the way hospitals were reimbursed because the old system of paying by patient days encouraged overuse and also motivated hospitals to avoid complex cases because the reimbursement was the same as for a simple case.

Access to Health Care

According to the World Health Organization (WHO), in 2008, 99.5 percent of births in Slovakia were attended by skilled personnel (for example, physicians, nurses, or midwives). The 2010 immunization rates for 1-year-olds were 98 percent for diphtheria and pertussis (DPT3), 99 percent for measles (MCV), and 98 percent for Hib (Hib3). In 2010, an estimated 81 percent of persons with advanced human immunodeficiency virus (HIV) infection were receiving antiretroviral therapy in accordance with the 2010 WHO guidelines. According to WHO, in 2010, Slovakia had 4.47 magnetic resonance imaging (MRI) machines per 1 million population and 12.41 computer tomography (CT) machines per 1 million.

Cost of Drugs

According to Douglas Ball, Slovakia charges a lower rate of 10 percent value-added tax (VAT) on medicines as opposed to the standard VAT rate of 19 percent. The prescription dispensing fee is set at SKK 5; this is split between the pharmacy (25 percent) and the insurance company (75 percent). The wholesale markup is 11 percent of the ex-factory price (the manufacturer's list price before discounts) for reimbursed medicines and nonreimbursed prescription-only medicines, 4 percent for very expensive medicines, 5 percent for vaccines and over-the-counter drugs, and 10 percent for hospital-only drugs. The pharmacy markup is 21 percent of the purchase price for reimbursed medicines and nonreimbursed prescription-only medicines, 10 percent for very expensive medicines, 7 percent for vaccines, 15 percent for over-the-counter drugs, and 10 percent for hospital-only drugs. Real annual growth in pharmaceutical expenditures in Slovakia grew 6.8 percent from 1997 to 2005, slower than the 8.4 percent growth of total health expenditure (minus pharmaceutical expenditures) over those years. According to Elizabeth Docteur, in 2004, generic drugs represented 30 percent of the market share by value and 43 percent of the market share by volume of the total pharmaceutical market.

Health Care Facilities

As of 2010, according to WHO, Slovakia had 0.29 health posts per 100,000 population, 0.11 district or rural hospitals per 100,000, 0.48 provincial hospitals per 100,000, and 0.95 specialized hospitals per 100,000. In 2008, Slovakia had 6.56 hospital beds per 1,000 population, among the 20 highest ratios in the world.

Major Health Issues

In 2008, WHO estimated that 6 percent of years of life lost in Slovakia were due to communicable diseases, 81 percent to noncommunicable diseases, and 13 percent to injuries. In 2008, the age-standardized estimate of cancer deaths was 219 per 100,000 for men and 110 per 100,000 for women; for cardiovascular disease and diabetes, 431 per 100,000 for men and 259 per 100,000 for women; and for chronic respiratory disease, 22 per 100,000 for men and eight per 100,000 for women.

The maternal mortality rate (death from any cause related to or aggravated by pregnancy) in Slovakia in 2008 was six maternal deaths per 100,000 live births, among the lowest in the world. The infant mortality rate, defined as the number of deaths of infants younger than 1 year, was 6.47 per 1,000 live births as if 2012. In 2010, tuberculosis incidence was 8.0 per 100,000 population, tuberculosis prevalence 9.6 per 100,000, and deaths due to tuberculosis among HIV-negative people 0.47 per 100,000. As of 2009, an estimated 0.1 percent of adults age 15 to 49 were living with HIV or acquired immune deficiency syndrome (AIDS).

Health Care Personnel

Slovakia has three medical schools: the Lekarska Fakulta of the Univerzita Komenskeho in Bratislava, the Lekarska Fakulta of the Univerzity P. J. Safarika in Kosice, and the Jeseniova Lekarska Fakulta of the Universita Komenskeho in Bratislava. The basic medical training course lasts six years, and the degree awarded is Medicinae Universae Doctor (doctor of medicine). The license to practice is granted to graduates of recognized medical schools who hold specialization diplomas. Foreigners also require a residence permit and work permit.

Slovakia, as a member of the EU, cooperates with other countries in recognizing physicians qualified to practice in other EU countries, as specified by Directive 2005/36/EC of the European Parliament. This allows qualified professionals to practice their profession in other EU states on a temporary basis and requires that the host country automatically recognize qualifications for certain professions, including physicians, nurses, dentists, midwives, and pharmacists, if certain conditions have been met (for instance, facility in the language of the host country may be required). In 2007, Slovakia had 3.00 physicians per 1,000 population, 0.47 pharmaceutical personnel per 1,000, 0.50 dentistry personnel per 1,000, and 6.58 nurses and midwives per 1,000.

Government Role in Health Care

According to WHO, in 2010, Slovakia spent $7.7 billion on health care, an amount that comes to $1,413 per capita. All health care funding came from domestic sources. Almost two-thirds (66 percent) of health care spending was paid for through government expenditures, with the remainder provided through household expenditures (31 percent) and other sources (4 percent). In 2010, Slovakia allocated 14 percent of its total government expenditures to health, in the median range for high-income European countries; government expenditures on health came to 6 percent of GDP, in the low range for high-income European countries.

Public Health Programs

In 2010, almost 100 percent of the population of Slovakia had access to improved sanitation facilities (99 percent in rural areas and 100 percent in urban), and access to improved sources of drinking water was essentially universal. According to the World Higher Education Database (WHED), three universities in Slovakia offer programs in epidemiology or public health: the Catholic University in Ruzomberok, the University of Trnava in Trnava, and the University of Veterinary Medicine in Kosice.

SLOVENIA

Slovenia is a southern European country, sharing borders with Austria, Croatia, Hungary, and Italy and

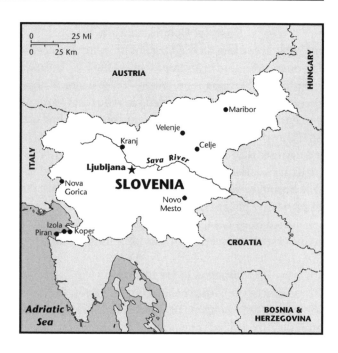

having a short (29-mile or 46.6-kilometer) coastline on the Gulf of Venice. The area of 7,827 square miles (20,273 square kilometers) makes Slovenia about the size of New Jersey, and the July 2012 population was estimated at 2.0 million. In 2010, 50 percent of the population lived in urban areas, and the 2010 to 2015 annual rate of urbanization was estimated at 0.2 percent. Ljubljana is the capital and largest city (with a 2009 population estimated at 260,000). The population growth rate in 2012 was negative 0.2 percent, the net migration rate 0.4 migrants per 1,000 population, the birth rate 9.9 births per 1,000, and the total fertility rate 1.3 children per woman.

Slovenia was part of the Austro-Hungarian Empire and became part of the new country of Yugoslavia in 1918. In 1991, Slovenia became an independent country, following a 10-day war fought against the Serbs. Slovenia ranked 35th among 183 countries on the *Corruption Perceptions Index 2011,* with a score of 5.9 (on a scale where 0 indicates highly corrupt and 10 very clean).

In 2011, Slovenia was classified as a country with very high human development (the highest of four categories) on the United Nations Development Programme's (UNDP's) Human Development Index (HDI), with a score of 0.884 (on a scale where 1 denotes high development and 0 low development). Life expectancy at birth in 2012 was estimated at 77.48 years, and per capita gross domestic product (GDP) in 2011 was estimated at $29,100. Income distribution is among the most equal in the world: In 2008, the Gini Index (a measure of dispersion, in which perfect equality is denoted by 0 and maximum inequality is denoted by 100) for family income was 28.4. According to the World Economic Forum's *Global Gender Gap Index 2011*, Slovenia ranks 41st out of 135 countries on gender equality, with a score of 0.704 (on a scale with a theoretical range of 1 for equality to 0 for inequality and an actual range in 2011 from 0.8530 to 0.4873).

Emergency Health Services

Slovenia's laws governing its emergency health system date from the 2000s, as does recognition of emergency medicine as a medical specialty; by law, free access to hospitals for emergency care is provided for all persons, including the uninsured. Funding for the emergency system is provided by multiple sources. Slovenia has one national telephone number for medical emergencies, 112 (the European Union, or EU, standard); the country has 12 dispatch centers that are interconnected.

Insurance

Slovenia has a social insurance system providing medical benefits to broad classes of the population and cash benefits to a smaller set of groups. The employed and self-employed, professional athletes, and farmers are covered under both systems; residents without social insurance coverage, war veterans and invalids, military personnel, refugees, prisoners, and recipients of cash benefits are entitled to only medical benefits. The system is funded through contributions from wages (6.36 percent of gross earnings for medical and sickness benefits and 0.1 percent for maternity benefits), contributions from earnings for the self-employed (12.92 percent of assessed income for sickness and medical benefits and 0.1 percent for maternity benefits; farmers contributed 6.36 percent of assessed income or 18.78 percent of income from agricultural and forest lands), and employer contributions (6.56 percent of payroll for sickness and medical benefits and 0.1 percent for maternity benefits).The government funds the health care of refugees, prisoners, and military personnel and the emergency care of uninsured people, and finances most (92 percent) of the cost of maternity care. According to Ke Xu and colleagues, in 2003, less than 0.1 percent of households in Slovenia experienced catastrophic health expenditures annually; "catastrophic" was defined as exceeding 40 percent of household income remaining after basic needs were met.

The Health Insurance Institute provides medical services, including hospitalization, surgery, medical and dental care, rehabilitation, medicines, and transportation; a waiting period is required for some benefits, and copayments vary according to the specific service. Some classes of the population receive services free or at a reduced rate, including the disabled, children, and young people; some services and diseases are also covered for free, including organ transplants, emergency care, family planning, and diagnosis and treatment of communicable diseases. The maternity benefit is 100 percent of earnings for 28 days before and 77 days after the due date. The paternity benefit is 100 percent of earnings for 15 days. The sickness benefit is 90 percent of earnings for illness, 80 percent for injury, and 100 percent for organ donation, quarantine, or if the person is a war invalid. The Health Insurance Institute administers the cash sickness and medical benefits program through 10 regional units and 45 local offices, the Ministry of Health provides general supervision, and the Ministry of Labor, Family, and Social Affairs administers parental benefits.

Costs of Hospitalization

In 2008, according to the Organisation for Economic Co-operation and Development (OECD), hospital spending in Slovenia represented 41.6 percent of total spending on health, and per capita spending was $918; hospitals were paid based on global budgets and case-based payments. As of 2002, hospital staff were salaried.

Access to Health Care

According to the World Health Organization (WHO), in 2008, 99.9 percent of births in Slovenia were attended by skilled personnel (for example, physicians, nurses, or midwives). The 2010 immunization rates for 1-year-olds were 96 percent for diphtheria and pertussis (DPT3), 95 percent for measles (MCV), and 96 percent for Hib (Hib3).

Cost of Drugs

No data available.

Health Care Facilities

As of 2010, according to WHO, Slovenia had 3.15 health posts per 100,000 population, 0.49 provincial

Selected Health Indicators: Slovenia Compared With the Organisation for Economic Co-operation and Development (OECD) Country Average

	Slovenia	OECD average (2010 or nearest year)
Male life expectancy at birth, 2010	76.3	77
Female life expectancy at birth, 2010	82.7	82.5
Total expenditure on health (percent of GDP), 2010	9	9.5
Total expenditure on health (per capita, USD purchasing power parity), 2009	2,428.5	3,265
Public expenditure on health (per capita, USD purchasing power parity), 2010	1,768.4	2,377.8
Public expenditure on health (percent total expenditure on health), 2010	72.8	72.2
Doctor consultations (number per capita), 2010	6.4	6.4
Practicing physicians (per 1,000 population), 2010	2.4	3.1
Practicing nurses (per 1,000 population), 2010	8.2	8.6
CT scanners (per 1,000,000 population), 2011	13.8	22.6
Hospital beds (per 1,000 population), 2010	4.6	4.9

Source: OECD Health Data 2012 (Organisation for Economic Co-operation and Development, 2012).

hospitals per 100,000, and 0.10 specialized hospitals per 100,000. In 2008, Slovenia had 4.70 hospital beds per 1,000 population, among the 50 highest rates in the world.

Major Health Issues

In 2008, WHO estimated that 4 percent of years of life lost in Slovenia were due to communicable diseases, 80 percent to noncommunicable diseases, and 16 percent to injuries. In 2008, the age-standardized estimate of cancer deaths was 207 per 100,000 for men and 113 per 100,000 for women; for cardiovascular disease and diabetes, 210 per 100,000 for men and 128 per 100,000 for women; and for chronic respiratory disease, 22 per 100,000 for men and seven per 100,000 for women.

The maternal mortality rate (death from any cause related to or aggravated by pregnancy) in Slovenia in 2008 was 18 maternal deaths per 100,000 live births. The infant mortality rate, defined as the number of deaths of infants younger than 1 year, was 4.12 per

1,000 live births as of 2012. In 2010, tuberculosis incidence was 11.0 per 100,000 population, tuberculosis prevalence 14.0 per 100,000, and deaths due to tuberculosis among human immunodeficiency virus (HIV)-negative people 0.78 per 100,000. As of 2009, an estimated 0.1 percent of adults age 15 to 49 were living with HIV or acquired immune deficiency syndrome (AIDS).

Health Care Personnel

Slovenia has one medical school, the Medicinska Fakulteta of the Univerza v Ljubljani in Ljubljana, which has been offering instruction since 1919. The basic medical training course lasts six years, and an additional two years of supervised work in a teaching hospital is required for the degree Doktor Medicine (doctor of medicine). Graduates must pass a licensure exam as well as complete the two-year internship to receive their medical licenses; graduates of foreign medical schools must have their degrees validated, and foreigners must have an adequate command of

Slovenian and become Slovenian citizens (except for citizens of other EU countries).

Slovenia, as a member of the EU, cooperates with other countries in recognizing physicians qualified to practice in other EU countries, as specified by Directive 2005/36/EC of the European Parliament. This allows qualified professionals to practice their profession in other EU states on a temporary basis and requires that the host country automatically recognize qualifications for certain professions, including physicians, nurses, dentists, midwives, and pharmacists, if certain conditions have been met (for instance, facility in the language of the host country may be required). In 2008, Slovenia had 2.47 physicians per 1,000 population, 0.50 pharmaceutical personnel per 1,000, 0.62 dentistry personnel per 1,000, and 8.16 nurses and midwives per 1,000.

Government Role in Health Care

According to WHO, in 2010, Slovenia spent $4.4 billion on health care, an amount that comes to $2,154 per capita. All health care funding came from domestic sources. Almost three-quarters (74 percent) of health care spending was paid for through government expenditures, with the remainder provided through household expenditures (13 percent) and other sources (14 percent). In 2010, Slovenia allocated 14 percent of its total government expenditures to health, in the median range for high-income European countries; government expenditures on health came to 7 percent of GDP, in the median range for high-income European countries.

Public Health Programs

The National Institute of Public Health for Slovenia is located in Ljubljana and directed by Marija Seljak. It is the primary institute in Slovenia involved with epidemiological research, disease prevention, and health promotion. Major current areas of research include drug and alcohol abuse, suicide, and psychiatry. Slovenia has modern infrastructure, and in 2010, access to improved sanitation facilities and access to improved sources of drinking water were essentially universal.

According to the World Higher Education Database (WHED), four universities in Slovenia offer programs in epidemiology or public health: the European Center in Maribor, the University of Ljubljana, Jesenice College of Nursing, and the Novo Mesto School of Health Sciences.

SOLOMON ISLANDS

The Solomon Islands is an island nation in the south Pacific Ocean, east of Papua New Guinea. The area of 11,156 square miles (28,896 square kilometers) makes the Solomon Islands about the size of Maryland, and the July 2012 population was estimated at 584,578. In 2010, 19 percent of the population lived in urban areas, and the 2010 to 2015 annual rate of urbanization was estimated at 4.2 percent. Honiara is the capital and largest city (with a 2009 population estimated at 72,000). The population growth rate in 2012 was 2.2 percent, the net migration rate negative 1.9 migrants per 1,000 population, the birth rate 27.5 births per 1,000, and the total fertility rate 3.5 children per woman. The Solomon Islands was seriously damaged by an earthquake and tsunami in 2007.

The Solomon Islands became a British protectorate in the 1890s and became an independent country in 1978. Ethnic violence, crime, and government corruption have undermined the civil society; in 2003, at the request of Prime Minister Sir Allan Kemakeza, a multinational force led by Australia restored law and order to the Solomon Islands. The Solomon Islands ranked tied for 120th among 183 countries on the *Corruption Perceptions Index 2011*, with a score of 2.7 (on a scale where 0 indicates highly corrupt and 10 very clean).

In 2011, the Solomon Islands was classified as a country with low human development (the lowest of four categories) on the United Nations Development Programme's (UNDP's) Human Development Index (HDI), with a score of 0.510 (on a scale where 1 denotes high development and 0 low development). Life expectancy at birth in 2012 was estimated at 74.42 years, and estimated gross domestic product (GDP) per capita in 2011 was $3,300.

Emergency Health Services

According to the World Health Organization (WHO), as of 2007, the Solomon Islands did not have a formal and publicly available system for providing prehospital care (emergency care).

Insurance

Most health services on the Solomon Islands are provided by the Ministry of Health and Medical Services, with less than 15 percent of services provided by religious organizations and nongovernmental organizations (NGOs). There are a few private service providers in the country, providing an estimated 2 to 3 percent of health care services. Employers in the Solomon Islands are required, under the Labor Act, to give female employees at least 12 weeks of maternity leave.

Costs of Hospitalization

No data available.

Access to Health Care

According to WHO, in 2007, 8.5 percent of births in the Solomon Islands were attended by skilled personnel (for example, physicians, nurses, or midwives), and 65 percent of pregnant women received at least four prenatal care visits. The 2010 immunization rates for 1-year-olds were 79 percent for diphtheria and pertussis (DPT3), 68 percent for measles (MCV), and 79 percent for Hib (Hib3).

Cost of Drugs

Essential drugs are provided free of charge in public health care facilities, although the transportation infrastructure has made it difficult to keep all locations supplied. A 2003 report found that access to essential drugs varied from 80 to 94 percent in the Solomon Islands; in fairness, this survey was conducted after a period of civil unrest on the islands, which may have hampered the distribution process.

Health Care Facilities

In 2005, the Solomon Islands had 1.40 hospital beds per 1,000 population.

Major Health Issues

In 2008, WHO estimated that 51 percent of years of life lost in the Solomon Islands were due to communicable diseases, 41 percent to noncommunicable diseases, and 8 percent to injuries. In 2008, the age-standardized estimate of cancer deaths was 86 per 100,000 for men and 86 per 100,000 for women; for cardiovascular disease and diabetes, 425 per 100,000 for men and 304 per 100,000 for women; and for chronic respiratory disease, 75 per 100,000 for men and 41 per 100,000 for women.

In 2008, the age-standardized death rate from malaria was 29.0 per 100,000 population. In 2010, tuberculosis incidence was 108.0 per 100,000 population, tuberculosis prevalence 178.0 per 100,000,

and deaths due to tuberculosis among human immunodeficiency virus (HIV)-negative people 17.0 per 100,000.

Compared to other countries at a similar level of development, the Solomon Islands ranked ninth (tied with Comoros) among 43 least-developed countries on the 2011 Mothers' Index, produced by the international nongovernmental organization (NGO) Save the Children, based on a number of health and social factors relating to women, children, and maternal and child care. The Solomon Islands' maternal mortality rate (death from any cause related to or aggravated by pregnancy) was estimated in 2008 as 100 maternal deaths per 100,000 live births. The infant mortality rate, defined as the number of deaths of infants younger than 1 year, was estimated at 17.25 per 1,000 live births as of 2012. In 2007, 11.5 percent of children under age 5 were underweight (defined as 2 kilograms [kg] below standard weight-for-age at age 1, 3 kg below for ages 2 to 3, and 4 kg below for ages 4 to 5).

Health Care Personnel

The Solomon Islands has no medical school. Physicians wishing to practice must register with the Medical and Dental Board of the Ministry of Health and Medical Services, must hold a degree from a

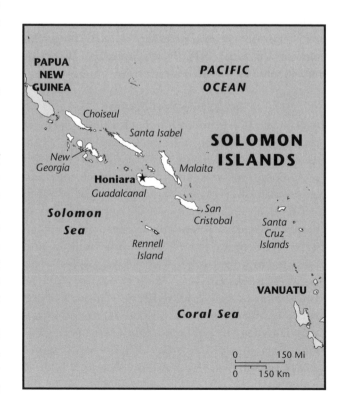

recognized medical school, and must not have a criminal record. Foreigners also need work permits to practice in the Solomon Islands. In 2005, the Solomon Islands had 0.19 physicians per 1,000 population, 0.11 pharmaceutical personnel per 1,000, 0.11 dentistry personnel per 1,000, and 145 nurses and midwives per 1,000.

Government Role in Health Care

According to WHO, in 2010, the Solomon Islands spent $57 million on health care, an amount that comes to $107 per capita. Just over two-thirds (68 percent) of health care funding came from domestic sources, with 32 percent coming from abroad. Most (93 percent) of health care spending was paid for through government expenditures, with the remainder provided through household expenditures (4 percent) and other sources (3 percent). In 2010, the Solomon Islands allocated 23 percent of its total government expenditures to health, in the high range for lower-middle-income western Pacific region countries; government expenditures on health came to 8 percent of GDP, in the high range for lower-middle-income western Pacific region countries. In 2009, according to WHO, official development assistance (ODA) for health in the Solomon Islands came to $30.56 per capita.

Public Health Programs

In 2005, 32 percent of the population of the Solomon Islands had access to improved sanitation facilities (18 percent in rural areas and 98 percent in urban), and 70 percent had access to improved sources of drinking water (65 percent in rural areas and 94 percent in urban).

SOMALIA

Somalia is an east African country, sharing borders with Djibouti, Ethiopia, and Kenya and having coastlines on the Indian Ocean and the Gulf of Aden. The area of 246,201 square miles (637,657 square kilometers) makes Somalia about the size of Texas, and the July 2012 population was estimated at 10.1 million. In 2010, 37 percent of the population lived in urban areas, and the 2010 to 2015 annual rate of urbanization was estimated at 4.1 percent. Mogadishu is the capital and largest city (with a 2009 population estimated at 1.4 million). The population growth rate in 2012 was 1.6 percent, the net migration rate negative 11.6 migrants per 1,000 population (among the 10 highest emigration rates in the world), the birth rate 42.1 births per 1,000 (the seventh-highest in the world), and the total fertility rate 6.3 children per woman (the fourth-highest in the world). The United Nations High Commissioner for Refugees (UNHCR) estimated that, in 2010, there were 1,937 refugees and persons in refugee-like situations in Somalia.

In 1960, British Somaliland joined with Italian Somaliland to form the nation of Somalia. The country has been marked by disorder, violence, and dictatorship for much of its history, and in 1991, after the collapse of Mohamed Siad Barre's government, the country descended into anarchy. In 1991, clans in the northern part of Somalia formed the Republic of Somaliland that, although not recognized by any government, is a stable region.

According to the Ibrahim Index, in 2011, Somalia ranked last out of 53 African countries in terms of governance performance, with a score of 8 (out of 100). The Somali government is perceived to be among the most corrupt in the world, ranking tied for 182nd among 183 countries in terms of perceived public-sector corruption on the *Corruption Perceptions Index 2011,* with a score of 1.0 (on a scale where 0 indicates highly corrupt and 10 very clean).

Living conditions in Somalia are very poor for most individuals, and due to the chaotic state of the government, up-to-date information about Somalia can be difficult to attain. Life expectancy at birth in 2012 was estimated at 50.80 years, among the 10 lowest in the world, and estimated gross domestic product (GDP) per capita in 2010 was $600, among the 10 lowest in the world. In 2011, the World Food Programme estimated that 4 million people in Somalia were food insecure, but that this situation somewhat improved in 2012, leaving about 2.5 million people food insecure.

Emergency Health Services

Doctors Without Borders (Médecins Sans Frontières, or MSF) began working in Somalia in 1991 and had 1,461 staff members in the country at the close of 2010. Due to continuing violence, the time MSF staff can stay in the country is limited, and they provide specialty support from a base in Nairobi; several MSF facilities have closed due to the continued fighting.

MSF operates a hospital near Mogadishu, providing free emergency care and treatment for war injuries, and supplies the community in Afgooye, on the southern coast. MSF runs a number of clinics and hospitals in southern Somalia, provides telemedicine consultations with Istarlin Hospital in central Somalia, provided emergency relief after severe flooding in Belet Weyne and drought in Galgaduud, and provided measles and tetanus vaccinations in the country.

In July 2011, the World Health Organization (WHO), United Nations Children's Fund (UNICEF), and the Kenyan Ministry of Health launched an emergency vaccination campaign in Dadaab, a camp for Somali refugees located in northeastern Kenya; the campaign included administration of vitamin A and deworming tablets as well as the measles and polio vaccines. WHO is also involved in providing training in trauma surgery in Somalia, providing medicines and supplies to Somali facilities, and training staff in emergency procedures, including cesarean sections and blood transfusions.

Insurance

Somalia has no statutory system of cash benefits for sickness or maternity. Medical care is provided in government dispensaries and hospitals, and the Labor Code of 1972 requires that employers give at least 14 weeks of maternity leave, at 50 percent of pay, to employees with at least six months of employment.

Costs of Hospitalization

No data available.

Access to Health Care

Health care in Somalia is provided almost entirely by nongovernmental organizations (NGOs). According to WHO, in 2006, 33 percent of births in Somalia were attended by skilled personnel (for example, physicians, nurses, or midwives), and 6 percent of pregnant women received at least for prenatal care visits. The 2010 immunization rates four 1-year-olds were 45 percent for diphtheria and pertussis (DPT3) and 46 percent for measles (MCV). In 2010, an estimated 3 percent of persons with advanced human immunodeficiency virus (HIV) infection were receiving antiretroviral therapy in accordance with the 2010 WHO guidelines.

Cost of Drugs

No data available.

Health Care Facilities

No data available.

Major Health Issues

In 2008, WHO estimated that 74 percent of years of life lost in Somalia were due to communicable diseases, 14 percent to noncommunicable diseases, and 11 percent to injuries. In 2008, the age-standardized estimate of cancer deaths was 105 per 100,000 for men and 97 per 100,000 for women; for cardiovascular disease and diabetes, 571 per 100,000 for men and 573 per 100,000 for women; and for chronic respiratory disease, 88 per 100,000 for men and 58 per 100,000 for women.

In 2008, the age-standardized death rate from malaria was 16.0 per 100,000 population. In 2010, tuberculosis incidence was 286.0 per 100,000 population, tuberculosis prevalence 513.0 per 100,000, and deaths due to tuberculosis among HIV-negative people 56.0 per 100,000. As of 2009, an estimated 0.7 percent of adults age 15 to 49 were living with HIV or acquired immune deficiency syndrome (AIDS). In 2008, the age-standardized death rate from childhood-cluster diseases (pertussis, polio, diphtheria, measles, and tetanus) was 68.6 per 100,000 population, the highest in the world.

Somalia's maternal mortality rate (death from any cause related to or aggravated by pregnancy) is the second-highest in the world, estimated at 1,200 per 100,000 live births as of 2008. A 2006 survey estimated

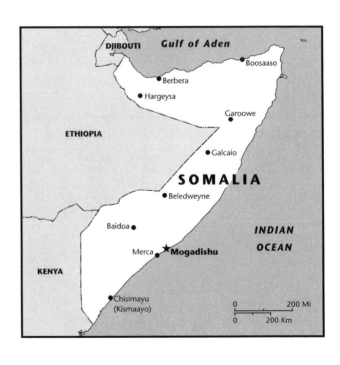

the prevalence of female genital mutilation at 97.9 percent. The infant mortality rate, defined as the number of deaths of infants younger than 1 year, is the fourth-highest in the world, at 103.72 per 1,000 live births as of 2012. Child malnutrition is a serious problem: In 2006, 36.8 percent of children under age 5 were underweight (defined as 2 kilograms [kg] below standard weight-for-age at age 1, 3 kg below for ages 2 to 3, and 4 kg below for ages 4 to 5), one of the 20 highest rates in the world.

Health Care Personnel

In 2006, WHO identified Somalia as one of 57 countries with a critical deficit in the supply of skilled health workers. Somalia has one medical school, Benadir University Medical College in Mogadishu, which was founded in 2002. The course of study lasts six years, including one year pre-med (chemistry, biology, English, and so on), two years preclinical, and 3 years clinical instruction. In 2006, Somalia had 0.04 physicians per 1,000 population, 0.01 pharmaceutical personnel per 1,000, and 0.11 nurses and midwives per 1,000. Michael Clemens and Bunilla Petterson estimate that 33 percent of Somalia-born physicians and 10 percent of Somalia-born nurses are working in one of nine developed countries, primarily in the United Kingdom and the United States.

Government Role in Health Care

In 2009, according to WHO, official development assistance (ODA) for health in Somalia came to $4.00 per capita.

Public Health Programs

According to WHO, in 2005, Somalia had 0.01 environmental and public health workers per 1,000 population. In 2010, 23 percent of the population had access to improved sanitation facilities (6 percent in rural areas and 52 percent in urban), and 29 percent had access to improved sources of drinking water (7 percent in rural areas and 66 percent in urban).

SOUTH AFRICA

South Africa is a country at the southern tip of Africa, sharing borders Botswana, Lesotho, Mozambique, Namibia, Swaziland, and Zimbabwe and having coastlines on the Indian Ocean and south Atlantic Ocean. The area of 470,693 square miles (1,219,090 square kilometers) makes South Africa about twice the size of Texas, and the July 2012 population was estimated at 48.8 million. In 2010, 62.2 percent of the population lived in urban areas, and the 2010 to 2015 annual rate of urbanization is estimated at 1.2 percent. Pretoria is the capital and Johannesburg and Cape Town the largest cities (with 2009 populations estimated at 3.6 million and 3.4 million, respectively). The population growth rate in 2012 was negative 0.4 percent, the net migration rate negative 6.2 migrants per 1,000 population, the birth rate 19.3 births per 1,000, and the total fertility rate 2.3 children per woman.

The Cape of Good Hope became an important stopover for international shipping in the 17th century, and colonial rule of the region that is now South Africa was contested by the British and the Dutch. In 1910, the Union of South Africa was formed, and in 1948, the policy of apartheid (racial separation) was instituted, favoring the white minority over the black majority. In 1994, the first multiracial elections were held; however, inequalities in income, education, and so on, remain.

According to the Ibrahim Index, in 2011, South Africa ranked fifth among 53 African countries in terms of governance performance, with a score of 71 (out of 100). South Africa ranked tied for 64th among 183 countries on the *Corruption Perceptions Index 2011* with a score of 4.1 (on a scale where 0 indicates highly corrupt and 10 very clean).

In 2011, South Africa was classified as a country with medium human development (the second from the lowest of four categories) on the United Nations Development Programme's (UNDP's) Human Development Index (HDI), with a score of 0.619 (on a scale where 1 denotes high development and 0 low development). Life expectancy at birth in 2012 was estimated at 49.41 years, among the five lowest in the world, and per capita gross domestic product (GDP) in 2011 was estimated at $11,000. Income distribution in South Africa is relatively unequal: In 2005, the Gini Index (a measure of dispersion, in which perfect equality is denoted by 0 and maximum inequality is denoted by 100) for family income was 65.0, among the highest in the world. Unemployment in 2011 was estimated at 23.9 percent.

According to the World Economic Forum's *Global Gender Gap Index 2011*, South Africa ranked 14th out of 135 countries on gender equality with a score of 0.748 (on a scale with a theoretical range of 1 for equality to 0 for inequality and an actual range in 2011 from 0.8530 to 0.4873).

Emergency Health Services

According to the World Health Organization (WHO), as of 2007, South Africa had a formal and publicly available emergency care (prehospital care) system accessible through a national access number.

Doctors Without Borders (Médecins Sans Frontières, or MSF) began working in South Africa in 1999 and had 154 staff members in the country at the close of 2010. MSF provided care for more than 16,400 migrants in Musina (northeastern South Africa), including care for more than 250 victims of sexual violence. MSF has provided integrated care for tuberculosis and human immunodeficiency virus/acquired immune deficiency syndrome (HIV/AIDS) in Khayelitsha, on the outskirts of Cape Town, since 1999, including antiretroviral treatment since 2001. This project has been instrumental in creating an effective environment for HIV/AIDS care in South Africa and has created many partnerships with community and other local organizations. In Johannesburg, MSF provided consultations for more than 26,100 patients in 2010 and also led projects to produce better living conditions in slum areas.

Insurance

South Africa had no National Health Insurance (NHI) plan as of 2010 but did have a plan to phase in a national system gradually over a 14-year period beginning in 2012. Implementation of the NHI plan is a key component of the Programme of Action for the health sector; other reforms include strengthening accreditation, and addressing infrastructure backlogs, poor quality of care, and workforce shortages. People in the middle- and upper-income classes sometimes have private insurance, but it generally provides limited coverage and requires high out-of-pocket payments. As of 2007, according to United States Agency for International Development (USAID), about 15 percent of the population was covered by voluntary private insurance, and the private insurance market was regulated by the Council for Medical Schemes.

South Africa has a social assistance system for medical benefits; cash maternity and sickness benefits are provided through unemployment legislation passed in 2001. The medical benefits system applies to people on disability or old-age pensions, while the cash benefits apply to workers (they must work at least 24 hours a month), the unemployed, and those with

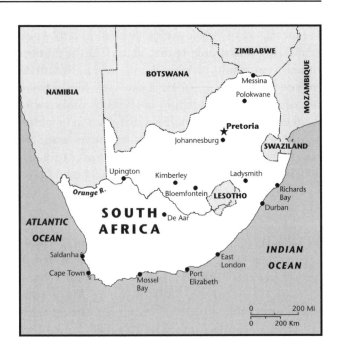

reduced earnings. Both the medical benefits and the cash benefits are funded entirely through government revenues. Persons on old-age and disability pensions receive subsidized medical care, including medicines and hospitalization, at provincial hospitals. The cash maternity benefit is 45 percent of earnings for 17 weeks; the cash sickness benefit provides 45 percent of earnings for 26 weeks. According to Ke Xu and colleagues, in 2003, less than 0.1 percent of households in South Africa experienced catastrophic health expenditures annually; "catastrophic" was defined as exceeding 40 percent of household income remaining after basic needs were met.

Costs of Hospitalization

No data available.

Access to Health Care

According to Donald West and colleagues, South Africa has 400 public hospitals, 205 private hospitals, and 4,100 public clinics and health care centers; the mining industry also runs a system of 60 hospitals and health clinics. There are large differences in quality and access depending on geographic location (cities are better served than rural areas, and quality also varies by province) and income (those who can afford private services can get excellent care, while public facilities are underfunded and inadequate for the number of people they must serve). However, even those with private insurance (18 percent of the population) frequently must make high out-of-pocket payments for services. Health care personnel are poorly distributed: For instance, Gauteng (the province including Johannesburg) has 21 percent of the nation's population but 45 percent of private-sector physicians, dentists, and pharmacists. The ratio of doctors and nurses to population is below international standards, in part because many choose to emigrate.

According to WHO, in 2003, 91 percent of births in South Africa were attended by skilled personnel (for example, physicians, nurses, or midwives). In 2003, 56 percent of pregnant women received at least four prenatal care visits. The 2010 immunization rates for 1-year-olds were 63 percent for diphtheria and pertussis (DPT3), 65 percent for measles (MCV), and 45 percent for Hib (Hib3). In 2010, an estimated 55 percent of persons with advanced HIV infection were receiving antiretroviral therapy in accordance with the 2010 WHO guidelines.

Cost of Drugs

According to Douglas Ball, increasing access to medicine was part of a national strategy, following independence in 1994, to increase health care access for the poor. In 1996, a National Medicines Policy (NMP) was published; one chapter contained a provision to provide safe and available drugs at low cost. Medicine pricing regulation in the private sector began in 2004. In 2010, South Africa created a structure for dispensing fees based on the cost of medicines, plus a flat fee, in an attempt to encourage the use of lower-priced drugs. Currently, the Directorate of Pharmaceutical Economic Evaluations establishes a single exit price (SEP) that represents the maximum price for medicines in the private sector; the SEP is based on average prices in 2003.

A 2004 survey conducted by the National Department of Health investigated the availability and cost of a market basket of medications in Gauteng province, a province including the national capital of Pretoria and the country's most populous city, Johannesburg. In retail pharmacies, the lowest-priced generic drugs have a median availability of 71.7 percent, the most-sold generic drugs a median availability of 46.7 percent, and innovator brands a median availability of 40.0 percent. In a few cases, including metformin (for diabetes mellitus), omeprazole (for ulcers), and phenytoin (for epilepsy), innovator brands were more available in

pharmacies than generics. Availability of antiretrovirals was below 40 percent in pharmacies. Prices were high, with a median price ratio (comparing the price to the international reference price) of 6.52 for the lowest-priced generics (so the median price in Gauteng was more than six times the international reference price), and even higher for the most-sold generics (6.82) and innovator brands (24.91).

In private hospital pharmacies, prices were high; the median price ratio for the lowest-price generics was 6.45, for the most-sold generics 6.82, and for innovator brands 26.35. Median availability for the lowest-price generics was 53.3 percent, for the most sold generics 30.0 percent, and for innovator brands 53.3 percent; some innovator brands were more available than either type of generic. Most private hospital pharmacies had antiretrovirals in stock. Availability was quite low for dispensing physicians, with a median availability of 25.0 percent for the lowest-priced generics, 7.7 percent for the most-sold generics, and 3.8 percent for innovator brands. None of those surveyed had the drugs in stock for a complete antiretroviral regimen, and only 3.8 percent had the drugs in stock for postexposure prophylaxis for HIV. Most dispensing doctors did not charge a separate fee for medicines, so the information about price ratios is calculated on a small sample. Very few stocked innovator brands and only 20 percent of the most-sold generics and 12.5 percent of the lowest-priced generics were sold at less than twice the international reference price.

Health Care Facilities

According to Donald West and colleagues, South Africa has about 400 public hospitals, 205 private hospitals, and 4,100 public clinics and health care centers; the mining industry also runs a system of 60 hospitals and health clinics. Most of the private hospitals are owned by three companies: Netcare (47 hospitals), Life (49 hospitals), and Mediclinic (21.1 percent of the beds). Currently, the government is making major efforts to build new facilities and upgrade those that already exist, and massive improvements are being made in five major public hospitals.

As of 2010, according to WHO, South Africa had 6.19 health posts per 100,000 population, 0.58 health centers per 100,000, 0.56 district or rural hospitals per 100,000, 0.13 provincial hospitals per 100,000, and 0.03 specialized hospitals per 100,000. In 2005, South Africa had 2.84 hospital beds per 1,000 population.

According to WHO, in 2010, South Africa had 2.58 magnetic resonance imaging (MRI) machines per 1 million population, 5.03 computer tomography (CT) machines per 1 million, 0.10 positron emission tomography (PET) machines per 1 million, 0.06 telecolbalt units per 1 million, and 0.06 radiotherapy machines per 1 million. According to Donald West and colleagues, this type of technology is primarily found in private-sector hospitals, and the private sector has a higher rate of MRI and CT scanners than do many high-income countries (including Canada, France, Germany, and the United Kingdom [UK]).

Major Health Issues

In 2008, WHO estimated that 79 percent of years of life lost in South Africa were due to communicable diseases, 15 percent to noncommunicable diseases, and 6 percent to injuries. In 2008, the age-standardized estimate of cancer deaths was 207 per 100,000 population for men and 124 per 100,000 for women; for cardiovascular disease and diabetes, 328 per 100,000 for men and 315 per 100,000 for women; and for chronic respiratory disease, 87 per 100,000 for men and 44 per 100,000 for women.

South Africa's maternal mortality rate (death from any cause related to or aggravated by pregnancy) is high by global standards, estimated at 410 maternal deaths per 100,000 live births as of 2008. The infant mortality rate, defined as the number of deaths of infants younger than 1 year, was estimated at 42.67 per 1,000 live births in 2012.

In 2010, tuberculosis incidence was 981.0 per 100,000 population, tuberculosis prevalence 795.0 per 100,000, and deaths due to tuberculosis among HIV-negative people 50.00 per 100,000. WHO estimated the 2010 case detection rate at 72 percent. As estimated, 1.8 percent of new tuberculosis cases and 6.7 percent of retreatment cases are multidrug resistant. As of 2009, South Africa had the third-highest HIV/AIDS rates in the world; in that year, an estimated 17.8 percent of adults age 15 to 49 were living with HIV or AIDS. As of 2009, an estimated 5.6 million people in South Africa were living with HIV or AIDS, by far the largest number in the world. In 2010, over 95 percent of pregnant women tested positive for HIV, one of the highest rates in the world. The mother-to-child transmission rate for HIV in 2010 was estimated at 18 percent, and in 2009, 34.8 percent of deaths to children under age 5 were attributed to HIV.

Health Care Personnel

South Africa has eight medical schools that offer instruction in English, Afrikaans, or both. The basic course of study lasts six years, and government service work is required after graduation. The license to practice medicine is granted after completion of a one-year internship and receipt of a certificate of competence. Foreigners may receive only temporary registration. South Africa has agreements with Belgium, Ireland, and the United Kingdom (UK).

In 2004, South Africa had 0.77 physicians per 1,000 population, 0.28 pharmaceutical personnel per 1,000, 0.04 laboratory health workers per 1,000, 0.51 health management and support workers per 1,000, 0.13 dentistry personnel per 1,000, 0.32 community and traditional health workers per 1,000, and 4.08 nurses and midwives per 1,000. Michael Clemens and Bunilla Petterson estimate that 21 percent of South Africa-born physicians and 5 percent of South Africa-born nurses are working in one of nine developed countries, primarily in the UK, Canada, the United States, and Australia. Because South Africa is a frequent site of migration for physicians and nurses born in other developed countries, the country actually receives more migrant medical professionals than it loses.

Government Role in Health Care

According to WHO, in 2010, South Africa spent $33 million on health care, an amount that comes to $649 per capita. Most (98 percent) of health care funding came from domestic sources, with 2 percent coming from abroad. Less than half (44 percent) of health care spending was paid for through government expenditures, with the remainder provided through household expenditures (17 percent) and other sources (39 percent). In 2010, South Africa allocated 12 percent of its total government expenditures to health, in the median range for upper-middle-income African countries; government expenditures on health came to 4 percent of GDP, in the median range for upper-middle-income African countries. In 2009, according to WHO, official development assistance (ODA) for health in South Africa came to $11.99 per capita.

Public Health Programs

The National Institute for Communicable Diseases (NICD) for South Africa is located in Sandringham (a suburb of Johannesburg) and directed by Shabir Madhi. The NICD was created in 2002 and is modeled on the U.S. Centers for Disease Control and Prevention (CDC), with particular focus on communicable diseases common in the country. The NICD has a staff of more than 300, including labs specializing in microbiology, parasitology, and entomology, and in 2008, the NICD established South Africa's first national lab devoted to studying tuberculosis. The NICD provides knowledge and expertise in communicable disease, assists with planning and policy creation, and helps develop responses to disease outbreaks.

About 11 percent of the national budget (8.7 percent of GDP) is allocated to public health, with these funds allocated to the country's provinces and municipalities; hospitals are managed at the state level, primary care at the municipal level. According to WHO, in 2004, South Africa had 0.06 environmental and public health workers per 1,000 population. In 2010, 79 percent of the population had access to improved sanitation facilities (67 percent in rural areas and 86 percent in urban), and 91 percent had access to improved sources of drinking water (79 percent in rural areas and 99 percent in urban). According to the World Higher Education Database (WHED), nine universities in South Africa offer programs in epidemiology or public health: the Cape Peninsula University of Technology, Stellenbosch University, the University of Johannesburg, the University of KwaZulu-Natal, the University of Limpopo, the University of Pretoria, the University of the Western Cape, the University of the Witwatersrand, and the University of Venda.

SOUTH KOREA

South Korea is a north Asian country, sharing a border with North Korea and having coastlines on the Yellow Sea and the Sea of Japan. The area of 38,502 square miles (99,720 square kilometers) makes South Korea about the size of Indiana, and the July 2012 population was estimated at 48.9 million. In 2010, 83 percent of the population lived in urban areas, and the 2010 to 2015 annual rate of urbanization was estimated at 0.6 percent. Seoul is the capital and largest city (with a 2009 population estimated at 9.8 million). The population growth rate in 2012 was 0.2 percent, the net migration rate 0.0 migrants per 1,000 population, the birth rate 8.4 births per 1,000 (among the 10 lowest in

the world), and the total fertility rate 1.2 children per woman (the third-lowest in the world).

The Korean peninsula was occupied by Japan from 1905 to 1945; North and South Korea became separate countries after the Korean War (1950–53). South Korea ranked 43rd among 183 countries on the *Corruption Perceptions Index 2011,* with a score of 5.4 (on a scale where 0 indicates highly corrupt and 10 very clean). In 2011, South Korea was classified as a country with very high human development (the highest of four categories) on the United Nations Development Programme's (UNDP's) Human Development Index (HDI), with a score of 0.897 (on a scale where 1 denotes high development and 0 low development). Life expectancy at birth in 2012 was estimated at 79.41 years, and per capita gross domestic product (GDP) in 2011 was estimated at $31,700. In 2010, the Gini Index (a measure of dispersion, in which perfect equality is denoted by 0 and maximum inequality is denoted by 100) for family income was 31.0. According to the World Economic Forum's *Global Gender Gap Index 2011*, South Korea ranked 107th out of 135 countries on gender equality with a score of 0.628 (on a scale with a theoretical range of 1 for equality to 0 for inequality and an actual range in 2011 from 0.8530 to 0.4873).

Emergency Health Services

South Korea recognized emergency medicine as a specialty in 1996, and as of 2007, about 300 emergency medicine specialists were working in South Korea. Dialing 119 accesses the Emergency Medical Services System; as of 2007, 119 rescue services affiliated with about 150 fire stations were prepared to answer emergency calls. The teams consist of ambulances, personnel (nurses, emergency medical technicians, and accredited specialists), and equipment (oxygen, fluids, and so on); in 2004, there were 943,378 rescue calls in South Korea, 35 percent of which came from Seoul. The most common causes for emergency medicine calls were internal medicine diseases (61.3 percent), injuries from accidents (23.1 percent), and traffic accidents (9.1 percent).

Insurance

South Korea has a social insurance system providing medical benefits and long-term care. All Korean citizens and employees are included in the system, except those with low income, who are covered by the medical aid program; foreigners residing in

Korea may join on a voluntary basis. The system is funded through contributions from employees (2.665 percent of gross monthly earnings for medical benefits and 0.175 percent for long-term care), the self-employed (rates are set based on a number of factors including income, age, gender, and property ownership), and employers (2.665 percent of payroll for medical benefits and 0.175 percent for long-term care). Medical services are provided by professionals, clinics, and hospitals under contract with the National Health Insurance Corporation; covered services include hospitalization, surgery, medical care, and medicines.

Copayments are required for most services, for example, 20 percent for hospitalization and 20 to 50 percent for outpatient care, with a maximum cap on copayments depending on income. Services provided by the long-term care benefits include institutional care, home visits, respite care, and equipment. The Health Insurance Review and Assessment Service evaluates the quality of medical and long-term care, the National Health Insurance Corporation collects contributions and pays service providers, and the Ministry of Health and Welfare supervises the system. According to Ke Xu and colleagues, in 2003, 1.7 percent of households in South

Korea experienced catastrophic health expenditures annually; "catastrophic" was defined as exceeding 40 percent of household income remaining after basic needs were met.

South Korea began extending its health insurance system in 1997, at a time when only 8 percent of the population was covered. The program gradually added different classes of workers, beginning with those employed in large enterprises and those with low incomes; civil servants and employees of small companies were added next. In 1989, South Korea passed a law providing universal national health insurance.

Costs of Hospitalization

A 20 percent copayment is required for hospital treatment, although there is a maximum cap on copayments.

Access to Health Care

According to the World Health Organization (WHO), in 2006, 100 percent of births in South Korea were attended by skilled personnel (for example, physicians, nurses, or midwives). The 2010 immunization rates for 1-year-olds were 94 percent for diphtheria and pertussis (DPT3) and 98 percent for measles (MCV). In 2010, an estimated 25 percent of persons with advanced human immunodeficiency virus (HIV) infection were receiving antiretroviral therapy in accordance with the 2010 WHO guidelines.

Cost of Drugs

According to Douglas Ball, South Korea charges the standard value-added tax (VAT) of 10 percent on medicines. Dispensing fees are set by a schedule that takes into account factors including the number of days covered by the prescription, and there is also a fixed management and administration fee of KRS 1,252. The wholesale margin is not fixed, but the average margin is 3.2 to 4.0 percent for prescription-only medicines and 2.0 to 3.0 percent for over-the-counter drugs. The pharmacy markup varies for over-the-counter drugs, while there is no official pharmacy markup for prescription-only medicines, although there are implicit margins. Real annual growth in pharmaceutical expenditures in South Korea grew 7.5 percent from 1997 to 2005, slower than the 9.0 percent growth of total health expenditure (minus pharmaceutical expenditures) over those years.

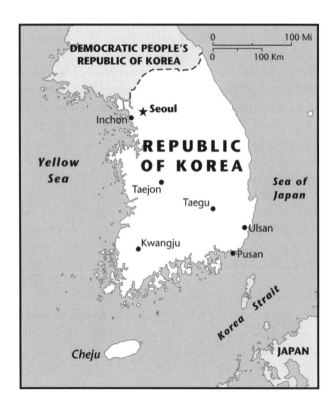

Selected Health Indicators: South Korea Compared With the Organisation for Economic Co-operation and Development (OECD) Country Average

	South Korea	OECD average (2010 or nearest year)
Out-of-pocket expenditure on health (percent total expenditure on health), 2010	32.1	19.5
Out-of-pocket expenditure on health (per capita, USD purchasing power parity), 2010	653.2	558.4
Total expenditure on health (percent of GDP), 2010	7.1	9.5
Total expenditure on health (per capita, USD purchasing power parity), 2010	2,035.4	3,265
Public expenditure on health (per capita, USD purchasing power parity), 2010	1,185.3	2,377.8
Public expenditure on health (percent total expenditure on health), 2010	58.2	72.2
Doctor consultations (number per capita), 2010	12.9	6.4
Hospital discharge rates, all causes (per 100,000 population), 2010	16,886	15,508
Average length of hospital stay, all causes (days), 2010	14.2	7.1
Causes of mortality: suicides (deaths per 100,000 population), 2010	33.5	12.9

Source: OECD Health Data 2012 (Organisation for Economic Co-operation and Development, 2012).

Health Care Facilities

As of 2010, according to WHO, South Korea had 57.73 health centers per 100,000, 2.83 district or rural hospitals per 100,000 population, 0.57 provincial hospitals per 100,000, and 0.09 specialized hospitals per 100,000. In 2008, South Korea had 12.28 hospital beds per 1,000 population, the third-highest ratio in the world.

Major Health Issues

In 2008, WHO estimated that 7 percent of years of life lost in South Korea were due to communicable diseases, 72 percent to noncommunicable diseases, and 21 percent to injuries. In 2008, the age-standardized estimate of cancer deaths was 191 per 100,000 population for men and 77 per 100,000 for women; and for cardiovascular disease and diabetes, 168 per 100,000 for men and 115 per 100,000 for women. Compared to other countries at a similar level of development,

South Korea ranked fifth (tied with Cyprus) among 80 less-developed countries on the 2011 Mothers' Index, produced by the international nongovernmental organization (NGO) Save the Children, based on a number of health and social factors relating to women, children, and maternal and child care. The maternal mortality rate (death from any cause related to or aggravated by pregnancy) in South Korea in 2008 was 18 maternal deaths per 100,000 live births. The infant mortality rate, defined as the number of deaths of infants younger than 1 year, was 4.08 per 1,000 live births as of 2012.

In 2010, tuberculosis incidence in South Korea was 97.0 per 100,000 population, tuberculosis prevalence 151.0 per 100,000, and deaths due to tuberculosis among HIV-negative people 5.40 per 100,000. As of 2009, an estimated 0.1 percent of adults age 15 to 49 were living with HIV or acquired immune deficiency syndrome (AIDS).

Health Care Personnel

As of June 2004, South Korea had 51 medical schools. The basic medical degree course lasts six years, and the degree awarded is Euihaksa (bachelor in medicine). Physicians must register with the Ministry of Health and Welfare, and graduates must pass the licensure exam before obtaining their medical licenses. In 2008, South Korea had 1.97 physicians per 1,000 population, 1.21 pharmaceutical personnel per 1,000, 0.50 dentistry personnel per 1,000, and 5.29 nurses and midwives per 1,000.

Government Role in Health Care

According to WHO, in 2010, South Korea spent $70 billion on health care, an amount that comes to $1,439 per capita. All health care funding came from domestic sources. Over half (59 percent) of health care spending was paid for through government expenditures, with the remainder provided through household expenditures (31 percent) and other sources (10 percent). In 2010, South Korea allocated 12 percent of its total government expenditures to health, in the median range for high-income western Pacific region countries; government expenditures on health came to 4 percent of GDP, in the median range for high-income western Pacific region countries.

Public Health Programs

In 2010, access to improved sanitation facilities was essentially universal in South Korea, and 98 percent of the population had access to improved sources of drinking water (88 percent in rural areas and 100 percent in urban). According to the World Higher Education Database (WHED), eight universities in South Korea offer programs in epidemiology or public health: Ajou University, Chungnam National University, the College of Medicine of Pochon CHA University, Daegu University, Daejeon University, Keimyung University, Kyungpook National University, and Seoul National University.

SPAIN

Spain is a western European country, sharing borders with Portugal, France, and Morocco and having coastlines on the Mediterranean Sea and the north Atlantic Ocean; Spain includes two cities, Ceuta and Melilla, on the continent of Africa and 17 autonomous communities, including the Canary Islands and the Balearic Islands. The area of 195,124 square miles (505,370 square kilometers) makes Spain about twice the size of Oregon, and the July 2012 population was estimated at 47.0 million. In 2010, 77 percent of the population lived in urban areas, and the 2010 to 2015 annual rate of urbanization was estimated at 1.0 percent. Madrid is the capital and largest city (with a 2009 population estimated at 5.8 million). The population growth rate in 2012 was 0.6 percent, the net migration rate 5.0 migrants per 1,000 population (the 19th-highest in the world), the birth rate 10.4 births per 1,000, and the total fertility rate 1.5 children per woman.

Spain was a colonial power in the 16th and 17th centuries but fell behind Britain, France, and Germany in economic development in the 18th and 19th centuries. Spain suffered a civil war from 1936 to 1939 but made a peaceful transition to democracy following the death of Francisco Franco in 1975. Spain ranked 31st among 183 countries on the *Corruption Perceptions Index 2011,* with a score of 6.2 (on a scale where 0 indicates highly corrupt and 10 very clean).

In 2011, Spain was classified as a country with very high human development (the highest of four categories) on the United Nations Development Programme's (UNDP's) Human Development Index (HDI), with a score of 0.878 (on a scale where 1 denotes high development and 0 low development). Life expectancy at birth in 2012 was estimated at 81.27 years, among the highest in the world, and per capita gross domestic product (GDP) in 2011 was estimated at $30,600. In 2005, the Gini Index (a measure of dispersion, in which perfect equality is denoted by 0 and maximum inequality is denoted by 100) for family income was 35.0. Spain was seriously affected by the Euro zone economic crisis, and in December 2011, the unemployment rate was 23 percent. According to the World Economic Forum's *Global Gender Gap Index 2011*, Spain ranked 12th out of 135 countries on gender equality with a score of 0.758 (on a scale with a theoretical range of 1 for equality to 0 for inequality and an actual range in 2011 from 0.8530 to 0.4873).

Emergency Health Services

Spain's laws governing the emergency health system date from the 2000s, as does recognition of emergency medicine as a medical specialty; by law, free access to hospitals for emergency care is provided for all persons, including the uninsured. Funding for inpatient care in the emergency system is provided from multiple sources. Spain has two national telephone numbers for medical emergencies, 112 (the European Union, or EU, standard) and 061; the country has 26 dispatch centers, which are not interconnected.

Insurance

Spain has a social insurance system covering the employed and self-employed; pensioners are covered for medical benefits, and voluntary coverage is available. The system is subsidized by general tax revenues and also funded through contributions from employees, the self-employed, and employers. Some occupational classes are covered under separate systems, including employees in the public sector, the military, some self-employed people, agricultural workers, and some farmers, seamen, coal miners, and household workers. Medical benefits are provided through National Health Management Institute facilities, by regional health services, or by hospitals and physicians under contract. Benefits covered include hospitalization, medications, medical and dental care, lab services, appliances, and transportation. Medications are free for pensioners when dispensed from social security facilities; for others, there is a cost of a 10 to 40 percent copayment, up to 2.64 euros. The national government defines the basic benefit package annually, and the 17 autonomous communities then design a service plan providing at least those services.

The maternity and adoption benefit is 100 percent of earnings for 16 weeks, and there is also a maternity benefit of 100 percent of the monthly minimum wage for six weeks. The father is entitled to a paternity benefit of 100 percent of earnings for 13 days and the mother to a nursing mother's allowance of 100 percent of average earnings until the child is nine months old. The cash sickness benefit is 60 percent of average earnings, and 75 percent from the 21st day, for up to 12 months; the benefit may be extended an additional six months. The National Health Management Institute and regional health services provide medical benefits, the National Institute of Social Security administers the cash benefit system, the General Treasury of Social Security collects contributions and registers insured people and employers, and the Ministry of Labor and Social Affairs supervises the system.

A 2004 study by the World Health Organization (WHO) found that 0.6 percent of the Spanish population had substitutive voluntary health insurance

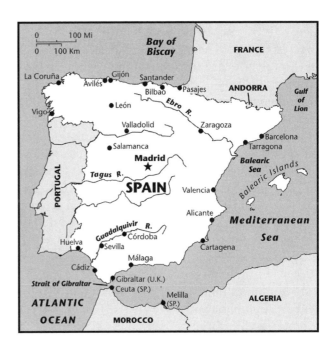

(covering services that would otherwise be available from the state), and 11.4 percent had complementary voluntary health insurance (covering services not covered or not fully covered by the state) or supplementary health insurance (providing increased choice or faster access to services). Ownership of voluntary policies is highly concentrated in the three richest parts of the country: the Balearic Islands (24 percent), Catalonia (22 percent), and Madrid (17 percent). Higher income, occupational status, and educational level are also positively associated with holding a voluntary policy. According to Ke Xu and colleagues, in 2003, 0.5 percent of households in Spain experienced catastrophic health expenditures annually; "catastrophic" was defined as exceeding 40 percent of household income remaining after basic needs were met.

Costs of Hospitalization

In general, hospitals in Spain are funded on a global budget basis, although each autonomous region can develop its own approach, and payments based on capitation, diagnosis-related groups (DRGs), or case-mix adjustments have become more common.

In 2008, according to the Organisation for Economic Co-operation and Development (OECD), hospital spending in Spain represented 39.8 percent of total spending on health. Per capita spending was $1,117; hospitals were paid based on a line-item budget.

Access to Health Care

Everyone in Spain has the right to a basic package of medical services defined annually by the national government; delivery of care is organized by Spain's 17 autonomous communities but must be at least to the standard specified by the national government. The basic benefit package includes health promotion, primary care, and chronic and acute medical care. The primary care system acts as a gatekeeper to specialist and hospital care; in 2008, Spain had 2,913 public primary care centers and 10,178 basic medical centers, nearly reaching the goal that every citizen should live within 15 minutes of a primary care center. Together, the primary and basic care centers provide more than 70 percent of Spain's annual health care visits. The 2010 immunization rates for 1-year-olds were 97 percent for diphtheria and pertussis (DPT3), 95 percent for measles (MCV), and 97 percent for Hib (Hib3). In 2010, an estimated 5 percent of persons with advanced human immunodeficiency virus (HIV) infection were receiving antiretroviral therapy in accordance with the 2010 WHO guidelines.

Cost of Drugs

According to Douglas Ball, Spain collects a lower value-added tax (VAT) of 4 percent on medicines than on most other purchases (the standard VAT is 16 percent). The wholesale margin is dependent on the cost of the drug: For drugs less than 89.62 euros, the margin is 7.6 percent; for more expensive drugs, a flat fee of 7.27 euros is allowed. The retail margin is 27.9 percent for generic drugs costing less than 89.62 euros and a flat fee of 37.54 euros for more expensive drugs. Real annual growth in pharmaceutical expenditures in Spain grew 6.6 percent from 1997 to 2005, faster than the 4.9 percent growth of total health expenditure (minus pharmaceutical expenditures) over those years. According to Elizabeth Docteur, in 2004, Spain ranked second-lowest among Organisation for Economic Co-operation and Development (OECD) countries in terms of the use of generics; generic drugs represented 5 percent of the market share by value and 9 percent of the market share by volume of the total pharmaceutical market.

Health Care Facilities

Most health care in Spain is provided through a network of more than 13,000 public primary and basic health care centers. Spain has about 800 hospitals, of which 120 are private, not-for-profit, and 349 private,

for-profit. Private hospitals serve individuals who have private health insurance, and many also contract with the government to provide services. Spain has a highly integrated system of electronic health insurance cards (used for 98 percent of primary care visits) and is planning to create an integrated electronic health record (EHR) system as well. As of 2002, hospitals were funded mostly on a global budget basis, although specific approaches vary by region (including case-mix adjustment and DRGs).

As of 2010, according to WHO, Spain had 1.19 district or rural hospitals per 100,000 population, 0.31 provincial hospitals per 100,000, and 0.16 specialized hospitals per 100,000. In 2008, Spain had 3.22 hospital beds per 1,000 population. According to WHO, in 2010, Spain had 8.59 magnetic resonance imaging (MRI) machines per 1 million population, 14.61 computer tomography (CT) machines per 1 million, 0.70 telecolbalt units per 1 million, and 0.70 radiotherapy machines per 1 million.

Major Health Issues

In 2008, WHO estimated that 7 percent of years of life lost in Spain were due to communicable diseases, 83 percent to noncommunicable diseases, and 10 percent to injuries. In 2008, the age-standardized estimate of cancer deaths was 168 per 100,000 population for men and 78 per 100,000 for women; for cardiovascular disease and diabetes, 140 per 100,000 for men and 86 per 100,000 for women; and for chronic respiratory disease, 44 per 100,000 for men and 16 per 100,000 for women.

The maternal mortality rate (death from any cause related to or aggravated by pregnancy) in Spain in 2008 was six maternal deaths per 100,000 live births, among the lowest in the world. The infant mortality rate, defined as the number of deaths of infants younger than 1 year, was 3.37 per 1,000 live births in 2012, the 10th-lowest in the world. In 2010, tuberculosis incidence was 16.0 per 100,000 population, tuberculosis prevalence 18.0 per 100,000, and deaths due to tuberculosis among HIV-negative people 0.69 per 100,000. As of 2009, an estimated 0.4 percent of adults age 15 to 49 were living with HIV or acquired immune deficiency syndrome (AIDS).

Health Care Personnel

Spain has 27 medical schools. The course of training for the basic medical degree lasts six years, and the degree granted is the Licenciado en Medicina y Cirugía (licentiate in medicine and surgery).

Spain, as a member of the EU, cooperates with other countries in recognizing physicians qualified to practice in other EU countries, as specified by Directive 2005/36/EC of the European Parliament. This allows qualified professionals to practice their profession in other EU states on a temporary basis and requires that the host country automatically recognize qualifications for certain professions, including physicians, nurses, dentists, midwives, and pharmacists, if certain conditions have been met (for instance, facility in the language of the host country may be required). In 2009, Spain had 3.71 physicians per 1,000 population, 1.07 pharmaceutical personnel per 1,000, and 5.16 nurses and midwives per 1,000, and in 2008 had 0.59 dentistry personnel per 1,000.

Government Role in Health Care

The Spanish constitution of 1978 established the right to health, including equal access to preventive, curative, and rehabilitative services. The national system is funded through general tax revenues. According to WHO, in 2010, Spain spent $133 billion on health care, an amount that comes to $2,883 per capita. All health care funding came from domestic sources. Almost three-quarters (73 percent) of health care spending was paid for through government expenditures, with the remainder provided through household expenditures (21 percent) and other sources (6 percent). In 2010, Spain allocated 15 percent of its total government expenditures to health, in the median range for high-income European countries; government expenditures on health came to 7 percent of GDP, in the median range for high-income European countries.

Public Health Programs

The primary goal of the Carlos II Health Institute, located in Madrid and directed by Joaquín Arenas Barbero, is to promote and assess health and medical research. The institute has more than 1,200 staff members working in a variety of areas, including cancer research, cardiovascular disease research, microbiology, epidemiology, environmental health, tropical disease, health technology, and bioinformatics. The National School of Public Health and the National School of Occupational Health are also located within the institute, as are the National Banks of Cell Lines and the National Health Library. Spain has a highly developed infrastructure, and in 2010, access to improved sanitary facilities and improved sources of drinking was essentially universal. According to the World Higher Education Database (WHED), 12 universities in Spain offer programs in epidemiology or public health.

SRI LANKA

Sri Lanka is a South Asian island nation in the Indian Ocean, southeast of India. The area of 25,332 square miles (65,610 square kilometers) makes Sri Lanka about the size of West Virginia, and the July 2012 population was estimated at 16.7 million. In 2010, 14 percent of the population lived in urban areas, and the 2010 to 2015 annual rate of urbanization was estimated at 1.1 percent. Columbo is the capital and largest city (with a 2009 population estimated at 681,000). The population growth rate in 2012 was 0.9 percent, the net migration rate negative 2.0 migrants per 1,000 population, the birth rate 17.0 births per 1,000, and the total fertility rate 2.2 children per woman. The United Nations High Commissioner for Refugees (UNHCR) estimated that, in 2010, there were 223 refugees and persons in refugee-like situations in Sri Lanka, and 161,128 internally displaced persons and persons in internally displaced-person-like situations.

Sri Lanka became a British crown colony in 1802; it became an independent country (as Ceylon) in 1948. From 1983 to 2002, the country was torn by war between Tamil separatists and the Sinhalese majority; violence broke out again in 2006 but was quelled in 2009. Sri Lanka ranked tied for 86th among 183 countries on the *Corruption Perceptions Index 2011*, with a score of 3.3 (on a scale where 0 indicates highly corrupt and 10 very clean).

In 2011, Sri Lanka was classified as a country with medium human development (the second from the lowest of four categories) on the United Nations Development Programme's (UNDP's) Human Development Index (HDI), with a score of 0.691 (on a scale where 1 denotes high development and 0 low development). Life expectancy at birth in 2012 was estimated at 75.94 years, and estimated gross domestic product (GDP) per capita in 2011 was $5,000. Income distribution in Sri Lanka is relatively unequal: In 2009, the Gini Index (a measure of dispersion, in which perfect equality is denoted by 0 and maximum inequality is denoted by 100) for family income was 49.0. According to the World Economic Forum's *Global Gender*

Gap Index 2011, Sri Lanka ranked 31st out of 135 countries on gender equality with a score of 0.721 (on a scale with a theoretical range of 1 for equality to 0 for inequality and an actual range in 2011 from 0.8530 to 0.4873).

Emergency Health Services

According to the World Health Organization (WHO), as of 2007, Sri Lanka did not have a formal and publicly available system for providing prehospital care (emergency care). Doctors Without Borders (Médecins Sans Frontières, or MSF) began working in Sri Lanka in 1991 and had 428 staff members in the country at the close of 2010. MSF adjusted its activities in Sri Lanka after the end of the Sri Lanka Civil War in May 2009, providing mental health services and rehabilitation care, as well as general medical services in the northern part of the country. In 2010, MSF provided mental health care and supplementary food rations to refugees at Menik Farm Camp, specialist support and staff training in Point Pedro Hospital, mental health services in Kilinochchi District Mental Health Unit, and rehabilitation services in Pampaimadhu hospital.

Insurance

Sri Lanka provides free medical care in government hospitals and health centers; there are no statutory maternity or sickness benefits. Plantations must provide medical care for their employees and have their own maternity wards and dispensaries. Employers are required by law to grant 84 days of maternity leave (42 days after the first two births) to female employees working on plantations, to some wage and salary earners, and to women covered under the Shop and Office Employees' Act. They are also required, under the Maternity Benefits Ordinance, to pay maternity benefits for 12 weeks (six weeks for the third and subsequent children). Low-income families (earning below LKR 1,000 per month) are eligible for Family Benefits under the social assistance system, which dates from 1995; these include family allowances, based on income and size, of LKR 100 to 1,000 monthly. According to Ke Xu and colleagues, in 2003, 1.2 percent of households in Sri Lanka experienced catastrophic health expenditures annually; "catastrophic" was defined as exceeding 40 percent of household income remaining after basic needs were met.

Costs of Hospitalization

No data available.

Access to Health Care

According to WHO, in 2007, 99 percent of births in Sri Lanka were attended by skilled personnel (for example, physicians, nurses, or midwives), and 93 percent of pregnant women received at least four prenatal care visits. The 2010 immunization rates for 1-year-olds were 99 percent for diphtheria and pertussis (DPT3), 99 percent for measles (MCV), and 99 percent for Hib (Hib3). According to WHO, in 2010, Sri Lanka had 0.45 magnetic resonance imaging (MRI) machines per 1 million population, 1.30 computer tomography (CT) machines per 1 million, 0.50 telecolbalt units per 1 million, and 0.50 radiotherapy machines per 1 million.

Cost of Drugs

No data available.

Health Care Facilities

As of 2010, according to WHO, Sri Lanka had 278.04 health posts per 100,000 population and, in 2004, had 3.10 hospital beds per 1,000.

Major Health Issues

In 2008, WHO estimated that 11 percent of years of life lost in Sri Lanka were due to communicable diseases, 39 percent to noncommunicable diseases, and

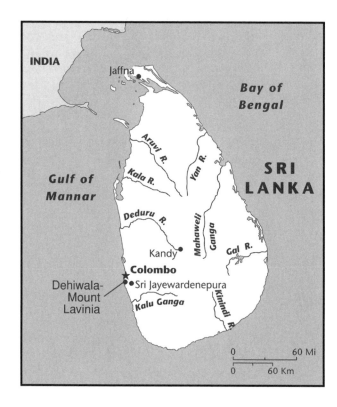

50 percent to injuries. In 2008, the age-standardized estimate of cancer deaths was 90 per 100,000 for men and 78 per 100,000 for women; for cardiovascular disease and diabetes, 385 per 100,000 for men and 241 per 100,000 for women; and for chronic respiratory disease, 101 per 100,000 for men and 58 per 100,000 for women. Sri Lanka's maternal mortality rate (death from any cause related to or aggravated by pregnancy) in 2008 was 39 maternal deaths per 100,000 live births. The infant mortality rate, defined as the number of deaths of infants younger than 1 year, was 9.47 per 1,000 live births in 2012. In 2007, 21.1 percent of children under age 5 were underweight (defined as 2 kilograms [kg] below standard weight-for-age at age 1, 3 kg below for ages 2 to 3, and 4 kg below for ages 4 to 5). In 2010, tuberculosis incidence was 66.0 per 100,000 population, tuberculosis prevalence 101.0 per 100,000, and deaths due to tuberculosis among human immunodeficiency virus (HIV)-negative people 9.10 per 100,000. As of 2009, an estimated 0.1 percent of adults age 15 to 49 were living with HIV or acquired immune deficiency syndrome (AIDS).

Health Care Personnel

Sri Lanka has six medical schools. The basic medical course lasts five years, and the degrees awarded are bachelor of medicine and bachelor of surgery. Graduates must also complete a one-year internship in general medicine before being licensed. Sri Lankan graduates of foreign medical schools must take a special exam to qualify, while foreigners require special invitation to practice in Sri Lanka. In 2006, Sri Lanka had 0.49 physicians per 1,000 population and, in 2007, had 0.04 pharmaceutical personnel per 1,000, 0.08 laboratory health workers per 1,000, 0.08 dentistry professionals per 1,000, and 1.93 nurses and midwives per 1,000. Using Fitzhugh Mullan's methodology, Sri Lanka has an emigration factor of 41.4, representing a high ratio of Sri Lankan physicians working outside the country (in the United States, the United Kingdom, Canada, or Australia) relative to those working in Sri Lanka. Alok Bhargava and colleagues place Sri Lanka 15th among countries most affected by the medical "brain drain" (international migration of skilled personnel) in 2004 and fourth among countries with a population of more than 4 million.

Government Role in Health Care

According to WHO, in 2010, Sri Lanka spent $1.5 billion on health care, an amount that comes to $70 per capita. Most (97 percent) of health care funding came from domestic sources, with 3 percent coming from abroad. Health care spending was primarily provided through government expenditures (45 percent) and household expenditures (45 percent), with the remainder (10 percent) coming from other sources. In 2010, Sri Lanka allocated 6 percent of its total government expenditures to health, in the median range for lower-middle-income southeast Asian region countries; government expenditures on health came to 1 percent of GDP, in the median range for lower-middle-income southeast Asian region countries. In 2009, according to WHO, official development assistance (ODA) for health in Sri Lanka came to $2.27 per capita.

Public Health Programs

According to WHO, in 2007, Sri Lanka had 0.11 environmental and public health workers per 1,000 population. In 2010, 92 percent of the population had access to improved sanitation facilities (93 percent in rural areas and 88 percent in urban), and 91 percent had access to improved sources of drinking water (90 percent in rural areas and 99 percent in urban). According to the World Higher Education Database (WHED), one university in Sri Lanka offers programs in epidemiology or public health: the University of Kelaniya.

SUDAN

Sudan is an east African country, sharing borders with the Central African Republic, Chad, Egypt, Eritrea, Ethiopia, and Libya, and having a coastline on the Red Sea. The area of 718,723 square miles (1,861,484 square kilometers) makes Sudan the 16th-largest country in the world, about one-fifth the size of the United States; the July 2012 population was estimated at 34.2 million. In 2010, 40 percent of the population lived in urban areas, and the 2010 to 2015 annual rate of urbanization was estimated at 3.7 percent. Khartoum is the capital and largest city (with a 2009 population estimated at 5.0 million). The population growth rate in 2012 was 1.9 percent, the net migration rate negative 4.5 migrants per 1,000 population, the birth rate 31.7 births per 1,000, and the total fertility rate 4.2 children per woman. The United Nations High Commissioner for Refugees (UNHCR) estimated that, in 2010, there were 109,391 refugees and persons in refugee-like situations in Sudan and 143,000 internally displaced persons and persons in internally displaced-person-like situations.

Sudan became independent from Great Britain in 1956. For much of the second half of the 20th century, Sudan was engaged in civil war between the northern and southern part of the country. In 2005, the southern part of the country was granted provisional independence for six years, and in 2011, South Sudan became an independent country; because of the recency of this separation, most published statistics refer to the country before separation. According to the Ibrahim Index, in 2011, Sudan ranked near the bottom (48th out of 53) among African countries in terms of governance performance, with a score of 33 (out of 100). Sudan's government is perceived as corrupt, ranking tied for 177th among 183 on the *Corruption Perceptions Index 2011,* with a score of 1.6 (on a scale where 0 indicates highly corrupt and 10 very clean).

In 2011, Sudan was classified as a country with low human development (the lowest of four categories) on the United Nations Development Programme's (UNDP's) Human Development Index (HDI), with a score of 0.408 (on a scale where 1 denotes high development and 0 low development). In 2011, the International Food Policy Research Institute (IFPRI) classified Sudan as a country with an "alarming" hunger problem, with a Global Hunger Index (GHI) score of 21.5 (where 0 reflects no hunger and higher scores more hunger). Life expectancy at birth in 2012 was estimated at 62.57 years, and estimated gross domestic product (GDP) per capita in 2011 was $3,000. The World Food Programme estimated in 2012 that an estimated 4.7 million people in South Sudan were food insecure, due in part to inflation, limited income opportunities, and disruption of trade with Sudan.

Emergency Health Services

According to the World Health Organization (WHO), as of 2007, Sudan did not have a formal and publicly available system for providing prehospital care (emergency care). Doctors Without Borders (Médecins Sans Frontières, or MSF) began working in Sudan in 1979 and had 2,226 staff members in the country at the close of 2010. In southern Sudan, MSF treated more than 2,500 people for *kala azar* (visceral leishmaniasis) in 2010, and in collaboration with the Ministry of Health, opened a kala azar treatment center in Al Gedaref, which treated more than 1,000

patients. MSF provides care in Aweil Civil Hospital in Northern Bahr El Ghazal, including provision of 37,000 prenatal visits and assistance in more than 3,000 births. In Western Equatoria, bordering on the Democratic Republic of the Congo, MSF provided medical and mental health services to refugees from the violence. In south Sudan, MSF provided more than 588,000 consultations. In Port Sudan, MSF staff provided maternal and reproductive services, including more than 14,000 prenatal visits and almost 2,000 births. MSF also helped raise awareness about the harm caused by genital cutting and the importance of seeking care during complicated deliveries; this project was transferred to the Ministry of Health at the end of 2010.

Insurance

The Health Insurance Fund, created under the 2004 Health Insurance Act, is a health insurance system for public-sector employees and insured pensioners. According to Sudan's Pharmaceutical Country profile, about 30 percent of the Sudanese population is covered by public health insurance.

Costs of Hospitalization

No data available.

Access to Health Care

According to WHO, in 2006, 49 percent of births in Sudan were attended by skilled personnel (for example, physicians, nurses, or midwives). The 2010 immunization rates for 1-year-olds were 90 percent for diphtheria and pertussis (DPT3), 90 percent for measles (MCV), and 75 percent for Hib (Hib3). In 2010, an estimated 5 percent of persons with advanced human immunodeficiency virus (HIV) infection were receiving antiretroviral therapy in accordance with the 2010 WHO guidelines. According to WHO, in 2010, Sudan had 0.29 magnetic resonance imaging (MRI) machines per 1 million population, 0.82 computer tomography (CT) machines per 1 million, 0.10 telecolbalt units per 1 million, and 0.10 radiotherapy machines per 1 million.

Cost of Drugs

In 2010, total pharmaceutical expenditures in Sudan came to SDG 2.83 billion ($1.35 billion); the per capita pharmaceutical expenditure was SDG 72.30 ($34.45). Pharmaceutical expenditures constituted 36 percent of health expenditures, and 2.2 percent of

GDP. The pharmaceutical market grew at an annual rate of 52 percent. Family planning medications are supported by the United Nations Population Fund, and a public program in Sudan provides free medicines to children younger than 5 years. Free medicines are provided for the first 24 hours of treating emergencies and for treating cancer, malaria, tuberculosis, sexually transmitted diseases, and human immunodeficiency virus/acquired immune deficiency syndrome (HIV/AIDS); vaccinations on WHO's Expanded Programme for Immunization (EPI) list are also provided free.

Funds for treating malaria, tuberculosis, and HIV/AIDS are provided by the Global Fund, and the Global Alliance for Vaccines and Immunization support the EPI vaccination program. Medications on the Essential Medicines List (EML) are at least partially subsidized by public and private insurance. Most (73 percent) medications prescribed in public health facilities are drawn from the EML.

A 2006 WHO and Health Action International study investigated availability, cost, and affordability of medicines in Sudan, collecting data in Khartoum, Cordovan, Gadara, and Northern State. About half (51 percent) of generic medicines were available in the public sector and 77 percent in the private sector. Prices were on the whole considerably higher than the international reference prices. For a basket of medicines, the median price ratio for generic drugs

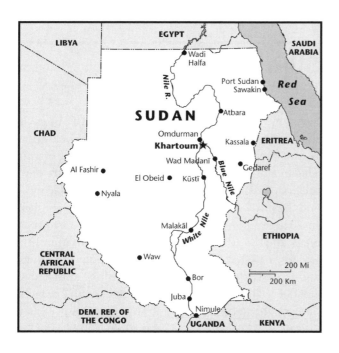

in Sudan was 4.4 in the public sector and 4.7 in the private sector, meaning in both cases that medicine prices in Sudan were more than four times the international reference price. For brand-name drugs, the median price ratio was 3.4 in the public sector and 11.5 in the private sector.

Affordability was measured by the number of days' wages the lowest-paid government employee would have to work to buy medicine (co-trimoxazole) for a child with a respiratory infection. To purchase generic medication in the public sector would require 0.28 day's wages; in the private sector, it would require 0.3 day's wages to buy the generic, while the brand-name medication would require 1.4 days'.

Health Care Facilities
As of 2010, according to WHO, Sudan had 9.39 health posts per 100,000 population, 3.21 health centers per 100,000, 0.56 district or rural hospitals per 100,000, 0.59 provincial hospitals per 100,000, and 0.03 specialized hospitals per 100,000. In 2008, Sudan had 0.70 hospital beds per 1,000 population, one of the 30 lowest rates in the world.

Major Health Issues
In 2008, WHO estimated that 59 percent of years of life lost in Sudan were due to communicable diseases, 24 percent to noncommunicable diseases, and 17 percent to injuries. In 2008, the age-standardized estimate of cancer deaths was 79 per 100,000 for men and 68 per 100,000 for women; for cardiovascular disease and diabetes, 550 per 100,000 for men and 546 per 100,000 for women; and for chronic respiratory disease, 85 per 100,000 for men and 55 per 100,000 for women.

In 2008, the age-standardized death rate from malaria was 15.9 per 100,000 population. In 2010, tuberculosis incidence was 119.0 per 100,000 population, tuberculosis prevalence 188.0 per 100,000, and deaths due to tuberculosis among HIV-negative people 19.0 per 100,000. As of 2009, an estimated 1.1 percent of adults age 15 to 49 were living with HIV or AIDS.

Sudan's maternal mortality rate (death from any cause related to or aggravated by pregnancy) is quite high by global standards, estimated at 750 maternal deaths per 100,000 live births as of 2008. A 2000 survey in northern Sudan (including approximately 80 percent of the population) estimated the prevalence of female genital mutilation at 90.0 percent. The infant mortality rate, defined as the number of deaths of infants younger than 1 year, is also high, at 55.63

per 1,000 live births as of 2012. Child malnutrition is a serious problem: In 2006, 31.7 percent of children under age 5 were underweight (defined as 2 kilograms [kg] below standard weight-for-age at age 1, 3 kg below for ages 2 to 3, and 4 kg below for ages 4 to 5), one of the 20 highest rates in the world.

Health Care Personnel

As of 2007, Sudan had 21 medical schools in operation. The basic medical degree course lasts five to six years, and the degrees awarded are the bachelor of medicine and bachelor of surgery. Three years of government service is required after graduation. The Provincial Ministry of Health grants the license to practice medicine to graduates of a recognized medical school. Graduates of foreign medical schools must have their degrees validated. Foreigners with work permits can be granted temporary registration.

In 2008, Sudan had 0.28 physicians per 1,000 population, 0.01 pharmaceutical personnel per 1,000, 0.02 dentistry personnel per 1,000, and 0.84 nurses and midwives per 1,000. Michael Clemens and Bunilla Petterson estimate that 13 percent of Sudan-born physicians and 1 percent of Sudan-born nurses are working in one of nine developed countries, primarily in the United Kingdom (physicians) and the United States (nurses).

Government Role in Health Care

Sudan has a National Health Policy (NHP), updated in 2007, and a National Medicines Policy (NMP), updated in 2005. The NMP covers the selection of essential medicines; the pricing, procurement, distribution and regulation of medicines; pharmacovigilance; human resource development; rational use of medicines; research; monitoring and evaluation; and traditional medicine. Pharmaceutical products must be assessed according to explicit criteria before being registered and allowed to be sold in Sudan; as of 2009, there were 3,072 pharmaceuticals registered in Sudan.

According to WHO, in 2010, Sudan spent $3.7 billion on health care, an amount that comes to $84 per capita. Most (97 percent) of health care funding came from domestic sources, with 3 percent coming from abroad. Two-thirds (67 percent) of health care spending was provided through household expenditures, with the remainder coming from government expenditures (30 percent) and other sources (3 percent). In 2010, Sudan allocated 10 percent of its total government expenditures to health, in the high range

for lower-middle-income eastern Mediterranean region countries; government expenditures on health came to 2 percent of GDP, in the median range for lower-middle-income eastern Mediterranean region countries. In 2009, according to WHO, official development assistance (ODA) for health in Sudan came to $3.32 per capita.

Public Health Programs

Sudan's Public Health Institute (PHI) is located in Khartoum and headed by Dr. Iqbal Ahmed Bashier; established in 2009, it is located within the National Ministry of Health for Sudan and employs more than 70 people. Its responsibilities include conducting scientific research, supporting decision making in public health, providing expert advice to the Ministry of Health, and providing specialized training in areas including public health, hospital management, health systems management, and disaster management.

According to the World Higher Education Database (WHED), four universities in Sudan offer programs in epidemiology or public health: Al-Zaiem Al-Azhari University, Bahr-Al-Ghazi University, Kordofan University, and Shendi University.

According to WHO, in 2006, Sudan had 0.08 environmental and public health workers per 1,000 population. In 2010, 26 percent of the population had access to improved sanitation facilities (14 percent in rural areas and 44 percent in urban), and 58 percent had access to improved sources of drinking water (52 percent in rural areas and 67 percent in urban).

SURINAME

Suriname is a country in northern South America, sharing borders with Guyana, French Guiana, and Brazil and having a coastline on the north Atlantic Ocean. The area of 63,251 square miles (163,820 square kilometers) makes Suriname about the size of Georgia, and the July 2012 population was estimated at 560,157. In 2010, 69 percent of the population lived in urban areas, and the 2010 to 2015 annual rate of urbanization was estimated at 1.5 percent. Paramaribo is the capital and largest city (with a 2009 population estimated at 259,000). The population growth rate in 2012 was 1.2 percent, the net migration rate 1.0 migrants per 1,000 population, the birth rate 17.4 births per 1,000, and the

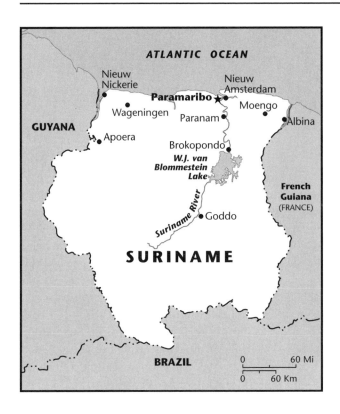

emergency medical care units in Paramaribo and in a remote western district.

Insurance

Suriname has several different types of insurance. The poor (31 percent of the population) are covered by the Ministry of Social Affairs and Housing, government employees are covered through the State Health Insurance Fund, residents of communities in the interior (8 percent) are covered by the Medical Mission (subsidized by the Ministry of Health), and 34 percent have private insurance, employer-sponsored plans, or pay for health care out of pocket. According to the Pan American Health Organization (PAHO), in 2007, about 64 percent of the population was covered by some kind of health insurance.

Costs of Hospitalization

In 2000, 55 percent of expenditures for health care in Suriname paid for secondary care, including hospital charges, medical specialists, and hospital drugs and services (for example, lab tests and X-rays).

Access to Health Care

Health is recognized in the Suriname constitution as a right of every citizen. The Ministry of Health is responsible for making policy and ensuring the availability and affordability of health care. Primary care is provided through the Regional Health Services and the Medical Mission, both subsidized by the government; the Regional Health Services provides care for the poor in the coastal area, while the Medical Mission provides care for Maroon (descendants of African slaves) and Amerindian populations in the interior. Private physicians also provide primary care, mostly in the capital; some nongovernmental organizations (NGOs) provide specific services (for example, family planning); and large firms have medical clinics to care for their employees and their families. Four of the five hospitals in Suriname are located in the capital, as is the psychiatric center; one hospital is located in Nickerie, in a rural coastal area.

According to WHO, in 2006, 90 percent of births in Suriname were attended by skilled personnel (for example, physicians, nurses, or midwives). The 2010 immunization rates for 1-year-olds were 88 percent for diphtheria and pertussis (DPT3), 89 percent for measles (MCV), and 88 percent for Hib (Hib3). In 2010, an estimated 45 percent of persons with advanced human immunodeficiency virus (HIV)

total fertility rate 2.1 children per woman. Suriname became a Dutch colony in 1667, and became an independent country in 1975. Suriname ranked tied for 100th among 183 countries on the *Corruption Perceptions Index 2011,* with a score of 3.0 (on a scale where 0 indicates highly corrupt and 10 very clean).

In 2011, Suriname was classified as a country with medium human development (the second from the lowest of four categories) on the United Nations Development Programme's (UNDP's) Human Development Index (HDI), with a score of 0.680 (on a scale where 1 denotes high development and 0 low development). Life expectancy at birth in 2012 was estimated at 71.12 years, and per capita gross domestic product (GDP) in 2011 was estimated at $9,500. According to the World Economic Forum's *Global Gender Gap Index 2011,* Suriname ranked 104th out of 135 countries on gender equality with a score of 0.640 (on a scale with a theoretical range of 1 for equality to 0 for inequality and an actual range in 2011 from 0.8530 to 0.4873).

Emergency Health Services

According to the World Health Organization (WHO), as of 2007, Suriname had a formal and publicly available emergency care (prehospital care) system accessible through a national access number. There are infection were receiving antiretroviral therapy in accordance with the 2010 WHO guidelines.

Cost of Drugs

The Drug Supply Company of Suriname, owned by the federal government, is the primary purchaser and importer of drugs for Suriname and distributes medicines on the National Essential Drug List to hospitals and private and public pharmacies. The Suriname government sets maximum sale prices and profits for pharmaceuticals; for instance, retail markup cannot be more than 35 percent over the wholesale price. Each new drug and its price must be approved by the Pharmaceutical Inspectorate.

Pharmaceutical expenditures in 2006 came to SRD 51.8 million ($18.8 million), and per capita expenditure was SRD 102.7 ($37.30). Pharmaceutical expenditures constituted 8.5 percent of health expenditures and 1.0 percent of GDP. Most (88 percent) of pharmaceutical expenditures were paid for from the private sector. Pharmaceuticals are provided free of charge in Medical Mission facilities, while pharmaceuticals are paid for out of pocket or by insurance plans at the Regional Health Services clinics. All health insurance plans cover the medicines on the Essential Medicines List (EML), although some charge copays. Free medicines are provided through public programs for tuberculosis, malaria, sexually transmitted diseases (STDs), and human immunodeficiency virus/acquired immune deficiency syndrome (HIV/AIDS); vaccines on WHO's Expanded Programme on Immunization (EPI) list are also provided free.

Health Care Facilities

A state foundation, the Regional Health Services, runs 40 clinics to provide primary health care in the coastal area for the poor and near poor; each clinic acts as a small pharmacy, supplied by a large pharmacy in Paramaribo. The Medical Mission operates about 40 clinics in the interior that provide health care and dispense drugs. Hospital care for Medical Mission patients is provided at the Deaconesses Hospital, with expenses paid by the Ministry of Social Affairs. Private-sector health care is provided primarily by private practitioners, and four public and two private hospitals provide secondary and specialized care. The Academic Hospital, a public training institution, provides most of the specialty care in the country. A military hospital provides care to members of the military and their dependents. In 2007, Suriname had 3.10 hospital beds

per 1,000 population. As of 2010, according to WHO, Suriname had 46.51 health posts per 100,000 population, 1.14 health centers per 100,000, 0.19 district or rural hospitals per 100,000, and 0.19 specialized hospitals per 100,000.

Major Health Issues

In 2008, WHO estimated that 30 percent of years of life lost in Suriname were due to communicable diseases, 52 percent to noncommunicable diseases, and 18 percent to injuries. In 2008, the age-standardized estimate of cancer deaths was 107 per 100,000 for men and 81 per 100,000 for women; for cardiovascular disease and diabetes, 426 per 100,000 for men and 276 per 100,000 for women; and for chronic respiratory disease, 28 per 100,000 for men and 14 per 100,000 for women.

In 2008, the age-standardized death rate from malaria was 2.6 per 100,000 population. Suriname's maternal mortality rate (death from any cause related to or aggravated by pregnancy) was estimated in 2008 as 100 maternal deaths per 100,000 live births. The infant mortality rate, defined as the number of deaths of infants younger than 1 year, was estimated at 28.94 per 1,000 live births in 2012. In 2010, tuberculosis incidence was 145.0 per 100,000 population, tuberculosis prevalence 238.0 per 100,000, and deaths due to tuberculosis among HIV-negative people 2.8 per 100,000. As of 2009, an estimated 1.0 percent of adults age 15 to 49 were living with HIV or AIDS.

Health Care Personnel

Suriname has one medical school, the Faculteit der Medische Wetenschappen of the Anton de Kom Universiteit van Suriname in Paramaribo, which has been offering instruction since 1892. The basic medical training course lasts seven years, and completion of a one-year internship is also required for the license to practice medicine. One year of work in government service is required after graduation. In 2004, Suriname had 0.45 physicians per 1,000 population, 0.01 dentistry personnel per 1,000, and 1.62 nurses and midwives per 1,000.

Government Role in Health Care

The right to health, including access to essential medicines and technologies, is recognized in national legislation. Suriname has a National Health Policy (NHP), updated in 2004, and a National Medicines Policy (NMP), updated in 2004. The NMP and other policies cover selection of essential medicines; pricing, procurement, distribution, and regulation of medicines; rational use of medicines; monitoring and evaluation; and traditional medicines.

According to WHO, in 2010, Suriname spent $258 million on health care, an amount that comes to $492 per capita. Most (91 percent) of health care funding came from domestic sources, with 9 percent coming from abroad. The largest share of health care spending was provided through government expenditures (48 percent), with the remainder coming from household expenditures (11 percent) and other sources (41 percent). In 2010, Suriname allocated 12 percent of its total government expenditures to health, in the median range for upper-middle-income Americas region countries; government expenditures on health came to 3 percent of GDP, in the median range for upper-middle-income Americas region countries. In 2009, according to WHO, official development assistance (ODA) for health in Suriname came to $32.11 per capita.

Public Health Programs

In 2010, 83 percent of the population in Suriname had access to improved sanitation facilities (66 percent in rural areas and 90 percent in urban), and 92 percent had access to improved sources of drinking water (81 percent in rural areas and 97 percent in urban). Large discrepancies exist between the coastal area and the interior; a 2007 report estimated that only 18 percent of households in the interior have running water, and only 31 percent have improved sanitary facilities.

SWAZILAND

Swaziland is a landlocked country in southern Africa, sharing borders with South Africa and Mozambique. The area of 6,704 square miles (17,364 square kilometers) makes Swaziland about the size of New Jersey, and the July 2012 population was estimated at 1.4 million. In 2010, 21 percent of the population lived in urban areas, and the 2010 to 2015 annual rate of urbanization was estimated at 1.5 percent. Mbabane is the capital and largest city (with a 2009 population estimated at 74,000). The population growth rate in 2012 was 1.2 percent, the net migration rate 0.0 migrants per 1,000 population, the birth rate 26.2 births per 1,000, and the total fertility rate 3.0 children per woman.

Swaziland, a former British colony, was granted autonomy in the late 19th century and independence in 1968. King Mswati III has ruled Swaziland as an absolute monarch since 1986. According to the Ibrahim Index, in 2011, Swaziland ranked 26th among 53 African countries in terms of governance performance, with a score of 51 (out of 100). Swaziland ranked tied for 95th among 183 countries on the *Corruption Perceptions Index 2011,* with a score of 3.1 (on a scale where 0 indicates highly corrupt and 10 very clean).

In 2011, Swaziland was classified as a country with medium human development (the second from the lowest of four categories) on the United Nations Development Programme's (UNDP's) Human Development Index (HDI), with a score of 0.522 (on a scale where 1 denotes high development and 0 low development). Life expectancy at birth in 2012 was estimated at 49.42 years, among the five lowest in the world. Estimated gross domestic product (GDP) per capita in 2011 was $5,200. Income distribution in Swaziland is relatively unequal: In 2001, the Gini Index (a measure of dispersion, in which perfect equality is denoted by 0 and maximum inequality is denoted by 100) for family income was 50.4. Unemployment in 2006 was estimated at 40.0 percent, among the highest rates in the world.

Emergency Health Services

According to the World Health Organization (WHO), as of 2007, Swaziland had a formal and publicly available emergency care (prehospital care) system accessible through a national access number. Doctors Without Borders (Médecins Sans Frontières, or MSF) began working in Swaziland in 2007 and had 160 staff members in the country at the close of 2010. MSF's primary focus is providing care for human immunodeficiency virus/acquired immune deficiency syndrome (HIV/AIDS) and tuberculosis patients through a community-based approach. People living in the community are trained to educate others and to test for HIV, while care is provided through dedicated HIV/AIDS clinics and decentralized tuberculosis clinics and hospitals.

Insurance

In February 2012, Swaziland launched its Essential Care Package, a set of health care interventions considered affordable and cost-effective that will be provided throughout the country.

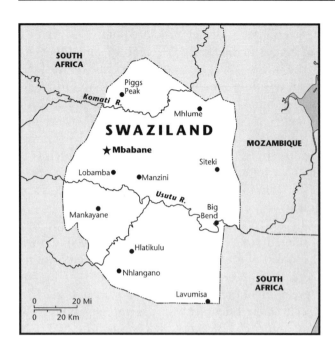

Costs of Hospitalization

No data available.

Access to Health Care

According to WHO, in 2007, 74 percent of births in Swaziland were attended by skilled personnel (for example, physicians, nurses, or midwives), and 79 percent of pregnant women received at least four prenatal care visits. The 2010 immunization rates for 1-year-olds were 89 percent for diphtheria and pertussis (DPT3), 94 percent for measles (MCV), and 89 percent for Hib (Hib3). In 2010, an estimated 72 percent of persons with advanced HIV infection were receiving antiretroviral therapy in accordance with the 2010 WHO guidelines. According to WHO, in 2010, Swaziland had fewer than 0.01 magnetic resonance imaging (MRI) machines per 1 million population and 2.57 computer tomography (CT) machines per 1 million.

Cost of Drugs

No data available.

Health Care Facilities

As of 2010, according to WHO, Swaziland had 13.66 health posts per 100,000 population, 0.67 health centers per 100,000, 0.17 district or rural hospitals per 100,000, 0.51 provincial hospitals per 100,000, and 0.17 specialized hospitals per 100,000. In 2006, Swaziland had 2.10 hospital beds per 1,000 population.

Major Health Issues

In 2008, WHO estimated that 72 percent of years of life lost in Swaziland were due to communicable diseases, 16 percent to noncommunicable diseases, and 12 percent to injuries. In 2008, the age-standardized estimate of cancer deaths was 93 per 100,000 for men and 71 per 100,000 for women; for cardiovascular disease and diabetes, 558 per 100,000 for men and 442 per 100,000 for women; and for chronic respiratory disease, 159 per 100,000 for men and 71 per 100,000 for women. In 2008, the age-standardized death rate from malaria was 0.3 per 100,000 population. Swaziland's maternal mortality rate (death from any cause related to or aggravated by pregnancy) is high by global standards, estimated at 420 maternal deaths per 100,000 live births as of 2008. The infant mortality rate, defined as the number of deaths of infants younger than 1 year, also has been high, at 59.57 per 1,000 live births as of 2012.

In 2010, tuberculosis incidence was 1,287.0 per 100,000 population, tuberculosis prevalence 704.0 per 100,000, and deaths due to tuberculosis among human immunodeficiency virus (HIV)-negative people 32.00 per 100,000. As of 2009, Swaziland had the highest human immunodeficiency virus/acquired immune deficiency syndrome (HIV/AIDS) rates in the world; in that year, an estimated 24.9 percent of adults age 15 to 49 were living with HIV or AIDS. In 2010, 83 percent of pregnant women tested positive for HIV. The mother-to-child transmission rate for HIV in 2010 was estimated at 14 percent, and in 2009, 29.5 percent of deaths to children under age 5 were attributed to HIV.

Health Care Personnel

In 2004, Swaziland had 0.16 physicians per 1,000 population, 0.06 pharmaceutical personnel per 1,000, 0.07 laboratory health workers per 1,000, 0.29 health management and support workers per 1,000, 0.03 dentistry personnel per 1,000, and, in 2000, had 1.62 nurses and midwives per 1,000. Michael Clemens and Bunilla Petterson estimate that 28 percent of Swaziland-born physicians and 3 percent of Swaziland-born nurses are working in one of nine developed countries, primarily South Africa (physicians) and South Africa, the United Kingdom, and the United States (nurses).

Government Role in Health Care

According to WHO, in 2010, Swaziland spent $241 million on health care, an amount that comes to $203 per capita. Most (83 percent) of health care funding came from domestic sources, with 17 percent coming from abroad. The largest share of health care spending was provided through government expenditures (64 percent), with the remainder coming from household expenditures (15 percent) and other sources (21 percent). In 2010, Swaziland allocated 10 percent of its total government expenditures to health, in the median range for lower-middle-income African countries; government expenditures on health came to 4 percent of GDP, in the high range for lower-middle-income African countries. In 2009, according to WHO, official development assistance (ODA) for health in Swaziland came to $34.57 per capita.

Public Health Programs

According to WHO, in 2004, Swaziland had 0.10 environmental and public health workers per 1,000 population. In 2010, 57 percent of the population had access to improved sanitation facilities (55 percent in rural areas and 64 percent in urban), and 71 percent had access to improved sources of drinking water (65 percent in rural areas and 91 percent in urban).

SWEDEN

Sweden is a northern European country, sharing borders with Norway and Finland and having a coastline on the Baltic Sea. The area of 173,860 square miles (450,295 square kilometers) makes Sweden about the size of California, and the July 2012 population was estimated at 9.1 million. In 2010, 85 percent of the population lived in urban areas, and the 2010 to 2015 annual rate of urbanization was estimated at 0.6 percent. Stockholm is the capital and largest city (with a 2009 population estimated at 1.3 million). The population growth rate in 2012 was 0.2 percent, the net migration rate 1.6 migrants per 1,000 population, the birth rate 10.2 births per 1,000, and the total fertility rate 1.7 children per woman.

Sweden has a 200-year history of neutrality and is often cited as a model of a country successfully combining a capitalist economic system with a generous package of social benefits. The Swedish government has a reputation for transparency and honesty, ranking fourth among 183 countries on the *Corruption Perceptions Index 2011,* with a score of 9.3 (on a scale where 0 indicates highly corrupt and 10 very clean).

Sweden ranked 10th in 2011 on the United Nations Development Programme's (UNDP's) Human Development Index (HDI), with a score of 0.904 (on a scale where 1 denotes high development and 0 low development). Life expectancy at birth in 2012 was estimated at 81.18 years, among the highest in the world, and per capita gross domestic product (GDP) in 2011 was estimated at $40,600. Income distribution is among the most equal in the world: In 2005 the Gini Index (a measure of dispersion, in which perfect equality is denoted by 0 and maximum inequality is denoted by 100) for family income was 23.0. Gender equality is also high: According to the World Economic Forum's *Global Gender Gap Index 2011*, Sweden ranked fourth out of 135 countries on gender equality with a score of 0.804 (on a scale with a theoretical range of 1 for equality to 0 for inequality and an actual range in 2011 from 0.8530 to 0.4873).

Emergency Health Services

Sweden's laws governing the emergency health system date from the 1980s, while recognition of emergency medicine as a medical specialty dates from the 2000s; by law, free access to hospitals for emergency care is provided for all persons, including the uninsured. Funding for both inpatient and outpatient care in the emergency system is provided entirely by public sources. Sweden has only one national telephone number for medical emergencies, 112 (the European Union or EU, standard); the country has 18 dispatch centers that are interconnected.

Insurance

Sweden has a national health service financed out of general tax revenues, which covers many health care services, including hospital care, primary health care, prescription drugs, preventive services, mental health care, and dental care for children. The national health service budget also includes public health services, rehabilitation services, disability support, home care, nursing home care, and patient transport. The system includes cost sharing for services including physician visits, prescription drugs, and hospital care; in 2005, out-of-pocket payments accounted for 13.9 percent of total health care expenditures. There is a cap of SEK 900 ($137) for health services and SEK 1,800 ($274) for drugs; children are exempt from most cost sharing. Most physicians are salaried, but private physicians are paid through a mix of capitation and fee for service. Hospital payments are based on global budgets plus case-based payments and include physician costs. Most patients, except in Stockholm, are required to register with a general practice physician.

A 2004 study by the World Health Organization (WHO) found that none of the Swedish population had substitutive voluntary health insurance (covering services that would otherwise be available from the state), and 1.0 to 1.5 percent had complementary voluntary health insurance (covering services not covered or not fully covered by the state) or supplementary health insurance (providing increased choice or faster access to services). Most voluntary policies are purchased by employers, most often for high-level management. According to Ke Xu and colleagues, in 2003, 0.2 percent of households in Sweden experienced catastrophic health expenditures annually; "catastrophic" was defined as exceeding 40 percent of household income remaining after basic needs were met.

Costs of Hospitalization

According to Organisation for Economic Co-operation and Development (OECD) data, in 2009, hospital spending per capita in Sweden was $1,637 (adjusted for differences in the cost of living), and hospital spending per discharge came to $9,870 in 2011. In 2008, according to the OECD, hospital spending in Sweden represented 46.9 percent of total spending on health; hospitals were paid based on payment per case or diagnosis-related group (DRG). The average length of stay in acute care was 4.5 days (in 2008), and there were 166 hospital discharges per 1,000 population. Sweden has limited cost sharing for medical services, with fees established by county councils; on average, the copayment in 2010 for hospitalization came to about $12 per day.

Access to Health Care

In 2009, according to OECD data, people in Sweden had an average of 2.9 physician visits. In 2010, over half (57 percent) reported that, when sick, they were able to get a medical appointment the same day or the next day, while just over two-thirds (68 percent) reported it was very or somewhat difficult to get medical care after usual office hours. For those who needed particular types of care, about one-third (31 percent) reported they waited two or more months to see a specialist (of those who needed to see a specialist in the prior two years), about one-quarter (22 percent) reported waiting four or more months for elective surgery (of those who required elective surgery

in the prior two years), and 10 percent reported they had experienced an access barrier due to cost in the previous two years; an access barrier was defined as failing to fill or refill a prescription, failing to visit a physician, or failing to get recommended care.

About 2.5 percent of the population has private insurance, which may provide quicker access to care than the public system; there is also limited cost sharing within the public system, with rates set by county councils; these fees tend to be quite modest, however, for instance, $23 to visit a primary care physician and $12 per day for inpatient care. Dental care is not part of the national health system but is partially subsidized by the government. National standards specify that nonacute patients should be able to obtain an appointment with a primary care physician within seven days and a specialist within 90 days after referral.

A 2011 Commonwealth Fund Survey compared access to health care for "sicker" adults (those 18 and older, in self-reported poor or fair health, who had been treated for a serious illness or injury in the past year or been hospitalized in the past two years) in 11 OECD countries. This survey found that 11 percent of sicker Swedish people surveyed reported having experienced an access problem related to cost in the previous year, the lowest proportion among the countries surveyed; the most common result was failing to fill a prescription or skipping doses of a prescribed drug. Other problems reported include having serious

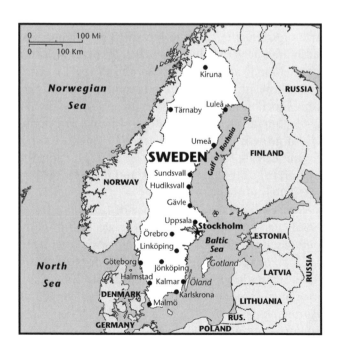

problems paying medical bills (4 percent), waiting six days or longer for needed care (22 percent), having difficulty getting after-hours care except in an emergency room (52 percent), and experiencing coordination gaps in care (39 percent).

Sweden ranked fourth among more developed countries in the 2011 Mothers' Index, produced by the international nongovernmental organization (NGO) Save the Children, based on a number of health and social factors relating to women, children, and maternal and child care. In 2010, the maternal mortality rate in Sweden was four deaths per 100,000 live births, and the infant mortality rate was two per 1,000 live births. Immunization rates in 2010 were 96 percent for measles, 98 percent for diphtheria and pertussis (DPT3), and 98 percent for Hib (Hib3).

Cost of Drugs

The Swedish Dental and Pharmaceutical Benefits (TLV) determines the price and reimbursement rates for prescription drugs based on health care needs and cost-effectiveness. Some county councils have created incentives to encourage physicians to control the amount of money spent on prescription drugs. The national health system includes cost sharing for prescription drugs: For outpatient drugs, patients pay the total cost up to SEK 900 ($127) annually, after which point costs are subsidized (from 50 to 100 percent) based on the level of out-of-pocket expenditure. A maximum of SEK 1,800 applies for children from the same family. In 2009, according to OECD data, pharmaceutical spending per capita in Sweden was $465 (adjusted for differences in the cost of living). Real annual growth in pharmaceutical expenditures in Sweden grew 4.1 percent from 1997 to 2005, slightly slower than the 4.5 percent growth of total health expenditure (minus pharmaceutical expenditures) over those years.

According to Douglas Ball, Sweden charges no value added-tax (VAT) for prescription-only medicine but the standard VAT of 25 percent for over-the-counter medicines. Wholesale markups are negotiated and average around 2.7 percent. Pharmacy markups are capped at SEK 167 (18 euros) for prescription-only medicines and are set by the distribution monopoly Apotek for over-the-counter drugs. According to Elizabeth Docteur, in 2004, generic drugs represented 12 percent of the market share by value and 39 percent of the market share by volume of the total pharmaceutical market.

Health Care Facilities

Most service delivery in Sweden is managed at the level of local county councils and municipalities, resulting in some variation in different parts of the country. Most hospitals in Sweden are publicly owned and operated; private hospitals work under contract to the same councils that operate public hospitals, and do primarily elective surgery. As of 2010, there were about 21,000 hospital beds in the private sector. Most (94 percent) of primary care physicians in Sweden used electronic medical records in 2009.

Major Health Issues

In 2008, WHO estimated that 5 percent of years of life lost in Sweden were due to communicable diseases, 83 percent to noncommunicable diseases, and 12 percent to injuries. In 2008, the age-standardized estimate of cancer deaths was 128 per 100,000 for men and 101 per 100,000 for women; for cardiovascular disease and diabetes, 179 per 100,000 for men and 103 per 100,000 for women; and for chronic respiratory disease, 17 per 100,000 for men and 13 per 100,000 for women.

The maternal mortality rate (death from any cause related to or aggravated by pregnancy) in Sweden in 2008 was five maternal deaths per 100,000 live births, among the lowest in the world. The infant mortality rate in Sweden was 2.74 per 1,000 live births as of 2012, the fifth-lowest in the world. In 2010, tuberculosis incidence was 6.8 per 100,000 population, tuberculosis prevalence 8.8 per 100,000, and deaths due to tuberculosis among human immunodeficiency virus (HIV)-negative people 0.28 per 100,000. As of 2009, an estimated 0.1 percent of adults age 15 to 49 were living with HIV or acquired immune deficiency syndrome (AIDS).

Health Care Personnel

Sweden has six medical schools. The basic medical degree course lasts 5.5 years, and the degree awarded is Läkarexamen (physician's examination). A 21-month internship is also required before granting the license to practice medicine. Graduates of foreign medical schools must pass an exam and language proficiency test and have knowledge of Swedish medical legislation.

Sweden, as a member of the EU, cooperates with other countries in recognizing physicians qualified to practice in other EU countries, as specified by Directive 2005/36/EC of the European Parliament. This allows qualified professionals to practice their profession in other EU states on a temporary basis and requires that the host country automatically recognize qualifications for certain professions, including physicians, nurses, dentists, midwives, and pharmacists, if certain conditions have been met (for instance, facility in the language of the host country may be required). Sweden also has an agreement with Iceland. In 2006, Sweden had 3.58 physicians per 1,000 population, 0.73 pharmaceutical personnel per 1,000, 0.83 dentistry personnel per 1,000, and 11.57 nurses and midwives per 1,000.

Government Role in Health Care

Several levels of government are involved in health care delivery in Sweden. Overall objectives and regulations are determined at the federal level, primary care is organized by the 21 Swedish county councils, and many details of service delivery are determined at the local level. Most health centers are owned and operated by county councils and historically have been responsible for providing primary care within specified regions. Most hospitals are still owned and operated by county councils and staffed by salaried physicians and staff. However, in 2010, a law took effect that privatized the provision of primary care and provided Swedes with more choices regarding their primary care providers. While there is no formal gatekeeping requirement, a person who does not visit a primary care provider before visiting a specialist or hospital can be charged higher copayments. Hospital payments are based on both global budgets and DRGs.

According to WHO, in 2010, Sweden spent $44 billion on health care, an amount that comes to $4,710 per capita. All health care funding came from domestic

Selected Health Indicators: Sweden Compared With the Organisation for Economic Co-operation and Development (OECD) Country Average

	Sweden	OECD average (2010 or nearest year)
Male life expectancy at birth, 2011	79.8	77
Female life expectancy at birth, 2011	83.7	82.5
Infant mortality (deaths per 1,000 live births), 2011	2.1	4.3
Total expenditure on health (percent of GDP), 2010	9.6	9.5
Total expenditure on health (per capita, USD purchasing power parity), 2010	3,757.7	3,265
Doctor consultations (number per capita), 2010	2.9	6.4
Hospital beds (per 1,000 population), 2010	2.7	4.9
Average length of hospital stay, all causes (days), 2010	5.7	7.1
Average length of hospital stay for a normal delivery (days), 2010	2.3	3.1
Cesarean sections (per 1,000 live births), 2010	168	261
Causes of mortality: Suicides (deaths per 100,000 population), 2010	11.7	12.9
Alcohol consumption (liters per capita [age 15+]), 2010	7.3	9.4
Tobacco consumption (percent of population 15+ who are daily smokers), 2010	14	21.1

Source: OECD Health Data 2012 (Organisation for Economic Co-operation and Development, 2012).

sources. The largest share of health care spending was provided through government expenditures (81 percent), with the remainder coming from household expenditures (17 percent) and other sources (2 percent). In 2010, Sweden allocated 15 percent of its total government expenditures to health, in the median range for high-income European countries; government expenditures on health came to 8 percent of GDP, in the high range for high-income European countries.

Public Health Programs

Sweden's National Institute of Public Health (SNIPH) is located in Östersund and headed by Sarah Wamala; it is located within the Ministry of Health and Social Affairs. The institute has a staff of approximately 160 organized into six departments: child and adolescent health and medical health; drug prevention; communications; health behaviors; policy analysis and monitoring; and community planning and health. It has three primary functions: to serve as a national center of knowledge in public health; to exercise supervision concerning illicit drugs, tobacco, and alcohol; and to monitor and implement the national health policy, adopted in 2003. Current priorities include promoting parenting skills; supporting the elderly; raising awareness about harmful drugs, alcohol, and tobacco; and encouraging physical activity. Sweden has a highly developed infrastructure, and access to improved sanitary facilities and improved sources of drinking water is essentially universal. According to the World Higher Education Database (WHED), six universities in Sweden offer programs in epidemiology or public health: Blekinge Institute of Technology, University College of Boras, the University of Skövde, Karlstad University, the Karolinska Institute, and Malmo University.

SWITZERLAND

Switzerland is a landlocked country in central Europe sharing borders with Austria, France, Italy, Liechtenstein, and Germany. The area of 15,937 square miles (41,277 square kilometers) makes Switzerland about twice the size of New Jersey, and the July 2012 population was estimated at 7.7 million. In 2010, 74 percent of the population lived in urban areas, and the 2010 to 2015 annual rate of urbanization was estimated at

0.5 percent. Berne is the capital and Zurich the largest city (with a 2009 population estimated at 1.1 million). The population growth rate in 2012 was 0.2 percent, the net migration rate 1.3 migrants per 1,000 population, the birth rate 9.5 births per 1,000, and the total fertility rate 1.5 children per woman.

Switzerland became independent of the Holy Roman Empire in 1499 and has a long history of neutrality. The Swiss government has a reputation for transparency, ranking tied for eighth among 183 countries on the *Corruption Perceptions Index 2011*, with a score of 8.8 (on a scale where 0 indicates highly corrupt and 10 very clean). In 2011, Switzerland was classified as a country with very high human development (the highest of four categories) on the United Nations Development Programme's (UNDP's) Human Development Index (HDI), with a score of 0.903 (on a scale where 1 denotes high development and 0 low development). Life expectancy at birth in 2012 was estimated at 81.17 years, among the highest in the world, and per capita gross domestic product (GDP) in 2011 in Switzerland was estimated at $43,400. In 2008, the Gini Index (a measure of dispersion, in which perfect equality is denoted by 0 and maximum inequality is denoted by 100) for family income was 33.7. According to the World Economic Forum's *Global Gender Gap Index 2011*, Switzerland ranked 10th out of 135 countries on gender equality, with a score of 0.763 (on a scale with a theoretical range of 1 for equality to 0 for inequality and an actual range in 2011 from 0.8530 to 0.4873).

Emergency Health Services

According to the World Health Organization (WHO), as of 2007, Switzerland had a formal and publicly available emergency care (prehospital care) system accessible through a national access number.

Insurance

Switzerland has a statutory health insurance system, with a universal mandate to purchase insurance provided through private companies in regional exchanges. The system is financed by general tax revenues and community-rated insurance premiums. The basic insurance package provided by all companies includes most physician services, preventive care, some prescription drugs, and out-of-canton services if medically necessary. Coinsurance of 10 percent is applied to most services, with additional charges for hospital treatment and prescription drugs, when a

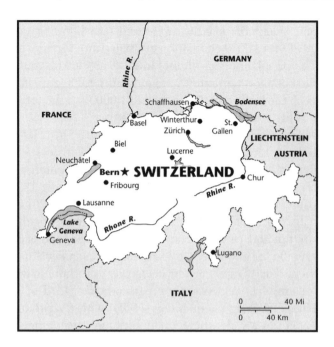

generic is available. Swiss citizens may buy additional private insurance, and about 70 percent do so. There is a cap on out-of-pocket expenses, and 30 percent of individuals receive premium assistance based on income; there are some cost sharing exemptions for children and pregnant women. Primary care is paid for primarily on a fee-for-service basis, with some capitation also used. Each canton decides how to handle hospital payments: Methods used include global budgets, per-diem payments, and case-based payments. Hospital payments include physician costs. Patients are not required to register with a general practice physician and are generally allowed to choose their own general practitioner and specialists, unless they have chosen to enroll in a managed care insurance plan. According to Ke Xu and colleagues, in 2003, 0.6 percent of households in Switzerland experienced catastrophic health expenditures annually; "catastrophic" was defined as exceeding 40 percent of household income remaining after basic needs were met.

Average premiums for insurance vary among cantons, from CHF 2,760 ($2,689) in Nidwalden to CHF 5,040 ($4,911) in Geneva as of 2010. Premiums are set for geographical regions and may vary only by age category (child, young adult, or adult) and choice of deductible level; premiums may thus vary widely within a region, for example, up to 90 percent in Zurich. Insurers offering supplemental coverage are

regulated at the national level; unlike basic insurers, they may refuse applicants and may operate for profit.

Costs of Hospitalization

Cantons are responsible for hospital planning and provide a substantial share of hospital funding; about 75 percent of acute inpatient care is provided in public or publicly subsidized hospitals. Insurers pay hospitals through per-diem rates or reimbursements based on diagnosis related groups (DRGs), with any deficits made up by the canton for public and publicly subsidized hospitals. In 2008, according to the Organisation for Economic Co-operation and Development (OECD), hospital spending in Switzerland represented 35.1 percent of total spending on health.

According to OECD data, in 2009, hospital spending per capita in Switzerland was $1,831 (adjusted for differences in the cost of living), and hospital spending per discharge came to $10,875 in 2011. The average length of stay in acute care was 7.5 days in 2008, and there were 168 hospital discharges per 1,000 population.

Access to Health Care

According to WHO, in 2006, 100 percent of births in Switzerland were attended by skilled personnel (for example, physicians, nurses, or midwives). The 2010 immunization rates for 1-year-olds were 96 percent for diphtheria and pertussis (DPT3), 90 percent for measles (MCV), and 94 percent for Hib (Hib3). In 2009, according to OECD data, the Swiss had an average of 4.0 physician visits. In 2010, almost all (93 percent) reported that, when sick, they were able to get a medical appointment the same day or the next day, although 43 percent reported it was very or somewhat difficult to get medical care after usual office hours. For those who needed particular types of care, only 5 percent reported they waited two or more months to see a specialist (of those who needed to see a specialist in the prior two years), only 7 percent reported waiting four or more months for elective surgery (of those who required elective surgery in the prior two years), and 10 percent reported they had experienced an access barrier due to cost in the previous two years; an access barrier was defined as failing to fill or refill a prescription, failing to visit a physician, or failing to get recommended care.

A 2011 Commonwealth Fund Survey compared access to health care for "sicker" adults (those 18 and older, in self-reported poor or fair health, who had been treated for a serious illness or injury in the past year or been hospitalized in the past two years) in 11 OECD countries. This survey found that 18 percent of sicker Swiss people surveyed reported having experienced an access problem related to cost in the previous year; the most common results were skipping a test, treatment, or follow-up, or having a medical problem but failing to visit a doctor. Other problems reported include having serious problems paying their medical bills (8 percent), waiting six days or longer for needed care (4 percent), having difficulty getting after-hours care except in an emergency room (26 percent), and experiencing coordination gaps in care (23 percent).

Cost of Drugs

According to Elizabeth Docteur, the Swiss Drug Commission evaluates new drugs based on therapeutic innovativeness and potential, and drugs are classified in five categories: therapeutic breakthrough, therapeutic progress, savings compared to other drugs, no therapeutic progress and no savings, and inappropriate for social health insurance. Drugs judged to be innovative or to reduce costs are eligible to be included in the positive list (eligible for reimbursement), and those judged to be innovative may charge a higher price than other drugs for the same condition. In general, the second drug in a therapeutic class entering the market within three years of the first drug may be allowed to charge a premium as well, with the logic that the short period of time did not allow for head-to-head trials comparing the two drugs; drugs entering the market later and offering no therapeutic advantage (me-too drugs) are generally not allowed to charge premiums.

As of 2009, Switzerland has used a reference pricing scheme for drugs based on prices in Germany, the Netherlands, the United Kingdom, Denmark, France, and Austria. Generic drugs are priced at least 50 percent below brand-name equivalents, and Swiss health plans charge 20 percent coinsurance on brand-name drugs if a generic equivalent is available, twice the level of coinsurance (10 percent) for most services. Pharmacists are paid a flat fee to dispense drugs. According to Elizabeth Docteur, in 2004, Switzerland ranked fourth-lowest among OECD countries in terms of the use of generics; generic drugs represented 6 percent of the pharmaceutical market share by value.

In 2009, according to OECD data, pharmaceutical spending per capita in Switzerland was $521 (adjusted for differences in the cost of living). Switzerland does not maintain an Essential Medicines List (EML) but instead a list of more than 2,500 drugs that are eligible for reimbursement. Social assistance offices provide medications free for those who cannot afford to pay and lower maximum copayments for children than for adults. Vaccines on WHO's Expanded Programme of Immunization (EPI) list are provided for free, as is the human papilloma virus (HPV) vaccine. According to Douglas Ball, Switzerland charges a reduced value-added tax (VAT) of 2.4 percent (the standard rate is 7.6 percent) on medicines. Pharmacist dispensing fees are paid according to a schedule. Distribution markups are shared between wholesalers and pharmacists and are defined by a scheme combining fixed markups (capped at CHF 240) and proportional markups (8 to 15 percent of ex-factory price, the manufacturer's list price before discounts); the distribution margin is also shared for over-the-counter drugs. Real annual growth in pharmaceutical expenditures in Switzerland grew 3.5 percent from 1997 to 2005, about the same as the 3.3 percent growth of total health expenditure (minus pharmaceutical expenditures) over those years.

Health Care Facilities

In 2008, Switzerland had 5.31 hospital beds per 1,000 population, among the 50 highest rates in the world.

Major Health Issues

In 2008, WHO estimated that 5 percent of years of life lost in Switzerland were due to communicable diseases, 82 percent to noncommunicable diseases, and 13 percent to injuries. In 2008, the age-standardized estimate of cancer deaths was 137 per 100,000 for men and 88 per 100,000 for women; for cardiovascular disease and diabetes, 143 per 100,000 for men and 86 per 100,000 for women; and for chronic respiratory disease, 19 per 100,000 for men and eight per 100,000 for women.

The maternal mortality rate (death from any cause related to or aggravated by pregnancy) in Switzerland in 2008 was 10 maternal deaths per 100,000 live births. The infant mortality rate, defined as the number of deaths of infants younger than 1 year, was 4.03 per 1,000 live births as of 2012. In 2010, tuberculosis incidence was 7.6 per 100,000 population, tuberculosis prevalence 9.4 per 100,000, and deaths due to tuberculosis among human immunodeficiency virus (HIV)-negative people 0.28 per 100,000. As of 2009, an estimated 0.4 percent of adults age 15 to 49 were living with HIV or acquired immune deficiency syndrome (AIDS).

Health Care Personnel

Switzerland has five medical schools, the oldest of which, the Medizinische Fakultët of the University of Basel, began offering instruction in 1460. The basic medical degree course lasts six years, and the degree awarded is Eidgenössisches Artzdiplom or Diplôme federal de médecin (federal diploma of physician). Physicians must register with the health authority of the canton in which they want to practice. The license to practice medicine is granted to holders of Swiss medical degrees who must also provide proof of their legal status and good conduct. Swiss nationals require special authorization to practice medicine, and foreigners may only enter private practice if they have qualified in Switzerland.

In 2009, Switzerland had 4.07 physicians per 1,000 population, and in 2008, had 0.58 pharmaceutical personnel per 1000, 0.55 dentistry personnel per 1,000, and 15.96 nurses and midwives per 1,000. In 2001, 19.1 percent of physicians practicing in Switzerland were trained abroad, primarily in Germany (59.7 percent).

Government Role in Health Care

Switzerland does not have a National Health Policy (NHP); instead, most health care decisions are handled at the canton level. Switzerland does have a National Medicines Policy (NMP), updated in 2007. Switzerland mandates universal health care coverage, and insurers are also regulated and supervised at the national level. A basic level of benefits is mandated, but insurers can offer different options: For instance, all plans must offer a minimum annual deductible (CHF 300, or $292, in 2010), but may also offer higher deductibles in return for lower premiums. Insurers are also allowed to waive the standard 10 percent coinsurance for people who enroll in managed care. A risk equalization scheme is used to redistribute costs among insurers, and cantons and confederations provide premium subsidies to low-income individuals as well as paying the premiums for the approximately 1.6 percent of residents who do not pay their own premiums.

According to WHO, in 2010, Switzerland spent $61 billion on health care, an amount that comes to $7,812 per capita. All health care funding came from domestic sources. The largest share of health care spending was provided through government expenditures (59 percent), with the remainder coming from household expenditures (31 percent) and other sources (10 percent). In 2010, Switzerland allocated 20 percent of its total government expenditures to health, in the high range for high-income European countries; government expenditures on health came to 7 percent of GDP, in the median range for high-income European countries.

Public Health Programs

In 2010, access to improved sanitary facilities and improved sources of drinking water was essentially universal in Switzerland.

SYRIA

Syria is a Middle Eastern country, sharing borders with Iraq, Israel, Jordan, Lebanon, and Turkey and having a coastline on the Mediterranean Sea. The area of 71,498 square miles (185,180 square kilometers) makes Syria about the size of North Dakota, and the July 2012 population was estimated at 22.5 million. In 2010, 56 percent of the population lived in urban areas, and the 2010 to 2015 annual rate of urbanization was estimated at 2.5 percent. Damascus is the capital and Aleppo the largest city (with a 2009 population estimated at 3.0 million). The population growth rate in 2012 was negative 0.8 percent, the net migration rate negative 27.8 migrants per 1,000 population (the second-highest emigration rate in the world), the birth rate 23.5 births per 1,000, and the total fertility rate 2.8 children per woman. The United Nations High Commissioner for Refugees (UNHCR) estimated that, in 2010, there were 140,677 refugees and persons in refugee-like situations in Syria. Civil unrest in 2011 and 2012 led to large numbers of people emigrating (the UNHCR estimated in 2012 that more than 60,000 had fled to neighboring countries) or becoming internally displaced; food prices increased in Syria due to the unrest as well as poor rainfall in the country's agricultural areas, creating the conditions for possible food shortages.

France acquired a mandate over Syria after World War I, and the country became independent in 1946. From 1958 to 1961, Syria joined with Egypt to form the United Arab Republic. Syria lost territory (the Golan Heights) to Israel following the 1967 Arab–Israeli War. Syria ranked tied for 129th among 183 countries on the *Corruption Perceptions Index 2011,* with a score of 2.6 (on a scale where 0 indicates highly corrupt and 10 very clean). In 2011, Syria was classified as a country with medium human development (the second from the lowest of four categories) on the United Nations Development Programme's (UNDP's) Human Development Index (HDI), with a score of 0.632 (on a scale where 1 denotes high development and 0 low development). Life expectancy at birth in 2012 was estimated at 74.92 years, and estimated gross domestic product (GDP) per capita in 2011 was $5,100. According to the World Economic Forum's *Global Gender Gap Index 2011,* Syria ranked 124th out of 135 countries on gender equality with a score of 0.590 (on a scale with a theoretical range of 1 for equality to 0 for inequality and an actual range in 2011 from 0.8530 to 0.4873).

Emergency Health Services

According to the World Health Organization (WHO), as of 2007, Syria had a formal and publicly available emergency care (prehospital care) system accessible through a national access number. Doctors Without Borders (Médecins Sans Frontières, or MSF) began working in Syria in 2009 and had five staff members in the country at the close of 2010. MSF established a Migrants Office in Damascus, the national capital, providing medical and mental care to migrants, refugees, and other vulnerable persons; more than 1,000 people received mental health counseling from this center in 2010, and more than 6,200 patients received medical care. As of January 2012, the United Nations Relief and Works Agency for Palestine Refugees (UNRWA) operated nine camps in Syria, with 510,444 registered persons, including 486,946 registered refugees.

Insurance

According to WHO, almost all (99.5 percent) of the Syrian population is covered by public health insurance, with the remaining 0.5 percent covered by private insurance.

Costs of Hospitalization

No data available.

Access to Health Care

According to WHO, in 2009, 95.3 percent of births in Syria were attended by skilled personnel (for example, physicians, nurses, or midwives). The 2010 immunization rates for 1-year-olds were 80 percent for diphtheria and pertussis (DPT3), 82 percent for measles (MCV), and 80 percent for Hib (Hib3).

Cost of Drugs

In 2010, total pharmaceutical expenditures in Syria came to SYP 29,785 million ($621 million), for a per capita expenditure of SYP 1,403 ($29.30). Pharmaceutical expenditures constitute 36.0 percent of health expenditures and 1.1 percent of GDP. Some population groups are entitled to free medicines; these include children younger than age 5, pregnant women, elderly people, and the poor. Some drugs are also provided free at public facilities, including those to treat malaria, tuberculosis, sexually transmitted disease (STDs), and human immunodeficiency virus/ acquired immune deficiency syndrome (HIV/AIDS); vaccines listed in the WHO's Expanded Programme on Immunization (EPI) list are provided for free, as are oral contraceptives, growth hormones, insulin, interferon, and immunosuppressants. Medicine prices are regulated by the government; about 5,000 medicines were registered as of 2008. Most medicines (90 percent) used in Syria are manufactured within the country rather than being imported.

A 2008 survey found that the median price ratio for public sector procurement was 1.54 for generic medicines, meaning that costs were on average 54 percent above the international reference price. For originator brands, the median price ratio was 7.0 (meaning costs were on average seven times the international reference price). Private-sector prices were much higher, with a median price ratio of 2.51 for generics and 9.6 for originator brands. Availability was quite high (98.2 percent) for the lowest-priced generics in the private sector. In public hospitals, median availability of generics was also high (93 percent). Few originator brands were marketed in Syria at the time of the survey.

Health Care Facilities

In 2009, Syria had 1.50 hospital beds per 1,000 population.

Major Health Issues

In 2008, WHO estimated that 23 percent of years of life lost in Syria were due to communicable diseases, 51 percent to noncommunicable diseases, and 16 percent to injuries. In 2008, the age-standardized estimate of cancer deaths was 66 per 100,000 for men and 47 per 100,000 for women; for cardiovascular disease and diabetes, 472 per 100,000 for men and 326 per 100,000 for women; and for chronic respiratory disease, 47 per 100,000 for men and 29 per 100,000 for women.

Syria's maternal mortality rate (death from any cause related to or aggravated by pregnancy) was estimated in 2008 as 46 maternal deaths per 100,000 live births. The infant mortality rate, defined as the number of deaths of infants younger than 1 year, was 15.12 per 1,000 live births as of 2012. In 2006, 10.0 percent of children under age 5 were underweight (defined as 2 kilograms [kg] below standard weight-for-age at age 1, 3 kg below for ages 2 to 3, and 4 kg below for ages 4 to 5). In 2010, tuberculosis incidence was 20.0 per 100,000 population, tuberculosis prevalence 23.0 per 100,000, and deaths due to tuberculosis among human immunodeficiency virus (HIV)-negative people 1.4 per 100,000. As of 2009, an estimated 0.1 percent of adults age 15 to 49 were living with HIV or acquired immune deficiency syndrome (AIDS).

Health Care Personnel

Syria has four medical schools. The basic medical degree course lasts six years, and the degree awarded is doctor of medicine. In 2008, Syria had 1.50 physicians

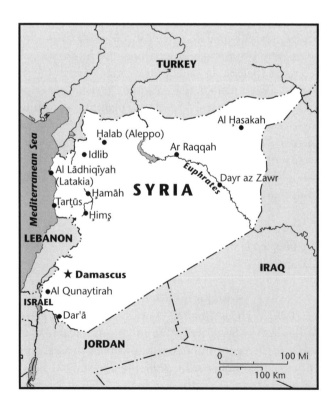

per 1,000 population, 0.81 pharmaceutical personnel per 1,000, 0.79 dentistry personnel per 1,000, and 1.86 nurses and midwives per 1,000, and in 2006, had 0.56 health management and support workers per 1,000.

Government Role in Health Care

The right to health, including access to essential medicines and medical technology, is recognized in national legislation. Syria has a National Health Plan (NHP) and National Medicines Plan (NMP) as well as implementation plans for both; the NHP, NMP, and their implementation plans all date from 2011. The NMP covers selection of essential medicines; financing, pricing, purchase, distribution, and regulation of drugs; pharmacovigilance; rational usage of medicines; human resource development; research; evaluation and monitoring; and traditional medicine. As of 2007, the Essential Medicines List (EML) for Syria included 312 medicines. Pharmaceutical products must be evaluated and registered before they can be sold in Syria; the list of registered pharmaceutical products is publicly available and, as of 2011, included 7,059 products.

According to WHO, in 2010, Syria spent $2.0 billion on health care, an amount that comes to $97 per capita. Most (99 percent) of health care funding came from domestic sources, with 1 percent coming from abroad. The largest share of health care spending was provided through household expenditures (54 percent), with the remainder coming from government expenditures (46 percent). In 2010, Syria allocated 6 percent of its total government expenditures to health, in the low range for lower-middle-income eastern Mediterranean region countries; government expenditures on health came to 2 percent of GDP, in the low range for lower-middle-income eastern Mediterranean region countries. In 2009, according to WHO, official development assistance (ODA) for health in Syria came to $1.02 per capita.

Public Health Programs

In 2010, 93 percent of the population in Syria had access to improved sanitation facilities (95 percent in rural areas and 96 percent in urban), and 90 percent had access to improved sources of drinking water (86 percent in rural areas and 93 percent in urban). According to the World Higher Education Database (WHED), three universities in Syria offer programs in epidemiology or public health: al-Baath University, the University of Aleppo, and Tishreen University.

TAIWAN

Taiwan is an island nation in the north Pacific Ocean. The area of 13,892 square miles (35,980 square kilometers) makes Taiwan about twice the size of Maryland and Delaware combined, and the July 2012 population was estimated at 23.1 million. Taipei is the capital. The population growth rate in 2012 was 0.2 percent, the net migration rate 0.0 migrants per 1,000 population, the birth rate 8.8 births per 1,000, and the total fertility rate 1.2 children per woman.

After Communist victory in China's civil war, about 2 million nationalists fled to Taiwan and established a government; however, China considers Taiwan one of its provinces rather than a separate country. Taiwan lost its seat in the United Nations (UN) in 1971, when the UN recognized China; Taiwan has regularly petitioned to be reinstated, but this had not been granted as of 2012. However, many health and other statistics are reported separately for Taiwan, and it has a different health care delivery system than does China, so it receives is own entry in this volume. Taiwan ranked tied for 32nd among 183 countries on the *Corruption Perceptions Index 2011,* with a score of 6.1 (on a scale where 0 indicates highly corrupt and 10 very clean).

Taiwan has a modern infrastructure and economy and a generally high standard of living. Life expectancy at birth in 2012 was estimated at 78.48 years, and per capita gross domestic product (GDP) in 2011 was estimated at $37,900; only 1.2 percent of the population lived below the poverty line in 2010. In 2000, the Gini Index (a measure of dispersion, in which perfect equality is denoted by 0 and maximum inequality is denoted by 100) for family income was 32.6.

Emergency Health Services

The National Taiwan University Hospital's Emergency Department was created in 1964, offering emergency care to the public, and became a division in 1972. In 1991, it was expanded and became the first emergency department in the country. The Taiwan Society of Emergency Medicine was founded in 1994, and in the same year, the first academic department of emergency medicine was established at National Taiwan University. Emergency medicine was recognized by the Department of Health as a medical specialty in 1997. Today, many hospitals in Taiwan have emergency medicine departments, including National Cheng Kung University in Tainan City, Cathay General Hospital, Chang Gung Memorial Hospital, Taiwan Adventist Hospital, and Chungshan Hospital in Taipei.

Insurance

Taiwan created its National Health Insurance (NHI) scheme in 1995; it is a single-payer social insurance program administered by the Bureau of National Health Insurance, but most medical services are delivered by private providers (that is, the providers are not employed by the NHI, but receive payments from it). Before creation of the NHI, only 59 percent of the Taiwanese population had insurance, with the uninsured being primarily children under age 14 and the elderly; before 1995, about half the medical expenditures were out of pocket. By the end of 1995, 92 percent of the Taiwanese population was insured, and out-of-pocket expenditures on medical care dropped to 30 percent of total expenditures; by 2010, 99 percent of the population was insured.

The NHI receives funding from mandated premiums paid by households and employers plus government funds to subsidize the contributions from some population groups. As of 2007, households (38 percent) and employers (37 percent) paid about equal shares of the system's costs, with government providing 25 percent of funding. For low-income households, military veterans and their survivors, and those serving in the military and their families, the government pays 100 percent of the costs of insurance.

Medical care is provided in clinics and hospitals paid directly by the Bureau of National Health Insurance; services provided include hospitalization, surgery, preventive care, medical care, medications, and prenatal care. Maternity care, preventive care, care of veterans and the poor, and care for certain illnesses are provided free; for other services, a copayment is required (for example, 20 percent of schedule fees for emergency care, 30 to 50 percent of scheduled fees for short-term inpatient care).

The maternity benefit is a lump sum payment equal to one month's average wages. The sickness benefit is 50 percent of average earnings for up to six months (up to 12 months if the person has been in the system for at least one year). The Bureau of National Health Insurance collects contributions and contracts with health care providers, the Bureau of Labor Insurance collects contributions and pays benefits, and the

Insurance Department of the Council of Labor Affairs supervises the system.

Costs of Hospitalization

Hospitals in Taiwan were traditionally paid on a fee-for-service basis, but a case-based, diagnosis-related group (DRG) system was introduced in 2002, and as of 2006, 53 DRGs were in use for inpatient care. Some pay-for-performance schemes have been introduced on an experimental basis beginning in 2001, and currently, hospitals in Taiwan have budget caps and receive a mix of case-based and per-diem payments. Patients pay extra fees for private and semiprivate rooms. Patients pay coinsurance for hospital stays, which average 5 to 10 percent, with higher charges for longer stays (a rule intended to discourage overuse).

Access to Health Care

Essentially, everyone in Taiwan is covered by the NHI plan, from cradle to grave, so issues such as health status or preexisting conditions do not interfere with a person having insurance and being able to receive care. Patients are free to choose their providers, and there is no mandatory gatekeeper system or waiting lists; however, a system was instituted in 2005 to offer financial incentives (lower copayments) for those who obtain referrals before seeking higher-level care. Fees for medical services are determined by the Bureau of National Health Insurance, and there is no balance billing allowed, so there is no reason for a physician to accept one patient while refusing another based on their ability to pay extra fees. One exception to this principle of equality is that people who require a medical device, such as an artificial knee, can choose between the standard device paid for by the NHI and a more expensive device and pay the difference out of pocket; for these devices, the Bureau of National Health Insurance publishes the prices of the different devices, so consumers can choose among them. Although bed occupancy in hospitals is about 67 percent, suggesting that hospital beds are oversupplied, this varies greatly by location. Many regional hospitals have low occupancy rates, while gaining a bed in one of the most popular urban hospitals, which offer the most up-to-date and high-tech care, may require spending several days waiting in the emergency room corridor before admittance.

Taiwan has an advanced information technology system for health care, which some consider the best in the world. Each resident has an NHI card with

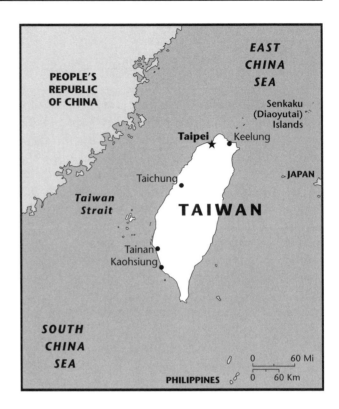

integrated circuitry that carries basic personal information (for example, name and date of birth); medical information about serious illnesses, prescriptions, allergies, and so on; records from their last six visits for care, including diagnosis; and premium payment history (as of 2007, 98 percent of Taiwanese were up to date on their insurance payments). This system records every medical care visit in real time, allowing national tracking of the volume of services delivered and monitoring of local disease outbreaks; patient-identifying information is scrambled to protect privacy.

Cost of Drugs

The cost of prescription drugs and Traditional Chinese Medicine (TCM) are covered under the NHI plan. Most types of drugs require copayments or coinsurance, but these are waived for some population classes (including low-income people, military veterans, and children up to 3 years) and for about 30 major diseases and conditions (including cancer, polio, hemophilia, and chronic mental illness).

Health Care Facilities

Most health care services in Taiwan are delivered through the private system; more than half (53 percent) of Taiwan's physicians work in private clinics, and 70 percent of hospital beds are in private institutions. Resources are concentrated in large hospitals and medical centers, where more high-tech care is available; in 2005, the 15 largest hospitals in the country performed 15 percent of all surgeries and employed 44 percent of hospital-based physicians and 32 percent of the total hospital-based workforce. Since institution of the NHI, the number of hospitals has decreased (a 29 percent drop between 1997 and 2007), while the number of clinics has increased (an increase of 16 percent from 1997 to 2007).

Major Health Issues

The leading causes of death in Taiwan in 2006 were malignant neoplasms, cerebrovascular disease, heart disease, diabetes mellitus, and accidents. The infant mortality rate, defined as the number of deaths of infants younger than 1 year, was 5.10 per 1,000 live births as of 2012 data.

Health Care Personnel

In 2006, Taiwan had 1.7 physicians per 1,000 population and 4.5 nurses per 1,000, a lower staffing level than many European countries (for example, Germany had 3.4 physicians per 1,000 and 9.7 nurses per 1,000), but comparable to other Asian countries, such as Korea. There are shortages of trained personnel in some specialties, including obstetrics and gynecology (OB/GYN), while higher-paying specialties such as cosmetic surgery and dermatology are attracting more practitioners.

Government Role in Health Care

Health care in Taiwan is paid for through the NHI program, funded by a combination of household, employer, and government contributions. Care is delivered primarily through private practitioners and providers; the government sets the fees that may be charged for services and also caps the budgets for hospitals and for the system as a whole. The delivery of services is monitored through an electronic data system, and reimbursement is based on a system of relative value units (RVUs). For instance, a particular service may be valued at 250 RVUs; the dollar amount of an RVU fluctuates based on the volume of services provided (more services on a national basis equal a lower dollar value for an RVU), and providers are paid based on the services provided and the value of an RVU during the time period when the services

were provided. This system allows the government to set a global budget for health care.

Public Health Programs

According to the World Higher Education Database (WHED), 13 universities in Taiwan offer programs in epidemiology or public health.

TAJIKISTAN

Tajikistan is a landlocked central Asian country sharing borders with Afghanistan, China, Kyrgyzstan, and Uzbekistan. The area of 55,251 square miles (143,100 square kilometers) makes Tajikistan about the size of Wisconsin, and the July 2012 population was estimated at 7.8 million. In 2010, 26 percent of the population lived in urban areas, and the 2010 to 2015 annual rate of urbanization was estimated at 2.2 percent. Dushanbe is the capital and largest city (with a 2009 population estimated at 1,704,000). The population growth rate in 2012 was 1.8 percent, the net migration rate negative 1.2 migrants per 1,000 population, the birth rate 25.9 births per 1,000, and the total fertility rate 2.8 children per woman. The United Nations High Commissioner for Refugees (UNHCR) estimated that, in 2010, there were 2,053 refugees and persons in refugee-like situations in Tajikistan.

Tajikistan came under Russian domination in the mid-19th century; that control was weakened during the Russian Revolution but was reestablished in 1925. Tajikistan contains a large Uzbek minority because, during the Soviet period, a large part of what is now Sughd province was transferred from the Uzbek SSR to the Tajik SSR. Tajikistan became an independent country in 1991; the country experienced a civil war from 1992 to 1997 and several security incidents in 2010. Tajikistan ranked tied for 152nd among 183 countries on the *Corruption Perceptions Index 2011*, with a score of 2.3 (on a scale where 0 indicates highly corrupt and 10 very clean).

In 2011, Tajikistan was classified as a country with medium human development (the second from the lowest of four categories) on the United Nations Development Programme's (UNDP's) Human Development Index (HDI), with a score of 0.607 (on a scale where 1 denotes high development and 0 low development). Life expectancy at birth in 2012 was estimated

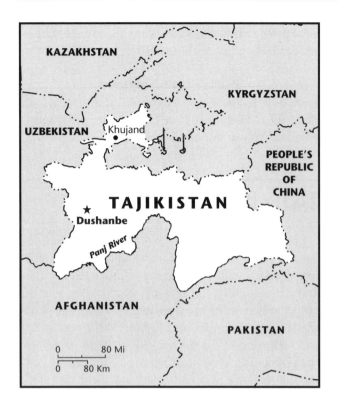

at 66.38 years, and estimated gross domestic product (GDP) per capita in 2011 was $2,000. In 2006, the Gini Index (a measure of dispersion, in which perfect equality is denoted by 0 and maximum inequality is denoted by 100) for family income was 32.6. According to the World Economic Forum's *Global Gender Gap Index 2011*, Tajikistan ranked 96th out of 135 countries on gender equality with a score of 0.653 (on a scale with a theoretical range of 1 for equality to 0 for inequality and an actual range in 2011 from 0.8530 to 0.4873).

Emergency Health Services

According to the World Health Organization (WHO), all national, district, and regional hospitals in Tajikistan have ambulance services, although many lack modern means of communication; the country also has specialized emergency hospitals. Emergency care is provided free of charge.

Insurance

Tajikistan does not have a national insurance plan, and private insurance plays a minor role; instead, subsidized services are provided at government facilities or paid for out of pocket. The government is the primary provider and funder of health care

in Tajikistan. National-level health care services are administered by the Ministry of Health, while local authorities are in charge of most health care services at the regional, district, and peripheral levels. Copayments for government-provided health care services were introduced in 2003, but many population groups were exempt, including pregnant women, children up to age 5, World War II veterans, and those suffering from specific diseases, including tuberculosis, cancer, asthma, diabetes, mental disorders, and some blood diseases. The national government has encouraged the development of private medical services, and the World Bank estimated, in 2007, that the majority of expenditures for health care were out of pocket rather than government expenditures. Many nongovernmental organizations (NGOs) also provide services in Tajikistan.

Costs of Hospitalization

According to Tajikistan's 1994 constitution, health care is a right for the population. However, copayments are required of most people, and informal payments also seem to be common (a 2007 study found a typical payment was $40 for a hospital patient).

Access to Health Care

The government is the primary provider and funder of health care in Tajikistan. National-level health care services are administered by the Ministry of Health, while local authorities are in charge of most health care services at the regional, district, and peripheral levels. Standards of care are generally higher in urban as opposed to rural areas, and access to care is also easier because less travel is required.

According to WHO, in 2007, 88.4 percent of births in Tajikistan were attended by skilled personnel (for example, physicians, nurses, or midwives), and 80 percent of pregnant women received at least four prenatal care visits. The 2010 immunization rates for 1-year-olds were 93 percent for diphtheria and pertussis (DPT3), 94 percent for measles (MCV), and 93 percent for Hib (Hib3). In 2010, an estimated 16 percent of persons with advanced human immunodeficiency virus (HIV) infection were receiving antiretroviral therapy in accordance with the 2010 WHO guidelines.

Cost of Drugs

A 2005 survey of the costs and availability of a market basket of core medicines concluded that the high cost of medicines in Tajikistan created a heavy burden on

Selected Health Indicators: Tajikistan Compared With the Global Average (2010)

	Tajikistan	Global Average
Male life expectancy at birth* (years)	66	66
Female life expectancy at birth* (years)	69	71
Under-5 mortality rate, both sexes (per 1,000 live births)	63	57
Adult mortality rate, both sexes* (probability of dying between 15 and 60 years per 1,000 population)	171	176
Maternal mortality ratio (per 100,000 live births)	65	210
HIV prevalence* (per 1,000 adults aged 15 to 49)	2	8
Tuberculosis prevalence (per 100,000 population)	382	178

Source: World Health Organization Global Health Observatory Data Repository.
*Data refers to 2009.

both the national health budget and individual family incomes. There is no national policy promoting the use of generics. The median price ratio (comparing the price in Tajikistan to the international reference price) in the private sector was 2.39 for the lowest-priced generics (meaning the price in Tajikistan was more than twice as high as the international reference price), 2.34 for the most-sold generics, and 42.58 for innovator brands. In the public sector, only a few innovator brands were available. The median price ratio for the lowest-priced generics was 2.36 and, for the most-sold generics, 2.33.

Mean availability in both the public and private sectors was more than 80 percent for some common drugs, including amoxicillin, ciprofloxacin, furosemide, ibuprofen, salbutamol, diclofenac, and metronidazole; however, other basic medicines had availabilities under 10 percent in one or both sectors, including metformin, amitryptline, and phenytoin. Even using generic drugs purchased in the public sector, treatment for many common conditions was not affordable. Using the standard of the lowest-paid government worker, it would require 3.15 days' wages to purchase amoxicillin for a course of treatment for pneumonia if the lowest-priced generics were purchased in the public sector; the same drugs in the private sector would cost 7.9 days' wages. To treat hypertension for a month would require 27 days' wages for generic drugs purchased in the public sector

or 30 days' wages for generic drugs purchased in the private sector.

Health Care Facilities

In 2006, Tajikistan had 426 hospitals and 3,003 outpatient care facilities; the latter include health posts, health centers, polyclinics, and specialized centers (providing services such as reproductive health, family medicine, or pediatrics). As of 2010, according to WHO, Tajikistan had 24.73 health posts per 100,000 population, 12.21 health centers per 100,000, 3.62 district or rural hospitals per 100,000, 1.92 provincial hospitals per 100,000, and 0.04 specialized hospitals per 100,000. In 2008, Tajikistan had 5.41 hospital beds per 1,000 population, among the 50 highest rates in the world.

Major Health Issues

In 2008, WHO estimated that 62 percent of years of life lost in Tajikistan were due to communicable diseases, 32 percent to noncommunicable diseases, and 6 percent to injuries. In 2008, the age-standardized estimate of cancer deaths was 84 per 100,000 for men and 81 per 100,000 for women; for cardiovascular disease and diabetes, 483 per 100,000 for men and 562 per 100,000 for women; and for chronic respiratory disease, 33 per 100,000 for men and 43 per 100,000 for women.

Tajikistan's maternal mortality rate (death from any cause related to or aggravated by pregnancy) was estimated in 2008 as 64 maternal deaths per 100,000 live births. The infant mortality rate, defined as the number of deaths of infants younger than 1 year, was estimated at 37.33 per 1,000 live births as of 2012. In 2005, 14.9 percent of children under age 5 were underweight (defined as 2 kilograms [kg] below standard weight-for-age at age 1, 3 kg below for ages 2 to 3, and 4 kg below for ages 4 to 5). In 2010, tuberculosis incidence was 206.0 per 100,000 population, tuberculosis prevalence 382.0 per 100,000, and deaths due to tuberculosis among HIV-negative people 41.0 per 100,000. As estimated, 17 percent of new tuberculosis cases and 62 percent of retreatment cases are multidrug resistant. As of 2009, an estimated 0.2 percent of adults age 15 to 49 were living with HIV or acquired immune deficiency syndrome (AIDS).

Health Care Personnel

Tajikistan has one medical school, the Tadzhik Medical Institute Im. Abu-Ali'ibn Sina in Dushanbe, which began offering instruction in 1939. In 2006, Tajikistan had 2.01 physicians per 1,000 population, 0.16 dentistry personnel per 1,000, and 5.03 nurses and midwives per 1,000, and in 2003, had 0.11 pharmaceutical personnel per 1,000. Most health care personnel are salaried state employees, and their average wages are lower than the national average wage, making it difficult to retain personnel in the state system (jobs with NGOs, for instance, pay much better). Low salaries have also encouraged medical personnel to collect informal payments from patients; a 2007 survey found that such payments totaled $40 per hospitalized patient and $10 per ambulatory payment, indicating that physicians and nurses may earn more of their incomes from these payments than from their official salaries.

Government Role in Health Care

According to WHO, in 2010, Tajikistan spent $338 million on health care, an amount that comes to $49 per capita. Most (94 percent) of health care funding came from domestic sources, with 6 percent coming from abroad. The largest share of health care spending was provided through household expenditures (67 percent), with the remainder coming from government expenditures (27 percent) and other sources (7 percent). In 2010, Tajikistan allocated 6 percent of its total government expenditures to health, in the low range for low-income Asian countries; government expenditures on health came to 2 percent of GDP, in the low range for low-income Asian countries. In

2009, according to WHO, official development assistance (ODA) for health in Tajikistan came to $4.51 per capita.

Public Health Programs

In 2010, 94 percent of the population in Tajikistan had access to improved sanitation facilities (94 percent in rural areas and 95 percent in urban), and 64 percent had access to improved sources of drinking water (54 percent in rural areas and 92 percent in urban).

TANZANIA

Tanzania is an east African country, sharing borders with Burundi, the Democratic Republic of the Congo, Kenya, Malawi, Mozambique, Rwanda, Uganda, and Zambia, and having a coastline on the Indian Ocean; Tanzania includes Mafia, Pemba, and Zanzibar. The area of 342,009 square miles (885,800 square kilometers) makes Tanzania about twice the size of California, and the July 2012 population was estimated at 43.6 million. In 2010, 26 percent of the population lived in urban areas, and the 2010 to 2015 annual rate of urbanization was estimated at 4.7 percent. Dar es Salaam is the capital and largest city (with a 2009 population estimated at 3.2 million). The population growth rate in 2012 was 2.0 percent, the net migration rate negative 0.3 migrants per 1,000 population, the birth rate 31.8 births per 1,000, and the total fertility rate 4.0 children per woman. The United Nations High Commissioner for Refugees (UNHCR) estimated that, in 2010, there were 109,286 refugees and persons in refugee-like situations in Tanzania.

The former British colony Tanganyika achieved independence in 1961 and merged with Zanzibar to form Tanzania in 1964. According to the Ibrahim Index, in 2011, Tanzania ranked 12th among 53 African countries in terms of governance performance, with a score of 58 (out of 100). Tanzania ranked tied for 100th among 183 countries on the *Corruption Perceptions Index 2011,* with a score of 3.0 (on a scale where 0 indicates highly corrupt and 10 very clean).

In 2011, Tanzania was classified as a country with low human development (the lowest of four categories) on the United Nations Development Programme's (UNDP's) Human Development Index (HDI), with a score of 0.466 (on a scale where 1 denotes high development and 0 low development). In 2011, the International Food Policy Research Institute (IFPRI) classified Tanzania as a country with an "alarming" hunger problem, with a Global Hunger Index (GHI) score of 20.5 (where 0 reflects no hunger and higher scores more hunger). Life expectancy at birth in 2012 was estimated at 53.14 years, among the 20 lowest in the world, and estimated gross domestic product (GDP) per capita in 2011 was $1,500, among the 30 lowest in the world. In 2007, the Gini Index (a measure of dispersion, in which perfect equality is denoted by 0 and maximum inequality is denoted by 100) for family income was 37.6. According to the World Economic Forum's *Global Gender Gap Index 2011*, Tanzania ranked 59th out of 135 countries on gender equality, with a score of 0.690 (on a scale with a theoretical range of 1 for equality to 0 for inequality and an actual range in 2011 from 0.8530 to 0.4873).

Emergency Health Services

According to the World Health Organization (WHO), as of 2007, Tanzania did not have a formal and publicly available system for providing prehospital care (emergency care). The Tanzanian Red Cross assisted more than 23,000 victims of the January 2010 floods in Tanzania, assisted by the International Federation of Red Cross and Red Crescent Societies.

Insurance

Tanzania has a social insurance system providing medical benefits and cash maternity benefits, as provided in the 1997 National Social Security Fund Act No. 28. The system includes private-sector workers, those working in cooperatives and other organized groups, public employees, and the self-employed; household workers are excluded, and some self-employed workers and employees of private companies are covered under a separate parastatal system. Voluntary coverage is possible. The system is funded through the same system that covers old-age and disability pensions and includes contributions from wages (10 percent of gross earnings), the self-employed and voluntary joiners (20 percent of declared income, with a floor of 20 percent of the legal minimum wage), and employers (10 percent of gross payroll). Medical benefits are provided through accredited hospitals under agreement with the National Social Security Fund and include inpatient and outpatient care.

Eligible dependents, including the insured's spouse and up to four children, are entitled to the same benefits as the insured; children are covered to age 18, or age 21 if enrolled full time in school. Maternity care is provided from the 24th week of pregnancy to two days after birth, with an extension to seven days after birth for a cesarean section and up to 12 weeks if necessary. Cash maternity benefits are 100 percent of average wages for up to 12 weeks. The system is administered by the National Social Security Fund under the general supervision of the Ministry of Labour and Employment. According to a 2009 South African Development Community survey, about 10 percent of the population of Tanzania was covered by public health insurance.

Costs of Hospitalization

No data available.

Access to Health Care

According to WHO, in 2010, 50.6 percent of births in Tanzania were attended by skilled personnel (for example, physicians, nurses, or midwives). In 2005, 62 percent of pregnant women received at least four prenatal care visits. The 2010 immunization rates for 1-year-olds were 91 percent for diphtheria and pertussis (DPT3), 92 percent for measles (MCV), and 91 percent for Hib (Hib3). In 2010, an estimated 42 percent of persons with advanced human immunodeficiency virus (HIV) infection were receiving antiretroviral therapy in accordance with the 2010 WHO guidelines. According to WHO, in 2010, Tanzania had 0.05 magnetic resonance imaging (MRI) machines per 1 million population, 0.14 computer tomography (CT) machines per 1 million, 0.02 positron emission tomography (PET) machines per 1 million, 0.07 telecolbalt units per 1 million, and 0.07 radiotherapy machines per 1 million.

Cost of Drugs

The Medical Stores department is in charge of procurement and distribution in the public sector for Tanzania. Most medicines require a copayment based on income, but medicines are provided free to certain populations groups, including children under age 5, pregnant women, the elderly, and the poor. Medicines to treat some conditions are also provided free, including medicines on the Essential Medicines List (EML) and those to treat malaria, tuberculosis, sexually transmitted disease (STD), and human immunodeficiency virus/acquired immune deficiency syndrome (HIV/AIDS); vaccines on WHO's Expanded Programme on Immunization (EPI) list are also provided free. In 2001, per capita public spending on medicine was approximately $6. A 2004 survey by the Tanzanian Ministry of Health of the cost and availability of a market basket of common medicines found that many had low availability or high prices or both and that, for the drugs necessary to treat many common conditions, the lowest-paid government worker would have to spend more than one day's wages, particularly if drugs had to be purchased in the private sector.

Procurement prices for the lowest-priced generic medicines in the public sector were generally low, with a median reference price of 0.69, meaning that, on average, the price in Tanzania was 31 percent below the international reference price. Patient prices in the public sector had a median price index of 1.33 (indicating an approximate 100 percent markup), with a wide range from 0.29 for omeprazole to 8.17 for albendazole. Innovator brands are not distributed in public-sector facilities, and only three innovator brands were found in private facilities. Prices for the lowest-priced generics were generally higher than in the public sector, with a median reference price of 2.67. In the nongovernmental (NGO) sector, the median reference price for the lowest-priced generic was 2.90. The median availability for the lowest-priced generics in private pharmacies was 47.9 percent and was 41.9 percent in NGO facilities.

Health Care Facilities

Health services in Tanzania are organized in a hierarchical structure, from the village health service through dispensaries, health centers, district hospitals, regional hospitals, and referral hospitals. In the public sector, in 2007, Tanzania had 78 hospitals, 409 health centers, and 2,450 dispensaries; in the private sector in 2007, there were 121 hospitals, 126 registered health centers, and 1,340 registered dispensaries. More than half the private hospitals and health centers were located in rural areas. In 2006, Tanzania had 1.10 hospital beds per 1,000 population.

Major Health Issues

In 2008, WHO estimated that 78 percent of years of life lost in Tanzania were due to communicable diseases, 13 percent to noncommunicable diseases, and 8 percent to injuries. In 2008, the age-standardized estimate of cancer deaths was 79 per 100,000 for men and 74 per 100,000 for women; for cardiovascular disease and diabetes, 473 per 100,000 for men and 382 per 100,000 for women; and for chronic respiratory disease, 130 per 100,000 for men and 52 per 100,000 for women. In 2008, the age-standardized death rate from malaria was 49.3 per 100,000 population.

Tanzania's maternal mortality rate (death from any cause related to or aggravated by pregnancy) is quite high by global standards, estimated at 790 maternal deaths per 100,000 live births as of 2008. A 2004 survey estimated the prevalence of female genital mutilation at 14.6 percent. The infant mortality rate, defined as the number of deaths of infants younger than 1 year, also has been high, at 65.74 per 1,000 live births in 2012. In 2005, 16.7 percent of children under age 5 were underweight (defined as 2 kilograms [kg] below standard weight-for-age at age 1, 3 kg below for ages 2 to 3, and 4 kg below for ages 4 to 5).

In 2010, tuberculosis incidence was 177.0 per 100,000 population, tuberculosis prevalence 183.0 per 100,000, and deaths due to tuberculosis among HIV-negative people 13.0 per 100,000. WHO estimated the 2010 case detection rate at 77 percent. As of 2009, an estimated 5.6 percent of adults age 15 to 49 were living with HIV or AIDS. As of 2009, an estimated 1.4 million people in Tanzania were living with HIV or AIDS, the fifth-largest number in the world. In 2010, 86 percent of pregnant women tested positive for HIV. The mother-to-child transmission rate for HIV in 2010 was estimated at 25 percent, and in 2009, 5.6 percent of deaths to children under age 5 were attributed to HIV.

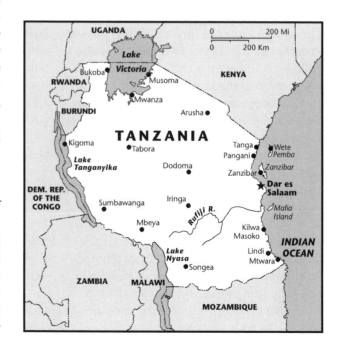

Health Care Personnel

Tanzania has two medical schools, the College of Health Sciences of the Institute of Public Health in the University of Dar es Salaam and Kilimanjaro Christian Medical College of Tumaini University in Moshi. The course of training for a basic medical degree lasts five years, and the degree awarded is doctor of medicine. In 2006, Tanzania had 0.01 physicians per 1,000 population, 0.01 laboratory health workers per 1,000, 0.01 dentistry personnel per 1,000, and 0.24 nurses and midwives per 1,000. Michael Clemens and Bunilla Petterson estimate that 52 percent of Tanzania-born physicians and 4 percent of Tanzania-born nurses are working in one of nine developed countries, primarily in the United Kingdom and the United States.

Government Role in Health Care

The right to health, including access to essential medicines and medical technologies, is recognized in national legislation. Tanzania has a National Health Policy (NHP), created in 2007, and a plan to implement the NHP, created in 2009; it also has a National Medicines Policy (NMP), created in 1991, and an implementation plan for the NMP, created in 1992. The NMP covers selection of essential medicines; financing, pricing, purchase, distribution, and regulation of drugs; pharmacovigilance; rational usage of medicines; human resource development; research; evaluation and monitoring; and traditional medicine. National law in Tanzania allows compulsory licensing of pharmaceutical products in the interests of public health.

According to WHO, in 2010, Tanzania spent $1.4 billion on health care, or $31 per capita. About half (51 percent) of health care funding came from domestic sources, with 49 percent coming from abroad. The largest share of health care spending was provided through government expenditures (67 percent), with the remainder coming from household expenditures (14 percent) and other sources (19 percent). In 2010, Tanzania allocated 14 percent of its total government expenditures to health, in the low range for low-income African countries; government expenditures on health came to 4 percent of GDP, in the low range for low-income African countries. In 2009, according to WHO, official development assistance (ODA) for health in Tanzania came to $17.92 per capita.

Public Health Programs

Tanzania's National Institute for Medical Research (NIMR) is located in Dar es Salaam and is headed by Mwele Ntuli Malecela. The NIMR is located within the Ministry of Health and, in 1980, took over Tanzania's health research institutions, which had been administered previously by the East African Medical Research Council. The goals of the NIMR are to improve disease control, prevention, and management; specific activities include researching diseases common in Tanzania, researching traditional medical practices, providing training for local personnel, and monitoring and evaluating medical research carried out within Tanzania.

According to WHO, in 2002, Tanzania had 0.05 environmental and public health workers per 1,000 population. In 2010, 10 percent of the population had access to improved sanitation facilities (7 percent in rural areas and 20 percent in urban), and 53 percent had access to improved sources of drinking water (44 percent in rural areas and 79 percent in urban). According to the World Higher Education Database (WHED), five universities in Tanzania offer programs in epidemiology or public health: the Hubert Kairuki Memorial University in Dar es Salaam, the Sokoine University of Agriculture in Morogoro, the International Medical and Technical University in Dar es Salaam, Kilimanjaro Christian Medical College in Moshi, and Muhimbili University of Health and Allied Sciences in Dar es Salaam.

THAILAND

Thailand is a southeastern Asian country, sharing borders with Myanmar, Cambodia, Laos, and Malaysia and having a coastline on the North Sea. The area of 198,117 square miles (513,120 square kilometers) makes Thailand about twice the size of Wyoming, and the July 2012 population was estimated at 67.1 million (the 20th-largest in the world). In 2010, 34 percent of the population lived in urban areas, and the 2010 to 2015 annual rate of urbanization was estimated at 1.8 percent. Bangkok is the capital and largest city (with a 2009 population estimated at 6.9 million). The population growth rate in 2012 was 0.5 percent, the net migration rate 0.0 migrants per 1,000 population, the birth rate 12.8 births per 1,000, and the total fertility rate 1.7 children per woman. The United Nations High Commissioner for Refugees (UNHCR) estimated that, in 2010, there were 96,675 refugees and persons in refugee-like situations in Thailand.

Thailand is the only country in southeast Asia to never have been colonized. Since 1932, Thailand has been a constitutional monarchy. Thailand ranked tied for 80th among 183 countries on the *Corruption Perceptions Index 2011*, with a score of 3.4 (on a scale where 0 indicates highly corrupt and 10 very clean). In 2011, Thailand was classified as a country with medium human development (the second from the lowest of four categories) on the United Nations Development Programme's (UNDP's) Human Development Index (HDI), with a score of 0.682 (on a scale where 1 denotes high development and 0 low development).

Life expectancy at birth in 2012 was estimated at 73.83 years, and per capita gross domestic product (GDP) in 2011 was estimated at $9,700. Income distribution in Thailand is relatively unequal: In 2009, the Gini Index (a measure of dispersion, in which perfect equality is denoted by 0 and maximum inequality is denoted by 100) for family income was 53.6, among the highest in the world. According to the World Economic Forum's *Global Gender Gap Index 2011*, Thailand ranked 60th out of 135 countries on gender equality, with a score of 0.689 (on a scale with a theoretical range of 1 for equality to 0 for inequality and an actual range in 2011 from 0.8530 to 0.4873).

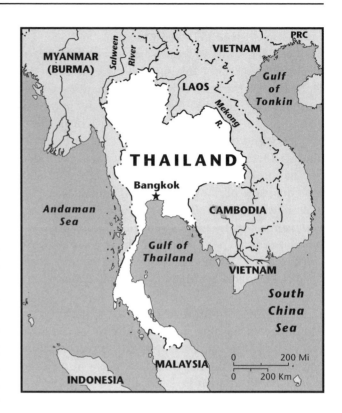

Emergency Health Services

According to the World Health Organization (WHO), as of 2007, Thailand had a formal and publicly available emergency care (prehospital care) system accessible through a national access number. Doctors Without Borders (Médecins Sans Frontières, or MSF) began working in Thailand in 1976 and had 41 staff members in the country at the close of 2010. MSF provides basic health care in Samut Sakhon province, an area where many undocumented migrants come to seek work, and in the Three Pagodas Pass area, where many migrant workers cross the Thailand–Myanmar border daily. Besides providing basic health care, MSF provided care to victims of postelection violence in Myanmar (in November 2010). MSF also trains "backpackers" from Myanmar to provide basic health services in Myanmar and provides support for malaria control in Myanmar from the Thai side of the border.

Insurance

Thailand has a social insurance system covering employees ages 15 to 60, with voluntary coverage for the self-employed. Temporary and seasonal workers are excluded, as are employees of foreign or international organizations and workers in agriculture, forestry, and fisheries. Judges, civil servants, employees of private schools, and employees of state enterprises are covered under separate systems. The system is funded by contributions from wage earners (1.5 percent of gross monthly earnings), voluntary contributors (an annual contribution of THB 3,360, which also funds disability and survivor benefits), employers (1.5 percent of monthly payroll), and the government (1.5 percent of gross monthly earnings).

To receive medical benefits, the insured must register with a hospital contracted with the health system and receive treatment in that hospital (emergency care and treatment for accidental injuries excepted); other care received outside the registered hospital is reimbursed following a fixed schedule. Covered services include medical treatment, hospitalization, medications, rehabilitation, and ambulance fees. A woman married to, or cohabiting with, an insured man is entitled to maternity care. The maternity benefit is 50 percent of average wages for up to 90 days; the cash sickness benefit is 50 percent of the average wage for up to 90 days; up to 180 days are covered per year, although in the case of a chronic condition, that may be increased to 365 days. The Social Security Office contracts with contractors to provide medical care, collects contributions, and administers cash benefits; the Ministry of Labor supervises the system.

Thailand introduced the so-called 30-bhat scheme, a plan for universal social coverage, in 2002. This plan offered basic care as well as services such as surgery, emergency care, and radiotherapy, but not dialysis; the latter was excluded due to the expense (dialysis cost about four times the quality-adjusted life year threshold then in force). However, many suffering renal failure were found to come from the poorest sector of society, and those individuals often exhausted their resources paying for treatment; in 2008, public pressure caused the government to add dialysis to the program. According to Ke Xu and colleagues, in 2003, 0.8 percent of households in Thailand experienced catastrophic health expenditures annually; "catastrophic" was defined as exceeding 40 percent of household income remaining after basic needs were met.

Costs of Hospitalization

No data available.

Access to Health Care

According to WHO, in 2009, 99.4 percent of births in Thailand were attended by skilled personnel (for example, physicians, nurses, or midwives), and 80 percent of pregnant women received at least four prenatal care visits. The 2010 immunization rates for 1-year-olds were 99 percent for diphtheria and pertussis (DPT3) and 98 percent for measles (MCV). In 2010, an estimated 67 percent of persons with advanced human immunodeficiency virus (HIV) infection were receiving antiretroviral therapy in accordance with the 2010 WHO guidelines. According to WHO, in 2010, Thailand had 0.89 magnetic resonance imaging (MRI) machines per 1 million population, 5.92 computer tomography (CT) machines per 1 million, 0.07 positron emission tomography (PET) machines per 1 million, 0.34 telecolbalt units per 1 million, and 0.34 radiotherapy machines per 1 million.

Cost of Drugs

According to Thailand's Drug Act, revised in 2003, manufacturers of medicines must have good management practices (GMP) certification, and generic drugs must provide evidence of bioequivalence. Drugs for each public hospital are selected by a Pharmacy and Therapeutic Committee, and the drugs may be obtained through group purchasing. Patients often buy prescription medicines from pharmacies located within hospitals rather than from drug stores or pharmacies in the community. Markups were variable and could be quite high: A 2006 survey found that cumulative markups for medicines ranged from 20 percent to more than 200 percent and, in the private sector, from 37 percent to 900 percent.

A 2006 survey found that medicines were not affordable for many Thai citizens using the standard that not more than 1 day's wages of the lowest-paid government worker should be required to purchase medicines to treat common illnesses. For acute diseases, purchase of generics to treat a respiratory infection would require 0.1 to 3.3 days' wages, depending on the specific medicine and where it was purchased, and originator brands would cost 0.2 to 5.0 days' wages. For common chronic conditions, a course of treatment required from 0.1 to 3.9 days' wages for generics purchased in the public sphere and from 0.1 to 5.3 days' wages for drugs purchased in the private sphere. The median price ratio in the public sector for the lowest-priced generic drugs was 1.46, meaning the procurement price was on average 46 percent higher than the international reference price. For the most-sold generics, the median price ratio was 3.3. Only a few originator brands were procured for the public sector, and their prices averaged 2.7 times the price of the lowest-priced generics to treat the same condition. Patient prices were higher: For the lowest-priced generics, the median price ratio was 2.55. The lowest-priced generics were more available in the public sphere (median availability 75 percent) than originator brands (median availability 10 percent). In the private sector, prices were much higher, with a median price ratio of 11.6, and availability was low at 28.6 percent for both the lowest-priced generics and originator brands.

Health Care Facilities

As of 2010, according to WHO, Thailand had 41.00 health posts per 100,000 population, 1.07 district or rural hospitals per 100,000, 0.60 provincial hospitals per 100,000, and 0.12 specialized hospitals per 100,000. In 2002, Thailand had 2.20 hospital beds per 1,000 population.

Major Health Issues

In 2008, WHO estimated that 24 percent of years of life lost in Thailand were due to communicable diseases,

55 percent to noncommunicable diseases, and 22 percent to injuries. In 2008, the age-standardized estimate of cancer deaths was 115 per 100,000 for men and 96 per 100,000 for women; for cardiovascular disease and diabetes, 343 per 100,000 for men and 280 per 100,000 for women; and for chronic respiratory disease, 114 per 100,000 for men and 30 per 100,000 for women.

In 2008, the age-standardized death rate from malaria was 0.5 per 100,000 population. In 2010, tuberculosis incidence was 137.0 per 100,000 population, tuberculosis prevalence 182.0 per 100,000, and deaths due to tuberculosis among HIV-negative people 16.00 per 100,000. WHO estimated the 2010 case detection rate at 70 percent. As of 2009, an estimated 1.3 percent of adults age 15 to 49 were living with HIV or acquired immune deficiency syndrome (AIDS).

Thailand's maternal mortality rate (death from any cause related to or aggravated by pregnancy) was estimated in 2008 as 48 maternal deaths per 100,000 live births. The infant mortality rate, defined as the number of deaths of infants younger than 1 year, was estimated at 15.90 per 1,000 live births in 2012.

Health Care Personnel

Thailand has 12 medical schools. The basic medical degree course lasts five or six years, and the degree granted is doctor of medicine. Three years of government service employment in a rural area is required after graduation. The Medical Office of the Ministry of Public Health grants graduates from public medical facilities the license to practice medicine, while graduates of private medical schools or foreign schools must take a licensing exam. In 2004, Thailand had 0.30 physicians per 1,000 population, 0.12 pharmaceutical personnel per 1,000, 0.07 dentistry personnel per 1,000, and 1.52 nurses and midwives per 1,000, and in 2000, had 1.93 health management and support workers and 0.65 community and traditional health workers per 1,000.

Government Role in Health Care

According to WHO, in 2010, Thailand spent $2.4 billion on health care, an amount that comes to $123 per capita. All health care funding came from domestic sources. The largest share of health care spending was provided through government expenditures (75 percent), with the remainder coming from household expenditures (14 percent) and other sources (11 percent). In 2010, Thailand allocated 13 percent of its total government expenditures to health, in the high range

for upper-middle-income southeast Asian region countries; government expenditures on health came to 3 percent of GDP, in the low range for upper-middle-income southeast Asian region countries. In 2009, according to WHO, official development assistance (ODA) for health in Thailand came to $0.96 per capita.

Public Health Programs

Thailand's National Institute of Health (NIH) is located in Nonthaburi and is headed by Pathorn Sawanpanyalert. The NIH focuses on infectious diseases, particularly influenza. It is located within the Ministry of Public Health and has approximately 450 staff members. The National Influenza Center (NIC) is engaged in improving the surveillance system and diagnostic process for influenza; it developed a rapid-response system for testing novel strains of the H1N1 virus and monitored drug-resistant strains of the flu virus during the 2009 pandemic.

According to WHO, in 2001, Thailand had 0.04 environmental and public health workers per 1,000 population. In 2010, 96 percent of the population had access to improved sanitation facilities (96 percent in rural areas and 95 percent in urban), and 96 percent had access to improved sources of drinking water (95 percent in rural areas and 97 percent in urban). According to the World Higher Education Database (WHED), 14 universities in Thailand offer programs in epidemiology or public health.

TIMOR-LESTE (EAST TIMOR)

Timor-Leste (East Timor) is a country in southeast Asia, occupying the eastern half of the island of Timor and sharing a border with Indonesia. The area of 5,743 square miles (14,874 square kilometers) makes East Timor slightly larger than Connecticut, and the July 2012 population was estimated at 1.2 million. In 2010, 28 percent of the population lived in urban areas, and the 2010 to 2015 annual rate of urbanization was estimated at 5.0 percent. Dili is the capital and largest city (with a 2009 population estimated at 166,000). The population growth rate in 2012 was 2.0 percent, the birth rate 25.4 births per 1,000 population, and the total fertility rate 3.1 children per woman.

East Timor was a Portuguese colony; following invasion and occupation by Indonesian forces in 1976, it was incorporated into Indonesia. Much of the country's infrastructure was destroyed during a two-decade struggle for independence, and an estimated 100,000 to 250,000 people were killed (with even more forced into exile). International peacekeepers helped end the conflict, and East Timor was internationally recognized as an independent country in 2002. East Timor ranked tied for 143rd among 183 countries on the *Corruption Perceptions Index 2011,* with a score of 2.4 (on a scale where 0 indicates highly corrupt and 10 very clean).

In 2011, East Timor was classified as a country with low human development (the lowest of four categories) on the United Nations Development Programme's (UNDP's) Human Development Index (HDI), with a score of 0.495 (on a scale where 1 denotes high development and 0 low development). In 2011, the International Food Policy Research Institute (IFPRI) classified East Timor as a country with an "alarming" hunger problem, with a Global Hunger Index (GHI) score of 27.1, the seventh-highest in the world. Life expectancy at birth in 2012 was estimated at 68.27 years, and estimated gross domestic product (GDP) per capita in 2011 was $3,100. In 2007, the Gini Index (a measure of dispersion, in which perfect equality is denoted by 0 and maximum inequality is denoted by 100) for family income was estimated at 31.9.

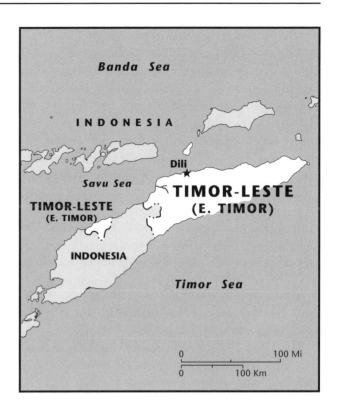

Emergency Health Services

According to the World Health Organization (WHO), as of 2007, East Timor had a formal and publicly available emergency care (prehospital care) system accessible through a national access number.

Insurance

No data available.

Costs of Hospitalization

No data available.

Access to Health Care

According to WHO, in 2010, 29.6 percent of births in East Timor were attended by skilled personnel (for example, physicians, nurses, or midwives), and 55 percent of pregnant women received at least four prenatal care visits. The 2010 immunization rates for 1-year-olds were 72 percent for diphtheria and pertussis (DPT3) and 66 percent for measles (MCV). Child malnutrition is a serious problem: In 2002, 40.6 percent of children under age 5 were underweight (defined as 2 kilograms [kg] below standard weight-for-age at age 1, 3 kg below for ages 2 to 3, and 4 kg below for ages 4 to 5), one of the highest rates in the world.

Cost of Drugs

No data available.

Health Care Facilities

Health care facilities under colonial rule were poorly developed, although this improved somewhat in 1951, when East Timor became an overseas province of Portugal; however, many of the improvements in medical care benefited primarily the Europeans in the country. In 1975, East Timor had only one hospital (in Dili), one surgeon, and one dentist, although some care was provided by physicians in the Portuguese army. The Indonesian government built many health facilities in part to counter the desire for independence; when the country became independent, many of these facilities were destroyed by the pro-Indonesian militia. Doctors Without Borders (Médecins Sans Frontières, or MSF) began providing medical services in the country beginning in September 1999 to provide immediate patient care and to help the country rebuild its medical infrastructure.

Major Health Issues

In 2008, WHO estimated that 76 percent of years of life lost in East Timor were due to communicable diseases, 18 percent to noncommunicable diseases, and 6 percent to injuries. In 2008, the age-standardized estimate of cancer deaths was 122 per 100,000 for men and 96 per 100,000 for women; for cardiovascular disease and diabetes, 359 per 100,000 for men and 276 per 100,000 for women; and for chronic respiratory disease, 78 per 100,000 for men and 50 per 100,000 for women.

In 2008, the age-standardized death rate from malaria was 94.4 per 100,000 population, the eighth-highest in the world. In 2010, tuberculosis incidence was 498.0 per 100,000 population, tuberculosis prevalence 643.0 per 100,000, and deaths due to tuberculosis among human immunodeficiency virus (HIV)-negative people 46.00 per 100,000.

East Timor's maternal mortality rate (death from any cause related to or aggravated by pregnancy) is high by global standards, estimated at 370 maternal deaths per 100,000 live births as of 2008. The infant mortality rate, defined as the number of deaths of infants younger than 1 year, is estimated at 36.78 per 1,000 live births as of 2012.

Health Care Personnel

In 2004, East Timor had 0.10 physicians per 1,000 population, 0.02 pharmaceutical personnel per 1,000, 0.04 laboratory health workers per 1,000, 0.22 health management and support workers per 1,000, 0.05 dentistry personnel per 1,000, 2.02 community and health workers per 1,000, and 2.19 nurses and midwives per 1,000.

Government Role in Health Care

According to WHO, in 2010, East Timor spent $64 million on health care, an amount that comes to $57 per capita. About two-thirds (66 percent) of health care funding was provided from domestic sources, with the remaining 34 percent provided by sources from abroad. The largest share (56 percent) of spending on health care was provided by government expenditures, with 11 percent provided by household spending and 33 percent from other sources. In 2010, East Timor allocated 5 percent of its total government expenditures to health, placing it in the low range when compared to other lower-middle-income southeast Asian region countries; government expenditures on health came to 5 percent of GDP, placing

East Timor in the high range when compared to other lower-middle-income southeast Asian region countries. In 2009, according to WHO, official development assistance (ODA) for health in East Timor came to $16.41 per capita.

Public Health Programs

According to WHO, in 2004, East Timor had 0.03 environmental and public health workers per 1,000 population. In 2010, 47 percent of the population had access to improved sanitation facilities (37 percent in rural areas and 73 percent in urban), and 69 percent had access to improved sources of drinking water (60 percent in rural areas and 91 percent in urban). According to the World Higher Education Database (WHED), no university in East Timor offers programs in epidemiology or public health.

TOGO

Togo is a west African country, sharing borders with Ghana, Burkina Faso, and Benin and having and having a coastline on the north Atlantic Ocean. The area of 214,976 square miles (556,785 square kilometers) makes Togo about the size of West Virginia, and the July 2012 population was estimated at 7.0 million. In 2010, 43 percent of the population lived in urban areas, and the 2010 to 2015 annual rate of urbanization was estimated at 3.9 percent. Lomé is the capital and largest city (with a 2009 population estimated at 1.6 million). The population growth rate in 2012 was 2.7 percent (the 19th-highest in the world), the net migration rate 0.0 migrants per 1,000 population, the birth rate 35.3 births per 1,000, and the total fertility rate 4.6 children per woman. The United Nations High Commissioner for Refugees (UNHCR) estimated that, in 2010, there were 4,155 refugees and persons in refugee-like situations in Togo.

Formerly a French colony, Togo became independent in 1960. The country was ruled by General Gnassingbé Eyadéma from 1967 to 2005, and he was succeeded by his son, Faure Gnassingbé. However, Togo held free elections in 2007. According to the Ibrahim Index, in 2011, Togo ranked 34th among 53 African countries in terms of governance performance, with a score of 46 (out of 100). Togo ranked tied for 143rd among 183 countries on the *Corruption*

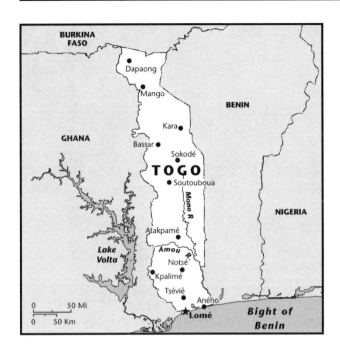

Perceptions Index 2011, with a score of 2.4 (on a scale where 0 indicates highly corrupt and 10 very clean).

In 2011, Togo was classified as a country with low human development (the lowest of four categories) on the United Nations Development Programme's (UNDP's) Human Development Index (HDI), with a score of 0.435 (on a scale where 1 denotes high development and 0 low development). In 2011, the International Food Policy Research Institute (IFPRI) classified Togo as a country with an "alarming" hunger problem, with a Global Hunger Index (GHI) score of 20.1 (where 0 reflects no hunger and higher scores more hunger). Life expectancy at birth in 2012 was estimated at 63.17 years, and estimated gross domestic product (GDP) per capita in 2011 was $900, among the 10 lowest in the world.

Emergency Health Services

According to the World Health Organization (WHO), as of 2007, Togo had a formal and publicly available emergency care (prehospital care) system accessible through a national access number.

Insurance

Togo has a social insurance system, providing maternity benefits only. The system covers the employed, the self-employed, and workers in the formal sector; students and apprentices are excluded. People working for the military and civil service are covered under separate systems. The system is funded through contributions from the self-employed (6 percent of declared earnings) and employers (6 percent of gross payroll) and is part of the same system as the Family Benefits program. The Labor Code requires employers to provide some medical services for their employees, along with paid sick leave. The maternity benefit is 100 percent of the average daily wage for up to eight weeks before and six weeks after the due date and may be extended three weeks for complications. The system of Family Benefits provides a prenatal allowance of XOF 500 monthly for up to nine months and a family allowance of XOF 2,000 monthly for each child up to four children; to receive the prenatal benefit, the woman must undergo required medical exams.

Costs of Hospitalization

No data available.

Access to Health Care

According to WHO, in 2006, 62 percent of births in Togo were attended by skilled personnel (for example physicians, nurses, or midwives). The 2010 immunization rates for 1-year-olds were 92 percent for diphtheria and pertussis (DPT3), 84 percent for measles (MCV), and 92 percent for Hib (Hib3). In 2010, an estimated 50 percent of persons with advanced human immunodeficiency virus (HIV) infection were receiving antiretroviral therapy in accordance with the 2010 WHO guidelines.

Cost of Drugs

No data available.

Health Care Facilities

As of 2010, according to WHO, Togo had 12.38 health centers per 100,000 population, 0.58 district or rural hospitals per 100,000, and 0.10 specialized hospitals per 100,000. In 2006, Togo had 0.85 hospital beds per 1,000 population, one of the 30 lowest rates in the world.

Major Health Issues

In 2008, WHO estimated that 76 percent of years of life lost in Togo were due to communicable diseases, 18 percent to noncommunicable diseases, and 6 percent to injuries. In 2008, the age-standardized estimate of cancer deaths was 86 per 100,000 for men and 91 per 100,000 for women; for cardiovascular disease and diabetes, 402 per 100,000 for men and 404 per 100,000

Health Expenditures: Togo Compared With the Global Average (2009)

	Togo	Global Average
Out-of-pocket expenditure as percent of private expenditure on health	84.2	50.2
Private prepaid plans as percent of private expenditure on health	4.3	38.9
Per capita total expenditure on health at average exchange rate (USD)	41	900
Per capita total expenditure on health (purchasing power parity, international dollars)	74	990
Per capita government expenditure on health at average exchange rate (USD)	18	549
Per capita government expenditure on health (purchasing power parity, international dollars)	32	584

Source: 2011 World Health Organization Global Health Expenditure Atlas.

for women; and for chronic respiratory disease, 109 per 100,000 for men and 60 per 100,000 for women.

In 2008, the age-standardized death rate from malaria was 40.5 per 100,000 population. In 2010, tuberculosis incidence was 455.0 per 100,000 population, tuberculosis prevalence 865.0 per 100,000, and deaths due to tuberculosis among HIV-negative people 106.0 per 100,000. As of 2009, an estimated 3.2 percent of adults age 15 to 49 were living with HIV or acquired immune deficiency syndrome (AIDS). Togo's maternal mortality rate (death from any cause related to or aggravated by pregnancy) is high by global standards, estimated at 350 maternal deaths per 100,000 live births as of 2008. A 2006 survey estimated the prevalence of female genital mutilation at 5.8 percent. The infant mortality rate, defined as the number of deaths of infants younger than 1 year, was estimated at 49.87 per 1,000 live births as of 2012. In 2008, 20.5 percent of children under age 5 were underweight (defined as 2 kilograms [kg] below standard weight-for-age at age 1, 3 kg below for ages 2 to 3, and 4 kg below for ages 4 to 5).

Health Care Personnel

Togo has one medical school, the Faculté mixte de Medecine et de Pharmacie of the University of Lomé (formerly the University of Bénin) in Lomé. The basic medical degree course lasts seven years, and the degree granted is Docteur en Médecine (Diplôme d'État), or doctor of medicine (state diploma). In 2008, Togo had 0.05 physicians per 1,000 population, 0.06 laboratory health workers per 1,000, 0.84 health management and support workers per 1,000, and 0.27 nurses and midwives per 1,000. Michael Clemens and Bunilla Petterson estimate that 40 percent of Togo-born physicians and 19 percent of Togo-born nurses are working in one of nine developed countries, primarily in France.

Government Role in Health Care

According to WHO, in 2010, Togo spent $245 million on health care, an amount that comes to $41 per capita. Most (85 percent) of health care funding came from domestic sources, with 15 percent coming from abroad. The largest share of health care spending was provided through household expenditures (47 percent), with the remainder coming from government expenditures (44 percent) and other sources (9 percent). In 2010, Togo allocated 15 percent of its total government expenditures to health, in the high range for low-income African countries; government expenditures on health came to 3 percent of GDP, in the high range for low-income African countries. In 2009, according to WHO, official development assistance (ODA) for health in Togo came to $6.15 per capita.

Public Health Programs

Togo's National Institute of Hygiene (Institut National d'Hygiene, or INH) is located in Lomé and headed by

Dr. Bangla Kere Abiba; it was established in 1967 and updated in 2002. The INH is an autonomous department within the Division of Laboratories and is the national reference lab for surveillance of potentially epidemic diseases. The INH includes five clinical labs for bacteriology, biochemistry, parasitology, hematology, and serology; two labs for food and water analysis; and a vaccination unit. According to WHO, in 2001, Togo had 0.01 environmental and public health workers per 1,000 population. In 2010, 13 percent of the population had access to improved sanitation facilities (3 percent in rural areas and 26 percent in urban), and 61 percent had access to improved sources of drinking water (40 percent in rural areas and 89 percent in urban).

TONGA

Tonga is an island nation in the south Pacific; the area of 288 square miles (747 square kilometers) makes Tonga about four times the size of Washington, D.C., and the July 2012 population was estimated at 106,146. In 2010, 23 percent of the population lived in urban

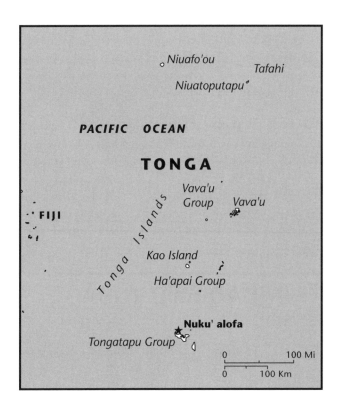

areas, and the 2010 to 2015 annual rate of urbanization was estimated at 0.8 percent. Nuku'alofa is the capital. The population growth rate in 2012 was 0.2 percent, the net migration rate negative 17.9 migrants per 1,000 population (the fourth-highest emigration rate in the world), the birth rate 24.7 births per 1,000, and the total fertility rate 3.6 children per woman.

Tonga is the only Pacific nation to have never lost its indigenous governance. In 1875, Tonga became a constitutional monarchy; in 1900, it became a British protectorate but left protectorate status in 1970. Tonga ranked tied for 95th among 183 countries on the *Corruption Perceptions Index 2011,* with a score of 3.1 (on a scale where 0 indicates highly corrupt and 10 very clean). In 2011, Tonga was classified as a country with high human development (the second-highest category) on the United Nations Development Programme's (UNDP's) Human Development Index (HDI), with a score of 0.704 (on a scale where 1 denotes high development and 0 low development). Life expectancy at birth in 2012 was estimated at 75.38 years, and estimated gross domestic product (GDP) per capita in 2011 was $7,500.

Emergency Health Services

According to the World Health Organization (WHO), as of 2007, Tonga did not have a formal and publicly available system for providing prehospital care (emergency care). However, all four hospitals (located in Nuku'alofa, Vava'u, Na'apai, and Eua) have emergency departments.

Insurance

Tonga's Ministry of Health is responsible for providing and monitoring health services in the country. Health care services are provided free by the government, and the system is funded primarily by government (54 percent) and donor (34 percent) expenditures. About 12 percent of the population, mostly government employees, had some type of insurance in 2011.

Costs of Hospitalization

No data available.

Access to Health Care

Government health care services are provided free of charge, and with the exception of small populations living on isolated islands, physical access to health care facilities is reasonable for most of Tonga's population. Tonga has four hospitals and a network of 14 health centers delivering preventive services and primary care. Treatment schemes funded by Tonga and New Zealand provide for patients to seek overseas care if necessary, and specialist teams regularly visit Tonga to provide care such as eye surgery and orthopedic surgery.

According to WHO, in 2005, 98 percent of births in Tonga were attended by skilled personnel (for example, physicians, nurses, or midwives). The 2010 immunization rates for 1-year-olds were 99 percent for diphtheria and pertussis (DPT3), 99 percent for measles (MCV), and 99 percent for Hib (Hib3).

Cost of Drugs

In 2011, 7.8 percent of health expenditures in Tonga went for drugs.

Health Care Facilities

As of 2010, according to WHO, Tonga had 14.42 health posts per 100,000 population, 13.45 health centers per 100,000, 2.88 district or rural hospitals per 100,000, and 0.96 provincial hospitals per 100,000. In 2008, Tonga had 2.44 hospital beds per 1,000 population.

Major Health Issues

In 2008, WHO estimated that 7 percent of years of life lost in Tonga were due to communicable diseases, 61 percent to noncommunicable diseases, and 8 percent to injuries. In 2008, the age-standardized estimate of cancer deaths was 67 per 100,000 for men and 94 per 100,000 for women; for cardiovascular disease and diabetes, 396 per 100,000 for men and 395 per 100,000 for women; and for chronic respiratory disease, 69 per 100,000 for men and 53 per 100,000 for women. Tonga has one of the highest adult obesity rates in the world, measured at 56.0 percent in 2000; obesity is defined as a body mass index (BMI) of 30 or above, and Type II diabetes has increased rapidly; in 2011, 18 percent of the adult population was diabetic, and a 2000 community survey indicated that many more may remain undiagnosed.

In 2008, the age-standardized death rate from malaria was 0.5 per 100,000 population. In 2010, tuberculosis incidence was 17.0 per 100,000 population, tuberculosis prevalence 29.0 per 100,000, and deaths due to tuberculosis among human immunodeficiency virus (HIV)-negative people 2.90 per 100,000. The infant mortality rate, defined as the number of deaths of infants younger than 1 year, was 13.21 per 1,000 live births in 2012. No information is available from WHO on the maternal mortality rate in Tonga.

Health Care Personnel

Tonga has no medical school, but many physicians train in Australia, Fiji, or New Zealand on WHO fellowships or bilateral scholarships. Nursing training is provided at the Queen Salote School of Nursing, which graduates about 30 nurses per year and also provides postgraduate training in midwifery, internal medicine, surgery, and public health. Physicians wishing to practice in Tonga must register with the Health Practitioners' Registration Council of the Ministry of Health and must have qualified at a recognized medical school. They must also be proficient in Tongan or English and provide evidence of professional competence and good character. In 2002, Tonga had 0.29 physicians per 1,000 population, and 0.04 pharmaceutical personnel per 1,000, and in 2007, had 0.56 dentistry personnel per 1,000 and 2.93 nurses and midwives per 1,000.

Government Role in Health Care

According to WHO, in 2010, Tonga spent $18 million on health care, an amount that comes to $172 per capita. Most (83 percent) of health care funding came from domestic sources, with 17 percent coming from abroad. The largest share of health care spending was provided through government expenditures (81 percent), with the remainder coming from household expenditures (13 percent) and other sources (6 percent). In 2010, Tonga allocated 13 percent of its total government expenditures to health, in the median range for lower-middle-income western Pacific region countries; government expenditures on health came to 4 percent of GDP, in the median range for lower-middle-income western Pacific region countries.

Public Health Programs

According to WHO, in 2009, Tonga had 0.24 environmental and public health workers per 1,000 population. In 2010, 96 percent of the population had access to improved sanitation facilities (96 percent in rural areas and 98 percent in urban), and access to improved sources of drinking water was essentially universal.

TRINIDAD AND TOBAGO

Trinidad and Tobago (Trinidad) is an island country in the Caribbean Sea; an area of 1,989 square miles (5,128 square kilometers) makes Trinidad about the size of Delaware, and the July 2012 population was estimated at 1.2 million. In 2010, 14 percent of the population lived in urban areas, and the 2010 to 2015 annual rate of urbanization was estimated at 3.0 percent. Port of Spain is the capital and largest city (with a 2009 population estimated at 57,000). The population growth rate in 2012 was negative 0.1 percent, the net migration rate negative 6.8 migrants per 1,000 population, the birth rate 14.2 births per 1,000, and the total fertility rate 1.7 children per woman. The United Nations High Commissioner for Refugees (UNHCR) estimated that, in 2010, there were 29 refugees and persons in refugee-like situations in Trinidad.

Trinidad came under British control in the 19th century and became independent in 1962. Thanks to oil and natural gas reserves, Trinidad is one of the most prosperous countries in the Caribbean. Trinidad ranked tied for 91st among 183 countries on the *Corruption Perceptions Index 2011,* with a score of 3.2 (on a scale where 0 indicates highly corrupt and 10 very clean). In 2011, Trinidad was classified as a country with high human development (the second-highest category) on the United Nations Development Programme's (UNDP's) Human Development Index (HDI), with a score of 0.760 (on a scale where 1 denotes high development and 0 low development). Life expectancy at birth in 2012 was estimated at 71.67 years, and per capita gross domestic product (GDP) in 2011 was estimated at $20,300. According to the World Economic Forum's *Global Gender Gap Index 2011,* Trinidad and Tobago ranked 21st out of 135 countries on gender equality with a score of 0.737 (on a scale with a theoretical range of 1 for equality to 0 for inequality and an actual range in 2011 from 0.8530 to 0.4873).

Emergency Health Services

According to the World Health Organization (WHO), as of 2007, Trinidad had a formal and publicly available emergency care (prehospital care) system accessible through a national access number. All three major care units provide emergency care, and in 2000, the Emergency Health Services was created to transfer patients to hospitals free of charge and under the supervision of trained staff; private transfer services are also available but must be paid for out of pocket.

Insurance

Trinidad has a social insurance and social assistance system funded by contributions from wages (0.22

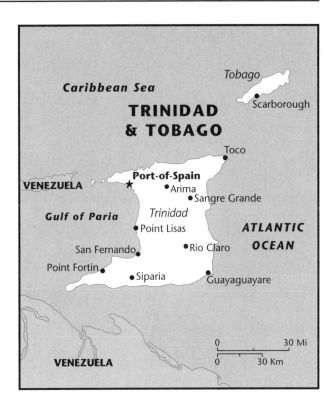

percent of covered earnings or one-third of the overall contribution rate) and employers (0.44 percent of covered earnings or two-thirds of the overall contribution rate); the contribution rates, which also fund the systems for pensions and work injury benefits, are determined by a schedule of wage classes. Means-tested medical benefits are provided for care in public hospitals and health centers. The maternity benefit is 60 percent of average earnings for up to 13 weeks; a maternity grant of TTD 2,500 is also paid. The cash sickness benefit is 60 percent of earnings for up to 52 weeks. Means-tested family benefits are provided to those determined to be needy; these include a dietary grant for individuals with sicknesses such as diabetes or heart disease, a medical equipment grant for purchases such as eyeglasses or hearing aids, a grant to pay for home health care, and a grant for the parents of a child with a physical or mental disability. The social assistance program is supervised by the Ministry of Social Development, and the social insurance program is administered by the National Insurance Board under the general supervision of the Ministry of Finance.

Costs of Hospitalization

No data available.

Access to Health Care

According to WHO, in 2006, 98 percent of births in Trinidad and Tobago were attended by skilled personnel (for example, physicians, nurses, or midwives). The 2010 immunization rates for 1-year-olds were 90 percent for diphtheria and pertussis (DPT3), 92 percent for measles (MCV), and 90 percent for Hib (Hib3). According to WHO, in 2010, Trinidad and Tobago had 3.00 magnetic resonance imaging (MRI) machines per 1 million population, 7.50 computer tomography (CT) machines per 1 million, 1.50 telecobalt units per 1 million, and 1.50 radiotherapy machines per 1 million.

Cost of Drugs

Trinidad's National Drug Policy acts as a formulary for both the public and private sectors, but there are no formal incentives to follow it, and many practitioners do not. Trinidad also has a Vital, Essential, and Necessary (VEN) drug list indicating which drugs will be purchased by the government as needed for public health facilities. Since 2005, prescription drugs have been provided free to patients with specific chronic diseases, including asthma, arthritis, diabetes, hypertension, glaucoma, prostate cancer, depression, some cardiac diseases, and benign prostatic hyperplasia. Vaccines are obtained through the Pan American Health Organization's (PAHO's) Revolving Fund for Vaccine Procurement.

Health Care Facilities

The public health system in Trinidad includes both public and private facilities. The public system includes a network of 36 outreach centers, 67 health centers, and three district health facilities, three specialized hospitals, three district hospitals, and three tertiary hospitals. The private sector includes physicians, hospitals, clinics, labs, pharmacies, and imaging services, and several private companies also provide health benefits, most commonly through employer-provided insurance. As of 2010, according to WHO, Trinidad had 7.83 health posts per 100,000 population and 0.30 health centers per 100,000. In 2008, Trinidad had 2.50 hospital beds per 1,000 population.

Major Health Issues

In 2008, WHO estimated that 22 percent of years of life lost in Trinidad were due to communicable diseases, 59 percent to noncommunicable diseases, and 19 percent to injuries. In 2008, the age-standardized estimate of cancer deaths was 157 per 100,000 for men and 89 per 100,000 for women; for cardiovascular disease and diabetes, 545 per 100,000 for men and 316 per 100,000 for women; and for chronic respiratory disease, 37 per 100,000 for men and 12 per 100,000 for women.

Trinidad's maternal mortality rate (death from any cause related to or aggravated by pregnancy) was estimated in 2008 as 55 maternal deaths per 100,000 live births. The infant mortality rate, defined as the number of deaths of infants younger than 1 year, was estimated at 26.73 per 1,000 live births in 2012. In 2010, tuberculosis incidence was 19.0 per 100,000 population, tuberculosis prevalence 21.0 per 100,000, and deaths due to tuberculosis among human immunodeficiency virus (HIV)-negative people 2.8 per 100,000. As of 2009, an estimated 1.5 percent of adults age 15 to 49 were living with HIV or acquired immune deficiency syndrome (AIDS).

Health Care Personnel

Trinidad and Tobago has one medical school, the Faculty of Medical Sciences of the University of the West Indies (UWI) in St. Augustine. Instruction has been offered since 1967, and the basic medical degree course lasts five years. The degrees granted are the bachelor of medicine and bachelor of surgery, and graduates must complete an 18-month internship to receive a license to practice medicine. Holders of government scholarships must work in government service after graduation. The UWI is supported by and serves students from 17 English-speaking Caribbean countries and territories. In 2007, Trinidad and Tobago had 1.18 physicians per 1,000 population, 0.49 pharmaceutical personnel per 1,000, 0.22 dentistry personnel per 1,000, and 3.56 nurses and midwives per 1,000.

Government Role in Health Care

According to WHO, in 2010, Trinidad spent $1.2 billion on health care, an amount that comes to $861 per capita. All health care funding came from domestic sources. The largest share of health care spending was provided through government expenditures (60 percent), with the remainder coming from household expenditures (33 percent) and other sources (7 percent). In 2010, Trinidad allocated 9 percent of total government expenditures to health, in the median range for high-income Americas region countries; government expenditures on health came to 3 percent of GDP, in the low range for high-income Americas region countries. In 2009, according to WHO, official development assistance (ODA) for health in Trinidad came to $0.97 per capita.

Public Health Programs

In 2010, 92 percent of the population in Trinidad had access to improved sanitation facilities (92 percent in rural areas and 92 percent in urban), and 94 percent had access to improved sources of drinking water (93 percent in rural areas and 98 percent in urban).

TUNISIA

Tunisia is a north African country, sharing borders with Algeria and Libya and having a coastline on the Mediterranean Sea. The area of 63,170 square miles (163,610 square kilometers) makes Tunisia about the size of Georgia, and the July 2012 population was estimated at 10.7 million. In 2010, 67 percent of the population lived in urban areas, and the 2010 to 2015 annual rate of urbanization was estimated at 1.5 percent. Tunis is the capital and largest city (with a 2009 population estimated at 759,000). The population growth rate in 2012 was 1.0 percent, the net migration rate negative 1.8 migrants per 1,000 population, the birth rate 17.3 births per 1,000, and the total fertility rate 2.0 children per woman. The United Nations High Commissioner for Refugees (UNHCR) estimated that, in 2010, there were 38 refugees and persons in refugee-like situations in Tunisia.

Tunisia was invaded by France in 1881 and made a French protectorate; the country became independent in 1956. According to the Ibrahim Index, in 2011, Tunisia ranked ninth among 53 African countries in terms of governance performance, with a score of 62 (out of 100). Tunisia ranked tied for 73rd among 183 countries on the *Corruption Perceptions Index 2011*, with a score of 3.8 (on a scale where 0 indicates highly corrupt and 10 very clean).

In 2011, Tunisia was classified as a country with high human development (the second-highest category) on the United Nations Development Programme's (UNDP's) Human Development Index (HDI), with a score of 0.698 (on a scale where 1 denotes high development and 0 low development). Life expectancy at birth in 2012 was estimated at 75.24 years, and per capita gross domestic product (GDP) in 2011 was estimated at $9,500. In 2005, the Gini Index (a measure of dispersion, in which perfect equality is denoted by 0 and maximum inequality is denoted by 100) for family income was estimated at 40.0. According to the World Economic Forum's *Global Gender Gap Index 2011*, Tunisia ranked 108th out of 135 countries on gender equality, with a score of 0.625 (on a scale with a theoretical range of 1 for equality to 0 for inequality and an actual range in 2011 from 0.8530 to 0.4873).

Emergency Health Services

According to the World Health Organization (WHO), as of 2007, Tunisia had a formal and publicly available emergency care (prehospital care) system accessible through a national access number.

Insurance

Tunisia has a social insurance system covering employees in the private and public sectors, the self-employed, artists, and fishermen; special systems cover civil servants, agricultural workers, members of parliament, and those in the military. Tunisians living abroad can join the system voluntarily. The system is financed through contributions from wages (2.75 percent of earnings), pensions (4.0 percent), the earnings of the self-employed (6.75 percent of gross earnings), and employers (4.0 percent of gross payroll). These contributions finance the death grant and death allowance as well as sickness and maternity

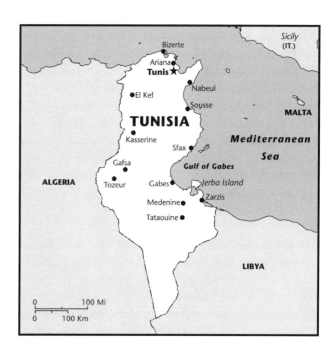

benefits; parental leave is financed under the Family Allowance plan.

For medical benefits, the insured have three options: services provided by government clinics and hospitals, operated by the social security system, or under contract with the National Health Insurance Fund; medical services coordinated by a private physician; or reimbursement by the National Health Insurance Fund for medical services, according to a specified schedule. Benefits include hospitalization, surgery, medical care, lab services, medications, dialysis, and appliances. Cost sharing is based on a specified schedule, and total cost sharing cannot be more than 1.5 times income or pension. Medicines are provided for free in the public sector, but may not always be available. The maternity benefit is two-thirds of the average wage, with a ceiling of twice the legal minimum wage, paid for 30 days, with a possible extension of 15 more days. The sickness benefit is two-thirds of the average daily wage, with a ceiling of twice the legal minimum wage for up to 180 days. For hospitalization of long-term illness, the benefit is 50 percent of the average daily wage. The National Health Insurance Fund administers the program under the general supervision of the Ministry of Social Affairs, Solidarity, and Tunisians Abroad.

Costs of Hospitalization

No data available.

Access to Health Care

According to WHO, in 2006, 94.6 percent of births in Tunisia were attended by skilled personnel (for example, physicians, nurses, or midwives), and 68 percent of pregnant women received at least four prenatal care visits. The 2010 immunization rates for 1-year-olds were 98 percent for diphtheria and pertussis (DPT3) and 97 percent for measles (MCV). In 2010, an estimated 10 percent of persons with advanced human immunodeficiency virus (HIV) infection were receiving antiretroviral therapy in accordance with the 2010 WHO guidelines.

Cost of Drugs

A 2004 survey conducted by the Union of Mutual Insurance Companies looked at the price and availability of a market basket of common drugs in Tunisia. The median reference procurement price for these drugs in the public sector was 1.26 for the lowest-priced generic versions, meaning they cost 26

percent more than the international reference price, and 7.44 for originator brands. There is no information about patient prices in the public sector because drugs are provided for free. Median availability for the lowest-priced generics in public-sector facilities was 64.3 percent, with a range (depending on the specific drug) from 2.4 to 95.2 percent. Very few originator brands were available in any public facilities. Patient prices were much higher in the private sector, with a median reference price of 6.82 for the lowest-priced generics and 11.89 for originator brands. However, availability was also higher in the private sector, with median availability of 95.1 percent for the lowest-priced generics and 76.8 percent for originator brands.

Although drugs are provided for free in the public sector, lack of availability means that sometimes they are purchased in the private sphere. Affordability of medicines used to treat various common conditions varied according to the condition, the drugs used, and whether generics or originator brands were used. For instance, to treat diabetes for 30 days would cost the lowest-paid government worker 0.3 day's salary to buy the lowest-price generic version of glibenclamide and 0.8 day's wages to purchase metformin; for originator brands, the costs would equal 1.2 and 1.1 days' wages, respectively. Amoxicillin to treat an adult respiratory infection would require 0.6 day's wages for the lowest-priced generic, while the lowest-priced generic version of ciprofloxacin would cost 1.7 days' wages. The lowest-priced generic to treat a peptic ulcer would cost the equivalent of 4.5 (ranitidine) or 7.0 (omeprazole) days' wages, while the brand-name version of ranitidine would cost 7.1 days' wages.

Health Care Facilities

As of 2010, according to WHO, Tunisia had 19.64 health posts per 100,000 population, 1.25 district or rural hospitals per 100,000, 0.91 provincial hospitals per 100,000, and 0.29 specialized hospitals per 100,000. In 2009, Tunisia had 2.10 hospital beds per 1,000 population.

Major Health Issues

In 2008, WHO estimated that 34 percent of years of life lost in Tunisia were due to communicable diseases, 53 percent to noncommunicable diseases, and 13 percent to injuries. In 2008, the age-standardized estimate of cancer deaths was 123 per 100,000 for men and 72 per 100,000 for women; for cardiovascular disease and diabetes, 268 per 100,000 for men and 245 per 100,000 for women; and for chronic respiratory disease, 30 per 100,000 for men and 21 per 100,000 for women. In 2008, the age-standardized death rate from malaria was 0.1 per 100,000 population.

Tunisia's maternal mortality rate (death from any cause related to or aggravated by pregnancy) was estimated in 2008 as 60 maternal deaths per 100,000 live births. The infant mortality rate, defined as the number of deaths of infants younger than 1 year, was estimated at 24.98 per 1,000 live births in 2012. In 2010, tuberculosis incidence was 25.0 per 100,000 population, tuberculosis prevalence 31.0 per 100,000, and deaths due to tuberculosis among HIV-negative people 2.20 per 100,000. As of 2009, an estimated 0.1 percent of adults age 15 to 49 were living with HIV or acquired immune deficiency syndrome (AIDS).

Health Care Personnel

Tunisia has four medical schools. The basic medical degree course lasts seven years, and the degree awarded is Doctorat en Médecine (doctor of medicine). Physicians must register with the Conseil National de l'Ordre des Médecins in Tunis, and graduates of foreign medical schools must have their degrees validated. Foreigners wishing to practice medicine in Tunisia must be authorized by the Ministry of Public Health. Tunisia has agreements with Algeria, Libya, Mauritania, and Morocco.

In 2009, Tunisia had 1.19 physicians per 1,000 population, 0.20 pharmaceutical personnel per 1,000, 0.24 dentistry personnel per 1,000, and 3.28 nurses and midwives per 1,000. Michael Clemens and Bunilla Petterson estimate that 33 percent of Tunisia-born physicians and 5 percent of Tunisia-born nurses are working in one of nine developed countries, primarily in France.

Government Role in Health Care

According to WHO, in 2010, Tunisia spent $2.5 billion on health care, an amount that comes to $238 per capita. All health care funding came from domestic sources. The largest share of health care spending was provided through government expenditures (54 percent), with the remainder coming from household expenditures (40 percent) and other sources (6 percent). In 2010, Tunisia allocated 11 percent of its total government expenditures to health, in the high range for upper-middle-income eastern Mediterranean region countries; government expenditures on health came to 3 percent of GDP, in the high range for upper-middle-income eastern Mediterranean region countries. In 2009, according to WHO, official development assistance (ODA) for health in Tunisia came to $0.59 per capita.

Public Health Programs

According to WHO, in 2009, Tunisia had 0.24 environmental and public health workers per 1,000 population. In 2010, 84 percent of the population had access to improved sanitation facilities (64 percent in rural areas and 96 percent in urban), and 94 percent had access to improved sources of drinking water (84 percent in rural areas and 99 percent in urban). According to C. B. Ijsselmuiden and colleagues, in 2007, Tunisia had six institutions offering postgraduate public health programs.

TURKEY

Turkey is a country in southeastern Europe and southwestern Asia, sharing borders with Armenia, Azerbaijan, Bulgaria, Georgia, Greece, Iran, Iraq, and Syria and having coastlines on the Black Sea and Mediterranean. The area of 302,535 square miles (783,562 square kilometers) makes Turkey about the size of Texas, and the July 2012 population was estimated at 79.7 million (the 17th-largest in the world). In 2010, 70 percent of the population lived in urban areas, and the 2010 to 2015 annual rate of urbanization was estimated at 1.7 percent. Ankara is the capital and Istanbul the largest city (with a 2009 population estimated at 10.4 million). The population growth rate in 2012 was 1.2 percent, the net migration rate 0.5 migrants per 1,000 population, the birth rate 17.6 births per 1,000, and the total fertility rate 2.1 children per woman. The United Nations High Commissioner for Refugees (UNHCR) estimated that, in 2010, there were 10,032 refugees and persons in refugee-like situations in Turkey.

The area that is Turkey today was part of the Ottoman Empire; modern Turkey was founded in 1923. The country was modernized by Mustafa Kemal (Ataturk); the country's first multiparty election was held in 1950. Turkey has suffered periods of instability and military coups since 1960. Turkey ranked tied for 61st among 183 countries, with a score of 4.2

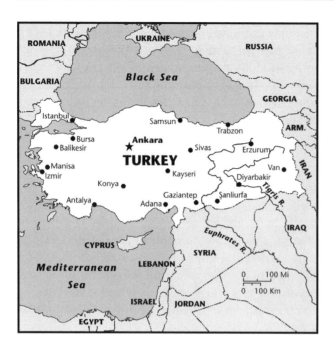

on the *Corruption Perceptions Index 2011* (on a scale where 0 indicates highly corrupt and 10 very clean). In 2011, Turkey was classified as a country with high human development (the second-highest category) on the United Nations Development Programme's (UNDP's) Human Development Index (HDI), with a score of 0.699 (on a scale where 1 denotes high development and 0 low development). Life expectancy at birth in 2012 was estimated at 72.77 years, and per capita gross domestic product (GDP) in 2011 was estimated at $14,600. In 2010, the Gini Index (a measure of dispersion, in which perfect equality is denoted by 0 and maximum inequality is denoted by 100) for family income was 40.2. According to the World Economic Forum's *Global Gender Gap Index 2011*, Turkey ranked 122nd out of 135 countries on gender equality with a score of 0.595 (on a scale with a theoretical range of 1 for equality to 0 for inequality and an actual range in 2011 from 0.8530 to 0.4873).

Emergency Health Services

According to the World Health Organization (WHO), as of 2007, Turkey had a formal and publicly available emergency care (prehospital care) system accessible through a national access number.

Insurance

Turkey has a universal medical benefits system, established in 2007, and a social insurance system to provide cash maternity and sickness benefits. The system is funded by contributions from wages (5 percent, up to a maximum), self-employed earnings (12.5 percent, up to a maximum), payroll (7.5 percent, up to a maximum), and the government. Medical benefits are provided to everyone living in Turkey. The cash benefit system includes people working under service contracts, including civil servants and the self-employed. Medical care is provided in health care facilities that have agreements with the Social Security Institution (SSI).

The maternity benefit, which covers insured women only (not spouses of insured men), pays 66 percent of earnings for up to eight weeks before and after the due date. A lump sum benefit is paid at childbirth and for a nursing grant. The cash sickness benefit is 50 percent of earnings for hospital treatment and 66 percent for outpatient treatments. The SSI provides medical care and medications through contracts with hospitals and pharmacies and administers cash benefits; the Ministry of Labour and Social Security Institution supervises the system.

Costs of Hospitalization

The dominant purchaser of hospital services in Turkey is the Ministry of Health, and in 2006, the SSI and Ministry of Health established a capped annual budget for all Ministry of Health hospitals. The SSI contracts with 350 private and university hospitals to deliver the benefits package; the system allows private providers to charge up to 30 percent above the SSI prices (extra billing), which the patient must pay out of pocket. All hospitals in Turkey, both public and private, participate in a management system to process claims for insurance funds. A certificate of need is required for new private hospitals, health care centers, and clinics.

Access to Health Care

Turkey has about 850 public hospitals and 260 private hospitals; public hospitals handle about 72 percent of cases. Turkey is in the process of implementing the Health Transformation Program (HTP), a program intended to address problems including unequal access to health care, poor health outcomes, fragmentation in the financing and delivery system, and poor quality and responsiveness in the health care system. Part of this program is establishing universal health insurance (described above) under the auspices of the SSI; other reforms include restructuring

Selected Health Indicators: Turkey Compared With the Organisation for Economic Co-operation and Development (OECD) Country Average

	Turkey	OECD average (2010 or nearest year)
Doctor consultations (number per capita), 2011	7.3	6.4
Professionally active physicians (per 1,000 population), 2010	1.7	3.1
Professionally active nurses (per 1,000 population), 2010	1.6	8.6
Medical graduates (per 100,000 population), 2010	7	10.3
Nursing graduates (per 100,000 population), 2010	6	39.8
MRI exams (per 1,000 population), 2010	79.5	46.3
CT exams (per 1,000 population), 2010	103.5	123.8

Source: OECD Health Data 2012 (Organisation for Economic Co-operation and Development, 2012).

the Ministry of Health, expanding the primary care delivery system, and improving the quality of care. A 2007 *Health Affairs* article (cited by Donald West) noted that navigating the Turkish health care delivery system often involved quite a few unofficial and unauthorized out-of-pocket payments, such as "donations" that were in fact required in order to receive services, "knife" payments required for surgery already covered under the national health plan, and the requirement to purchase drugs that should have been provided by the hospital.

According to WHO, in 2008, 91.3 percent of births in Turkey were attended by skilled personnel (for example, physicians, nurses, or midwives), and 74 percent of pregnant women received at least four prenatal care visits. The 2010 immunization rates for 1-year-olds were 96 percent for diphtheria and pertussis (DPT3), 97 percent for measles (MCV), and 96 percent for Hib (Hib3). In 2010, an estimated 56 percent of persons with advanced human immunodeficiency virus (HIV) infection were receiving antiretroviral therapy in accordance with the 2010 WHO guidelines. According to WHO, in 2010, Turkey had 6.22 magnetic resonance imaging (MRI) machines per 1 million population, 14.72 computer tomography (CT) machines per 1 million, 0.91 positron emission tomography (PET) machines per 1 million, 0.61 telecolbalt units per 1 million, and 0.61 radiotherapy machines per 1 million.

Cost of Drugs

According to Douglas Ball, Turkey charges a reduced rate of value-added tax (VAT), 8 percent for medicines versus the standard rate of 18 percent. Wholesale markups on drugs range from 2 to 9 percent, and retail markups range from 10 to 25 percent of the purchase price. According to Elizabeth Docteur, in 2004, generic drugs represented 40 percent of the market share by value (the second-highest among Organisation for Economic Co-operation and Development, or OECD, countries) and 55 percent of the market share by volume of the total pharmaceutical market.

Health Care Facilities

As of 2010, according to WHO, Turkey had 10.33 health posts per 100,000 population, 0.28 health centers per 100,000, 1.27 provincial hospitals per 100,000, and 0.33 specialized hospitals per 100,000.

Major Health Issues

In 2008, WHO estimated that 21 percent of years of life lost in Turkey were due to communicable diseases, 68 percent to noncommunicable diseases, and 11 percent to injuries. In 2008, the age-standardized estimate of cancer deaths was 158 per 100,000 for men and 78 per 100,000 for women; for cardiovascular disease and diabetes, 403 per 100,000 for men and 322 per 100,000 for women; and for chronic respiratory disease, 95 per 100,000 for men and 38 per 100,000 for women.

The maternal mortality rate (death from any cause related to or aggravated by pregnancy) in Turkey in 2008 was 23 maternal deaths per 100,000 live births. The infant mortality rate, defined as the number of deaths of infants younger than 1 year, was estimated at 23.07 per 1,000 live births in 2012. In 2010, tuberculosis incidence was 28.0 per 100,000 population, tuberculosis prevalence 24.0 per 100,000, and deaths due to tuberculosis among HIV-negative people 3.1 per 100,000. As of 2009, an estimated 0.1 percent of adults age 15 to 49 were living with HIV or acquired immune deficiency syndrome (AIDS).

Health Care Personnel

Turkey has 34 medical schools. The basic medical degree course lasts six or seven years, and the degree awarded is Tip Doktoru (doctor of medicine). Physicians wanting to go into private practice must register with the Turkish Medical Association, and graduates of foreign medical schools must have their degrees validated by the Ministry of Health. In 2008, Turkey had 1.45 physicians per 1,000 population, 0.33 pharmaceutical personnel per 1,000, 0.19 laboratory health workers per 1,000, and 1.89 nurses and midwives per 1,000.

Government Role in Health Care

According to WHO, in 2010, Turkey spent $50 billion on health care, an amount that comes to $678 per capita. All health care funding came from domestic sources. The largest share of health care spending was provided through government expenditures (75 percent), with the remainder coming from household expenditures (16 percent) and other sources (9 percent). In 2010, Turkey allocated 13 percent of its total government expenditures to health, in the high range for upper-middle-income European countries; government expenditures on health came to 5 percent of GDP, in the median range for upper-middle-income European countries. In 2009, according to WHO, official development assistance (ODA) for health in Turkey came to $0.16 per capita.

Public Health Programs

The Refik Saydam Hygiene Center, established in 1928, is located in Sihhiye (Ankara) and directed by Mustafa Ertek. The center includes a school of public health and departments of bacteriology, chemical analysis, pharmacology, and immunology, as well as labs devoted to hematology, pesticides, mycology, and drug control. According to WHO, in 2008, Turkey had 0.25 environmental and public health workers per 1,000 population. In 2010, 90 percent of the population had access to improved sanitation facilities (75 percent in rural areas and 97 percent in urban), and almost 100 percent had access to improved sources of drinking water (99 percent in rural areas and 100 percent in urban). According to the World Higher Education Database (WHED), 15 universities in Turkey offer programs in epidemiology or public health.

TURKMENISTAN

Turkmenistan is a European country, sharing borders with Afghanistan, Iran, Kazakhstan, and Uzbekistan and having a shoreline on the Caspian Sea. The area of 188,456 square miles (488,100 square kilometers) makes Turkmenistan about the size of California, and the July 2012 population was estimated at 5.0 million. In 2010, 50 percent of the population lived in urban areas, and the 2010 to 2015 annual rate of urbanization was estimated at 2.2 percent. Ashgabat is the capital and largest city (with a 2009 population estimated at 637,000). The population growth rate

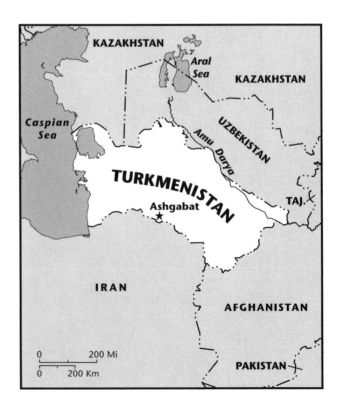

in 2012 was 1.1 percent, the net migration rate negative 1.9 migrants per 1,000 population, the birth rate 19.6 births per 1,000, and the total fertility rate 2.1 children per woman. The United Nations High Commissioner for Refugees (UNHCR) estimated that, in 2010, there were 62 refugees and persons in refugee-like situations in Turkmenistan.

The area that is now Turkmenistan was annexed by Russia and, in 1924, became a Soviet republic; Turkmenistan became an independent country in 1991. The government is perceived as corrupt, ranking tied for 177th among 183 countries in terms of perceived public-sector corruption, with a score of 1.6 (on a scale where 0 indicates highly corrupt and 10 very clean). In 2011, Turkmenistan was classified as a country with medium human development (the second from the lowest of four categories) on the United Nations Development Programme's (UNDP's) Human Development Index (HDI), with a score of 0.686 (on a scale where 1 denotes high development and 0 low development).

Life expectancy at birth in 2012 was estimated at 68.84 years, and estimated gross domestic product (GDP) per capita in 2011 was $7,500. In 1998, the Gini Index (a measure of dispersion, in which perfect equality is denoted by 0 and maximum inequality is denoted by 100) for family income was 40.8. Unemployment in 2004 was estimated at 60.0 percent, among the highest rates in the world.

Emergency Health Services

According to the World Health Organization (WHO), as of 2007, Turkmenistan had a formal and publicly available emergency care (prehospital care) system accessible through a national access number.

Insurance

Turkmenistan has a universal system providing medical care to everyone living in the country and a social insurance system providing maternity and sickness cash benefits. The system is funded by contributions from wages (1 percent), earnings of the self-employed (1 percent), and employers (20 percent of payroll), with government subsidies required. Medical care is provided through the public health system and includes hospitalization, medical care, dental care, maternity care, vaccination, lab services, and transportation. Medicines are free during hospitalization. The maternity benefit is 100 percent of earnings for 56 days before and after the due date, with extensions

for multiple births or complications. A birth grant is paid for the first four children, even if the parents do not work in covered employment: TMM 157.30 for the first two children, 302.50 for the third, and 605 for the fourth. A child care allowance of TMM 78 is paid for children over 18 months. The sickness benefit is 60 to 100 percent of earnings, depending on length of time contributing to the system and number of children at home. The medical benefits system is run by the Ministry of Health and Medical Industry, and the cash benefits system is run by the Ministry of Social Security.

Costs of Hospitalization

No data available.

Access to Health Care

According to WHO, in 2006, 100 percent of births in Turkmenistan were attended by skilled personnel (for example, physicians, nurses, or midwives). In 2000, 83 percent of pregnant women received at least four prenatal care visits. The 2010 immunization rates for 1-year-olds were 96 percent for diphtheria and pertussis (DPT3), 99 percent for measles (MCV), and 58 percent for Hib (Hib3).

Cost of Drugs

No data available.

Health Care Facilities

In 2007, Turkmenistan had 4.06 hospital beds per 1,000 population, among the 50 highest rates in the world.

Major Health Issues

In 2008, WHO estimated that 35 percent of years of life lost in Turkmenistan were due to communicable diseases, 52 percent to noncommunicable diseases, and 13 percent to injuries. In 2008, the age-standardized estimate of cancer deaths was 121 per 100,000 for men and 92 per 100,000 for women; for cardiovascular disease and diabetes, 881 per 100,000 for men and 668 per 100,000 for women; and for chronic respiratory disease, 49 per 100,000 for men and 32 per 100,000 for women. Turkmenistan's maternal mortality rate (death from any cause related to or aggravated by pregnancy) was estimated in 2008 as 77 maternal deaths per 100,000 live births. The infant mortality rate, defined as the number of deaths of infants younger than 1 year, was estimated at 40.89 per 1,000 live births in 2012.

In 2010, tuberculosis incidence was 66.0 per 100,000 population, tuberculosis prevalence 77.0 per 100,000, and deaths due to tuberculosis among human immunodeficiency virus (HIV)-negative people 20.00 per 100,000. As of 2009, an estimated 0.1 percent of adults age 15 to 49 were living with HIV or acquired immune deficiency syndrome (AIDS).

Health Care Personnel

Turkmenistan has one medical school, Turkmen Druzbi Narodov Medical Institute in Ashkhabat, which has been offering instruction since 1932. In 2007, Turkmenistan had 2.44 physicians per 1,000 population, 0.20 pharmaceutical personnel per 1,000, 0.14 dentistry personnel per 1,000, and 4.52 nurses and midwives per 1,000.

Government Role in Health Care

According to WHO, in 2010, Turkmenistan spent $535 million on health care, an amount that comes to $106 per capita. All health care funding came from domestic sources. The largest share of health care spending was provided through government expenditures (59 percent), with the remainder coming from household expenditures (41 percent). In 2010, Turkmenistan allocated 10 percent of its total government expenditures to health, in the high range for lower-middle-income European countries; government expenditures on health came to 1 percent of GDP, in the low range for lower-middle-income European countries. In 2009, according to WHO, official development assistance (ODA) for health in Turkmenistan came to $0.57 per capita.

Public Health Programs

In 2005, 98 percent of the population in Turkmenistan had access to improved sanitation facilities (97 percent in rural areas and 99 percent in urban), and 84 percent had access to improved sources of drinking water (72 percent in rural areas and 97 percent in urban).

TUVALU

Tuvalu is an island nation in the south Pacific Ocean; the area of 10 square miles (26 square kilometers) makes it about one-tenth the size of Washington, D.C., and one of the smallest independent countries in the world. The July 2012 population was estimated at 10,169, the smallest in the United Nations (UN); Funafuti is the capital. In 2010, 50 percent of the population lived in urban areas, and the 2010 to 2015 annual rate of urbanization was estimated at 1.4 percent. The population growth rate in 2012 was 0.7 percent, the net migration rate negative 7.0 migrants per 1,000 population, the birth rate 23.4 births per 1,000, and the total fertility rate 3.1 children per woman.

Tuvalu became in independent country in 1978; it was previously a British colony called the Ellice Islands and had also been part of the Gilbert and Ellice Islands (citizens of the Ellice Islands voted to separate from the Gilbert Islands in 1974). Because Tuvalu is composed of coral atolls, it is extremely sensitive to changes in sea level, and potable water must be collected through catchment systems or produced by desalination; almost all food and fuel must be imported, and Tuvalu receives much of its income from remittances, licensing of the Internet domain name ". tv," and income from a trust fund supported by Australia, New Zealand, Japan, and South Korea. Life expectancy at birth in 2012 was estimated at 65.11 years, and estimated gross domestic product (GDP) per capita in 2011 was $3,400.

Emergency Health Services

According to the World Health Organization (WHO), as of 2007, Tuvalu had a formal and publicly available emergency care (prehospital care) system accessible through a national access number.

Insurance

Tuvalu provides free health care services to its citizens; most care is provided through government institutions, while specialized care is provided by visiting teams of physicians and through referral to overseas care.

Costs of Hospitalization

No data available.

Access to Health Care

According to WHO, in 2007, 97.9 percent of births in Tuvalu were attended by skilled personnel (for example, physicians, nurses, or midwives), and 67 percent of pregnant women received at least four prenatal care visits. The 2010 immunization rates for 1-year-olds were 89 percent for diphtheria and pertussis (DPT3),

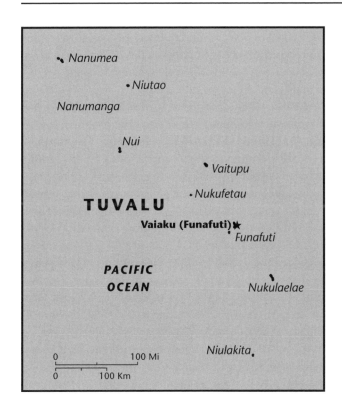

85 percent for measles (MCV), and 89 percent for Hib (Hib3).

Cost of Drugs

No data available.

Health Care Facilities

Tuvalu has one hospital, the Princess Margaret Hospital in Funafuti. In 2008, Tuvalu had 5.55 hospital beds per 1,000 population, among the 50 highest rates in the world.

Major Health Issues

In 2008, WHO estimated that 28 percent of years of life lost in Tuvalu were due to communicable diseases, 62 percent to noncommunicable diseases, and 10 percent to injuries. In 2008, the age-standardized estimate of cancer deaths was 107 per 100,000 for men and 154 per 100,000 for women; for cardiovascular disease and diabetes, 606 per 100,000 for men and 588 per 100,000 for women; and for chronic respiratory disease, 98 per 100,000 for men and 77 per 100,000 for women.

The infant mortality rate, defined as the number of deaths of infants younger than 1 year, was estimated at 33.55 per 1,000 live births in 2012. No

information was available on the maternal mortality rate. In 2010, tuberculosis incidence was 237.0 per 100,000 population, tuberculosis prevalence 366.0 per 100,000, and deaths due to tuberculosis among human immunodeficiency virus (HIV)-negative people 33.00 per 100,000.

Health Care Personnel

Tuvalu has no medical school. Physicians wishing to practice in Tuvalu must register with the Ministry of Health in Funafuti. In 2009, seven physicians from Tuvalu and four from Cuba were working in Tuvalu; medical teams from Taiwan and Australia also visit the country to provide specialist care (for example, surgery, cardiology, and eye surgery). In 2008, Tuvalu had 0.64 physicians per 1,000 population, 0.09 pharmaceutical personnel per 1,000, 0.18 dentistry personnel per 1,000, and 5.82 nurses and midwives per 1,000.

Government Role in Health Care

According to WHO, in 2010, Tuvalu spent $6 million on health care, an amount that comes to $568 per capita. Most (87 percent) of health care funding came from domestic sources, with 13 percent coming from abroad. All health care spending was provided through government expenditures. In 2010, Tuvalu allocated 14 percent of its total government expenditures to health, in the median range for lower-middle-income western Pacific region countries; government expenditures on health came to 17 percent of GDP, in the high range for lower-middle-income western Pacific region countries.

Public Health Programs

According to WHO, in 2008, Tuvalu had 1.09 environmental and public health workers per 1,000 population. In 2010, 85 percent of the population had access to improved sanitation facilities (81 percent in rural areas and 88 percent in urban), and 98 percent had access to improved sources of drinking water (97 percent in rural areas and 98 percent in urban).

UGANDA

Uganda is a landlocked central African country, sharing borders with the Democratic Republic of the

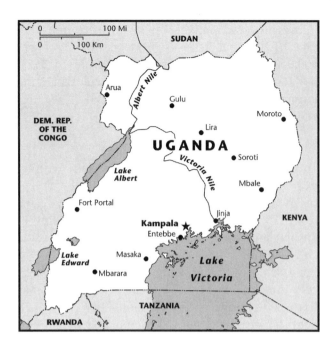

Congo, Kenya, Rwanda, South Sudan, and Tanzania and having a shoreline on Lake Victoria. The area of 93,065 square miles (241,038 square kilometers) makes Uganda about twice the size of New Jersey, and the July 2012 population was estimated at 35.9 million. In 2010, 13 percent of the population lived in urban areas, and the 2010 to 2015 annual rate of urbanization was estimated at 4.8 percent. Kampala is the capital and largest city (with a 2009 population estimated at 1.5 million). As of 2012, Uganda had second-highest birth rate in the world, at 47.38 births per 1,000 population; the second-highest fertility rate, at 6.65 children per woman; and the fourth-highest July 2012 population growth rate in the world, with 3.58 percent. The United Nations High Commissioner for Refugees (UNHCR) estimated that, in 2010, there were 135,801 refugees and persons in refugee-like situations in Uganda and 302,991 internally displaced persons and persons in internally displaced-person-like situations.

Uganda was a British colony before becoming independent in 1962. The country suffered under the dictatorial rule of Idi Amin from 1971 to 1979 and then Milton Obote from 1980 to 1995, considered jointly responsible for an estimated 400,000 deaths. The country has been ruled since 1986 by Yoweri Museveni and has enjoyed greater stability and economic growth under his leadership. According to the Ibrahim Index, in 2011, Uganda ranked 18th among 53 African countries in terms of governance performance, with a score of 55 (out of 100). Uganda ranks tied for 143rd among 183 countries on the *Corruption Perceptions Index 2011*, with a score of 2.4 (on a scale where 0 indicates highly corrupt and 10 very clean).

In 2011, Uganda was classified as a country with low human development (the lowest of four categories) on the United Nations Development Programme's (UNDP's) Human Development Index (HDI), with a score of 0.446 (on a scale where 1 denotes high development and 0 low development). Life expectancy at birth in 2012 was estimated at 53.45 years, among the 20 lowest in the world, and estimated gross domestic product (GDP) per capita in 2011 was $1,300, among the 30 lowest in the world. In 2009, the Gini Index (a measure of dispersion, in which perfect equality is denoted by 0 and maximum inequality is denoted by 100) for family income was 44.3. According to the World Economic Forum's *Global Gender Gap Index 2011*, Uganda ranked 29th out of 135 countries on gender equality, with a score of 0.722 (on a scale with a theoretical range of 1 for equality to 0 for inequality and an actual range in 2011 from 0.8530 to 0.4873).

Emergency Health Services

According to the World Health Organization (WHO), as of 2007, Uganda did not have a formal and publicly available system for providing pre-hospital care (emergency care). Doctors Without Borders (Médecins Sans Frontières, or MSF) began working in Uganda in 1980 and had 572 staff members in the country at the close of 2010. MSF services provide human immunodeficiency virus/acquired immune deficiency syndrome (HIV/AIDS) care, screening for and treatment of tuberculosis, care for malaria and sleeping sickness, and maternal health care.

Insurance

Government provision of health care has increased greatly since 1972, with a 400 percent increase in health facilities. However, the population also doubled during that time, and a 1993 survey found that less than half the population lives within 0.6 miles (5 kilometers) of a health facility. Access is particularly difficult in rural areas because health facilities are clustered in cities. As of 2004, about 60 percent of care was provided by the government sector and 40 percent by the mission sector.

Costs of Hospitalization

No data available.

Access to Health Care

According to WHO, in 2006, 42 percent of births in Uganda were attended by skilled personnel (for example, physicians, nurses, or midwives), and 48 percent of pregnant women received at least four prenatal care visits. The 2010 immunization rates for 1-year-olds were 60 percent for diphtheria and pertussis (DPT3), 55 percent for measles (MCV), and 60 percent for Hib (Hib3). In 2010, an estimated 47 percent of persons with advanced HIV infection were receiving antiretroviral therapy in accordance with the 2010 WHO guidelines. According to WHO, in 2010, Uganda had 0.03 magnetic resonance imaging (MRI) machines per 1 million population and 0.19 computer tomography (CT) machines per 1 million.

Cost of Drugs

The National Medical Stores obtains most of the medicines used within government health units, while the missionary hospitals obtain their drug supply from the Joint Medical Stores (partially financed by public funds). The National Drug Authority regulates importation, registration, and quality control for pharmaceuticals. Medicines are provided free at public health facilities; however, some public facilities have private wings as well, and within the private sector, there may be fees charged for medicines. Mission facilities charge for drugs. The estimated per capita pharmaceutical expenditures in the public sphere from 2004 to 2005 were $1.60 (excluding some vaccines and retrovirals provided by donors). In 2004, the Ministry of Health surveyed the price and availability of a market basket of common drugs in Uganda and found that availability was a serious problem and that unavailability had increased since 2001, when copayments for drugs were dropped.

From 2004 to 2005, public-sector procurement prices were found to be reasonable, with a median price ratio of 0.71 for the lowest-priced generic drug, meaning that Uganda obtained these drugs on average for 29 percent below the international reference price. Availability in public-sector facilities was 55 percent, although some of the drugs not available at lower-level facilities were available at the corresponding referral hospital. Innovator brands were not stocked at public facilities. The median price ratio for nongovernmental organization (NGO) procurement was 0.87 for the lowest-priced generics and 1.04 for the only innovator brand stocked; the patient price in the NGO sphere had a median price ratio of 2.69, and no innovator brands were available in the outlets surveyed. Median availability of the lowest-priced generics at NGO facilities was 45 percent. Drugs in private retail facilities had a median price ratio of 2.6 for the lowest-priced generic drugs and 13.6 for innovator brands, with a median availability of 80 percent for the lowest-priced generic drugs and very low availability of innovator brands. The availability of specific drugs varied widely across the sector, with many more available at private- and NGO-sector facilities than in public-sector facilities. The drugs necessary to treat many common conditions were unaffordable, given the standard that a course of drugs should not cost more than one day's wages for the lowest-paid government worker.

Health Care Facilities

Health care in Uganda is provided through a combination of public, private, and NGO facilities. Despite great expansion over the last 40 years, access to health care remains a problem, particularly outside cities. Uganda has two national referral hospitals, which are also teaching hospitals, in Mulago and Butabika; there are also 12 district hospitals, which also serve as referral hospitals. Nationally, medicines are dispensed mainly through public health facilities, with most private pharmacies located in Mbarara, Jinja, and Kampala.

As of 2010, according to WHO, Uganda had 8.99 health posts per 100,000 population, 3.77 health centers per 100,000, 0.34 district or rural hospitals per 100,000, 0.04 provincial hospitals per 100,000, and 0.01 specialized hospitals per 100,000. In 2009, Uganda had 0.39 hospital beds per 1,000 population, one of the 10 lowest rates in the world.

Major Health Issues

In 2008, WHO estimated that 76 percent of years of life lost in Uganda were due to communicable diseases, 13 percent to noncommunicable diseases, and 11 percent to injuries. In 2008, the age-standardized estimate of cancer deaths was 127 per 100,000 for men and 140 per 100,000 for women; for cardiovascular disease and diabetes, 562 per 100,000 for men and 384 per 100,000 for women; and for chronic respiratory disease, 159 per 100,000 for men and 53 per 100,000 for women.

In 2008, the age-standardized death rate from malaria was 50.2 per 100,000 population. In 2008, the age-standardized death rate from childhood-cluster diseases (pertussis, polio, diphtheria, measles, and tetanus) was 16.0 per 100,000 population, the ninth-highest in the world. In 2010, tuberculosis incidence was 209.0 per 100,000 population, tuberculosis prevalence 193.0 per 100,000, and deaths due to tuberculosis among HIV-negative people 15.00 per 100,000. WHO estimated the 2010 case detection rate at 61 percent. As of 2009, an estimated 6.5 percent of adults age 15 to 49 were living with HIV or AIDS. As of 2009, an estimated 1.2 million people in Uganda were living with HIV or AIDS, the seventh-largest number in the world. In 2010, 63 percent of pregnant women tested positive for HIV. The mother-to-child transmission rate for HIV in 2010 was estimated at 30 percent, and in 2009, 6.2 percent of deaths to children under age 5 were attributed to HIV.

Compared to other countries at a similar level of development, Uganda ranked fifth among 43 least-developed countries on the 2011 Mothers' Index, produced by the international NGO Save the Children, based on a number of health and social factors relating to women, children, and maternal and child care. Uganda's maternal mortality rate (death from any cause related to or aggravated by pregnancy) is high by global standards, estimated at 430 maternal deaths per 100,000 live births as of 2008. A 2006 survey estimated the prevalence of female genital mutilation at 0.8 percent. The infant mortality rate, defined as the number of deaths of infants younger than 1 year, also has been high, at 61.22 per 1,000 live births in 2012. In 2006, 16.4 percent of children under age 5 were underweight (defined as 2 kilograms [kg] below standard weight-for-age at age 1, 3 kg below for ages 2 to 3, and 4 kg below for ages 4 to 5).

Health Care Personnel

Uganda has three medical schools: Kigezi International School of Medicine in Kabale, the Faculty of Medicine of Makerere University Medical School in Kampala, and the Faculty of Medicine of Mbarara University of Science and Technology in Mbarara. The basic medical degree course lasts four or five years, and the degrees awarded are bachelor of medicine and bachelor of surgery. A one-year internship is also required before the license to practice medicine will be granted. Government service is obligatory for at least two years after graduation.

In 2005, Uganda had 0.12 physicians per 1,000 population, 0.03 pharmaceutical personnel per 1,000, 0.11 health management and support workers per 1,000, 0.02 dentistry personnel per 1,000, 0.19 community and traditional health workers per 1,000, and 1.31 nurses and midwives per 1,000. Michael Clemens and Bunilla Petterson estimate that 43 percent of Uganda-born physicians and 10 percent of Uganda-born nurses are working in one of nine developed countries, primarily in the United Kingdom. Alok Bhargava and colleagues place Uganda fifth among countries with populations of more than 4 million that were most affected by medical "brain drain" (international migration of skilled personnel) in 2004.

Government Role in Health Care

Uganda has a National Health Policy (NHP) and an implementation plan for it; both date from 2010. Uganda also has a National Medicines Policy (NMP), dating from 2002. The NMP covers selection of essential medicines; financing, pricing, purchase, distribution, and regulation of drugs; pharmacovigilance; rational usage of medicines; human resource development; research; evaluation and monitoring; and traditional medicine.

According to WHO, in 2010, Uganda spent $1.6 million on health care, an amount that comes to $47 per capita. About three-quarters (74 percent) of health care funding came from domestic sources, with 26 percent coming from abroad. The largest share of health care spending was provided through household expenditures (50 percent), with the remainder coming from government expenditures (22 percent) and other sources (28 percent). In 2010, Uganda allocated 12 percent of its total government expenditures to health, in the median range for low-income African countries; government expenditures on health came to 2 percent of GDP, in the low range for low-income African countries. In 2009, according to WHO, official development assistance (ODA) for health in Uganda came to $14.72 per capita.

Public Health Programs

The Uganda Virus Research Institute (UVRI) is located in Entebbe and headed by Edward Mbidde; it is a semiautonomous department within the Ministry of Health. The UVRI has a core staff of approximately 200, organized into departments of immunology; arbovirology, emerging, and reemerging diseases; ecology and zoology; virology; entomology and vector biology; epidemiology; an EPI laboratory; clinical research; and training. The UVRI works with many international organizations, including the Wellcome

Trust, the African AIDS Vaccine Program, and the European and Developing Countries Clinical Trials Partnership, and is expanding its traditional focus on viral diseases to include noncommunicable diseases, malaria, and tuberculosis. UVRI conducts disease surveillance and control projects (most recently, for yellow fever and Ebola), conducts research that has influenced policy on issues such as male circumcision and the use of Bactrin to protect against HIV, and provides training and other capacity-building activities for other countries in Africa.

According to WHO, in 2004, Uganda had 0.04 environmental and public health workers per 1,000 population. In 2010, 34 percent of the population had access to improved sanitation facilities (34 percent in rural areas and 34 percent in urban), and 72 percent had access to improved sources of drinking water (68 percent in rural areas and 95 percent in urban). According to the World Higher Education Database (WHED), two universities in Uganda offer programs in epidemiology or public health: Makerere University in Kampala and the Mountains of the Moon University in Fort Portal.

UKRAINE

Ukraine is an eastern European country, sharing borders with Belarus, Hungary, Moldova, Poland, Romania, Russia, and Slovakia and having a coastline on the Black Sea. The area of 233,032 square miles (603,550 square kilometers) makes Ukraine about the size of Texas, and the July 2012 population was estimated at 44.8 million (the 29th-largest in the world). In 2010, 69 percent of the population lived in urban areas, and the 2010 to 2015 annual rate of urbanization is estimated at negative 0.1 percent. Kyiv is the capital and largest city (with a 2009 population estimated at 2.8 million). The population growth rate in 2012 was negative 0.6 percent, the net migration rate negative 0.1 migrants per 1,000 population, the birth rate 9.6 births per 1,000, and the total fertility rate 1.3 children per woman. The United Nations High Commissioner for Refugees (UNHCR) estimated that, in 2010, there were 318 refugees and persons in refugee-like situations in Ukraine.

Most of Ukraine was absorbed by Russia in the 18th century; the country was independent from 1917 to 1920 before being reconquered by the Soviet Union;

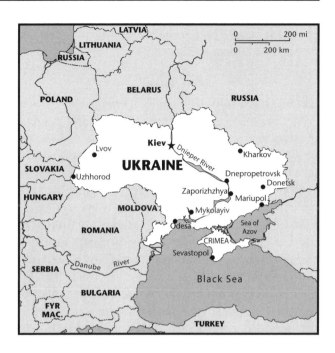

an estimated 8 million Ukrainians died in famines under Soviet rule from 1921 to 1922 and from 1932 to 1933. Ukraine became independent in 1991. Ukraine ranked tied for 152nd among 183 countries on the *Corruption Perceptions Index 2011,* with a score of 2.3 (on a scale where 0 indicates highly corrupt and 10 very clean). In 2011, Ukraine was classified as a country with high human development (the second-highest category) on the United Nations Development Programme's (UNDP's) Human Development Index (HDI), with a score of 0.729 (on a scale where 1 denotes high development and 0 low development). Life expectancy at birth in 2012 was estimated at 68.74 years, and estimated gross domestic product (GDP) per capita in 2011 was $7,200. Income distribution is among the most equal in the world: In 2008, the Gini Index (a measure of dispersion, in which perfect equality is denoted by 0 and maximum inequality is denoted by 100) for family income was 27.5. According to the World Economic Forum's *Global Gender Gap Index 2011*, Ukraine ranked 64th out of 135 countries on gender equality, with a score of 0.686 (on a scale with a theoretical range of 1 for equality to 0 for inequality and an actual range in 2011 from 0.8530 to 0.4873).

Emergency Health Services

According to the World Health Organization (WHO), as of 2007, Ukraine had a formal and publicly available emergency care (prehospital care) system accessible through a national access number.

Insurance

Ukraine has a universal medical benefits system covering everyone residing in the country and a social insurance system providing cash sickness and maternity benefits. Individuals may also purchase voluntary medical insurance. The medical benefits system is funded out of general tax revenues, while the cash benefits system is funded through wage contributions (0.25 to 0.5 percent of earnings), earnings of the self-employed (3 percent of declared income), and employer contributions (2.5 percent of payroll); the government subsidizes maternity cash benefits for those without insurance. Medical benefits are provided through government health care providers; services covered include hospitalization, medical care, maternity care, dental care, lab services, and transportation. Some cost sharing is involved, but free medicines are provided for pensioners receiving the minimum pension, children younger than 1 year, and disabled children younger than 16. Care in sanatoriums and rest homes may be provided, but those who can pay part of the cost are given preference.

The maternity benefit is 100 percent of earnings for 70 days before and 56 days after the due date, with extensions for multiple births or complications. The sickness benefit is 60 to 100 percent of earnings, depending on the length of time working and other circumstances, for up to six months. The Ministry of Health coordinates medical benefits, along with local government health departments, and the Ministry of Labor and Social Policy administers benefits, along with local government social protection departments. According to Ke Xu and colleagues, in 2003, 3.9 percent of households in Ukraine experienced catastrophic health expenditures annually; "catastrophic" was defined as exceeding 40 percent of household income remaining after basic needs were met.

Costs of Hospitalization

No data available.

Access to Health Care

According to WHO, in 2007, 99 percent of births in Ukraine were attended by skilled personnel (for example, physicians, nurses, or midwives), and 75 percent of pregnant women received at least four prenatal care visits. The 2010 immunization rates for 1-year-olds were 90 percent for diphtheria and pertussis (DPT3), 94 percent for measles (MCV), and 81 percent for Hib (Hib3). In 2010, an estimated 13 percent of persons with advanced human immunodeficiency virus (HIV) infection were receiving antiretroviral therapy in accordance with the 2010 WHO guidelines.

Cost of Drugs

Drugs in Ukraine are exempt from taxes and custom fees, and markups are set as low as 10 to 12 percent for distributors and 25 to 35 percent for pharmacies. A 2007 survey by the Open Public Health Institute, located in Kiev, examined the price and availability of a market basket of common drugs. Lowest-priced generic drugs were procured in the public sphere with a median price ratio of 3.5, meaning they cost, on average, 3.5 times the international reference price. The most-sold generics had a median price ratio of 3.1, while originator brands had a median price ratio of 7.8. Often, the same institution procured both the originator brand and generic version of a drug, sometimes paying more than 30 times as much for the originator as for the generic version. Public-sector prices (to patients) had a median price ratio of 4.0 for the lowest-priced generics, with higher median price ratios for the most-sold generics at 4.8 and originator brands at 9.9. Availability was good in the public sector, with median availability of 83.3 percent for the lowest-priced generics, 72.2 percent for the most-sold generics, and 55.1 percent for originator brands. The median price ratio in the private sector was higher for originator brands (13.8) but lower for the lowest-priced generics (3.7) and for the most-sold generics (3.8). The median availability for the lowest-priced generics in the private sector was 79.5 percent, for the most-sold generics 68.8 percent, and for originator brands 47 percent.

Many drugs to treat common conditions were not affordable using the standard that the lowest-paid government worker should not pay for than 1 day's wages for a course of drugs. For instance, generics to treat hypercholesterolemia would cost 3.5 days' wages in the public sphere and 7.0 or 7.1 days' wages in the private sphere. However, some courses of treatment met the standard: For instance, a course of treatment with generic atenolol for hypertension would cost 0.4 day's wages in either the public or private sphere.

Health Care Facilities

In 2008, Ukraine had 8.73 hospital beds per 1,000 population, the sixth-highest ratio in the world.

Major Health Issues

In 2008, WHO estimated that 14 percent of years of life lost in Ukraine were due to communicable diseases, 70 percent to noncommunicable diseases, and 17 percent to injuries. In 2008, the age-standardized estimate of cancer deaths was 159 per 100,000 for men and 79 per 100,000 for women; for cardiovascular disease and diabetes, 772 per 100,000 for men and 441 per 100,000 for women; and for chronic respiratory disease, 43 per 100,000 for men and eight per 100,000 for women.

Compared to other countries at a similar level of development, Ukraine ranked low (39th out of 43 countries) on the 2011 Mothers' Index, produced by the international nongovernmental organization (NGO) Save the Children, based on a number of health and social factors relating to women, children, and maternal and child care. Ukraine's maternal mortality rate (death from any cause related to or aggravated by pregnancy) in 2008 was 26 maternal deaths per 100,000 live births. The infant mortality rate, defined as the number of deaths of infants younger than 1 year, was 8.38 per 1,000 live births in 2012.

In 2010, tuberculosis incidence was 101.0 per 100,000 population, tuberculosis prevalence 60.0 per 100,000, and deaths due to tuberculosis among HIV-negative people 3.00 per 100,000. As estimated 16 percent of new tuberculosis cases and 44 percent of retreatment cases are multidrug resistant. As of 2009, an estimated 1.1 percent of adults age 15 to 49 were living with HIV or acquired immune deficiency syndrome (AIDS).

Health Care Personnel

Ukraine has 17 medical schools. The basic medical degree course lasts six to eight years, and the degree awarded is Vra c-spetsialist (doctor of medicine). Work in government service is required during specialist training. Physicians must register with the Health Administration of the province in which they wish to work, and the license to practice medicine is granted to graduates of recognized medical schools with training in a specialization. Ukraine has bilateral agreements with a number of countries. In 2006, Ukraine had 3.13 physicians per 1,000 population, 0.48 pharmaceutical personnel per 1,000, 0.42 dentistry personnel per 1,000, and 8.45 nurses and midwives per 1,000.

Government Role in Health Care

According to WHO, in 2010, Ukraine spent $11 billion on health care, an amount that comes to $234 per capita. All health care funding came from domestic sources. The largest share of health care spending was provided through government expenditures (57 percent), with the remainder coming from household expenditures (41 percent) and other sources (3 percent). In 2010, Ukraine allocated 9 percent of its total government expenditures to health, in the median range for lower-middle-income European countries; government expenditures on health came to 4 percent of GDP, in the high range for lower-middle-income European countries. In 2009, according to WHO, official development assistance (ODA) for health in Ukraine came to $1.46 per capita.

Public Health Programs

In 2010, 94 percent of the population of Ukraine had access to improved sanitation facilities (89 percent in rural areas and 96 percent in urban), and 98 percent had access to improved sources of drinking water (98 percent in rural areas and 98 percent in urban). According to the World Higher Education Database (WHED), four universities in Ukraine offer programs in epidemiology or public health: the Dnipropetrovsk State Agrarian University, Kharkiv National Medical University, Lviv National Medical University Danylo Halyckyj, and Odessa National Medical University.

UNITED ARAB EMIRATES

The United Arab Emirates (UAE) is a Middle Eastern country, sharing borders with Oman and Saudi Arabia and having a coastline on the Persian Gulf and the Gulf of Oman. The area of 32,278 square miles (83,600 square kilometers) makes the UAE about the size of Maine, and the July 2012 population was estimated at 5.3 million. In 2010, 84 percent of the population lived in urban areas, and the 2010 to 2015 annual rate of urbanization was estimated at 2.3 percent. Abu Dhabi is the capital and largest city (with a 2009 population estimated at 666,000). The population growth rate in 2012 was 3.0 percent (the 10th-highest in the world), the net migration rate 15.8 migrants per 1,000 population (the fifth-highest in the world), the birth rate 10.9 births per 1,000, and the total fertility rate 2.4

children per woman. The United Nations High Commissioner for Refugees (UNHCR) estimated that, in 2010, there were 538 refugees and persons in refugee-like situations in the UAE.

The UAE was formed in 1971, when six states (Abu Zaby, Ajman, Al Fujayrah, Ash Shariqah, Dubai, and Umm al Qaywain) merged; a seventh state, Ra's al Khaimah, joined in 1972. The UAE ranked 28th among 183 countries on the *Corruption Perceptions Index 2011,* with a score of 6.8 (on a scale where 0 indicates highly corrupt and 10 very clean). In 2011, the UAE was classified as a country with very high human development (the highest of four categories) on the United Nations Development Programme's (UNDP's) Human Development Index (HDI), with a score of 0.846 (on a scale where 1 denotes high development and 0 low development).

Life expectancy at birth in 2012 was estimated at 76.71 years, and per capita gross domestic product (GDP) in 2011 in the UAE was estimated at $48,500, among the highest in the world. According to the World Economic Forum's *Global Gender Gap Index 2011,* the UAE ranked 103rd out of 135 countries on gender equality, with a score of 0.645 (on a scale with a theoretical range of 1 for equality to 0 for inequality and an actual range in 2011 from 0.8530 to 0.4873).

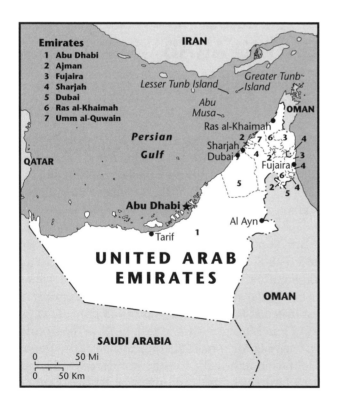

Emergency Health Services

According to the World Health Organization (WHO), as of 2007, the UAE had a formal and publicly available emergency care (prehospital care) system accessible through a national access number.

Insurance

In 2008, the UAE began a Strategic Framework for the years 2008 through 2010 in order to improve health facilities, improve regulation, and improve the qualifications of health care personnel and administrators. The framework is also focused on improving access and quality of care, with particular emphasis on preventive care. A basic, compulsory insurance scheme for residents of Abu Dhabi has already been instituted, and there are plans to introduce a national health insurance scheme throughout the country by 2012. Free medical and pharmaceutical services are provided for all nationals at facilities run by the Ministry of Health and local authorities, but non-nationals must have health insurance provided by their home countries or employers or pay out of pocket.

Costs of Hospitalization

No data available.

Access to Health Care

According to WHO, in 2008, 100 percent of births in the UAE were attended by skilled personnel (for example, physicians, nurses, or midwives). The 2010 immunization rates for 1-year-olds were 94 percent for diphtheria and pertussis (DPT3), 94 percent for measles (MCV), and 94 percent for Hib (Hib3).

Cost of Drugs

Drug prices in the UAE are set by the Ministry of Health, based on the international reference prices. Generics are priced 30 percent below the international reference cost, and a 2009 law requires prescriptions be written by generic name. A 2006 survey of the price and availability of a market basket of common drugs found that many drugs would be unaffordable, using the standard of the wages of the lowest-paid government worker, if purchased in the private sphere, but that drugs were available for free to UAE nationals in government facilities. The median price ratio for the public procurement price for the lowest-priced generic versions of drugs was 1.25, meaning that the price paid was on average 25 percent over the international reference price. Originator brands were more expensive, with an international reference price of 4.92. Availability for generics (61.1 percent) was much higher than availability for originator brands (16.7 percent). Prices in the private sector (from retail pharmacies) are much higher than in the public sector, with a median reference price of 13.8 for the lowest-priced generics and 23.5 for originator brands. Median availability for the lowest-priced generics in the private sector was 73.9 percent and 100 percent for originator brands.

Health Care Facilities

In 2008, the UAE had 1.90 hospital beds per 1,000 population.

Major Health Issues

In 2008, WHO estimated that 14 percent of years of life lost in the UAE were due to communicable diseases, 57 percent to noncommunicable diseases, and 30 percent to injuries. In 2008, the age-standardized estimate of cancer deaths was 63 per 100,000 for men and 64 per 100,000 for women; for cardiovascular disease and diabetes, 309 per 100,000 for men and 204 per 100,000 for women; and for chronic respiratory disease, 12 per 100,000 for men and 23 per 100,000 for women. The UAE has one of the highest adult obesity rates in the world, estimated at 33.7 percent in 2008; obesity is defined as a body mass index (BMI) of 30 or above.

The maternal mortality rate (death from any cause related to or aggravated by pregnancy) in the UAE in 2008 was 10 maternal deaths per 100,000 live births. The infant mortality rate, defined as the number of deaths of infants younger than 1 year, was 11.59 per 1,000 live births in 2012. In 2010, tuberculosis incidence was 3.1 per 100,000 population, tuberculosis prevalence 6.2 per 100,000, and deaths due to tuberculosis among human immunodeficiency virus (HIV)-negative people 0.30 per 100,000. As of 2001, an estimated 0.2 percent of adults age 15 to 49 were living with HIV or acquired immune deficiency syndrome (AIDS).

Health Care Personnel

The UAE has three medical schools: the Faculty of Medicine and Health Sciences of the UAE University in Abu Dhabi, Dubai Medical College for Girls in Dubai, and Gulf Medical University (formerly Gulf Medical College) in Ajman. The basic medical course requires six or seven years to complete. In 2007, the UAE had

1.93 physicians per 1,000 population, 0.59 pharmaceutical personnel per 1,000, 0.43 dentistry personnel per 1,000, and 4.09 nurses and midwives per 1,000.

Government Role in Health Care

According to WHO, in 2010, the UAE spent $11 billion on health care, an amount that comes to $1,450 per capita. All health care funding came from domestic sources. The largest share of health care spending (74 percent) was provided through government expenditures, with the remainder coming from household expenditures (19 percent) and other sources (7 percent). In 2010, the UAE allocated 9 percent of its total government expenditures to health, in the high range for high-income eastern Mediterranean region countries; government expenditures on health came to 3 percent of GDP, in the high range for high-income eastern Mediterranean region countries.

Public Health Programs

In 2010, 98 percent of the population of the UAE had access to improved sanitation facilities (95 percent in rural areas and 98 percent in urban), and access to improved sources of drinking water was essentially universal. According to the World Higher Education Database (WHED), two universities in the UAE offer programs in epidemiology or public health: the Boston University Institute for Dental Research and Education in Dubai, and the University of Sharjah.

UNITED KINGDOM

The United Kingdom (UK) is composed of four constituent countries: England, Scotland, Wales, and Northern Ireland. Although these four countries form one nation, there are also important differences among them, not only historically and culturally but also in terms of how they organize health care delivery. All four are part of the National Health Service (NHS), but health care delivery is managed separately in each. Sometimes, statistics are collected and reported at the national level and sometimes specifically within one of the four constituent parts. For this reason, the name *the UK* will be used when discussing information about the entire nation, while if only one of the four areas is discussed, it will be identified by name (for example, England or Scotland).

The UK is an island in the north Atlantic, consisting of all of the island of England and part of the island of Ireland as well as numerous smaller islands. The area of 94,058 square miles (243,610 square kilometers) makes the UK about the size of Oregon, and the July 2012 population was estimated at 63.0 million (the 22nd largest in the world). In 2010, 80 percent of the population lived in urban areas, and the 2010 to 2015 annual rate of urbanization was estimated at 0.7 percent. London is the capital and largest city (with a 2009 population estimated at 8.6 million). The population growth rate in 2012 was 0.6 percent, the net migration rate 2.6 migrants per 1,000 population (the 30th-highest in the world), the birth rate 12.3 births per 1,000, and the total fertility rate 1.9 children per woman.

The British Empire in the 19th century covered one-quarter of the world's surface; almost all British colonies became independent in the 20th century. However, the UK remains a world leader in international affairs, economic development, and education and research. The UK has a reputation for transparency and honesty, ranking tied for 16th among 183 countries on the *Corruption Perceptions Index 2011,* with a score of 7.8 (on a scale where 0 indicates highly corrupt and 10 very clean). In 2011, the UK was classified as a country with very high human development (the highest of four categories) on the United Nations Development Programme's (UNDP's) Human Development Index (HDI), with a score of 0.863 (on a scale

where 1 denotes high development and 0 low development). Life expectancy at birth in 2012 was estimated at 80.17 years, among the highest in the world, and per capita gross domestic product (GDP) in 2011 was estimated at $35,900. In 2005, the Gini Index (a measure of dispersion, in which perfect equality is denoted by 0 and maximum inequality is denoted by 100) for family income was 34.0. According to the World Economic Forum's *Global Gender Gap Index 2011*, the UK ranked 16th out of 135 countries on gender equality, with a score of 0.646 (on a scale with a theoretical range of 1 for equality to 0 for inequality and an actual range in 2011 from 0.8530 to 0.4873).

Emergency Health Services

The UK's laws regulating emergency care date from the 1990s, while recognition of emergency care as a specialty dates from the 1980s (second after Hungary among European Union, or EU, countries); by law, everyone, including the uninsured and unidentified, is entitled to emergency access to hospitals. Both inpatient and outpatient emergency care is funded entirely by the state budget, but ambulance services are organized at the regional level. The emergency call number is 999, and the country has 33 noninterconnected dispatch centers. A secure Internet connection provides information about the availability of intensive care beds.

Insurance

Britain's National Health Service (NHS) was designed by William Beveridge, and systems modeled after it (for example, by T.R. Reid) are sometimes called "Beveridge systems." The characteristics of a Beveridge system include government-provided and government-financed health care and a dual system in which most hospitals are owned by the government, but there are also private hospitals, and some physicians are employed by the government, while others are paid through government fees. The UK has an NHS, created in 1948, that provides universal access to health care. The system is funded through national taxation, but the service is managed separately in England, Scotland, Wales, and Northern Ireland. The NHS in England (officially the only system called the National Health Service) is the largest, employing about 1.4 million people as of 2012; NHS Scotland employs more than 155,000; NHS Wales more than 85,000; and Health and Social Care (HSC) in Northern Ireland more than 65,000. Although there are many similarities in how each NHS operates, there are

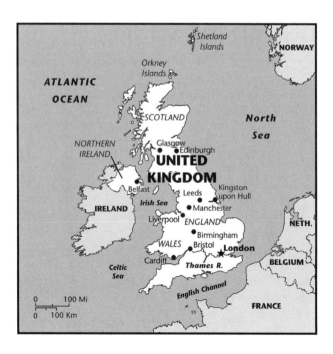

Selected Health Indicators: United Kingdom Compared With the Organisation for Economic Co-operation and Development (OECD) Country Average

	United Kingdom	OECD average (2010 or nearest year)
Male life expectancy at birth, 2010	78.6	77
Female life expectancy at birth, 2010	82.6	82.5
Total expenditure on health (percent of GDP), 2010	9.6	9.5
Total expenditure on health (per capita, USD purchasing power parity), 2010	3,433.2	3,265
Public expenditure on health (per capita, USD purchasing power parity), 2010	2,857.3	2,377.8
Public expenditure on health (percent total expenditure on health), 2010	83.2	72.2
Out-of-pocket expenditure on health (percent total expenditure on health), 2010	8.9	19.5
Out-of-pocket expenditure on health (per capita, USD purchasing power parity), 2010	305.7	558.4
Hospital discharge rates, all causes (per 100,000 population), 2010	13,596	15,508
Average length of hospital stay, all causes (days), 2010	7.7	7.1
Hospital beds (per 1,000 population), 2010	3	4.9

Source: OECD Health Data 2012 (Organisation for Economic Co-operation and Development, 2012).

also important differences. For instance, while England since 2000 has deliberately introduced market competition into the delivery of health care services, reducing wait times and allowing patients to choose from a variety of hospitals and clinics, in Scotland, waiting times have been reduced without introducing market competition; instead, the responsibility to allocate resources and deliver services is decided by networks of physicians. Scotland also provides free personal care (for example, assistance in dressing and bathing) to the elderly without requiring means testing, while in England, provision of this care is means tested.

A 2004 study by the World Health Organization (WHO) found that none of the UK population had substitutive voluntary health insurance (covering services that would otherwise be available from the state), and 11.5 percent had complementary voluntary health insurance (covering services not covered or not fully covered by the state) or supplementary health insurance (providing increased choice or faster access to services). Policyholders were most likely to be middle-aged professionals, managers, or employers and based in London or the southern region. According to Ke Xu and colleagues, in 2003, less than 0.1 percent of households in the UK experienced catastrophic health expenditures annually; "catastrophic" was defined as exceeding 40 percent of household income remaining after basic needs were met.

Costs of Hospitalization

Hospital care is provided free in NHS hospitals for anyone "considered ordinarily resident" in England, meaning anyone living lawfully in the UK with an identifiable purpose for their residence; those not considered ordinarily resident are subject to the Charges to Overseas Visitors (NHS Regulations 2011). England has bilateral health care agreements with many countries, including those in the European Economic

Area, many other European countries, and residents of some other countries, including Australia, the British Virgin Islands, and the Falkland Islands. According to Organisation for Economic Co-operation and Development (OECD) data, in England in 2008, the average length of stay in acute care was 6.8 days, and there were 138 hospital discharges per 1,000 population. In 2008, according to the OECD, hospitals in the UK were funded 70 percent through payments per case or diagnosis-related group (DRG) and 30 percent through global budgets.

Access to Health Care

In 2009, according to OECD data, people in England had an average of 5.0 physician visits. In 2010, almost three-quarters (70 percent) reported that, when sick, they were able to get medical appointments the same day or the next day. Just over one-third (38 percent) reported it was very or somewhat difficult to get medical care after usual office hours. For those who needed particular types of care, less than two-fifths (19 percent) reported they waited two or more months to see a specialist (of those who needed to see a specialist in the prior two years), a similar proportion (21 percent) reported waiting four or more months for elective surgery (of those who required elective surgery in the prior two years), but only 5 percent reported they had experienced an access barrier due to cost in the previous two years; an access barrier was defined as failing to fill or refill a prescription, failing to visit a physician, or failing to get recommended care.

In 2010, less than one in 10 (8 percent) of people in England reported experiencing a medical, medication, or lab test error in the previous two years, and 14 percent of those who needed to visit a specialist in the previous two years reported that the specialist did not have information about their medical history at the time of the appointment. Half (50 percent) reported experiencing a gap in hospital discharge planning in the previous two years (due to any of the following: did not receive a written plan for care, did not have arrangements made for follow-up visits, did not know whom to contact with questions, or did not receive instruction about when to seek further care).

A 2011 Commonwealth Fund Survey compared access to health care for "sicker" adults (those 18 and older, in self-reported poor or fair health, who had been treated for a serious illness or injury in the past year or been hospitalized in the past two years) in 11 OECD countries. This survey found that 11 percent of sicker residents of the UK surveyed reported having experienced an access problem related to cost in the previous year, the lowest proportion among the 11 countries surveyed; the most common result was having a medical problem but failing to visit a doctor. Other problems reported include having serious problems paying their medical bills (1 percent, the lowest proportion in the survey), waiting six days or longer for needed care (2 percent, the lowest proportion in the survey), having difficulty getting after-hours care except in an emergency room (21 percent, the lowest proportion in the survey), and experiencing coordination gaps in care (20 percent, the lowest proportion in the survey).

According to WHO, in 2008, 99 percent of births in the UK in were attended by skilled personnel (for example, physicians, nurses, or midwives). The 2010 immunization rates for 1-year-olds were 96 percent for diphtheria and pertussis (DPT3), 93 percent for measles (MCV), and 97 percent for Hib (Hib3).

Cost of Drugs

According to data reported by the office for National Statistics, in 2009 in England, an average of 17.1 prescription items were dispensed per person; in Wales, an average of 22.5 items; in Scotland, an average of 16.6 items; and in Northern Ireland, an average of 18.9 items. The average net ingredient cost (not including dispensing fees or costs) per person was £164.8 in England, £194.1 in Wales, £187.5 in Scotland, and £232.4 in Northern Ireland, an average net prescription (not including dispensing fees or costs) was £9.6 in England, £8.6 in Wales, £11.2 in Scotland, and £12.3 in Northern Ireland.

Real annual growth in pharmaceutical expenditures in the UK grew 3.9 percent from 1997 to 2005, much slower than the 7.3 percent growth of total health expenditure (minus pharmaceutical expenditures) over those years. According to Elizabeth Docteur, in 2004, generic drugs represented 21 percent of the market share by value and 49 percent of the market share by volume of the total pharmaceutical market.

According to Douglas Ball, the standard value-added tax (VAT) of 17.5 percent is charged for both prescription-only and over-the-counter medicines, but for prescription-only medicines the rate is essentially 0 percent, as these are paid for by the government. The wholesalers' distribution margin is included in the NHS list price; manufacturers and wholesalers may negotiate discounts, as may pharmacists and wholesalers; the pharmacists' markup is the difference between the NHS reimbursement price and the selling price in the pharmacy.

Health Care Facilities

From 2008 to 2009, according to data reported by the Office of National Statistics, the UK had 206,900 hospital beds, or 3.4 per 1,000 population: 160,300 in England (3.1 per 1,000), 13,100 in Wales (4.4 per 1,000), 25,800 in Scotland (5.0 per 1,000), and 7,700 in Northern Ireland (4.3 per 1,000). Most hospital beds were in the acute sector, with smaller proportions for maternity, mental illness, learning disability, geriatrics, and general beds. In the UK overall, there were 2.1 acute beds per 1,000 population (61.8 percent of the total), in England 2.0 per 1,000, in Wales 2.8 per 1,000, in Scotland 2.4 per 1,000, and in Northern Ireland 2.4 per 1,000.

Major Health Issues

In 2008, WHO estimated that 8 percent of years of life lost in the UK were due to communicable diseases, 83 percent to noncommunicable diseases, and 9 percent to injuries. In 2008, the age-standardized estimate of cancer deaths was 155 per 100,000 for men and 114 per 100,000 for women; for cardiovascular disease and diabetes, 166 per 100,000 for men and 102 per 100,000 for women; and for chronic respiratory disease, 39 per 100,000 for men and 27 per 100,000 for women. In 2002, an estimated 22.7 percent of adults in the UK were obese (defined as a body mass index, or BMI, of 30 or greater).

The maternal mortality rate (death from any cause related to or aggravated by pregnancy) in the UK in 2008 was 12 maternal deaths per 100,000 live births. The infant mortality rate, defined as the number of deaths of infants younger than 1 year, was 4.56 per 1,000 live births in 2012. In 2010, tuberculosis incidence was 13.0 per 100,000 population, tuberculosis prevalence 15.0 per 100,000, and deaths due to tuberculosis among human immunodeficiency virus (HIV)-negative people 0.64 per 100,000. As of 2009, an estimated 0.2 percent of adults age 15 to 49 were living with HIV or acquired immune deficiency syndrome (AIDS).

Health Care Personnel

The UK has 27 medical schools. The basic course of training lasts five to seven years, and the degrees granted are the bachelor of medicine and bachelor of surgery. In 2005, an investigation revealed that several unaccredited squatter medical schools, including St. Christopher's College of Medicine in Luton, were operating in the UK and using NHS facilities for training, although the schools' degree-awarding powers came from other countries (Senegal, in the case of St. Christopher's), and the UK ceased recognizing degrees from these schools (St. Christopher's left the UK and now operates only in Senegal).

The UK, as a member of the EU, cooperates with other countries in recognizing physicians qualified to practice in other EU countries, as specified by Directive 2005/36/EC of the European Parliament. This allows qualified professionals to practice their profession in other EU states on a temporary basis and requires that the host country automatically recognize qualifications for certain professions, including physicians, nurses, dentists, midwives, and pharmacists, if certain conditions have been met (for instance, facility in the language of the host country may be required).

In 2009, the UK had 2.74 physicians per 1,000 population, 0.66 pharmaceutical personnel per 1,000, and 10.30 nurses and midwives per 1,000. In 2001, 12.6 percent of practicing physicians in the UK were trained in another country, primarily India and Ireland. In 2001, 37.3 percent of physicians in postgraduate training in the UK had received their medical education in another country. Overall, the UK exports about 10 times as many physicians (primarily to Australia and the United States, among other countries) as it imports.

Government Role in Health Care

According to WHO, in 2010, the UK spent $217 billion on health care, an amount that comes to $3,503 per capita. All health care funding came from domestic sources. The largest share of health care spending was provided through government expenditures (84 percent), with the remainder coming from household expenditures (10 percent) and other sources (6 percent). In 2010, the UK allocated 16 percent of its total government expenditures to health, in the median range for high-income European countries; government expenditures on health came to 8 percent of GDP, in the high range for high-income European countries.

According to the UK Office for National Statistics, total identifiable expenditures on health and personal social services from 2008 to 2009 came to £113,809,000 in England (£2,212 per capita), £7,466,000 in Wales (£2,494 per capita), £13,148,000 in Scotland (£2,544 per capita), and £4,136,000 in Northern Ireland (£2,330 per capita).

Public Health Programs

The Health Protection Agency (HPA) for the United Kingdom is located in London and headed by Justin McCracken. The HPA employs more than 3,000 staff members and operates three main centers, in Salisbury (the Centre for Emergency Preparedness and Response), North London (the Centre for Infections), and Chilton (the Centre for Radiation, Chemicals, and Environmental Hazards) as well as the National Institute of Biological Standards and Control (in Hertfordshire). Its goal is to protect the health of the UK population, including setting standards for health protection, and identifying and responding to health threats from both infectious diseases and environmental standards. The HPA played a key role in preparing for potential threats involved with the 2012 Olympics; other recent projects include introduction of the human papilloma virus (HPV) vaccine for girls aged 12 to 13 years, investigating an outbreak of pseudomonas in neonatal units in Northern Ireland, studying hospital-related infections, studying the health effects of air pollution, and creating a real-time surveillance system to track health threats across the country.

According to WHO, in 1997 (the most recent year for which data was available), the UK had 0.25 environmental and public health workers per 1,000 population. In 2010, access to improved sanitary facilities and improved sources of drinking water was essentially universal. According to the World Higher Education Database (WHED), 24 universities in the UK offer programs in epidemiology or public health.

UNITED STATES

The United States is a North American country, sharing borders with Canada and Mexico and having coastlines on the north Atlantic and north Pacific Oceans. The area of 3,794,100 square miles (9,826,675 square kilometers) makes the United States the third-largest country in the world; the July 2012 population was estimated at 313.8 million (the 3rd largest in the

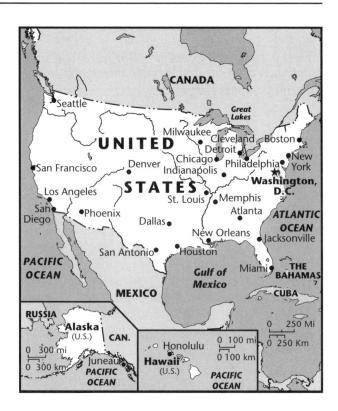

world). Washington, D.C., is the capital and New York City the largest city (with a 2009 population of the metropolitan area estimated at 19.3 million). In 2010, 82 percent of the population lived in urban areas, and the 2010 to 2015 annual rate of urbanization was estimated at 1.2 percent. The population growth rate in 2012 was 0.9 percent, the net migration rate 3.6 migrants per 1,000 population (the 26th-highest in the world), the birth rate 13.4 births per 1,000, and the total fertility rate 2.1 children per woman.

The United States became independent from Great Britain in 1776 and gradually expanded westward across the North American continent. The United States benefited greatly by avoiding the destruction of World War I and World War II and became the world's dominant economic and military force in the 20th century.

The United States ranked 24th among 183 countries on the *Corruption Perceptions Index 2011,* with a score of 7.1 (on a scale where 0 indicates highly corrupt and 10 very clean). The United States was ranked tied for third (with the Netherlands) in 2011 on the United Nations Development Programme's (UNDP's) Human Development Index (HDI), with a score of 0.910 (on a scale where 1 denotes high development and 0 low development). Life expectancy at birth in

2012 was estimated at 78.49 years, and per capita gross domestic product (GDP) in 2011 in the United States was estimated at $48,100, among the highest in the world. In 2007, the Gini Index (a measure of dispersion, in which perfect equality is denoted by 0 and maximum inequality is denoted by 100) for family income was 45.0. According to the World Economic Forum's *Global Gender Gap Index 2011*, the United States ranked 17th out of 135 countries on gender equality, with a score of 0.741 (on a scale with a theoretical range of 1 for equality to 0 for inequality and an actual range in 2011 from 0.8530 to 0.4873).

Emergency Health Services

The United States has an organized system of emergency care accessible through the national access telephone number 911. Since passage of the Emergency Medical Treatment and Active Labor Act in 1986, hospitals who accept Medicaid and Medicare payments (virtually all the hospitals in the United States) are required to provide emergency care to anyone who requests it, regardless of ability to pay. However, the costs of providing this care is not reimbursed by the federal government, and it has become an issue because the costs must be covered out of the general hospital budget (in essence, unreimbursed care is paid for by the people who do pay their bills).

In addition to true emergencies, some individuals use the emergency room (ER) for care that could have been provided in a physician's office or medical clinic because the individual does not have a regular physician or that physician is not available for after-hours care. A 2012 Commonwealth Fund study reported that, among Medicaid recipients, about one-third of visits to the ER could have been avoided were other sources of care available: Nonemergent cases constituted 13 percent of ER visits, and emergent conditions that could have been treated by primary care constituted another 20 percent. Avoidable ER use varied by region, from 129 visits per 1,000 Medicare recipients to 294 visits per 1,000.

Insurance

As of 2012, the United States does not have a system of national health care or national health insurance in the sense that many other industrialized countries do. Instead, health care is provided and paid for by a variety of mechanisms, including employer-based insurance, privately purchased insurance, government insurance and health care programs, and out-of-pocket purchases by individuals. There is wide variety among the various insurance plans regarding premiums, services covered, and cost sharing; however, most plans cover physician services and hospital care, and many also include prescription drugs and preventive health care.

As of 2012, about 56 percent of the population had private insurance, and 16 percent of the population was uninsured. Insurance rates vary widely among geographic region; for instance, a 2012 Commonwealth Fund Study found that the insured rate for adults age 18 to 64 varied among the 306 hospital referral regions in the United States from almost universal coverage (94.6 percent) to less than half (46.8 percent); the rates of insurance for children ages 0 to 17 ranged from 98.8 to 79.8. Health care expenditures are a leading cause of bankruptcy in the United States. According to a study by David Himmelstein and colleagues, in 2007, 62.1 percent of bankruptcies in the United States were caused by medical expenses and increased from 2001, when 46.2 percent of bankruptcies were caused by medical expenses. Most of those declaring bankruptcy due to medical expenses in 2007 had health insurance.

According to a Robert Wood Johnson 2009 report, about 45 million Americans were covered by Medicare, a federal program for the elderly (age 65 and older) and disabled. About 61 million Americans were covered by Medicaid, a program for low-income Americans paid for jointly by the federal government and the government of the state in which the individual resides. The federal government also pays for a large share of the health care of about 9 million federal employees and their dependents (through subsidized insurance), and the Veterans Health Administration provides care directly to about 7.8 million veterans. The Indian Health Service, a federal program, provides direct care to about 1.9 million Native Americans and Alaska Natives.

According to the Center for Medicaid and Medicare Services (CMS), CMS is the largest U.S. purchaser of health care, with Medicare and Medicaid accounting for about one-third of U.S. health care expenditures. In 2012, Medicaid and Medicare provided care for about one-third of the U.S. population, about 105 million individuals. Medicare is financed through a payroll tax and premiums, while Medicaid is financed through federal and state tax revenues. There are no general caps on out-of-pocket expenses (different insurance plans may have different caps). Primary care is paid for primarily on a fee-for-service basis, with some insurance plans using a capitation system instead or as well. Hospital payments are handled through a combination of per-diem and case-based payments and generally do not include physician costs. Most patients are not required to register with a general practice physician, although this is required in some insurance programs.

Costs of Hospitalization

U.S. hospitals may be public, nonprofit, or for-profit and are reimbursed in a variety of ways, including payments based on diagnosis-related groups (DRGs) or per-diem charges. According to Organisation for Economic Co-operation and Development (OECD) data, in 2009, hospital spending per capita in the United States was $2,475 (adjusted for differences in the cost of living), and hospital spending per discharge came to $18,142 in 2011 The average length of stay in acute care was 5.4 days in 2008, and there were 131 hospital discharges per 1,000 population.

Access to Health Care

In 2009, according to OECD data, people in the United States had an average of 3.9 physician visits. In 2010, over half (57 percent) reported that, when sick, they were able to get medical appointments the same day or the next day, although a higher percentage (63 percent) reported it was very or somewhat difficult to get medical care after usual office hours. For those who needed particular types of care, less than one in 10 (9 percent) reported they waited two or more months to see a specialist (of those who needed to see a specialist in the prior two years), only 7 percent reported waiting four or more months for elective surgery (of those who required elective surgery in the prior two years), but 33 percent reported they had experienced an access barrier due to cost in the previous two years; an access barrier was defined as failing to fill or refill a prescription, failing to visit a physician, or failing to get recommended care. In 2010, almost two in 10 (18 percent) people in the United States reported experiencing a medical, medication, or lab test error in the previous two years, and 22 percent of those who needed to visit a specialist in the previous two years reported that the specialist did not have information about their medical history at the time of the appointment. More than one-third (38 percent) reported experiencing a gap in hospital discharge planning in the previous two years (due to any of the following:

did not receive a written plan for care, did not have arrangements made for follow-up visits, did not know whom to contact with questions, or did not receive instruction about when to seek further care).

Access to care varies widely, depending on income, the type of insurance coverage, and other factors. A 2012 Commonwealth Fund study found that, comparing the 306 hospital referral regions in the United States, the number of adults with a usual source of care ranged from 93.0 percent to 58.7 percent, and the percent of adults age 50 and older who received recommended preventive care and screenings ranged from 58.8 percent to 26.0 percent. The number of adults who reported that cost did not prevent them from accessing needed medical services ranged from 95.3 percent to 66.9 percent.

A 2011 Commonwealth Fund Survey compared access to health care for "sicker" adults (those 18 and older, in self-reported poor or fair health, who had been treated for a serious illness or injury in the past year or been hospitalized in the past two years) in 11 OECD countries. This survey found that 42 percent of sicker residents of the United States surveyed reported having experienced an access problem related to cost in the previous year, the highest proportion among the 11 countries surveyed; the most common result was skipping a test, treatment, or follow-up. Other problems reported include having serious problems paying their medical bills (27 percent, the highest proportion in the survey), waiting six days or longer for needed care (16 percent), having difficulty getting after-hours care except in an emergency room (55 percent), and experiencing coordination gaps in care (42 percent). According to the World Health Organization (WHO), in 2006, 99.4 percent of births in the United States were attended by skilled personnel (for example, physicians, nurses, or midwives). The 2010 immunization rates for 1-year-olds were 95 percent for diphtheria and pertussis (DPT3), 92 percent for measles (MCV), and 93 percent for Hib (Hib3).

Cost of Drugs

In 2009, according to OECD data, pharmaceutical spending per capita in the United States was $956 (adjusted for differences in the cost of living). Wholesale and resale markups of drugs are both unregulated; wholesale markups average 2 to 4 percent, according to Douglas Ball, and retail markups average 22 to 25 percent. The United States is by far

Selected Health Indicators: United States Compared With the Organisation for Economic Co-operation and Development (OECD) Country Average

	United States	OECD average (2010 or nearest year)
Male life expectancy at birth, 2009	76	77
Female life expectancy at birth, 2009	80.9	82.5
Total expenditure on health (percent of GDP), 2010	17.6	9.5
Total expenditure on health (per capita, USD purchasing power parity), 2010	8,232.9	3,265
Public expenditure on health (per capita, USD purchasing power parity), 2010	3,966.7	2,377.8
Public expenditure on health (percent total expenditure on health), 2010	48.2	72.2
Out-of-pocket expenditure on health (percent total expenditure on health), 2010	11.8	19.5
Out-of-pocket expenditure on health (per capita, USD purchasing power parity), 2010	969.7	558.4
Total expenditure on pharmaceuticals and other medical nondurables (percent total expenditure on health), 2010	11.9	16.6
Total expenditure on pharmaceuticals and other medical nondurables (per capita, USD purchasing power parity), 2010	983.1	495.4
Obesity (percent of female population with a BMI>30 kg/m2, self-reported), 2010	27.8	14.8
Obesity (percent of male population with a BMI>30 kg/m2, self-reported), 2010	28.3	15.1

Source: OECD Health Data 2012 (Organisation for Economic Co-operation and Development, 2012).

the greatest purchaser of pharmaceuticals among countries, accounting for a 45 percent global share of the world market (the second-largest is Japan, with 9 percent of the world market). Real annual growth in pharmaceutical expenditures in the United States grew 8.3 percent from 1997 to 2005, much faster than the 4.7 percent growth of total health expenditure (minus pharmaceutical expenditures) over those years. The United States is also a major manufacturer of pharmaceuticals, with global pharmaceutical sales of $290 billion in 2006 (at ex-manufacturer prices, that is, the list price from the manufacturer before any discounts are taken), accounting for 47.7 percent of sales production. According to Elizabeth Docteur, in 2004, generic drugs represented 12 percent of the

market share by value and 53 percent of the market share by volume of the total pharmaceutical market.

The price for prescription drugs may be totally or partially covered by an individual's insurance plan. When drugs are covered, they may be divided into tiers so that different copayments are required for different tiers; for instance, generics may require only a small copayment or no copayment, while brand-name drugs may require higher copayments. Different brand-name drugs treating the same condition may require different copayments, depending on arrangements negotiated between the insurer and the pharmaceutical manufacturers. Medicare began offering prescription drug coverage (Medicare Part D) in January 2006; however, Medicare does not negotiate with manufacturers over the price of drugs, so covered individuals must pick among a number of competing plans offered by insurers, who provide different benefits at different copayment levels. In addition, Medicare Part D features a "doughnut hole" of coverage, such that no subsidy was offered for the portion of prescription expenditures for an individual that fell between $2,700 and $6,154 annually.

Health Care Facilities

In 2008, the United States had 3.10 hospital beds per 1,000 population. In 2009, the United States had 25.9 magnetic resonance imaging (MRI) machines per 1 million population, and 91.2 MRI exams were performed per 100,000 population. Just under half (46 percent) of primary care physicians used electronic medical records in 2009.

Major Health Issues

In 2008, WHO estimated that 9 percent of years of life lost in the United States were due to communicable diseases, 72 percent to noncommunicable diseases, and 19 percent to injuries. In 2008, the age-standardized estimate of cancer deaths was 141 per 100,000 for men and 104 per 100,000 for women; for cardiovascular disease and diabetes, 190 per 100,000 for men and 122 per 100,000 for women; and for chronic respiratory disease, 38 per 100,000 for men and 28 per 100,000 for women. The United States has one of the highest adult obesity rates in the world, estimated at 33.9 percent in 2000; obesity is defined as a body mass index (BMI) of 30 or above.

The maternal mortality rate (death from any cause related to or aggravated by pregnancy) in the United States in 2008 was 24 maternal deaths per 100,000 live births; in Puerto Rico, it was 18 deaths per 100,000 live births. The infant mortality rate, defined as the number of deaths of infants younger than 1 year, was 5.98 per 1,000 live births in 2012 in the United States and 7.90 per 1,000 live births in Puerto Rico.

In 2010, tuberculosis incidence was 4.1 per 100,000 population, tuberculosis prevalence 4.8 per 100,000, and deaths due to tuberculosis among human immunodeficiency virus (HIV)-negative people 0.18 per 100,000. As of 2009, an estimated 0.6 percent of adults age 15 to 49 were living with HIV or acquired immune deficiency syndrome (AIDS). As of 2009, an estimated 1.2 million people in the United States were living with HIV or AIDS, the seventh-largest number in the world.

Health Care Personnel

As of 2007, there were 141 medical schools operating in the United States. The course of training for the basic medical degree lasts four to eight years and the degree granted is doctor of medicine or doctor of osteopathy. Licensing is handled at the state level and requires an acceptable degree, accredited residency training, and completion of an examination. In some states, licensing of osteopathic physicians is handled separately. Graduates of foreign medical schools must be certified by the Educational Commission for Foreign Medical Graduates to be eligible for licensing in most states and to enter programs of graduate medical education.

In 2004, the United States had 2.67 physicians per 1,000 population; in 2005, had 9.82 nurses and midwives per 1,000; and in 2000, had 0.88 pharmaceutical personnel per 1,000, 2.28 laboratory health workers per 1,000, 24.76 health management and support workers per 1,000, and 1.63 dentistry personnel per 1,000.

In 2001, 27.0 percent of practicing physicians in the United States were trained in another country (primarily India, Pakistan, and the Philippines), and 13.1 percent of physicians attending postgraduate training in the United States had graduated from medical school in another country. About 3 percent of physicians were U.S. citizens who received their medical education abroad and then returned to the United States to practice. Overall, the United States imports about 20 times as many physicians as it exports.

Government Role in Health Care

According to WHO, in 2010, the United States spent $2.58 trillion on health care, an amount that comes to $8,362 per capita. All health care funding came from domestic sources. The largest share of health care spending was provided through government expenditures (53 percent), with the remainder coming from household expenditures (12 percent) and other sources (35 percent). In 2010, the United States allocated 22 percent of its total government expenditures to health, in the high range for high-income Americas region countries; government expenditures on health came to 9 percent of GDP, in the high range for high-income Americas region countries.

As of 2012, the U.S. government is a major purchaser of health care through programs such as

Medicaid, Medicare, and the Veterans Health Administration, among others.

In 2006, Massachusetts became the first U.S. state to require residents to have at least minimal health insurance coverage. All large and medium-sized employers were also required to contribute toward the insurance premiums of their employees or pay a financial penalty. As of 2008, Massachusetts had an uninsured rate of 4.1 percent, among the lowest among U.S. states. From 2009 to 2010, based on information from the Current Population Study, the uninsured rate in Massachusetts was 5 percent, still lowest among U.S. states, while the state with the next-lowest uninsured rate was Hawaii (8 percent). By way of comparison, the states with the highest uninsured rates were Texas (25 percent), Florida (21 percent), Nevada (21 percent), New Mexico (21 percent), and Georgia (20 percent).

In 2010, the Patient Protection and Affordable Care Act was signed into law. This bill contains a number of provisions that would change aspects of the way health insurance is currently provided in the United States, with the changes phased in over a series of years. The most major changes were scheduled to become effective in 2014, including a universal mandate to acquire health insurance and a prohibition on insurers' discrimination against individuals with pre-existing medical conditions.

Public Health Programs

The United States has a highly developed network for education in public health, with many institutions offering degree programs and conducting research in public health and related fields. In 2012, according to the Association of Schools of Public Health, there were 50 schools offering programs of public health in the United States (including one in Puerto Rico) accredited by the Council on Education of Public Health. These schools offered a variety of programs, including certificates and bachelor's, master's, and doctoral degrees, in traditional disciplines such as biostatistics and epidemiology as well as more specialized areas such as population and reproductive health and preparedness response and recovery.

Briefer, focused training is available through the Public Health Training Centers (PHTC), which were established by the federal Health Resources and Services Administration (HRSA). PHTCs are located throughout the country to provide quick training and refresher courses in core areas of public health and public health management. The courses offered

through PHTCs are bundled into eight areas: program evaluation, Public Health 101, epidemiology, health literacy, environmental public health, Cultural Competency and Diversity 101, communication, and health disparities.

The U.S. Centers for Disease Control and Prevention (CDC) has established Preparedness and Emergency Response Learning Centers (PERLC) within 14 schools of public health across the country, offering competency-based training in core areas of public health in order to enhance the ability of the public health workforce to respond to the needs of the population. In 2008, the Coordinating Office for Terrorism Preparedness and Emergency Response of the CDC created Preparedness and Emergency Response Research Centers (PERRC) in seven U.S. schools of public health; the purpose of the PERRCs is to develop further capacity of the public health system to respond to emergencies, and current activities include improving emergency communications, enhancing training, creating response systems, and developing metrics to evaluate the effectiveness of activities related to preparedness and response.

Public health services provided at the local level vary considerably across the United States, as does spending on public health: A 2009 study by Glen Mays and Sharla Smith found that communities in the top quintile for public health spending per capita (that is, the 20 percent who spent the most relative to their population) spent more than 13 times as much on public health as the lowest quintile (the 20 percent who spent the least) and that most of this could not be explained by differences in service mix or demographics. Median per capita community spending was $29.57 in 2005, with the lowest quintile averaging less than $8 per capita in 2005 and the top quintile almost $102 per capita. About 15 percent of the variation among communities could be explained by the services provided, another 8 percent by agency structures, and another 8 percent by population characteristics; the remaining unexplained variation (about two-thirds) is similar to the unexplained variation in spending found in studies of medical care spending in different geographical areas (approximately 50 to 75 percent).

In 2010, access to improved sanitary facilities was nearly universal (99 percent in rural areas and 100 percent in urban), and access to improved sources of drinking water was also close to universal (99 percent overall, 94 percent in rural areas, and 100 percent in urban). According to the World Higher Education

Database (WHED), more than 100 universities in the United States offer programs in epidemiology or public health: 49 were accredited members of the Association of Schools of Public Health.

URUGUAY

Uruguay is a country in southeastern South America, sharing borders with Argentina and Brazil and having a coastline on the south Atlantic Ocean. The area of 68,037 square miles (176,215 square kilometers) makes Uruguay about the size of the state of Washington, and the July 2012 population was estimated at 3.3 million. In 2010, 92 percent of the population lived in urban areas, and the 2010 to 2015 annual rate of urbanization was estimated at 0.4 percent. Montevideo is the capital and largest city (with a 2009 population estimated at 1.6 million). The population growth rate in 2012 was 0.2 percent, the net migration rate negative 1.4 migrants per 1,000 population, the birth rate 13.4 births per 1,000, and the total fertility rate 1.9 children per woman. The United Nations High Commissioner for Refugees (UNHCR) estimated that, in 2010, there were 105 refugees and persons in refugee-like situations in Uruguay.

A former Spanish colony, Uruguay became an independent country in 1828. Uruguay ranked tied for 25th among 183 countries on the *Corruption Perceptions Index 2011,* with a score of 7.0 (on a scale where 0 indicates highly corrupt and 10 very clean). In 2011, Uruguay was classified as a country with high human development (the second-highest category) on the United Nations Development Programme's (UNDP's) Human Development Index (HDI), with a score of 0.783 (on a scale where 1 denotes high development and 0 low development). Life expectancy at birth in 2012 was estimated at 76.41 years, and per capita gross domestic product (GDP) in 2011 was estimated at $19,600. In 2010, the Gini Index (a measure of dispersion, in which perfect equality is denoted by 0 and maximum inequality is denoted by 100) for family income was 45.3. According to the World Economic Forum's *Global Gender Gap Index 2011*, Uruguay ranked 58th out of 135 countries on gender equality with a score of 0.691 (on a scale with a theoretical range of 1 for equality to 0 for inequality and an actual range in 2011 from 0.8530 to 0.4873).

Emergency Health Services

According to the World Health Organization (WHO), as of 2007, Uruguay did not have a formal and publicly available system for providing prehospital care (emergency care). Mobile emergency systems provide ambulance services as part of some private insurance packages.

Insurance

Uruguay has a social insurance system providing cash maternity and sickness benefits. The sickness benefits system covers the employed and their dependents (up to age 18), the self-employed, pensioners, small employers (up to three employees), and people on unemployment. Workers who earn less than UYU 2,782 per month or work less than 13 days of covered work per month are excluded. Police and the military are covered under separate systems. The system is financed by contributions from wages (3 to 6 percent of gross earnings), small business owners (UYU 1,374 or UYU 1,591; the higher amount is for those with children), the self-employed (UYU 1,374 or UYU 1,591; the higher amount is for those with children), and employers (5 percent of payroll); the government makes up deficits. The maternity benefit is part of the Family Benefits system and

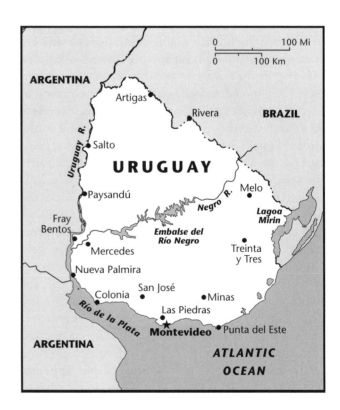

is funded entirely by the government. The maternity benefit is 100 percent of earnings for six weeks before and six weeks after the due date, and children are provided with free medical care (to age 6), dental care (to age 9), and specialist care (to age 14). The family allowance is based on income, and ranges from UYU 356 to UYU178; the allowance is doubled for a disabled child or multiple births. The sickness benefit is 70 percent of earnings for up to a year, with possible extensions to two years. Medical benefits are provided through mutual health institutions; services provided include surgery, medical assistance, and medicines, while health institutions provide grants for appliances, such as eyeglasses and prostheses, and for psychiatric hospitalization. The Social Insurance Bank contracts with collective medical assistance or mutual health institutions to provide medical care and supervises and administers the cash benefits. As of 2007, six companies sold private insurance plans in Uruguay, providing care to 55,000 subscribers.

Costs of Hospitalization

No data available.

Access to Health Care

According to Latinobarometer, an annual public opinion survey conducted in Latin America, 69 percent of citizens in Uruguay are satisfied with the level of health care available to them (the regional average is 51.9 percent). According to WHO, in 2006, 99 percent of births in Uruguay were attended by skilled personnel (for example, physicians, nurses, or midwives). The 2010 immunization rates for 1-year-olds were 95 percent for diphtheria and pertussis (DPT3), 95 percent for measles (MCV), and 95 percent for Hib (Hib3). In 2010, an estimated 71 percent of persons with advanced human immunodeficiency virus (HIV) infection were receiving antiretroviral therapy in accordance with the 2010 WHO guidelines.

Cost of Drugs

The Ministry of Public Health authorizes the registration of drugs considered necessary, efficacious, and safe, and controls production and distribution of drugs.

Health Care Facilities

Uruguay has a variety of health care institutions. The State Health Services Administration has the largest network, providing care to low-income people (about 40 percent of the population) through physician services, polyclinics, health centers, and hospitals (about 8,000 beds); the Scientific Hospital of the University of the Republic also serves this population. The Armed Forces Health Services has its own infrastructure, including about 450 hospital beds in Montevideo and nursing services throughout the country. The Police Health Service has a hospital infrastructure (132 beds) in Montevideo and contracts with private providers and the State Health Services Administration to provide services elsewhere in the country. The State Insurance Fund operates a hospital in Montevideo and contracts for service in the rest of the country. The private sector includes 41 medical centers providing comprehensive, prepaid services. As of 2010, according to WHO, Uruguay had 17.81 health posts per 100,000 population, 3.56 health centers per 100,000, 0.10 provincial hospitals per 100,000, and 0.42 specialized hospitals per 100,000. In 2007, Uruguay had 2.90 hospital beds per 1,000 population.

Major Health Issues

In 2008, WHO estimated that 12 percent of years of life lost in Uruguay were due to communicable diseases, 74 percent to noncommunicable diseases, and 14 percent to injuries. In 2008, the age-standardized estimate of cancer deaths was 217 per 100,000 for men and 118 per 100,000 for women; for cardiovascular disease and diabetes, 264 per 100,000 for men and 161 per 100,000 for women; and for chronic respiratory disease, 60 per 100,000 for men and 20 per 100,000 for women.

Uruguay's maternal mortality rate (death from any cause related to or aggravated by pregnancy) in 2008 was 27 maternal deaths per 100,000 live births. The infant mortality rate, defined as the number of deaths of infants younger than 1 year, was 9.44 per 1,000 live births in 2012. In 2010, tuberculosis incidence was 21.0 per 100,000 population, tuberculosis prevalence 22.0 per 100,000, and deaths due to tuberculosis among HIV-negative people 1.1 per 100,000. As of 2009, an estimated 0.5 percent of adults age 15 to 49 were living with HIV or acquired immune deficiency syndrome (AIDS).

Health Care Personnel

Uruguay has one medical school, the Facultad de Medicina of the Universidad de la Republica del Uruguay in Montevideo, which began offering instruction in 1875. The basic medical degree course lasts

8.5 years, and the degree awarded is doctor of medicine. In 2008, Uruguay had 3.74 physicians per 1,000 population, 0.53 pharmaceutical personnel per 1,000, 0.17 laboratory health workers per 1,000, 0.70 health management and support workers per 1,000, 0.70 dentistry personnel per 1,000, and 5.55 nurses and midwives per 1,000.

Government Role in Health Care

According to WHO, in 2010, Uruguay spent $3.4 billion on health care, an amount that comes to $998 per capita. All health care funding came from domestic sources. The largest share of health care spending was provided through government expenditures (67 percent), with the remainder coming from household expenditures (13 percent) and other sources (20 percent). In 2010, Uruguay allocated 20 percent of its total government expenditures to health, in the high range for upper middle-income Americas region countries; government expenditures on health came to 6 percent of GDP, in the high range for upper middle-income Americas region countries. In 2009, according to WHO, official development assistance (ODA) for health in Uruguay came to $0.66 per capita.

Public Health Programs

In 2006, Uruguay passed a national law making all public places, including workplaces, bars, and restaurants, tobacco-free. In 2010, access to improved sanitation facilities was nearly universal (99 percent in rural areas and 100 percent in urban), as was access to improved sources of drinking water (essentially 100 percent in both rural and urban areas); the main exception are people living in informal settlements around Montevideo, where an estimated 80 percent receive sanitary services.

UZBEKISTAN

Uzbekistan is a doubly landlocked country in central Asia, sharing borders with Afghanistan, Kazakhstan, Kyrgyzstan, Tajikistan, and Turkmenistan; Uzbekistan has 261 miles (420 kilometers) of shoreline on the Aral Sea. The area of 172,742 square miles (447,400 square kilometers) makes Uzbekistan about the size of California, and the July 2012 population was estimated at 28.4 million. In 2010, 36 percent of the population

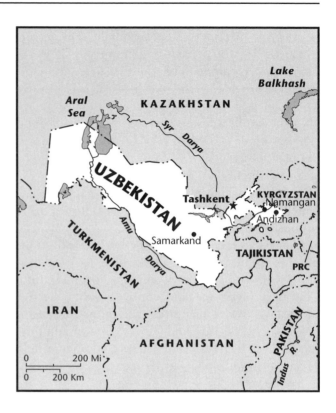

lived in urban areas, and the 2010 to 2015 annual rate of urbanization was estimated at 1.4 percent. Tashkent is the capital and largest city (with a 2009 population estimated at 2.2 million). The population growth rate in 2012 was 0.9 percent, the net migration rate negative 2.6 migrants per 1,000 population, the birth rate 17.3 births per 1,000, and the total fertility rate 1.9 children per woman. The United Nations High Commissioner for Refugees (UNHCR) estimated that, in 2010, there were 311 refugees and persons in refugee-like situations in Uzbekistan.

The territory that is now Uzbekistan was conquered by Russia in the late 19th century, and Uzbekistan became part of the Soviet Union in 1924. The country suffered extreme environmental damage during the Soviet period due to overuse of agricultural chemicals and depletion of water supplies in order to grow cotton. The current government is perceived as corrupt, ranking 177th among 183 countries on the *Corruption Perceptions Index 2011*, with a score of 1.6 (on a scale where 0 indicates highly corrupt and 10 very clean). In 2011, Uzbekistan was classified as a country with medium human development (the second from the lowest of four categories) on the United Nations Development Programme's (UNDP's) Human Development Index (HDI), with a score of 0.641 (on a scale where 1 denotes high development and 0 low development). Life expectancy at birth in 2012 was estimated at 72.77 years, and estimated gross domestic product (GDP) per capita in 2011 was $3,300. In 2003, the Gini Index (a measure of dispersion, in which perfect equality is denoted by 0 and maximum inequality is denoted by 100) for family income was 36.8.

Emergency Health Services

According to the World Health Organization (WHO), as of 2007, Uzbekistan had a formal and publicly available emergency care (prehospital care) system accessible through a national access number. Doctors Without Borders (Médecins Sans Frontières, or MSF) began working in Uzbekistan in 1997 and had 117 staff members in the country at the close of 2010. MSF's primary focus is diagnosis and treatment of drug-resistant tuberculosis, and it currently provides care in four districts; MSF also provides social and psychological counseling for family members of tuberculosis patients and promotes innovative approaches to tuberculosis treatment and care. MSF also provided counseling and relief to refugees from the conflict in Kyrgyzstan.

Insurance

Uzbekistan has a universal medical system covering everyone residing in the country and a social insurance system providing cash sickness and maternity benefits. The medical benefits system is entirely funded by general tax revenues, while the cash benefits system is part of the same system that provides pensions and is financed through contributions from wages (4 percent), self-employed income (at least the same amount as a person earning the minimum wage), and employers (25 percent of payroll); the government covers the cost of social pensions and makes up deficits. Medical benefits are provided directly through government health care providers; benefits include hospitalization, medical care, medicines, and prostheses.

The maternity benefit is 100 percent of wages for 70 days before and 56 days after childbirth, with extensions for multiple births or complications. Mothers remaining at home to care for children younger than age 2 are entitled to paid leave (20 percent of wages) and unpaid leave to care for a child between the ages of 2 and 3. The sickness benefit is 60 to 100 percent of wages, depending on the length of employment and number of children. The Ministry of Health and local

health departments provide medical services through government hospitals, clinics, and other facilities; the Extrabudgetary Pension Fund administers the maternity benefits; the Department of Social Protection pays the cash benefits, and the system is coordinated and supervised by the Ministry of Labor and Social Protections.

Costs of Hospitalization

No data available.

Access to Health Care

According to WHO, in 2006, 100 percent of births in Uzbekistan were attended by skilled personnel (for example, physicians, nurses, or midwives). The 2010 immunization rates for 1-year-olds were 99 percent for diphtheria and pertussis (DPT3), 98 percent for measles (MCV), and 99 percent for Hib (Hib3). In 2010, an estimated 28 percent of persons with advanced human immunodeficiency virus (HIV) infection were receiving antiretroviral therapy in accordance with the 2010 WHO guidelines.

Cost of Drugs

According to WHO, in 2004, the median availability of selected generic drugs in the private sector in Uzbekistan was 82.5 percent; the median price ratio (comparing the price in Uzbekistan to the international reference price) was 2.0 in the private sphere for selected generic medicines, indicating that median prices in the public sphere were twice as high as the international reference price.

Health Care Facilities

In 2007, Uzbekistan had 4.83 hospital beds per 1,000 population, among the 50 highest rates in the world.

Major Health Issues

In 2008, WHO estimated that 34 percent of years of life lost in Uzbekistan were due to communicable diseases, 55 percent to noncommunicable diseases, and 10 percent to injuries. In 2008, the age-standardized estimate of cancer deaths was 77 per 100,000 for men and 66 per 100,000 for women; for cardiovascular disease and diabetes, 718 per 100,000 for men and 564 per 100,000 for women; and for chronic respiratory disease, 33 per 100,000 for men and 22 per 100,000 for women.

Uzbekistan's maternal mortality rate (death from any cause related to or aggravated by pregnancy) in

2008 was 30 maternal deaths per 100,000 live births. The infant mortality rate, defined as the number of deaths of infants younger than 1 year, was estimated at 21.20 per 1,000 live births in 2012. In 2010, tuberculosis incidence was 128.0 per 100,000 population, tuberculosis prevalence 227.0 per 100,000, and deaths due to tuberculosis among HIV-negative people 20.00 per 100,000. As estimated 14 percent of new tuberculosis cases and 49 percent of retreatment cases are multidrug resistant. As of 2009, an estimated 0.1 percent of adults age 15 to 49 were living with HIV or acquired immune deficiency syndrome (AIDS).

Health Care Personnel

As of 2007, Uzbekistan had nine medical schools. The basic medical degree course lasts six to seven years and a year of supervised clinical practice in a specialty is also required. The degree granted is general practitioner. Uzbekistan has agreements with other members of the Commonwealth of Independent States (countries formerly part of the Soviet Union). In 2007, Uzbekistan had 2.62 physicians per 1,000 population, 0.03 pharmaceutical personnel per 1,000, 0.17 dentistry personnel per 1,000, and 10.81 nurses and midwives per 1,000.

Government Role in Health Care

According to WHO, in 2010, Uzbekistan spent $2.3 billion on health care, an amount that comes to $82 per capita. Most (99 percent) of health care funding came from domestic sources, with 1 percent coming from abroad. The largest share of health care spending was provided through government expenditures (47 percent), with the remainder coming from household expenditures (43 percent) and other sources (10 percent). In 2010, Uzbekistan allocated 9 percent of its total government expenditures to health, in the median range for lower-middle-income Asian countries; government expenditures on health came to 3 percent of GDP, in the median range for lower-middle-income Asian region countries. In 2009, according to WHO, official development assistance (ODA) for health in Uzbekistan came to $1.05 per capita.

Public Health Programs

In 2010, access to improved sanitation facilities was essentially universal in Uzbekistan, and 87 percent had access to improved sources of drinking water (81 percent in rural areas and 98 percent in urban).

VANUATU

Vanuatu is an island nation in the south Pacific Ocean, including more than 85 islands. The area of 4,706 square miles (12,189 square kilometers) makes Vanuatu about the size of Connecticut, and the July 2012 population was estimated at 227,574. In 2010, 26 percent of the population lived in urban areas, and the 2010 to 2015 annual rate of urbanization was estimated at 4.2 percent. Port-Vila is the capital. The population growth rate in 2012 was 1.3 percent, the net migration rate 0.0 migrants per 1,000 population, the birth rate 20.6 births per 1,000, and the total fertility rate 2.4 children per woman. The United Nations High Commissioner for Refugees (UNHCR) estimated that, in 2010, there were four refugees and persons in refugee-like situations in Vanuatu.

The New Hebrides were administered by France and Britain in the 19th and early 20th centuries; the country became independent and adopted the name of Vanuatu in 1980. Vanuatu ranked tied for 77th among 183 countries on the *Corruption Perceptions Index 2011*, with a score of 3.5 (on a scale where 0 indicates highly corrupt and 10 very clean). In 2011, Vanuatu was classified as a country with medium human development (the second from the lowest of four categories) on the United Nations Development Programme's (UNDP's) Human Development Index (HDI), with a score of 0.617 (on a scale where 1 denotes high development and 0 low development). Life expectancy at birth in 2012 was estimated at 65.06 years, and estimated gross domestic product (GDP) per capita in 2011 was $4,900.

Emergency Health Services

According to the World Health Organization (WHO), as of 2007, Vanuatu had a formal and publicly available emergency care (prehospital care) system accessible through a national access number.

Insurance

Vanuatu has no system providing statutory medical, sickness, or maternity benefits. Employers are required, under the 1983 Employment Act (amended in 2008), to provide medical care for workers and dependents if they live on the employer's property; to provide sick leave for employees who have been working for at least one year, for up to 21 days at 100 percent of pay; to provide maternity leave for women who have been working for at least six months, for up to three months at 100 percent of wages; and to allow nursing women two breaks of one hour daily in order to feed their children.

Costs of Hospitalization
No data available.

Access to Health Care
According to WHO, in 2007, 74 percent of births in Vanuatu were attended by skilled personnel (for example, physicians, nurses, or midwives). The 2010 immunization rates for 1-year-olds were 68 percent for diphtheria and pertussis (DPT3) and 52 percent for measles (MCV).

Cost of Drugs
No data available.

Health Care Facilities
As of 2010, according to WHO, Vanuatu had 125.18 health posts per 100,000 population, 16.27 health centers per 100,000, 1.67 district or rural hospitals per 100,000, 0.42 provincial hospitals per 100,000, and 0.42 specialized hospitals per 100,000. In 2008, Vanuatu had 1.69 hospital beds per 1,000 population.

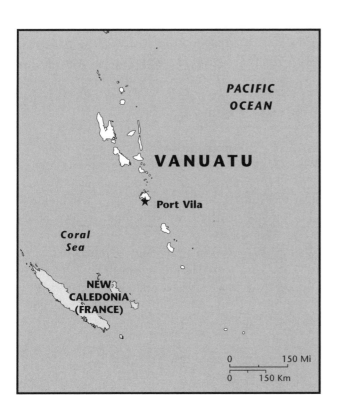

Major Health Issues
In 2008, WHO estimated that 35 percent of years of life lost in Vanuatu were due to communicable diseases, 56 percent to noncommunicable diseases, and 10 percent to injuries. In 2008, the age-standardized estimate of cancer deaths was 95 per 100,000 for men and 94 per 100,000 for women; for cardiovascular disease and diabetes, 462 per 100,000 for men and 333 per 100,000 for women; and for chronic respiratory disease, 80 per 100,000 for men and 45 per 100,000 for women.

In 2008, the age-standardized death rate from malaria was 11.4 per 100,000 population. In 2010, tuberculosis incidence was 69.0 per 100,000 population, tuberculosis prevalence 78.0 per 100,000, and deaths due to tuberculosis among human immunodeficiency virus (HIV)-negative people 5.8 per 100,000. The infant mortality rate, defined as the number of deaths of infants younger than 1 year, was estimated at 45.57 per 1,000 live births in 2012.

Health Care Personnel
Vanuatu has no medical school. Physicians wishing to practice in Vanuatu must register with the Ministry of Health, and a medical license is granted to graduates of a recognized medical school who are qualified to practice in the country in which the degree was awarded. Foreigners may be granted a two-year license to practice medicine. In 2008, Vanuatu had 0.12 physicians per 1,000 population, 0.01 pharmaceutical personnel per 1,000, 0.01 dentistry personnel per 1,000, 0.95 community and traditional health workers per 1,000, and 1.70 nurses and midwives per 1,000.

Government Role in Health Care
According to WHO, in 2010, Vanuatu spent $38 million on health care, an amount that comes to $157 per capita. More than two-thirds (77 percent) of health care funding came from domestic sources, with 23 percent coming from abroad. The largest share of health care spending was provided through government expenditures (91 percent), with the remainder coming from household expenditures (5 percent) and other sources (4 percent). In 2010, Vanuatu allocated 18 percent of its total government expenditures to health, in the high range for lower-middle-income western Pacific region countries; government expenditures on health came to 5 percent of GDP, in the median range for lower-middle-income western Pacific region countries.

Public Health Programs

According to WHO, in 2007, Vanuatu had 0.05 environmental and public health workers per 1,000 population. In 2010, 57 percent of the population of Vanuatu had access to improved sanitation facilities (54 percent in rural areas and 64 percent in urban), and 90 percent had access to improved sources of drinking water (87 percent in rural areas and 98 percent in urban).

VENEZUELA

Venezuela is a country in northern South America, sharing borders with Colombia, Brazil, and Guyana and having a coastline on the Caribbean Sea. The area of 352,144 square miles (912,050 square kilometers) makes Venezuela about twice the size of California, and the July 2012 population was estimated at 28.0 million. In 2010, 93 percent of the population lived in urban areas, and the 2010 to 2015 annual rate of urbanization was estimated at 1.7 percent. Caracas is the capital and largest city (with a 2009 population estimated at 3.0 million). The population growth rate in 2012 was 1.5 percent, the net migration rate 0.0 migrants per 1,000 population, the birth rate 19.9 births per 1,000, and the total fertility rate 2.4 children per woman. The United Nations High Commissioner for Refugees (UNHCR) estimated that, in 2010, there were 21,145 refugees and persons in refugee-like situations in Venezuela.

Venezuela was a Spanish Colony before it formed Gran Colombia with Ecuador and New Granada (Colombia); it became an independent country in 1830. After Chavez died in 2013, his hand-picked successor, Nicolas Madura, was elected president. Venezuela was ruled by military strongmen in the first half of the 20th century but has had elected governments since 1959. In 1999, Hugo Chavez was elected president and began a reform campaign to address social conditions. Venezuela ranked tied for 172nd among 183 countries on the *Corruption Perceptions Index 2011,* with a score of 1.9 (on a scale where 0 indicates highly corrupt and 10 very clean). In 2011, Venezuela was classified as a country with high human development (the second-highest category) on the United Nations Development Programme's (UNDP's) Human Development Index (HDI), with a score of 0.735 (on a scale where 1 denotes high development and 0 low development). Life expectancy at birth in 2012 was estimated at 74.08 years, and

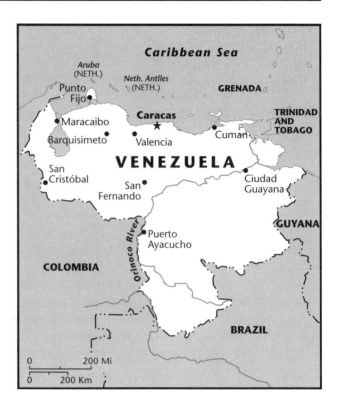

per capita gross domestic product (GDP) in 2011 was estimated at $12,400. In 2011, the Gini Index (a measure of dispersion, in which perfect equality is denoted by 0 and maximum inequality is denoted by 100) for family income was 39.0. According to the World Economic Forum's *Global Gender Gap Index 2011,* Venezuela ranked 63rd out of 135 countries on gender equality with a score of 0.686 (on a scale with a theoretical range of 1 for equality to 0 for inequality and an actual range in 2011 from 0.8530 to 0.4873).

Emergency Health Services

According to the World Health Organization (WHO), as of 2007, Venezuela had a formal and publicly available emergency care (prehospital care) system accessible through a national access number. In 2006, about 100 comprehensive diagnostic centers provided emergency care as well as intermediate and intensive care. In 2005, the Ministry of Health created an Emergency and Disaster Coordination Office and Caracas established a Health Risk Management Unit to prepare for and manage natural and man-made disasters.

Insurance

Venezuela has a social insurance system covering employees in the public and private sectors, members

Health Expenditures: Venezuela Compared With the Global Average (2009)

	Venezuela	Global Average
Out-of-pocket expenditure as percent of private expenditure on health	90.6	50.2
Private prepaid plans as percent of private expenditure on health	3.4	38.9
Per capita total expenditure on health at average exchange rate (USD)	688	900
Per capita total expenditure on health (purchasing power parity, international dollars)	734	990
Per capita government expenditure on health at average exchange rate (USD)	275	549
Per capita government expenditure on health (purchasing power parity, international dollars)	294	584

Source: 2011 World Health Organization Global Health Expenditure Atlas.

of cooperatives, pensioners, some dependents, and household, seasonal, and casual workers; the self-employed are excluded. The system is funded through contributions from wages (4 percent in the private sector and 2 percent in the public sector and for members of cooperatives), employers (9 to 11 percent of covered payroll in the private sector and 4.75 percent in the public sector), and the government (covering administrative costs); the same funds are used to finance pensions. Medical benefits are provided through medical facilities run by the Social Security Institute and are generally free; services covered include hospitalization, medical care, lab services, dental care, medicines, appliances, transportation, and maternity care. The maternity benefit is 66.7 percent of earnings for six weeks before and 12 weeks after the due date. The sickness benefit is 66.7 percent of earnings for up to 52 weeks, with the payment reduced by half during hospitalization. The system is administered by the Social Insurance Institute, with general supervision provided by the Ministry of the People's Power for Labor and Social Security.

Costs of Hospitalization

No data available.

Access to Health Care

Venezuela's health services system includes both public and private sectors and is complex and segmented;

decentralization began in the 1990s but was not completed, so both centralized and decentralized services exist. The Misión Barrio Adentro program provides free medical services to the poor. According to Latinobarometer, an annual public opinion survey conducted in Latin America, 64 percent of citizens in Venezuela are satisfied with the level of health care available to them (the regional average is 51.9 percent). According to WHO, in 2005, 95 percent of births in Venezuela were attended by skilled personnel (for example, physicians, nurses, or midwives). The 2010 immunization rates for 1-year-olds were 78 percent for diphtheria and pertussis (DPT3), 79 percent for measles (MCV), and 78 percent for Hib (Hib3). In 2010, an estimated 57 percent of persons with advanced human immunodeficiency virus (HIV) infection were receiving antiretroviral therapy in accordance with the 2010 WHO guidelines.

Cost of Drugs

The Ministry of Health regulates which medicines may be sold in Venezuela; as of 2007, more than 4,300 medicines were available, of which about two-thirds required a prescription. Institutions within the National Public Health System (SPNS) are allowed only to purchase drugs listed on the national list of essential medicines; as of 2007, this list included 534 drugs. Health clinics provide 103 drugs for free to treat the most common diseases. Antiretroviral drugs, diagnostic tests, and monitoring services are provided free of charge to people with human immunodeficiency virus/acquired immune deficiency syndrome (HIV/AIDS).

Health Care Facilities

As of 2005, Venezuela had 4,804 ambulatory centers providing primary care, of which 96 percent were operated by the Ministry of Health, and 296 public hospitals. The private sector included 315 for-profit care centers and 29 centers run by benevolent institutions. In 2007, Venezuela had 1.30 hospital beds per 1,000 population.

Major Health Issues

In 2008, WHO estimated that 20 percent of years of life lost in Venezuela were due to communicable diseases, 42 percent to noncommunicable diseases, and 38 percent to injuries. In 2008, the age-standardized estimate of cancer deaths was 102 per 100,000 for men and 92 per 100,000 for women; for cardiovascular disease and diabetes, 266 per 100,000 for men and 207 per 100,000 for women; and for chronic respiratory disease, 25 per 100,000 for men and 20 per 100,000 for women.

In 2008, the age-standardized death rate from malaria was 0.1 per 100,000 population. In 2010, tuberculosis incidence was 33.0 per 100,000 population, tuberculosis prevalence 48.0 per 100,000, and deaths due to tuberculosis among HIV-negative people 2.8 per 100,000. Venezuela's maternal mortality rate (death from any cause related to or aggravated by pregnancy) was estimated in 2008 as 68 maternal deaths per 100,000 live births. The infant mortality rate, defined as the number of deaths of infants younger than 1 year, was estimated at 20.18 per 1,000 live births in 2012.

Health Care Personnel

Venezuela has nine medical schools. The basic degree course requires 6.5 to seven years to complete, and a period of a year to practice in a rural area is also required before the degree (Médico Cirujano, or physician and surgeon) is awarded. Physicians must register with the Ministerio de Sanidad y Asistencia Social in Caracas and the Colegio de Medicos in the state in which they wish to practice. Foreigners may practice medicine in Venezuela only if they have permanent residence status. Venezuela has agreements with Bolivia, Colombia, Ecuador, and Peru. In 2001,

Venezuela had 1.94 physicians per 1,000 population, 0.55 dentistry personnel per 1,000, and 1.13 nurses and midwives per 1,000.

Government Role in Health Care

According to WHO, in 2010, Venezuela spent $19 billion on health care, an amount that comes to $663 per capita. All health care funding came from domestic sources. The largest share of health care spending was provided through household expenditures (59 percent), with the remainder coming from government expenditures (35 percent) and other sources (6 percent). In 2010, Venezuela allocated 8 percent of its total government expenditures to health, in the low range for upper-middle-income Americas region countries; government expenditures on health came to 2 percent of GDP, in the low range for upper-middle-income Americas region countries. In 2009, according to WHO, official development assistance (ODA) for health in Venezuela came to $0.12 per capita.

Public Health Programs

In 2005, 91 percent of the population of Venezuela had access to improved sanitation facilities (57 percent in rural areas and 94 percent in urban), and 92 percent had access to improved sources of drinking water (75 percent in rural areas and 94 percent in urban). According to the World Higher Education Database (WHED), one university in Venezuela offers programs in epidemiology or public health: Lisandro Alvarado Central Western University in Barquisimeto.

VIETNAM

Vietnam is a southeastern Asian country, sharing borders with Laos, China, and Cambodia and having coastline on the south China Sea. The area of 127,881 square miles (331,210 square kilometers) makes Vietnam about the size of New Mexico, and the July 2012 population was estimated at 91.6 million (the 14th-largest in the world). In 2010, 30 percent of the population lived in urban areas, and the 2010 to 2015 annual rate of urbanization was estimated at 3.0 percent. Hanoi is the capital and Ho Chi Minh City the largest city (with a 2009 population estimated at 6.0 million). The population growth rate in 2012 was 1.0 percent, the net migration rate negative 0.3 migrants per 1,000 population, the birth rate 16.8 births per 1,000, and the total fertility rate 1.9 children per woman.

Vietnam was conquered by France in 1884, and the country became part of French Indochina in 1887. After World War II, Vietnam declared itself independent, but France continued to rule the country until defeated in 1954 by forces led by Ho Chi Minh. The Geneva Accord of 1954 divided the country into North and South Vietnam; the United States provided military and economic aid to South Vietnam but withdrew in 1973; forces from the North overran South Vietnam in 1975 and reunited the country. Vietnam ranked tied for 112th among 183 countries on the *Corruption Perceptions Index 2011*, with a score of 2.9 (on a scale where 0 indicates highly corrupt and 10 very clean).

In 2011, Vietnam was classified as a country with medium human development (the second from the lowest of four categories) on the United Nations Development Programme's (UNDP's) Human Development Index (HDI), with a score of 0.593 (on a scale where 1 denotes high development and 0 low development). Life expectancy at birth in 2012 was estimated at 72.41 years, and estimated gross domestic product (GDP) per capita in 2011 was $3,300. In 2008, the Gini Index (a measure of dispersion, in which perfect equality is denoted by 0 and maximum inequality is denoted by 100) for family income was 37.6. According to the World Economic Forum's *Global Gender Gap Index 2011*, Vietnam ranked 79th out of 135 countries on gender equality with a score of 0.673 (on a scale with a theoretical range of 1 for equality to 0 for inequality and an actual range in 2011 from 0.8530 to 0.4873).

Emergency Health Services

According to the World Health Organization (WHO), as of 2007, Vietnam had a formal and publicly available emergency care (prehospital care) system accessible through a national access number.

Insurance

Vietnam has a social insurance system providing health insurance and cash sickness and maternity benefits. People in the health insurance system include civil servants, salaried employees, the disabled, the unemployed, pensioners, war veterans, children young than age 6, the poor, recipients of social welfare, and students. The cash benefits system includes employers with contracts longer than

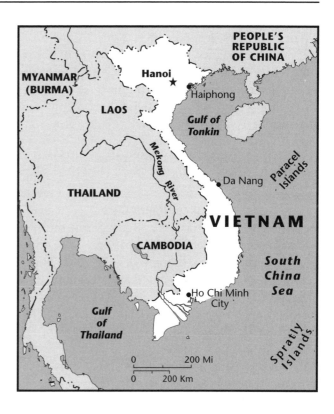

three months (including household workers); workers in salt production, agriculture, and fishing; civil servants; policemen; military officers; and employees of unions and cooperatives. The medical benefits system is financed by contributions from wages (1.5 percent of gross earnings, with a minimum and maximum), earnings of the self-employed (4.5 percent of the minimum wage), and employers (3 percent of monthly payroll); the government pays the contributions of some classes of people and provides subsidies for the system. The cash benefits system is financed by employers (3 percent of payroll).

Medical benefits covered include medical care, examinations, preventive care, maternity benefits, rehabilitation, and transfers; the amount of copayment required depends on the type of insurance and service used. Free medical benefits are provided for dependents of people in the army or security services, and students and the poor pay lower rates; coverage of dependents from other insured households requires payment of an additional premium, depending on the size of the family. Vietnam Social Security collects contributions, pays benefits, implements policy, and manages the health insurance fund; the Ministry of Health supervises health insurance; and the Ministry of Labor, Invalids, and Social

Affairs provides general supervision. According to Ke Xu and colleagues, in 2003, 10.4 percent of households in Vietnam experienced catastrophic health expenditures annually; "catastrophic" was defined as exceeding 40 percent of household income remaining after basic needs were met.

Costs of Hospitalization

No data available.

Access to Health Care

According to WHO, in 2006, 88 percent of births in Vietnam were attended by skilled personnel (for example, physicians, nurses, or midwives). In 2002, 29 percent of pregnant women received at least four prenatal care visits. The 2010 immunization rates for 1-year-olds were 93 percent for diphtheria and pertussis (DPT3), 98 percent for measles (MCV), and 63 percent for Hib (Hib3). In 2010, an estimated 52 percent of persons with advanced human immunodeficiency virus (HIV) infection were receiving antiretroviral therapy in accordance with the 2010 WHO guidelines.

Cost of Drugs

According to Anh Tuan Nguyen and colleagues, in 2005, more than half (53.3 percent) of Vietnam's health expenditures went for medicines. Soaring prices (fourfold between 2003 and 2004 alone) have created difficulties in assuring access to essential medicines, and prices for some common medications are higher than in nearby countries such as Pakistan, Australia, and New Zealand. Nguyen's 2009 survey of the availability and price of common medicines found that both availability and access constituted barriers. Paradoxically, drugs were sometimes available more cheaply in the private than in the public sector. The median price ratio in the public procurement sector for the lowest-priced generics was 1.82, meaning that, on average, these drugs were procured at a price almost twice that of the international reference price; the median price ratio for innovator brands in the public sector was 8.29, or more than eight times as high as the international reference price. Prices varied dramatically for generics, while they were more stable for innovator brands. The median patient price in the public sector was 11.41 for the lowest-priced generics and 46.58 for innovator brands; in the private sector, the median price ratio was 8.59 for insured patients for the lowest-priced generics and 38.88 for innovator brands. In the public sector, the median availability was 33.6 percent for the lowest-price generics and 19.6 percent for innovator brands, while in the private sector, the availability of the lowest-priced generics for insured patients was 40.4 percent, and the availability of innovator brands was 10.9 percent. Availability differed substantially by region, with Hanoi and Ho Chi Minh City having the highest availability.

Drugs to treat chronic illnesses were particularly unaffordable, using the standard that a drug regimen to treat a common illness should cost no more than 1 day's wages of the lowest-paid government worker. One month's worth of treatment for a peptic ulcer, using generic ranitidine, cost 1.3 days' wages if purchased in the private sector versus 13.9 days' wages if purchased in the public sector; if the innovator brand of omeprazole were used instead, it would have cost 48.9 days' wages in the private sector and 50.9 days' wages in the public sector. Drugs to treat an adult acute respiratory infection would have cost 0.7 day's wages if the lowest-price generic amoxicillin were used and the purchase made in the public sector, while if generic ceftriaxone were used instead and purchased in the public sector, it would have required 15.9 days' wages.

Health Care Facilities

In 2008, Vietnam had 2.87 hospital beds per 1,000 population.

Major Health Issues

In 2008, WHO estimated that 29 percent of years of life lost in Vietnam were due to communicable diseases, 56 percent to noncommunicable diseases, and 15 percent to injuries. In 2008, the age-standardized estimate of cancer deaths was 137 per 100,000 for men and 94 per 100,000 for women; for cardiovascular disease and diabetes, 382 per 100,000 for men and 298 per 100,000 for women; and for chronic respiratory disease, 77 per 100,000 for men and 45 per 100,000 for women.

In 2008, the age-standardized death rate from malaria was 0.1 per 100,000 population. In 2010, tuberculosis incidence was 199.0 per 100,000 population, tuberculosis prevalence 334.0 per 100,000, and deaths due to tuberculosis among HIV-negative people 34.0 per 100,000. As estimated 2.7 percent of new tuberculosis cases and 19 percent of retreatment cases are multidrug resistant. WHO estimated the 2010 case detection rate at 54 percent. As of 2009, an estimated 0.4 percent of adults age 15 to 49 were living with HIV or acquired immune deficiency syndrome (AIDS). Vietnam's maternal mortality rate (death from any cause related to or aggravated by pregnancy) was estimated in 2008 as 56 maternal deaths per 100,000 live births. The infant mortality rate, defined as the number of deaths of infants younger than 1 year, was estimated at 20.24 per 1,000 live births in 2012. In 2008, 20.2 percent of children under age 5 were underweight (defined as 2 kilograms [kg] below standard weight-for-age at age 1, 3 kg below for ages 2 to 3, and 4 kg below for ages 4 to 5).

Health Care Personnel

Vietnam has nine medical schools. The course of training for the basic degree lasts six years, and the degree granted is doctor of medicine. Five years' work in government service is required after graduation. Licensing is handled at the provincial level with licenses granted according to local needs. In 2008, Vietnam had 1.22 physicians per 1,000 population, 0.32 pharmaceutical personnel per 1,000, and 1.01 nurses and midwives per 1,000.

Government Role in Health Care

According to WHO, in 2010, Vietnam spent $7.2 billion on health care, an amount that comes to $83 per capita. Most (97 percent) of health care funding came from domestic sources, with 3 percent coming from abroad. The largest share of health care spending was provided through household expenditures (58 percent), with the remainder coming from government expenditures (38 percent) and other sources (5 percent). In 2010, Vietnam allocated 8 percent of its total government expenditures to health, in the low range for lower-middle-income western Pacific region countries; government expenditures on health came to 3 percent of GDP, in the low range for lower-middle-income western Pacific region countries. In 2009, according to WHO, official development assistance (ODA) for health in Vietnam came to $3.31 per capita.

Public Health Programs

The National Institute of Hygiene and Epidemiology (NIHE) is located in Hanoi and directed by Nguyen Tran Hien. It was founded in 1928 and became a national public health institute in 1997, currently employing about 1,000 people. The focus of the NIHE is on the control and prevention of communicable diseases, including national surveillance, development of vaccines (the NIHE produces about 80 percent of the vaccines used in Vietnam), and offering public health education at the undergraduate and postgraduate levels. The Pasteur Institute, founded in 1891, is located in Ho Chi Minh City (formerly Saigon) and is the center for the study of infectious disease and infection control in southern Vietnam; it offers lab analysis, produces vaccines, conducts scientific research, and offers postgraduate training in microbiology, immunology, and epidemiology. In 2010, 94 percent of the population of Vietnam had access to improved sanitation facilities (76 percent in rural areas and 94 percent in urban), and 95 percent had access to improved sources of drinking water (93 percent in rural areas and 99 percent in urban).

According to the World Higher Education Database (WHED), five universities in Vietnam offer programs in epidemiology or public health: the Hanoi University of Odonto-Stomatology, the Hanoi School of Public Health, the Ho Chi Minh City University of Medicine and Pharmacy, Hanoi Medical University, and Thai Binh Medical University.

YEMEN

Yemen is a Middle Eastern country, sharing borders with Saudi Arabia and Oman and having a coastline on the Red Sea and the Gulf of Aden. The area of 203,850 square miles (527,968 square kilometers) makes Yemen about twice the size of Wyoming, and the July 2012 population was estimated at 24.8 million. In 2010, 32 percent of the population lived in urban areas, and the 2010 to 2015 annual rate of urbanization was estimated at 4.6 percent. Sana'a is the capital and largest city (with a 2009 population estimated at 2.2 million). The population growth rate in 2012 was 2.6 percent (the 26th-highest in the world), the net migration rate 0.0 migrants per 1,000 population, the birth rate 32.6 births per 1,000, and the total fertility rate 4.4 children per woman (the 30th-highest in the world). The United Nations High Commissioner for Refugees (UNHCR) estimated that, in 2010, there were 109,102 refugees and persons in refugee-like situations in Yemen, and 94,712 internally displaced persons and persons in internally displaced-person-like situations.

North Yemen was part of the Ottoman Empire before becoming independent in 1918; North and South Yemen (a former British protectorate) were unified as the Republic of Yemen in 1990. Yemen ranked tied for 164th among 183 countries on the *Corruption Perceptions Index 2011,* with a score of 2.1 (on a scale where 0 indicates highly corrupt and 10 very clean). In 2011, Yemen was classified as a country with low human development (the lowest of four categories) on the United Nations Development Programme's (UNDP's) Human Development Index (HDI), with a score of 0.462 (on a scale where 1 denotes high development and 0 low development). In 2011, the International Food Policy Research Institute (IFPRI) classified Yemen as a country with an "alarming" hunger problem, with a Global Hunger Index (GHI) score of 39.0, and in 2012, the World Food Programme estimated that 44.5 percent of the population was food insecure.

Life expectancy at birth in 2012 was estimated at 64.11 years, and the estimated gross domestic product (GDP) per capita in 2011 was $2,500. In 2005, the Gini Index (a measure of dispersion, in which perfect equality is denoted by 0 and maximum inequality is denoted by 100) for family income was 37.7. Unemployment in 2003 was estimated at 35.0 percent, among the highest rates in the world. According to the World Economic Forum's *Global Gender Gap Index 2011*, Yemen ranked last out of 135 countries on gender equality with a score of 0.487 (on a scale with a theoretical range of 1 for equality to 0 for inequality and an actual range in 2011 from 0.8530 to 0.4873).

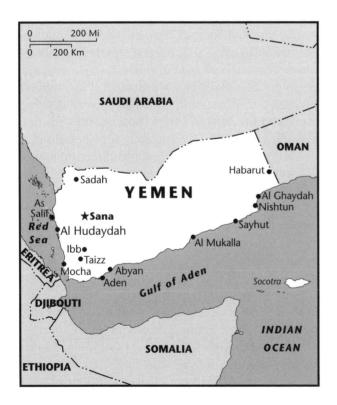

Emergency Health Services

According to the World Health Organization (WHO), as of 2007, Yemen had a formal and publicly available emergency care (prehospital care) system accessible through a national access number. Doctors Without Borders (Médecins Sans Frontières, or MSF) began working in Yemen in 2007 and had 467 staff members in the country at the close of 2010. MSF expanded its activities in Yemen in 2010 in response to a number of emergencies, including violent conflict and increased migration. Despite having to cease operations for several months, MSF provided more than 32,000 consultations in northern Yemen. MSF began a nutrition program in Saada, treating 820 malnourished children, and provided medical care and humanitarian aid to refugees displaced by the conflict. MSF staff provided general health care and provided psychological counseling to displaced persons camps near Al Mazraq. In South Yemen, MSF provided emergency treatment to more than 5,000 people in the public hospital in Radfan. MSF also provided medical care to migrants from the horn of Africa, a program transferred to the UNHCR in April 2010. MSF provided human immunodeficiency virus (HIV) testing and counseling in Sana'a, the national capital, and offered a program to prevent mother-to-child transmission of HIV.

Insurance

Yemen has a National Health Strategy for the years 2011 to 2025 with the goals of providing high-quality, equitable preventive, curative, and rehabilitative health services to its population. According to Ke Xu and colleagues, in 2003, 1.7 percent of households in Yemen experienced catastrophic health expenditures annually; "catastrophic" was defined as exceeding 40 percent of household income remaining after basic needs were met.

Costs of Hospitalization

No data available.

Access to Health Care

According to WHO, in 2006, 36 percent of births in Yemen were attended by skilled personnel (for example, physicians, nurses, or midwives). In 2003,

14 percent of pregnant women received at least four prenatal care visits. The 2010 immunization rates for 1-year-olds were 87 percent for diphtheria and pertussis (DPT3), 73 percent for measles (MCV), and 87 percent for Hib (Hib3). According to WHO, in 2010, Yemen had 0.70 magnetic resonance imaging (MRI) machines per 1 million population, 2.18 computer tomography (CT) machines per 1 million, 0.04 telecolbalt units per 1 million, and 0.04 radiotherapy machines per 1 million.

Cost of Drugs

According to WHO, in 2006, the median availability of selected generic drugs in the public sector in Yemen was 5.0 percent; in the private sector, the mean availability was 90.0 percent. The median price ratio (comparing the price in Yemen to the international reference price) was 1.1 in the public sector for selected generic medicines, indicating that median prices were 10 percent higher than the international reference price; in the private sector, the median reference price was 3.5, indicating costs more than three times as high as the international reference price.

Health Care Facilities

As of 2010, according to WHO, Yemen had 11.53 health posts per 100,000 population, 4.82 health centers per 100,000, 2.09 district or rural hospitals per 100,000, 0.91 provincial hospitals per 100,000, and 0.01 specialized hospitals per 100,000. In 2009, Yemen had 0.70 hospital beds per 1,000 population, one of the 30 lowest rates in the world.

Major Health Issues

In 2008, WHO estimated that 61 percent of years of life lost in Yemen were due to communicable diseases, 26 percent to noncommunicable diseases, and 13 percent to injuries. In 2008, the age-standardized estimate of cancer deaths was 87 per 100,000 for men and 81 per 100,000 for women; for cardiovascular disease and diabetes, 542 per 100,000 for men and 446 per 100,000 for women; and for chronic respiratory disease, 63 per 100,000 for men and 43 per 100,000 for women.

In 2008, the age-standardized death rate from malaria was 4.2 per 100,000 population. In 2010, tuberculosis incidence was 49.0 per 100,000 population, tuberculosis prevalence 71.0 per 100,000, and deaths due to tuberculosis among HIV-negative people 5.9 per 100,000. Yemen's maternal mortality rate

(death from any cause related to or aggravated by pregnancy) was estimated in 2008 as 210 maternal deaths per 100,000 live births. A 2003 survey estimated the prevalence of female genital mutilation at 38.2 percent. The infant mortality rate, defined as the number of deaths of infants younger than 1 year, was estimated at 53.50 per 1,000 live births in 2012. Child malnutrition is a serious problem: In 2003, 43.1 percent of children under age 5 were underweight (defined as 2 kilograms [kg] below standard weight-for-age at age 1, 3 kg below for ages 2 to 3, and 4 kg below for ages 4 to 5), one of the highest rates in the world.

Health Care Personnel

In 2006, WHO identified Yemen as one of 57 countries with a critical deficit in the supply of skilled health workers. Yemen has four medical schools: the Faculty of Medicine and Pharmacy of the University of Aden, the Faculty of Medicine and Health Sciences of the University of Sana'a, the College of Medical Sciences of the University of Science and Technology in Sana'a, and the College of Medicine and Health Sciences of Hadhramout University of Science and Technology in Mukalla City. The basic course of training lasts sixor 6.5 years, and the degrees awarded are bachelor of medicine and surgery or doctor of medicine.

In 2009, Yemen had 0.30 physicians per 1,000 population and 0.10 dentistry personnel per 1,000, and in 2004, had 0.13 pharmaceutical personnel per 1,000, 0.23 laboratory health workers per 1,000, 0.53 health management and support workers per 1,000, 0.29 community and traditional health workers per 1,000, and 0.66 nurses and midwives per 1,000.

Government Role in Health Care

According to WHO, in 2010, Yemen spent $1.5 billion on health care, an amount that comes to $63 per capita. Most (96 percent) of health care funding came from domestic sources, with 4 percent coming from abroad. The largest share of health care spending was provided through household expenditures (75 percent), with the remainder coming from government expenditures (24 percent) and other sources (1 percent). In 2010, Yemen allocated 4 percent of its total government expenditures to health, in the low range for lower-middle-income eastern Mediterranean region countries; government expenditures on health came to 1 percent of GDP, in the low range for lower-middle-income eastern Mediterranean region countries. In 2009, according to WHO, official development assistance (ODA) for health in Yemen came to $3.84 per capita.

Public Health Programs

According to WHO, in 2004, Yemen had 0.04 environmental and public health workers per 1,000 population. In 2010, 53 percent of the population of Yemen had access to improved sanitation facilities (34 percent in rural areas and 93 percent in urban), and 55 percent had access to improved sources of drinking water (47 percent in rural areas and 92 percent in urban).

ZAMBIA

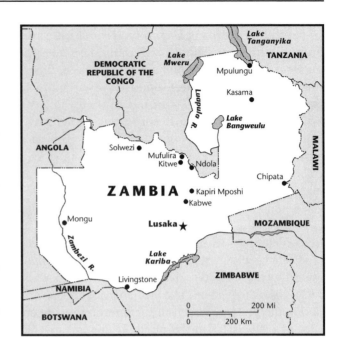

Zambia is a landlocked southern African country sharing borders with Angola, the Democratic Republic of the Congo, Malawi, Mozambique, Namibia, Tanzania, and Zimbabwe. The area of 290,587 square miles (752,618 square kilometers) makes Zambia about the size of Texas, and the July 2012 population was estimated at 14.3 million. In 2010, 36 percent of the population lived in urban areas, and the 2010 to 2015 annual rate of urbanization was estimated at 3.2 percent. Lusaka is the capital and largest city (with a 2009 population estimated at 1.4 million). The population growth rate in 2012 was 3.0 percent, the net migration rate negative 0.7 migrants per 1,000 population, the birth rate 43.5 births per 1,000 (the fourth-highest in the world), and the total fertility rate 5.9 children per woman (the eighth-highest in the world. The United Nations High Commissioner for Refugees (UNHCR) estimated that, in 2010, there were 6,550 refugees and persons in refugee-like situations in Zambia.

A former British colony (Northern Rhodesia), Zambia became independent in 1964. According to the Ibrahim Index, in 2011, Zambia ranked 15th among 53 African countries in terms of governance performance, with a score of 57 (out of 100). Zambia ranked tied for 91st among 183 countries on the *Corruption Perceptions Index 2011,* with a score of 3.2 (on a scale where 0 indicates highly corrupt and 10 very clean). In 2011, Zambia was classified as a country with low human development (the lowest of four categories) on the United Nations Development Programme's (UNDP's) Human Development Index (HDI), with a score of 0.430 (on a scale where 1 denotes high development and 0 low development). In 2011, the International Food Policy Research Institute (IFPRI) classified Zambia as a country with an "alarming" hunger problem, with a Global Hunger Index (GHI) score of 24.0 (where 0 reflects no hunger, and higher scores more hunger). Life expectancy at birth in 2012 was estimated at 52.97 years, among the 20 lowest in the world, and estimated gross domestic product (GDP) per capita in 2011 was $1,600, among the 30 lowest in the world. Income distribution in Zambia is relatively unequal: In 2004, the Gini Index (a measure of dispersion, in which perfect equality is denoted by 0 and maximum inequality is denoted by 100) for family income was 50.8. According to the World Economic Forum's *Global Gender Gap Index 2011*, Zambia ranked 106th out of 135 countries on gender equality with a score of 0.630 (on a scale with a theoretical range of 1 for equality to 0 for inequality and an actual range in 2011 from 0.8530 to 0.4873).

Emergency Health Services

According to the World Health Organization (WHO), as of 2007, Zambia had a formal and publicly available emergency care (prehospital care) system accessible through a national access number. Doctors Without Borders (Médecins Sans Frontières, or MSF) began working in Zambia in 199 and had 51 staff members in the country at the close of 2010. MSF provides maternal, reproductive, and obstetric care in Luwingu (northern Zambia), including human immunodeficiency virus (HIV) testing and preventing mother-to-child transmission (PMTCT) treatment. MSF also provided emergency services during the March 2010 cholera outbreak in Lusaka and has been working with Zambian authorities since 2004 to help prevent future outbreaks (cholera outbreaks are common during Zambia's rainy season).

Insurance

The public health system in Zambia provides health services to the population; medicines are provided free, including antiretrovirals, but some services require a copayment. As of 2010, about 5 percent of the population was covered by private insurance as well, generally through their employers. According to Ke Xu and colleagues, in 2003, 2.3 percent of households in Zambia experienced catastrophic health expenditures annually; "catastrophic" was defined as exceeding 40 percent of household income remaining after basic needs were met.

Costs of Hospitalization

No data available.

Access to Health Care

Health services in Zambia are provided primarily through the public sector; the private sector is concentrated primarily in cities. Many Zambians use the services of traditional healers as well as or in place of Western medical services.

According to WHO, in 2007, 46 percent of births in Zambia were attended by skilled personnel (for example, physicians, nurses, or midwives), and 60 percent of pregnant women received at least four prenatal care visits. The 2010 immunization rates for 1-year-olds were 82 percent for diphtheria and pertussis (DPT3), 91 percent for measles (MCV), and 82 percent for Hib (Hib3). In 2010, an estimated 72 percent of persons with advanced HIV infection were receiving antiretroviral therapy in accordance with the 2010 WHO guidelines. According to WHO, in 2010, Zambia had 0.08 magnetic resonance imaging (MRI) machines per 1 million population, 0.24 computer tomography (CT) machines per 1 million, 0.08 telecolbalt units per 1 million, and 0.08 radiotherapy machines per 1 million.

Cost of Drugs

Zambia's public health system provides medicines for free, including all the medicines on the Essential Medicines List (EML), which contained 404 medicines as of 2008, including formulations for children. Private health plans offer some coverage for medicines as well. Total pharmaceutical expenditures in Zambia in 2011 came to ZMK 117,745 million ($23.3 million), which comes to ZMK 9,025.40 ($1.80) per capita. Pharmaceutical expenditures represented 3.0 percent of total health expenditures and 0.1 percent of GDP.

Health Care Facilities

As of 2010, according to WHO, Zambia had 1.31 health posts per 100,000 population, 9.25 health centers per 100,000, 0.33 district or rural hospitals per 100,000, 0.14 provincial hospitals per 100,000, and 0.04 specialized hospitals per 100,000. In 2008, Zambia had 1.90 hospital beds per 1,000 population.

Major Health Issues

In 2008, WHO estimated that 75 percent of years of life lost in Zambia were due to communicable diseases, 15 percent to noncommunicable diseases, and 10 percent to injuries. In 2008, the age-standardized estimate of cancer deaths was 105 per 100,000 for men and 108 per 100,000 for women; for cardiovascular disease and diabetes, 563 per 100,000 for men and 473 per 100,000 for women; and for chronic respiratory disease, 159 per 100,000 for men and 75 per 100,000 for women.

In 2008, the age-standardized death rate from malaria was 55.2 per 100,000 population. In 2010, tuberculosis incidence was 462.0 per 100,000 population, tuberculosis prevalence 345.0 per 100,000, and deaths due to tuberculosis among HIV-negative people 20.0 per 100,000. Zambia has one of the highest human immunodeficiency virus/acquired immune deficiency syndrome (HIV/AIDS) rates in the world; as of 2009, an estimated 13.5 percent of adults age 15 to 49 were living with HIV or AIDS. In 2010, 94 percent of pregnant women tested positive for HIV. As of 2009, an estimated 980,000 people in Zambia were living with HIV or AIDS, the 10th-largest number in the world.

Zambia's maternal mortality rate (death from any cause related to or aggravated by pregnancy) is high by global standards, estimated at 470 maternal deaths per 100,000 live births as of 2008. The infant mortality rate, defined as the number of deaths of infants younger than 1 year, also has been high, at 64.61 per 1,000 live births as of 2012. In 2007, 14.9 percent of children under age 5 were underweight (defined as 2 kilograms [kg] below standard weight-for-age at age 1, 3 kg below for ages 2 to 3, and 4 kg below for ages 4 to 5). As of December 2010, an estimated 84 percent of adults and 26 percent of children who needed antiretroviral therapy were receiving it. The mother-to-child transmission rate for HIV in 2010 was estimated at 20 percent, and in 2009, 11.7 percent of deaths to children under age 5 were attributed to HIV.

Health Care Personnel

Zambia has one medical school, the School of Medicine of the University of Zambia in Lusaka. The course of training for the basic medical degree lasts seven years, and the degrees awarded are bachelor of medicine and bachelor of surgery. Physicians must register with the Medical Council of Zambia, and a temporary license is granted after completion of a one-year internship. One year of government service is required after graduation. Zambia has agreements with China, Cuba, the Netherlands, and the United Kingdom (UK). In 2006, Zambia had 0.06 physicians per 1,000 population, 0.01 pharmaceutical personnel per 1,000, 0.05 laboratory health workers per 1,000, 0.93 health management and support workers per 1,000, 0.01 dentistry personnel per 1,000, and 0.71 nurses and midwives per 1,000. Michael Clemens and Bunilla Petterson estimate that 57 percent of Zambia-born physicians and 9 percent of Zambia-born nurses are working in one of nine developed countries, primarily in the UK.

Government Role in Health Care

The right to health, including access to essential medicines and medical technologies, is recognized in national legislation. Zambia has a National Health Policy (NHP) and a plan to implement it, both created in 2011; Zambia also has a National Medicines Policy (NMP) and a plan to implement it, both created in 2010. The NMP covers selection of essential medicines; financing, purchase, distribution, and regulation of drugs; pharmacovigilance; rational usage of medicines; human resource development; research; evaluation and monitoring; and traditional medicine. Pharmaceutical policy implementation is regularly monitored by the Ministry of Health. Zambia is a World Trade Organization (WTO) member and recognizes patent protection for pharmaceuticals but also has national legislation allowing compulsory licensing for reasons of public health. In 2009, according

to WHO, official development assistance (ODA) for health in Zambia came to $32.83 per capita.

According to WHO, in 2010, Zambia spent $954 million on health care, an amount that comes to $73 per capita. More than half (61 percent) of health care funding came from domestic sources, with 39 percent coming from abroad. The largest share of health care spending was provided through government expenditures (60 percent), with the remainder coming from household expenditures (26 percent) and other sources (13 percent). In 2010, Zambia allocated 16 percent of its total government expenditures to health, in the high range for lower-middle-income African countries; government expenditures on health came to 4 percent of GDP, in the high range for lower-middle-income African countries.

Public Health Programs

According to WHO, in 2006, Zambia had 0.07 environmental and public health workers per 1,000 population. In 2010, 48 percent of the population of Zambia had access to improved sanitation facilities (43 percent in rural areas and 57 percent in urban), and 61 percent had access to improved sources of drinking water (46 percent in rural areas and 87 percent in urban). According to C. B. Ijsselmuiden and colleagues, in 2007, Zambia had one institution offering postgraduate public health programs.

ZIMBABWE

Zimbabwe is a landlocked country in southern Africa sharing borders with Botswana, Mozambique, South African, and Zambia. The area of 150,872 square miles (390,757 square kilometers) makes Zimbabwe about the size of Montana, and the July 2012 population was estimated at 12.7 million. In 2010, 38 percent of the population lived in urban areas, and the 2010 to 2015 annual rate of urbanization was estimated at 3.4 percent. Harare is the capital and largest city (with a 2009 population estimated at 1.6 million). The population growth rate in 2012 was 4.4 percent (the second-highest in the world), the net migration rate 23.8 migrants per 1,000 population (the second-highest in the world), the birth rate 32.2 births per 1,000, and the total fertility rate 3.6 children per woman. The United Nations High Commissioner for Refugees (UNHCR) estimated that, in 2010, there were 4,435 refugees and persons in refugee-like situations in Zimbabwe.

A former British colony (Southern Rhodesia), Zimbabwe became independent in 1965. Robert Mugabe has been the only ruler of Zimbabwe (first as prime minister then as president); a land redistribution campaign, which began in 2000, created widespread shortages of basic commodities. According to the Ibrahim Index, in 2011, Zimbabwe ranked near the bottom (51st out of 53) among African countries in terms of governance performance, with a score of 31 (out of 100). Zimbabwe ranked tied for 152nd among 183 countries on the *Corruption Perceptions Index 2011,* with a score of 2.2 (on a scale where 0 indicates highly corrupt and 10 very clean).

In 2011, Zimbabwe was classified as a country with low human development (the lowest of four categories) on the United Nations Development Programme's (UNDP's) Human Development Index (HDI), with a score of 0.376 (on a scale where 1 denotes high development and 0 low development). In 2012, the World Food Programme estimated that 1 million people in Zimbabwe would be food insecure due to poor harvests and increased prices. Life expectancy at birth in 2012 was estimated at 51.82 years, among the 10 lowest in the world, and estimated gross domestic product (GDP) per capita in 2011 was $500, among the 10 lowest in the world. Income distribution in Zimbabwe is relatively unequal: In 2008, the Gini Index (a measure of dispersion, in which perfect equality is denoted by 0 and maximum inequality is denoted by 100) for family income was 50.1. According to the World Economic Forum's *Global Gender Gap Index 2011*, Zimbabwe ranked 88th out of 135 countries on gender equality with a score of 0.681 (on a scale with a theoretical range of 1 for equality to 0 for inequality and an actual range in 2011 from 0.8530 to 0.4873).

Emergency Health Services

According to the World Health Organization (WHO), as of 2007, Zimbabwe had a formal and publicly available emergency care (prehospital care) system accessible through a national access number. Doctors Without Borders (Médecins Sans Frontières, or MSF) began working in Zimbabwe in 2000 and had 895 staff members in the country at the close of 2010. MSF provided antiretroviral treatment to more than 34,000 human immunodeficiency virus/acquired immune deficiency syndrome (HIV/AIDS) patients

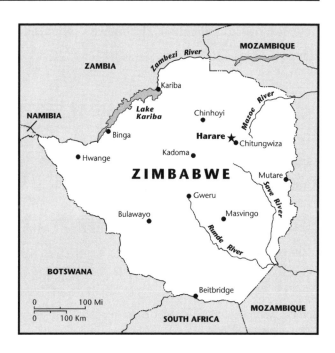

in 2010, trained nurses in routine HIV care, created a program to treat the special needs of pediatric and adolescent patients with HIV/AIDS, and began a treatment to treat drug-resistant tuberculosis in December 2010. All MSF HIV/AIDS programs also treat victims of sexual violence and provide outreach and educational services regarding sexual violence.

Insurance

As of 2011, Zimbabwe was in the process of creating a social insurance scheme to provide universal access to health care. Already, some essential primary services are provided free to certain population groups, including children under the age of 5, pregnant women, the elderly, and the poor. Drugs to treat malaria, tuberculosis, and HIV/AIDS are also provided free, as are vaccines on WHO's Expanded Programme on Immunization (EPI) list. Private insurance, mostly employer-based, also covers some of the population. Health care provided in the public sector does not require copayment, but treatment in the private sector generally does.

Costs of Hospitalization

No data available.

Access to Health Care

According to WHO, in 2009, 60 percent of births in Zimbabwe were attended by skilled personnel (for

Selected Health Indicators: Zimbabwe Compared With the Global Average (2010)

	Zimbabwe	Global Average
Male life expectancy at birth* (years)	47	66
Female life expectancy at birth* (years)	50	71
Under-5 mortality rate, both sexes (per 1,000 live births)	80	57
Adult mortality rate, both sexes* (probability of dying between 15 and 60 years per 1,000 population)	606	176
Maternal mortality ratio (per 100,000 live births)	570	210
HIV prevalence* (per 1,000 adults aged 15 to 49)	143	8
Tuberculosis prevalence (per 100,000 population)	402	178

Source: World Health Organization Global Health Observatory Data Repository.
*Data refers to 2009.

example, physicians, nurses, or midwives). In 2006, 72 percent of pregnant women received at least four prenatal care visits. The 2010 immunization rates for 1-year-olds were 83 percent for diphtheria and pertussis (DPT3), 84 percent for measles (MCV), and 83 percent for Hib (Hib3). In 2010, an estimated 59 percent of persons with advanced HIV infection were receiving antiretroviral therapy in accordance with the 2010 WHO guidelines. According to WHO, in 2010, Zimbabwe had 0.32 magnetic resonance imaging (MRI) machines per 1 million population, 0.48 computer tomography (CT) machines per 1 million, 0.24 telecolbalt units per 1 million, and 0.24 radiotherapy machines per 1 million.

Cost of Drugs

Zimbabwe has no regulations or price controls affecting pharmaceuticals.

Health Care Facilities

As of 2010, according to WHO, Zimbabwe had 10.59 health centers per 100,000 population, 0.41 district or rural hospitals per 100,000, 0.09 provincial hospitals per 100,000, and 0.09 specialized hospitals per 100,000. In 2006, Zimbabwe had 3.00 hospital beds per 1,000 population.

Major Health Issues

In 2008, WHO estimated that 87 percent of years of life lost in Zimbabwe were due to communicable diseases,

9 percent to noncommunicable diseases, and 4 percent to injuries. In 2008, the age-standardized estimate of cancer deaths was 112 per 100,000 for men and 115 per 100,000 for women; for cardiovascular disease and diabetes, 357 per 100,000 for men and 291 per 100,000 for women; and for chronic respiratory disease, 96 per 100,000 for men and 41 per 100,000 for women.

In 2008, the age-standardized death rate from malaria was 45.8 per 100,000 population, and the age-standardized death rate from childhood-cluster diseases (pertussis, polio, diphtheria, measles, and tetanus) was 23.1 per 100,000 population, the fifth-highest in the world. In 2010, tuberculosis incidence was 633.0 per 100,000 population, tuberculosis prevalence 402.0 per 100,000, and deaths due to tuberculosis among HIV-negative people 27.00 per 100,000. WHO estimated the 2010 case detection rate at 56 percent. As of 2009, Zimbabwe had the fifth-highest HIV/AIDS rate in the world; in that year, an estimated 14.3 percent of adults age 15 to 49 were living with HIV or AIDS. As of 2009, an estimated 1.2 million people in Zimbabwe were living with HIV or AIDS, the seventh-largest number in the world. In 2010, 90 percent of pregnant women tested positive for HIV. The mother-to-child transmission rate for HIV in 2010 was estimated at 25 percent, and in 2009, 24.7 percent of deaths to children under age 5 were attributed to HIV.

Zimbabwe's maternal mortality rate (death from any cause related to or aggravated by pregnancy) is quite high by global standards, estimated at 790 maternal deaths per 100,000 live births as of 2008. The infant mortality rate, defined as the number of deaths of infants younger than 1 year, was estimated at 28.23 per 1,000 live births in 2012. In 2006, 14.0 percent of children under age 5 were underweight (defined as 2 kilograms [kg] below standard weight-for-age at age 1, 3 kg below for ages 2 to 3, and 4 kg below for ages 4 to 5).

Health Care Personnel

Zimbabwe has one medical school, the Godfrey Huggins School of Medicine of the University of Zimbabwe in Harare, which has offered instruction since 1963. The basic medical degree course lasts five years, and the degrees granted are bachelor of medicine and bachelor of surgery. Licensing is handled by the Health Professions Council and requires two years of work as an intern as well as graduation from a recognized medical school.

In 2004, Zimbabwe had 0.16 physicians per 1,000 population, 0.07 pharmaceutical personnel per 1,000, 0.07 laboratory health workers per 1,000, 0.02 dentistry personnel per 1,000, 0.04 community and traditional health workers, and 0.72 nurses and midwives per 1,000. Michael Clemens and Bunilla Petterson estimate that 51 percent of Zimbabwe-born physicians and 24 percent of Zimbabwe-born nurses are working in one of nine developed countries, primarily in the United Kingdom (UK) and South Africa (physicians) and the UK (nurses). Alok Bhargava and colleagues place Zimbabwe ninth among countries most affected by the medical "brain drain" (international migration of skilled personnel) in 2004 and first among countries with populations greater than 4 million.

Government Role in Health Care

Zimbabwe has a National Health Policy (NHP) and a plan to implement it, both created in 2009; the NHP's primary goal from 2009 to 2013 is to increase equality and equity in health. Zimbabwe has a National Medicines Policy (NMP), created in 1995, a plan to implement it, created in 2006, and a body of legislation addressing pharmaceuticals, most recently updated in 2011. Together, they cover selection of essential medicines; financing, pricing, purchase, distribution, and regulation of drugs; pharmacovigilance; rational usage of medicines; human resource development; research; evaluation and monitoring; and traditional medicine.

Zimbabwe is a member of the World Trade Organization (WTO) and observes patent law, but national law also includes some elements of the Trade-Related Aspects of Intellectual Property Rights (TRIPS) that provide exceptions to patent law. These exceptions include compulsory licensing for reasons of public health, the Bolar exception that allows manufacturers to perform research and testing to create generic drugs before a patent has expired, and parallel importing provisions (allowing import of drugs created for sale in a different country).

Total health expenditures in Zimbabwe in 2007 came to ZWD 9,463,652.5 million ($978.1 million) and per capita health expenditures to ZWD 751,381.7 ($77.70). Almost half (46.2 percent) of health expenditures came from the government, and health expenditures represented 8.9 percent of the total government budget. In 2009, according to WHO, official development assistance (ODA) for health in Zimbabwe came to $8.85 per capita.

Public Health Programs

According to WHO, in 2004, Zimbabwe had 0.14 environmental and public health workers per 1,000 population. In 2010, 40 percent of the population of Zimbabwe had access to improved sanitation facilities (32 percent in rural areas and 52 percent in urban), and 80 percent had access to improved sources of drinking water (69 percent in rural areas and 98 percent in urban). According to the World Higher Education Database (WHED), one university in Zimbabwe offers programs in epidemiology or public health: Africa University in Mutare.

BIBLIOGRAPHY

Ameli, Omid and William Newbrander. "Contracting for Health Services: Effects of Utilization and Quality on the Costs of the Basic Package of Health Services in Afghanistan." *Bulletin of the World Health Organization*, v.86/12 (December 2008). http://www.who.int/bulletin/volumes/86/12/08-053108.pdf (Accessed June 2012).

Ball, Douglas. "The Regulation of Mark-Ups in the Pharmaceutical Supply Chain." WHO/HAI Project on Medicine Prices and Availability: Review Series on Pharmaceutical Pricing Policies and Interventions Working Paper 3. Geneva, Switzerland: World Health Organization and Health Action International, 2011. http://www.haiweb.org/medicineprices/05062011/Mark-ups%20final%20May2011.pdf (Accessed April 2012).

Bhargava, Alok, Frederic Docquier, and Yasser Moullan. "Modeling the Effects of Physician Emigration on Human Development." *Economics and Human Biology*, v.9/2 (March 2011). http://www.cepr.org/meets/wkcn/2/2414/papers/Moullan.pdf (Accessed May 2012).

Blank, Robert H. and Viola Burau. *Comparative Health Policy*. 3rd ed. New York: Palgrave Macmillan, 2010.

Central Intelligence Agency. The World Factbook. https://www.cia.gov/library/publications/the-world-factbook/index.html (Accessed May 2012).

Choi, Sung-Hyuk, Yun-Sik Hong, Sung-Woo Lee, In-Chul Jung, and Chul-Su Kim. "Prehospital and Emergency Department Care in South Korea." *Canadian Journal of Emergency Medicine*, v.9/3 (May 2007).

Clemens, Michael A. and Bunilla Petterson. "New Data on Health Professionals Abroad." Center for Global Development Working Paper 95 (August 11, 2006). http://www.cgdev.org/content/publications/detail/9267 (Accessed June 2012).

Cylus, Jonathan and Rachel Irwin. "The Challenges of Hospital Payment Systems." *Euro Observer*, v.12/3 (Autumn 2010). http://www.euro.who.int/__data/assets/pdf_file/0018/121743/EuroObserver_Autumn2010.pdf (Accessed April 2012).

Docteur, Elizabeth. "Pharmaceutical Pricing Policy in a Global Market." Workshop on Current Pharmaceuticals Challenges, European Health Forums, Gastein, Austria (October 1, 2008). http://www.ehfg.org/fileadmin/ehfg/Website/Archiv/2008/Powerpoints/WS2/08_WS2_Docteur.pdf (Accessed June 2012).

Doctors Without Borders. http://www.doctorswithoutborders.org (Accessed May 2012).

Forcier, Melanie Bourassa, Steven Simoens, and Antonio Giuffrida. "Impact, Regulation and Health Policy

Implications of Physician Migration in OECD Countries." *Human Resources for Health,* v.2 (2004). http://www.ncbi.nlm.nih.gov/pmc/articles/PMC493284 (Accessed May 2012).

Froystad, Mona, Ottar Maestad, and Nohra Villamil. "Health Services in Angola: Availability, Quality, and Utilisation." *CMI Report* (2011). http://www.cmi.no/publications/file/4319-health-services-in-angola.pdf (Accessed April 2012).

German, Fikre. "The Development of Emergency Medicine in Ethiopia." *Canadian Journal of Emergency Medicine,* v.13/6 (2011).

Glied, Sherry and Peter C. Smith, eds. *The Oxford Handbook of Health Economics.* New York: Oxford University Press, 2011.

Gobah, Freeman Kobla and Liang Zhang. "The National Health Insurance Scheme in Ghana: Prospects and Challenges: A Cross-Sectional Evidence." *Global Journal of Health Science,* v.3/2 (2011). http://www.ccsenet.org/journal/index.php/gjhs/article/view/9911 (Accessed May 2012).

Gould, Eric and Omer Moav. "The Israeli Brain Drain." The Shalem Center: The Institute for Economic and Social Policy (July 2006). http://www.shalemcenter.org.il/FileServer/df4b061c96a6fbceb95026260cb4de8a.pdf (Accessed June 2012).

Graig, Laurene A. *Health of Nations: An International Perspective on U.S. Health Care Reform.* 3rd ed. Washington, DC: Congressional Quarterly, 1999.

Hausmann, Ricardo, Laura D. Tyson, and Saadia Zahidi. *The Global Gender Gap Report 2011.* Geneva, Switzerland: World Economic Forum, 2011.

Himmelstein, David U., Deborah Thorne, Elizabeth Warren, and Steffie Woolhandler. "Medical Bankruptcy in the United States, 2007: Results of a National Study." *The American Journal of Medicine,* v.122/8 (August 2009). http://download.journals.elsevierhealth.com/pdfs/journals/0002-9343/PIIS0002934309004045.pdf (Accessed April 2012).

Ijsselmuiden, C. B., T. C. Nchinda, S. Duala, N. M. Tumwesigye, and D. Serwadda. "Mapping Africa's

Advanced Public Health Education Capacity: The AfriHealth Project." *Bulletin of the World Health Organization,* v.85/12 (December 2007). http://www.who.int/bulletin/volumes/85/12/07-045526.pdf (Accessed May 2012).

International Association of National Public Health Institutes. http://www.ianphi.org (Accessed April 2012).

International Association of Universities. *The World Higher Education Database.* 23rd ed. London: Palgrave Macmillan, 2011.

International Red Cross. http://www.ifrc.org/ (Accessed April 2012).

International Social Security Association. "Country Profiles." http://www.issa.int/Observatory/Country-Profiles (Accessed May 2012).

Jaffe, Susan. "Health Policy Brief: Key Issues in Health Reform." *Health Affairs* (August 20, 2009). http://www.rwjf.org/files/research/82409healthaffairs7.pdf (Accessed April 2012).

Jowett, Matthew and Elizabeth Danielyan. "Is There a Role for User Charges? Thoughts on Health System Reform in Armenia." *Bulletin of the World Health Organization,* v.88 (2010). http://www.who.int/bulletin/volumes/88/6/09-074765.pdf (Accessed May 2012).

Kaiser Family Foundation. "Your Source for State Health Data." http://www.statehealthfacts.org (Accessed June 2012).

Kaushik, Manas, Abihishek Jaiswal, Naseem Shah, and Ajay Mahal. "High-End Physician Migration From India." *Bulletin of the World Health Organization,* v.86/1 (January 2008). http://www.who.int/bulletin/volumes/86/1/07-041681.pdf (Accessed June 2012).

Kutzin, Joseph, Cheryl Cashin, and Melitta Jakab, eds. *Implementing Health Financing Reform.* Observatory Studies Series 21. Copenhagen, Denmark: WHO Regional Office for Europe, 2010.

Lateef, Fatimah and V. Anantharaman. "Emergency Medical Services in Singapore." *Canadian Journal of Emergency Medicine,* v.2/4 (October 2000).

Mays, Glenn P. and Sharla A. Smith. "Geographic Variation in Public Health Spending: Correlates and Consequences." *Health Services Research,* v.44/5/2 (October 2009).

McDonald, Archibald, Jean Williams-Johnson, Eric Williams, and Simone French. "Emergency Medicine in Jamaica." *Canadian Journal of Emergency Medicine,* v.7/5 (2005). http://www.cjem-online.ca/v7/n5/p340 (Accessed May 2012).

McKee, Martin and Judith Healy, eds. *Hospitals in a Changing Europe.* Philadelphia: Open University Press, 2002. http://www.euro.who.int/__data/assets/pdf_file/0004/98401/E74486.pdf (Accessed May 2012).

Mo Ibrahim Foundation. *2011 Ibrahim Governance of African Governance.* London: Ibrahim Foundation, 2011. http://www.moibrahimfoundation.org/en/media/get/20111003_ENG2011-IIAG-Summary Report-sml.pdf (Accessed April 2012).

Mossialos, Elias and Sarah Thomson. "Voluntary Health Insurance in the European Union." Brussels, Belgium: European Observatory on Health Systems and Policies, 2004. http://www.euro.who.int/__data/assets/pdf_file/0006/98448/E84885.pdf (Accessed May 2012).

Mullan, Fitzhugh. "The Metrics of the Physician Brain Drain." *The New England Journal of Medicine,* v.353 (October 2005). http://www.arp.harvard.edu/AfricanHigherEducation/Braindrain_medicine.pdf (Accessed June 2012).

Pan American Health Organization. http://new.paho.org/index.php (Accessed May 2012).

Radley, David C., Sabrina K. H. How, Ashley-Kay Fryer, Douglas McCarthy, and Cathy Schoen. *Rising to the Challenge: Results From a Scorecard on Local Health Systems Performance, 2012.* New York: The Commonwealth Fund, 2012. http://www.commonwealthfund.org/Publications/Fund-Reports/2012/Mar/Local-Scorecard.aspx (Accessed May 2012).

Reid, T. R. *The Healing of America; A Global Question for Better, Cheaper, and Fairer Health Care.* New York: Penguin Press, 2009.

Roberts, Graham, et al. "The Fiji Islands Health System Review." *Health Systems in Transition,* v.1/1 (2011). http://www2.wpro.who.int/asia_pacific_observatory/resources/FijiIslandsHealthSystemsReview-FINAL.pdf (Accessed June 2012).

Sanchez-Serrano, Ibis. *The World's Health Care Crisis: From the Laboratory Bench to the Patient's Bedside.* New York: Elsevier, 2011.

Save the Children. *State of the World's Mothers 2012.* Westport, CT: Save the Children, 2012. http://www.savethechildren.org/atf/cf/{9def2ebe-10ae-432c-9bd0-df91d2eba74a}/STATEOFTHEWORLDS MOTHERSREPORT2012.PDF (Accessed April 2012).

Schoen, Cathy and Robin Osborn. "New 2011 Survey of Patients with Complex Care Needs in Eleven Countries Finds That Care is Often Poorly Coordinated." *Health Affairs,* v.30/12 (December 2011).

Thomson, S., R. Osborn, D. Squires, and S. J. Reed. *International Profiles of Health Care Systems, 2011.* New York: The Commonwealth Fund, 2011. http://www.commonwealthfund.org/Publications/Fund-Reports/2011/Nov/International-Profiles-of-Health-Care-Systems-2011.aspx (Accessed June 2012).

Transparency International. *Corruption Perceptions Index 2011.* Berlin, Germany: Author, 2012. http://cpi.transparency.org/cpi2011 (Accessed April 2012).

Triggle, Nick. "The Carve-Up of the NHS." *BBC News* (January 2, 2008). http://news.bbc.co.uk/2/hi/health/7140980.stm (Accessed May 2012).

Tsounta, Evridiki. "Universal Health Care 101: Lesson for the Eastern Caribbean and Beyond." IMF Working Paper WP/09/61 (March 2009). http://www.imf.org/external/pubs/ft/wp/2009/wp0961.pdf (Accessed June 2012).

United Nations Development Programme. *Human Development Report 2011: Sustainability and Equity: A Better Future for All.* New York: United Nations Development Programme, 2011. http://hdr.undp.org/en/reports/global/hdr2011/download (Accessed May 2012).

United Nations Relief and Works Agency for Palestine Refugees. http://unrwa.org (Accessed May 2012).

United States Agency for International Development. *Guyana Health System Assessment 2010*. Bethesda, MD: Abt Associates, 2011. http://www.healthsystems 2020.org/content/resource/detail/85822/ (Accessed April 2012).

United States Agency for International Development. *Health Systems 20/20*. http://www.healthsystems2020 .org/ (Accessed May 2012).

"Universal Health Coverage Still Rare in Africa." *Canadian Medical Association Journal*, v.184/2 (February 7, 2012).

West, Donald J., Jr., Gary Filerman, Bernardo Ramirez, and Jill Steinkogler. *CAHME: International Healthcare Management Education Final Report*, 2011. http:// www.cahme.org/Resources/FINAL%20REPORT %20_%20International%20Study%20.pdf (Accessed June 2012).

World Food Programme. Global Update: Food Security Monitoring 7, June 2012. http://documents.wfp.org/ stellent/groups/public/documents/ena/wfp247978 .pdf (Accessed June 2012).

World Health Organization. "Countries." http://www .who.int/countries/en/ (Accessed May 2012).

World Health Organization. "Female Genital Mutilation and Other Harmful Practices: Prevalence of FGM." http://www.who.int/reproductivehealth/top ics/fgm/prevalence/en/index.html (Accessed April 2012).

World Health Organization. *Global Atlas of the Health Workforce*. Geneva, Switzerland: World Health Organization, 2012. http://apps.who.int/globalatlas/default .asp (Accessed June 2012).

World Health Organization. "Global Health Observatory." http://www.who.int/gho/en (Accessed May 2012).

World Health Organization. "Global Health Workforce Alliance. Human Resources of Health Country Plans." http://www.who.int/workforcealliance/coun tries/hrhcountryplans/en/index.html (Accessed May 2012).

World Health Organization. *Global HIV/AIDS Response: Epidemic Update and Health Sector Progress Toward Universal Access*. Geneva, Switzerland: WHO, 2011. http://www.who.int/hiv/pub/progress _report2011/hiv_full_report_2011.pdf (Accessed May 2012).

World Health Organization. *Health Systems Financing: The Path to Universal Coverage*. Geneva, Switzerland: WHO, 2010. http://www.who.int/whr/2010/en/ index.html (Accessed May 2012).

World Health Organization. "Medicines: Development of Country Profiles and Monitoring of the Pharmaceutical Situation in Countries." http:// www.who.int/medicines/areas/coordination/coor dination_assessment/en/index.html (Accessed June 2012).

World Health Organization. "Policies and Practices of Countries that Are Experiencing a Crisis in Human Resources for Health: Tracking Survey." *Human Resources for Health Observer*, v.6 (December 2010). http://www.who.int/hrh/resources/observer6/en/ index.html (Accessed June 2012).

World Health Organization. Regional Office for Africa. http://www.afro.who.int/ (Accessed May 2012).

World Health Organization. Regional Office for the Eastern Mediterranean. http://www.emro.who.int/ (Accessed May 2012).

World Health Organization, Regional Office for Europe. "Disaster Preparedness and Response." http://www.euro.who.int/en/what-we-do/health-top ics/emergencies/disaster-preparedness-and-response/ country-work (Accessed May 2012).

World Health Organization, Regional Office for Europe. *Emergency Medical Services Systems in the European Union: Report of an Assessment Project Co-ordinated by the World Health Organization*. Copenhagen, Denmark: WHO, 2008. http://www .euro.who.int/__data/assets/pdf_file/0016/114406/ E92038.pdf (Accessed April 2012).

World Health Organization. Regional Office for South-East Asia. http://www.searo.who.int (Accessed June 2012).

World Health Organization, Regional Office for South-East Asia, Regional Office for the Western Pacific. *Social Health Insurance: Selected Case Studies from Asia and the Pacific.* SEARO Regional Publication No. 42. New Delhi, India: SEARO, 2005. http://www.wpro.who.int/publications/docs/searpno42.pdf (Accessed May 2012).

World Health Organization. Regional Office for the Western Pacific Region. http://www.wpro.who.int/en/ (Accessed April 2012).

World Health Organization. *WHO 2011 Global Tuberculosis Control.* Geneva, Switzerland: WHO, 2011. http://www.who.int/tb/publications/global_report/en (Accessed April 2012).

World Health Organization. *WHO's Activities in Emergencies and Humanitarian Action.* Geneva, Switzerland: WHO, 2010. http://www.who.int/hac/publications/hac_overview2010_may11.pdf (Accessed June 2012).

World Health Organization. World Directory of Medical Schools (with 2007 updates). http://www.who.int/hrh/wdms/en (Accessed June 2012).

World Health Organization. *World Health Statistics 2011.* Geneva, Switzerland: WHO, 2011. http://www.who.int/whosis/whostat/2011/en/index.html (Accessed April 2012).

Xu, Ke, David B. Evans, Kei Kawabata, Riadh Zeramdini, Jan Klavus, and Christopher J. L. Murray. "Household Catastrophic Health Expenditure: A Multicountry Analysis." *The Lancet,* v.362 (July 12, 2003).

RESOURCE GUIDE

Blank, Robert H. and Viola Burau. *Comparative Health Policy.* **3rd ed. New York: Palgrave Macmillan, 2010.**

Intended primarily for students, *Comparative Health Policy* provides a relatively brief (310 pages) and readable introduction to major issues in health care policy. The book focuses on the health care systems of Australia, Germany, Japan, New Zealand, the Netherlands, Sweden, Singapore, Taiwan, the United Kingdom, and the United States, so it is most useful for those interested in health care organization in countries that have already achieved a high level of development and less so for developing countries. Chapters are organized around topics, including the context of health care; funding, provision, and governance; priorities and resource allocation; the medical profession; home health care; and public health.

The Commonwealth Fund
http://www.commonwealthfund.org

The Commonwealth Fund is a private foundation created by Anna M. Harkness in 1918 to "enhance the common good" (according to the fund's Web page). The fund's focus today is on creating health care systems that are more efficient and higher quality and offer better access than existing systems, particularly for vulnerable populations, such as low-income people and the uninsured; topics covered by Commonwealth Fund reports include health policy reform, health care delivery, health care quality, health insurance,

payment reform, and vulnerable populations. The fund's emphasis is on the United States, but it also produces reports and studies on international health policy. Commonwealth Fund publications, surveys, and so on, are available for viewing or download from the Web site, as is information about fellowships and grants available from the Commonwealth Fund.

Glied, Sherry and Peter C. Smith, eds. *The Oxford Handbook of Health Economics.* **New York: Oxford University Press, 2011.**

The Oxford handbook includes 38 essays written by international guest contributors covering a broad range of topics relevant to the many ways health care may be organized and delivered. Some essays provide overviews of broad topics, such as "Health Systems in Industrialized Countries" (by Bianca K. Frogner, Peter S. Hussey, and Gerard F. Anderson) and "Socioeconomic Status and Health: Dimensions and Mechanisms" (by David M. Cutler, Adriana Lleras-Muney, and Tom Vogl), while others are more specific, for example, "Health Utility Measurement" (by Donna Rowen and John Brazier) and "Provider Payment and Incentives" (by John B. Christianson and Douglas Conrad).

Health Affairs
http://www.healthaffairs.org

This monthly peer-reviewed journal, founded in 1981, focuses on health care policy and research.

Some issues are focused on particular topics (for example, cancer care, substance abuse treatment, or health disparities), while others carry articles on a variety of topics. The focus is primarily on the United States, but international issues are also covered, and some international articles compare health systems or outcomes across countries. Some free content is available from the *Health Affairs* Web site, including a general blog, another covering grants, and "Health Policy Briefs" (summaries of relevant information on topics such as workplace wellness programs and the influence of public reporting of quality and costs on consumer choice).

International Association of National Public Health Institutes
http://www.ianphi.org

The International Association of National Public Health Institutes (IANPHI) is an international organization dedicated to promoting stronger national public health institutes and more coordinated public health systems globally while also serving as a professional organization for the directors of national public health institutes. It was created in 2006, has 79 members (from 74 countries, representing all regions of the world), and is supported through dues and a grant from the Bill and Melinda Gates Foundation. The IANPHI Web site includes profiles of member organizations, descriptions of IANPHI projects, news and events relevant to international public health, resources including case studies of how different national public health institutes were created, the IANPHI's *Framework for the Creation and Development of National Public Health Institutes* (a 2007 publication downloadable in PDF format), public health multimedia resources, and links to other relevant Web sites.

The International Social Security Association
http://www.issa.int/Observatory/Country-Profiles

The International Social Security Association (ISSA) is an international organization dedicated to promoting social security systems through providing information and encouraging networking among those involved in social security. The ISSA was founded in 1927 in response to the rapid growth of social insurance after the conclusion of World War I and is headquartered at the International Labour Office in Geneva, Switzerland. As of 2012, the ISSA had 335 member organizations in 157 countries, including institutions, government departments, and agencies. The observatory provides profiles of national social security programs in more than 170 countries and territories; most data is collected by surveys carried out by the ISSA and the U.S. Social Security Administration, with other information provided by the Organisation for Economic Co-operation and Development (OECD), the International Organization of Pension Supervisors, and national social security officials. Reports are organized within geographic regions (Africa, the Americas, Asia and the Pacific, and Europe) for each country. Separate sections provide basic statistical information on each country and its social security scheme, a more detailed description of the country's schemes (divided into Family Benefits; Old Age, Disability, and Survivors; Sickness and Mortality; Unemployment; and Work Injury), a timeline of reforms, and links to further resources.

Joint United Nations Programme on HIV/AIDS
http://www.unaids.org/en

The mission of the Joint United Nations Programme on HIV/AIDS (UNAIDS) is to promote universal access to human immunodeficiency virus (HIV) prevention, care, support, and treatment and to achieve these goals by 2015. Specific goals include reducing sexual transmission, eliminating new infections among children, preventing transmission among drug users, avoiding acquired immune deficiency syndrome (AIDS)-related tuberculosis deaths, eliminating inequalities in access to preventive and treatment services, eliminating travel restrictions, and eliminating discrimination against people who are HIV positive. The Web site includes a searchable database of HIV- and AIDS-related indicators with the ability to create customized, graphical displays. It also includes press releases, statistical reports, country reports, fact sheets, and multimedia presentations about HIV and AIDS.

Organisation for Economic Co-operation and Development
http://www.oecd.org

The Organisation for Economic Co-operation and Development (OECD) is an international organization dedicated to providing a forum for governments to share information and seek common solutions and to promoting policies to improve the well-being of people in all countries through economic growth and social development, while also being mindful of the environmental results of development. The

OECD was founded in 1961, is headquartered in Paris, and as of 2012, had a membership of 34 countries in all regions of the world, controlled a budget of 347 million euros, and produced about 250 publications a year. The OECD regularly monitors national and global events (in both member and nonmember countries), collects and analyzes data, and issues recommendations. Regular OECD publications include the *OECD Economic Outlook* (four issues per year), the *OECD Factbook*, *OECD Economic Surveys* (produced every two years for OECD countries plus Brazil, Russia, India, Indonesia, China, and South Africa), and the *OECD Yearbook*. The OECD also produces numerous special reports and books, and most OECD information is available in a variety of formats, including free access on the Web site, free downloads, and hard copy (for purchase).

PLoS Medicine
http://www.plosmedicine.org

A peer-reviewed, open-access journal published by the Public Library of Science, the focus is on articles that are likely to influence public health policy or clinical health practice and on the diseases and risk factors that, on a global basis, cause the greatest loss of years of healthy life. Articles are published under a Creative Commons Attribution License, so they may be freely downloaded. Articles cover a broad range of topics from molecular biology to nutrition to public health and nutrition, and many have an international focus.

Save the Children
http://www.savethechildren.org

Save the Children is an independent organization dedicated to improving children's lives, both in the United States and around the world. It was founded in 1932 in the United States, modeled after an English organization of the same name founded after World War I; it currently operates in more than 50 countries. Of particular interest in comparative health studies are Save the Children's annual *State of the World's Mothers* report, which highlights the conditions faced by women, children, and mothers in different countries around the world. Data on a number of international indicators relevant to the health and status of women and children is included in the report, and countries are ranked on three composite scales (the women's index, the mother's index, and the children's index) within three development groups (more developed, less developed, and least developed) according to the conditions presented for each demographic group.

United Nations Development Project Human Development Reports
http://hdr.undp.org/en

The goal of the Human Development Reports produced by the United Nations Human Development Report Office (HDRO) is to advance human development, freedom, and opportunities globally. The HDRO challenges policies that constrain human development, advocates for practical policy changes, and promotes new ideas to advance human development. Data for the International Human Development Indicators (used in the Human Development Index, or HDI, as well as other indices) is available from the Web site, along with various data tools to visualize the data, compare trends over time, and contrast human development in different countries. The Human Development Reports are available for the years 1990 to 2012; some are country specific, while others cover many countries, and they address a variety of topics, including democratic governance; economic reform and public finance; gender; environment and energy; education, knowledge, and culture; human security and conflicts; millennial goals and international cooperation; poverty and inequality; public health; and societal groups and social inclusions. Information on the Web site may be searched by key word or accessed through indices arranged by country or topic.

World Health Organization Countries
http://www.who.int/countries/en

This section of the World Health Organization's (WHO) Web site organizes information alphabetically by country. The specific information available for each country differs, and much of the information is also available from other sources, but this is a handy way to get an overview of each country and to access the available information from various WHO reports and sources. For each country, basic statistics and a map are presented, as well as the country health profile comparing the country to the average for its region on statistics such as immunization rates, the health workforce, and adult risk factors. Other information typically available includes the country's regional profile, information about disease crises and outbreaks, collaborating centers, data about mortality and the burden of disease, the national health accounts (expenditures for health), and information about immunizations, nutrition, and risk factors such as alcohol, road injuries, and tobacco use.

World Health Organization Global Health Observatory Data Repository
http://apps.who.int/ghodata
This convenient online interface accesses WHO's *World Health Statistics 2011* and more than 50 data sets on a variety of global health topics, including mortality, burden of disease, health systems, environmental health, and the Millennium Development Goals. The interface includes a free-text search as well as a hierarchical index organized by topics (for example, HIV/AIDS, immunization, neglected tropical diseases, tobacco control). The default search on any topic retrieves all countries and all related indicators; users can then filter the data by region and years and also export data sets as an Excel spreadsheet, CSV file, or HTML file. Definitions are provided for many of the statistics, and many of the individual data points include explanatory notes as well, making this Web site a rich resource for anyone interested in global health.

GLOSSARY

Active immunity: Immunity provided through vaccination or by contracting the disease; with active immunity, a person's immune system produces antibodies against a disease, and the protection is generally permanent.

Acute disease: A disease that is short-lived and generally develops quickly; examples include strep throat and influenza.

Adolescent fertility rate: The annual number of births for women aged 15 to 19 years divided by the number of women aged 15 to 19 years in a population; usually expressed per 1,000.

Adverse selection: The tendency of an individual or group to choose to join a health care utilization pool only when they expect their utilization to be above average for the group; the classic example is a healthy person who does not buy insurance until he or she has a need for services.

Age rating: A method used by insurance companies (when legal) to charge different rates for individuals of different ages.

Age-adjusted mortality rate: A mortality rate statistically adjusted to facilitate comparison of mortality across populations by removing the effect of differing age distributions in the different populations.

Age-specific mortality rate: A mortality rate for a particular age group, such as persons aged 20 to 29 years.

Aid effectiveness: As defined by the Paris Declaration, a measure of how well development aid succeeds in achieving targets.

Aid in kind: Aid by provision of goods or services (for example, food) rather than money.

Appropriate care: Medical care that is safe and effective, based on the best available evidence, which meets priorities for the allocation of resources with the needs of the entire population taken into account.

Arbovirus: A virus transmitted by an arthropod, such as a tick or mosquito; examples include yellow fever, dengue fever, and West Nile virus.

Attack rate: The proportion of a population that develops an acute condition (for example, a specified disease) during a specified time period; the attack rate is calculated by the number of new cases during the time period divided by the population at the start of the period and is usually expressed per 1,000 or per 100,000.

Births attended by skilled personnel: A measure of health service coverage in a country, calculated by dividing the number of births in a time period attended by doctors, nurses, or midwives by the total number of live births in the same period.

Body mass index (BMI): An index used to calculate rates of the underweight, overweight, and obese; calculated by dividing weight in kilograms by squared height in meters.

Burden of disease: The difference between a situation in which everyone in a country lives into old age without illness or disability and the current situation in the country.

Capitation: A method of funding hospitals or health care providers based on the number and types of services provided or the number of patients on the patient list for the provider.

Case management: A method of organizing and coordinating medical and other services required by a person; normally provided to people with complex social and health needs who require expensive care or who are members of a vulnerable population subgroup.

Catastrophic health insurance plan: A type of insurance that typically has a high deductible or only covers expensive types of treatment (for example, hospitalization).

Cause-specific mortality rate: The mortality rate from some specific cause, such as lung cancer or an automobile accident.

Centers for Medicare and Medicaid Services: In the United States, the federal agency that manages the Medicare and Medicaid programs; it was formerly known as the Health Care Financing Administration (HCFA).

Children's Health Insurance Program (CHIP): A U.S. program to provide insurance to children (and in some states, pregnant women) whose families cannot afford private coverage but earn too much to qualify for Medicare.

Chronic disease: A disease that lasts for a long time and typically has a slow onset, such as arthritis or cancer.

Clinical practice guidelines: Recommendations based on scientific evidence to guide patients and health care professionals in selecting appropriate treatment or intervention for a condition.

COBRA: A U.S. law that allows an employee to keep an employer-provided health plan after the conclusion of employment; usually the employee pays the full cost of the plan plus an administrative fee.

Cohort: A group of individuals who have some well-defined common experience. Examples include being born in a particular year or being exposed to some health risk.

Common source outbreak: An outbreak of disease due to individuals being exposed to the same source of harmful influence (rather than spreading from person to person).

Communicable disease: An infectious disease that can be passed from one person to another or from an animal to a person.

Community immunity: *See* herd immunity.

Community rating: In insurance, charging the same premiums to everyone within a geographic area without differences due to health status, age, gender, and so on.

Consensus building: A method of achieving overall agreement on some issue or policy among the stakeholders involved.

Corruption Perceptions Index: An index published by Transparency International, assigning each country a score based on the perception of corruption in the public sector; scores range from 0 (very corrupt) to 10 (very clean).

Cost sharing: Various methods by which an individual pays part of the costs of medical treatment covered by insurance; cost sharing includes coinsurance (paying a percentage of the cost), deductibles (paying the costs up to a certain total), and copayments (paying a specified cost per service).

Cost-benefit analysis: A type of economic analysis in which the costs and benefits of some course of action (such as a type of surgery or other treatment) are expressed in monetary terms; often used to compare different courses of action or to decide if a particular course of action is worth taking.

Crude birth rate: The number of live births during a time period divided by the population during the period (usually the population at the period midpoint) and expressed per 1,000.

Deductible: In insurance, the amount that a person must pay for medical treatment before the insurance policy begins to pay for the care.

Demand for health services: The willingness to use (and perhaps pay for) health care services.

Demographic information: Information describing a person or group of persons (for example, a community), which may include both inherent (for example, race or gender) and descriptive (for example, income or geographic location) factors.

Dengue fever: A viral disease transmitted by mosquitoes (*Aedes aegypti*) and characterized by fever and severe headache, leading to death in approximately 5 percent of cases.

Dependent: A person related to another and for whom insurance coverage may be extended; examples include partners, spouses, and children.

Diagnosis-related group (DRG): A method of funding hospitals for care based on services provided based on a list of closely defined diseases, injuries, procedures, and so on.

Disability adjusted life year (DALY): A measure of disease burden in which the years of life lost due to premature mortality (YLL) and the years of life lost due to disability (YLD) are added together; the sum of DALYs across a population is the burden of disease.

Disease management: A method for coordinating services for a specific medical condition, with the focus on the disease rather than on the individual patient (the latter would be *case management*).

Donut hole: A colloquial term for the fact that, in Medicare Part D (in the United States), there is a gap in the coverage for prescription drugs so that an insured person must pay all the costs within a certain range. The insurance provides coverage up to a certain annual amount, and after a higher annual amount is reached; the part between those two amounts is the donut hole.

DPT3: A combination diptheria and pertussis vaccine on the list of recommended child vaccines.

Economy of scale: A principle in economics in which the cost of a production of a unit of something (for example, a medication) declines as output decreases because the fixed costs are relatively constant for larger or smaller production runs.

Effectiveness: A measure of how well an intervention (such as a prescription drug or course of therapy) produces the desired effect in the intended conditions of use (as opposed to a clinical trial or other artificial situation).

Efficiency: A measure of how well an intervention or procedure produces the intended results under ideal conditions (for example, during a clinical trial).

Emergency Medical Treatment and Active Labor Act (EMTALA): A 1986 U.S. federal law requiring hospitals to treat patients with medical emergencies without regard to their insurance status or ability to pay.

Endemic: The constant presence of a health condition (for example, malaria) or risk factor in a geographic area or population.

Entitlement program: A program in which everyone meeting specified standards (for example, age or disability) is legally entitled to benefits provided by the program.

Epidemic: An occurrence of a higher than usual number of cases of a health condition, often disease or injury, in an area or population.

Epidemic triad: The three components of infectious disease: an agent, a host, and an environment bringing the agent and host together.

Epidemiology: The study of disease occurrence (or occurrence of other health events) in populations, including the factors related to the occurrence of disease and methods to control it.

Evaluation: A systematic, objective method of determining how well a course of action succeeded in its goals.

Exclusive provider organization (EPO): A type of health insurance plan that only reimburses care received from providers within its network.

Expressed demand for health services: The willingness to use (and perhaps pay for) health care services as measured by actual use, contrasted with potential demand.

Fee for service: A method of paying for medical care in which providers are paid according to the number of services (for example, office visits) they perform.

Fetal mortality rate: The number of fetal deaths in a geographic area in a given period divided by the number of live births and fetal deaths for the same area and year; usually expressed as per 1,000.

Flexible spending account (FSA): A type of health insurance program in which a specified amount of money from an individual's paycheck is deposited in an account to be used for medical expenses.

Gatekeeper: A person, often a primary care physician, who is the first point of contact for an individual seeking care and has the authority to refer the person to specialist care.

Gender Inequality Index: An index calculated by the United Nations Development Programme including three dimensions: reproductive health (maternal mortality and adolescent fertility), empowerment (parliamentary representation and educational attainment), and labor market (labor force participation).

Gini coefficient (Gini index): A measure of the distribution of income in a country; a lower Gini index means greater income equality (a country with perfect equality would have a Gini index of 0) and a higher Gini index greater inequality (a country with perfect inequality would have a Gini index of 100).

Global burden of disease (GBD): An estimate, on a global level, of the difference between a situation in which everyone in the world lives to old age without illness or disability and the current global situation;

the World Healch Organization reports the GBD based on the disability and mortality from 107 diseases and 10 risk factors.

Global Gender Gap Index: An index published annually by the World Economic Forum evaluating the status of women in each country in terms of economic, political, educational, and health criteria and ranging in theory from 1.0 (most equal) to 0.0 (least equal); it is focused on gaps between men and women rather than levels, and on outcomes rather than inputs.

Gross domestic product (GDP): The value of all final goods and services produced by a country in a year.

Gross domestic product (GDP) per capita: GDP divided by the population at midyear.

Harmonization: One of the principles of aid effectiveness; it means that donor activities and contributions are coordinated, that information is shared, and that donors attempt to avoid duplication and achieve collective effectiveness.

Health expenditures: Expenditures to promote, restore, or maintain human health through the application of medical, nursing, or related knowledge and technology.

Health indicator: A statistic, such as the mortality rate, used to evaluate the health of a population, the effectiveness of a health care system, and so on.

Health insurance: A type of insurance in which the insurer pledges to compensate either the insured person or the provider of health services if specific conditions occur (for example, the person has an illness or injury that is covered by the health insurance policy).

Health services: Services meant to contribute to improved health, including diagnostic, treatment, and rehabilitation services (not limited to medical services).

Hepatitis A: A viral disease spread through fecal-contaminated food and water, which causes jaundice, fever, and diarrhea.

Herd immunity: The ability of a community or other group of people to resist infection with a particular disease (for example, measles) because most of the population is immune to the disease.

Hib3: The immunization for *haemophilus influenzae* type b, a bacterial disease that is a particular threat to children under age 5.

Hospital bed density: The number of hospital beds per 1,000 population, used as a measure of the availability of inpatient care.

Human capital: The skills and capabilities of individuals in a country, including those gained by training and education.

Human Development Index (HDI): An index developed by the UNDP and combining measures of education, living standards, and health; scores rank from 0 (low) to 1 (high).

Human immunodeficiency virus/acquired immune deficiency syndrome (HIV/AIDS) adult prevalence rate: The percentage of persons aged 15 to 19 years in a country who are HIV positive or have AIDS.

Ibrahim Index: An index produced by the Mo Ibrahim Foundation that evaluates the quality of governance of African countries using 84 indicators in the categories of safety and rule of law, human rights and participation, human development, and sustainable economic opportunity; the theoretical range is from 100 (best) to 0 (worst).

Immunity: Protection from infection with a disease.

Improved sanitary facilities: Use of facilities such as flush toilets to a piped sewer system, septic tank, or pit latrine; a composting toilet; a ventilated, improved latrine; or a pit latrine with a slab.

Improved sources of drinking water: Water from sources likely to guarantee its quality, including water piped into a home; drawn from a public tap; drawn from a tube well, borehole, or protected dug well; drawn from a protected spring; and collected rainwater.

Incidence: A measure of the new cases of a condition, such as a specific illness or injury, in a specified period and in a specified population.

Infant mortality rate: The rate of death for children aged less than 1 year; a statistic often used as a measure of the quality of a national health care system. Infant mortality is calculated as the number of deaths in this age group over a specified period of time (usually one year) divided by the number of live births in the same period and expressed per 1,000.

Internally displaced person: A person who has left his or her home for reasons similar to those of a refugee (for example, a well-founded fear of prosecution for reasons such as race, religion, or political opinion) but remains within his or her own country.

Irrational demand for health services: Demand for health services not corresponding to an actual need; contrasted with rational demand, which does correspond to an actual need for health services.

Japanese encephalitis: A viral disease spread by mosquitoes (*Culex tritaeniorhynchus*) that leads to fatality in approximately 30 percent of cases.

Leishmaniasis: A disease transmitted by sand flies, which transmit the parasite *leishmania*, resulting in chronic skin lesions; endemic in 88 countries, with most cases occurring in Brazil, Afghanistan, Iran, Peru, Syria, and Saudi Arabia.

Life course approach: A method of looking at the results of a health system over the course of a lifetime and with regard to the interaction of risk and protective factors at different stages of life.

Life expectancy at birth: An estimate of the average number of years a person is expected to live based on current age and assuming that the mortality rates current when the life expectancy is calculated continue to apply.

Lifetime limit: The maximum amount that an insurance policy will pay over the course of a person's lifetime or the number of times a service will be covered; not all policies include lifetime limits, but those that do may specify limits in different categories (for example, $1 million total claims or a single gastric bypass).

Long-term care: Services provided to people who cannot perform activities of daily living (ADLs) such as bathing or dressing themselves; long-term care includes medical and nonmedical services and may be provided in a variety of settings, including the individual's home or in a nursing home or other care facility.

Marginal cost: In economics, the cost of producing one more unit of something.

Maternal mortality index: The rate of maternal deaths (death while pregnant or within 42 days of pregnancy termination for any reason related to or aggravated by the pregnancy or pregnancy management) in a country in a given period of time divided by the number of live births in the country in the same period; usually expressed per 100,000 live births. Measuring maternal mortality is difficult in many countries and may be estimated using multiple sources of information, including household surveys, verbal autopsy, and records review.

MCV: The vaccine for measles, a highly infectious viral disease characterized by red spots on the skin.

Microinsurance: Insurance developed for low-income people who are not covered by conventional insurance policies; microinsurance policies are usually characterized by low premiums and low levels of coverage.

Mortality rate: A statistic expressing the frequency of death during some time period (often a year), calculated by dividing the number of deaths in that period by the population during that period (the latter is often the population at the midpoint of the period).

Mumps: A contagious viral illness characterized by swelling of the salivary glands.

National health accounts: Information about the health expenditures in a country; this often includes facts such as total health expenditures, private and public health expenditures, out-of-pocket expenditures, and so on.

Neonatal mortality rate: The mortality rate for children less than 28 days old, calculated by dividing the number of deaths in this age group over a specified period by the number of live births in the same period and expressed per 1,000.

Net migration rate: The difference between the number of people immigrating to and emigrating from a country in a given year and generally expressed as per 1,000 population; a positive rate means more people are entering the country than leaving it, a negative rate that more people are leaving than entering.

Notifiable disease: A disease that must be reported to public health authorities, as prescribed by law.

Opportunity cost: In economics, the value of opportunities not taken as the result of choosing a particular choice of action; sometimes defined as the cost of not taking the next best alternative course of action.

Organisation for Economic Co-operation and Development (OECD): An international organization promoting policies that will improve human economic and social well-being.

Outbreak: A term sometimes used in preference to epidemic in order to prevent public panic; an outbreak is the occurrence of more than the expected number of cases of a health condition (for example, disease or injury) in a population or geographic area in a given period.

Out-of-pocket limits: The maximum that an individual or family will be required to pay for medical services in a given year, including deductibles, copayments, and coinsurance.

Out-of-pocket payments: Payments by the person receiving a good or service; in health care, services or products (for example, a physician visit or prescription drug) often require an out-of-pocket payment as well as partial subsidy by an insurer or the government.

Pandemic: An epidemic that occurs in multiple countries.

Paris Declaration on Aid Effectiveness: A 2005 international agreement specifying five principles intended to promote effective aid: (1) ownership of development policies by the partner countries, (2) alignment between the donors' support and the development policies of the partner countries, (3) harmonization among the donor countries, (4) managing for results (that is, the focus is on measurable development results, and these results are evaluated), and (5) mutual accountability among donors, partners, and countries.

Passive immunity: Immunity acquired by antibodies produced by another person or animal (for example, babies are protected by maternal antibodies during their first months of life); protection is usually limited and diminishes over time.

People-centered care: Care centered around the needs of individual patients and communities rather than on treating a disease in the abstract.

Percent urbanization: The projected rate of change in urbanization; a positive rate means more people are expected to live in urban areas in the future, while a negative rate means that fewer are expected to live in urban areas.

Performance-based payments: Sometimes called P4P or pay for performance, a method of paying health service providers based on their meeting particular standards (or paying bonuses based on meeting a standard); may also apply to health systems or entire countries.

Pertussis: A bacterial disease sometimes called whooping cough due to the convulsive cough associated with it.

Point of service (POS): A type of insurance plan in which the patient chooses a primary care provider from within the insurer's network; that provider can make referrals to specialists within or outside the network, but the patient typically pays more for care received outside the network.

Population growth rate: The average annual percentage change estimated for a country's population, calculated using the birth and death rates and the net migration rate.

Postneonatal mortality rate: The mortality rate for children from age 28 days to less than 1 year, calculating by dividing the number of deaths in this age group for a specified period (usually one year) by the number of live births in the same period and expressed per 1,000.

Preferred provider organization (PPO): A type of health insurance in which you pay less for treatment received from providers and hospitals within a network, as opposed to providers and hospitals outside the network.

Prevalence rate: The number of total cases of a disease in a population and time period; contrasted with incidence, which is the number of new cases.

Preventive services: Medical services intended to prevent illness or detect it at an early stage, including immunizations, screenings, and patient education.

Primary care: Medical care and preventive services for common illnesses, usually provided by general practice physicians, nurses, and so on.

Primary prevention: Measures intended to help a person avoid a health problem; examples include immunization against a disease and education to encourage the use of automobile safety belts.

Private health insurance: A type of health insurance in which the cost of a policy is based on either individual or group risks; an example of group risk would be the risk for all the employees of a particular company, who are provided with insurance as a benefit of their employment.

Propagated outbreak: An outbreak of disease that is spread from one person to another.

Public health services: Services intended to benefit an entire population, such as the provision of a municipal sewage and water system; contrasted with medical care, which is focused on benefiting the individual patient.

Purchasing power parity (PPP): A method of comparing costs or prices across countries, based on the international dollar, an economic construct whose purchasing power in the country in question equals the purchasing power of one U.S. dollar in the United States. It is used to account for differences in cost levels across countries and for fluctuations in exchange rates.

Race-specific mortality rate (ethnic-specific mortality rate): The mortality rate for a particular racial or ethnic group, for example, African Americans or Hispanic Americans.

Rational demand for health services: *See* irrational demand for health services.

Recurrent costs: Costs for items that are regularly purchased and last less than a year; in a health care system, recurrent costs could include (among other things) salaries, pharmaceuticals, and other supplies.

Refugee: According to the United Nations (UN), a person living outside his or her habitual residence due to a well-founded fear of persecution due to reasons including race, religion, nationality, social group, or political opinion and who is unable to return home for that reason.

Rescission: Cancelling a health insurance policy retroactively, whether for intentional fraud or for unintentional errors in the application process.

Risk adjustment: A method used by insurers (where legal) to consider previous patterns of health care utilization, health history, and current health when enrolling individuals in a health insurance plan.

Risk pooling: In insurance, the practice of spreading risk across members of a group (for example, persons employed by a company or residents of a country).

Secondary attack rate: The frequency of new cases of a disease among persons who are contacts of persons known to have the disease.

Secondary care: Standard hospital care, including general medicine and surgery, pediatrics, and obstetrics.

Secondary prevention: Measures intended to detect a disease before clinical symptoms have developed, such as screening tests for tuberculosis or prostate cancer.

Stakeholder: Someone or something (for example, an organization) who has an interest in the outcome of some situation.

Tertiary care: Advanced and specialized hospital care and posthospital rehabilitation.

Tertiary prevention: Measures intended to minimize the effects of an already-established disease and to restore the patient to the highest possible level of functioning.

Total fertility rate: The average number of children a cohort of women would have if the fertility rate for a given period applied throughout their entire reproductive period; expressed as the number of children per woman and used to estimate future population growth in a country.

Transparency International: An international organization with chapters in more than 100 countries, which promotes corruption-free government, business, and civil society and publishes the Corruption Perceptions Index.

United States Agency for International Development (USAID): A federal agency that administers civilian foreign aid.

Universal coverage: In health insurance, the guaranteed provision of specified benefits for everyone within a population (for example, the citizens or residents of a country).

Urban population: The percentage of the population of a country living in urban areas, using the definition of "urban" provided by the country.

USD: U.S. dollars; this is the ISO 4127 currency code. When other currencies are cited, the ISO 4127 code is also used, and the currency is generally that of the country in question (for example, AFN = Afghanistan Afghani, EUR = euro).

Years of life lost (YLL): A measure of the impact of premature death on a population, calculated as the difference between current life expectancy or a particular age (for example, 55 years) and the actual age of death.

Yellow fever: A viral disease spread by mosquitoes and prevalent only in sub-Saharan Africa and tropical South America.

INDEX

Index note: Volume numbers are in **boldface**. Article titles and their page numbers are in **boldface**.